WITHDRAWN
WRIGHT STATE UNIVERSITY LIBRARIES

DISORDERS OF THE SPLEEN

HEMATOLOGY

Series Editor

Kenneth M. Brinkhous, M.D.
*Department of Pathology
University of North Carolina
School of Medicine
Chapel Hill, North Carolina*

Volume 1   Prostaglandins and Leukotrienes: Blood and Vascular Cell Function, *Jonathan M. Gerrard*

Volume 2   Hematopoietic Stem Cells, *edited by David W. Golde and Fumimaro Takaku*

Volume 3   Bone Marrow Transplantation: Biological Mechanisms and Clinical Practice, *edited by Dirk W. van Bekkum and Bob Löwenberg*

Volume 4   Myelofibrosis: Pathophysiology and Clinical Management, *edited by S. M. Lewis*

Volume 5   Plasma Fibronectin: Structure and Function, *edited by Jan McDonagh*

Volume 6   The Acute Leukemias: Biologic, Diagnostic, and Therapeutic Determinants, *edited by Sanford A. Stass*

Volume 7   Hemostasis and Animal Venoms, *edited by Hubert Pirkle and Francis S. Markland, Jr.*

Volume 8   Hematopoiesis: Long-Term Effects of Chemotherapy and Radiation, *edited by Nydia G. Testa and Robert Peter Gale*

Volume 9   Coagulation and Bleeding Disorders, *edited by Theodore S. Zimmerman and Zaverio M. Ruggeri*

Volume 10　　Disorders of the Spleen, *edited by Carl Pochedly, Richard H. Sills, and Allen D. Schwartz*

Additional Volumes in Preparation

Red Blood Cell Membranes: Structure, Function, and Clinical Implications, *edited by Peter Agre and John C. Parker*

DISORDERS OF THE SPLEEN
Pathophysiology and Management

edited by

CARL POCHEDLY
University of Chicago
Chicago, Illinois

RICHARD H. SILLS
Children's Hospital of New Jersey
and University of Medicine and
Dentistry – New Jersey Medical
School, Newark, New Jersey

ALLEN D. SCHWARTZ
University of Maryland
Baltimore, Maryland

MARCEL DEKKER, INC.   New York and Basel

1989

Library of Congress Cataloging in Publication Data

Disorders of the spleen : pathophysiology and management / edited by
   Carl Pochedly, Richard H. Sills, Allen D. Schwartz.
      p.   cm. -- (Hematology ; v. 10)
   Includes bibliographies and index.
   ISBN 0-8247-7933-9
   1. Spleen--Pathophysiology. 2. Spleen-Diseases. 3. Spleen-
-Physiology. I. Pochedly, Carl. II. Sills, Richard H.,
III. Schwartz, Allen D., IV. Series: Hematology (New York,
N.Y.) ; v. 10.
   [DNLM: 1. Splenic Diseases--physiopathology. 2. Splenic Diseases-
-therapy. W1 HE873 v. 10 / WH 600 D612]
   RC654.D57   1989
   616.4'1--dc19   88-20354

Copyright © 1989 by MARCEL DEKKER, INC.   All Rights Reserved

Neither this book nor any part may be reproduced or transmitted in any form
or by any means, electronic or mechanical, including photocopying, microfilm-
ing, and recording, or by any information storage and retrieval system, without
permission in writing from the publisher.

MARCEL DEKKER, INC.
270 Madison Avenue, New York, New York 10016

Current printing (last digit):
10 9 8 7 6 5 4 3 2 1

PRINTED IN THE UNITED STATES OF AMERICA

Series Introduction

For most of this century hematology has followed a pattern of major scientific discoveries, improved understanding of disease, and rapid application of new knowledge in the clinic. The rate of advance continues at an accelerating pace, so that all but the most zealous have difficulty in keeping up with the literature in even a limited area of specialized interest. As the explosive development of knowledge continues apace, it is a continuing challenge to keep abreast of significant new developments as they impact on clinical and laboratory hematology. The Hematology series is designed to help in this respect, by providing up-to-date and expert presentations on important subject areas in our field. It is hoped that these works, both individually and collectively, will become important volumes for updating information and for reference for the clinician, investigator, teacher, and student, and in this manner contribute to the advancement of hematology.

This volume of the series provides a comprehensive overview of the spleen and its disorders. As with previous volumes, this presentation embodies the current state of the art, bringing together both the basic and clinical advances. The structure and function of the spleen remained enigmatic in many respects until recent times. With improved understanding of the immune function of the spleen, its unique vasculature with alternate blood flow through the splenic cords and sinusoids, its role in the clearance, storage, and degradation of blood and other elements, and its limited hematopoeitic function, a more rational approach to splenic disorders and their diagnosis and management became possible. The splenic disorders of both pediatric and adult medicine are covered. Taking advantage of this setting, the editors and authors have contributed a volume that should be a valuable addition to the field.

Kenneth M. Brinkhous
Series Editor

Foreword

For years I have been an aficionado of books about the spleen. Whoever wrote or published a spleen book could be sure of one purchaser. I have a shelf of them, some in languages I cannot read. His five poems titled "Spleen" attracted my attention to Charles Baudelaire, and, thus caught, I spent ten years translating *Les Fleurs du Mal*. There was a time when I contemplated writing a spleen book myself, but we must draw the line somewhere: romancing the spleen has been a pleasure, but marriage was out of the question. I have, however, from time to time written essays and fielded opinions on the spleen, and I have gradually learned a bit about its medical history. A historical vantage point provides a perspective, not only of the importance of splenic function but also of splenic research.

In 1948 the spleen was still supposed to be "an organ filled with mystery," and anyone who wrote about the spleen demonstrated his erudition by a reference to Galen's epigram. It is a source of wonder that in 1948 it could still be stated—seriously—that the function of the spleen was mysterious. For hundreds of years the evidence of splenic functions had been accumulating.

The spleen's apparent independence was puzzling. It was attached to the rest of the body only by its blood supply. Malpighi (17th century), the first great histologist, was puzzled. He perceived the white pulp of the spleen (the malpighian corpuscles) as glandular, and he was puzzled because, unlike the other glands he described, there were no channels for drainage of a secretion. He proposed that the spleen's secretion might be carried by the blood to act at distant parts and thus Malpighi was the first to propose the existence of endocrine activity. The *Oxford English Dictionary* (OED) describes the spleen as a ductless gland, and *Dorland's* calls it a gland-like but ductless organ. Malpighi casts a long shadow.

Hewson (18th century) associated the spleen with the thymus and the lymph nodes because all three accumulated "central particles," later called lymphocytes. Thus even before the phenomena of immunity were recognized, its anatomical system had been identified.

Kolliker (19th century) was author of the first textbook of histology. In 1847 he discovered the phenomenon of erythrophagocytosis while studying the spleen and proposed that it provided the normal disposal of the red cells. It was an indication of the phenomenon of normal cell turnover. Thereafter, very slowly it was perceived that not only red cells but all cells—except nerve cells—have a finite life span and that populations are continually renewed. Study of the spleen had provided the first intimation of this.

"Ague-cake," described by the OED as a vulgarism, refers to the splenomegaly of malaria. Ague is the malarial paroxysm; cake is the large, hard spleen. In times past in England, even the common folk knew of the spleen's involvement with infection. When in the latter 19th century the bacterial basis of infections was established, investigators set to work at once to examine the behavior of the spleen. Organisms injected intravenously disappeared promptly from the blood and appeared in great numbers in the spleen. A small dose of intravenous anthrax bacillus that could not kill normal dogs did kill splenectomized dogs. Small doses of tetanus bacillus that did not kill splenectomized rabbits could not immunize them. They could be killed by a challenge dose that did not kill immunized controls. The inability of asplenic humans (and animals) to cope with pneumococcus--the overwhelming postsplenectomy infection--recalls these 100-year-old experiments. The spleen demonstrates a difference in responses to particulate and to soluble antigen, a difference that seems somehow related to the unique circulation of the intact spleen. Consider the "reborn" spleen of splenosis. Fragments of autogenous spleen can reestablish themselves using blood supply that penetrates from contiguous organs. But such splenic tissue does not protect against organisms (particulate challenge) as does the original organ that receives blood through its hilus.

In the capacity of a filter the spleen disposes of much debris. To this end it is well provided with macrophages. In the spleen's participation in iron metabolism, two varieties of macrophages are evident. At the end of the human red blood cells' life cycle most of them are disposed of by erythrophagocytosis in the spleen. About 20 mg of iron per day is recovered from degraded hemoglobin and surrendered to the plasma. The disposal is efficient: the normal spleen does not accumulate iron. The splenic cells involved are the perisinal phagocytes. The other population is the tissue macrophages in the red pulp. Abnormal red blood cells (sickle cells or antibody-sensitized cells, for example) are to some extent destroyed by the cordal phagocytes, which seem incapable of surrendering iron to plasma. Dense siderosis of the red pulp results.

When the body burden of iron is grossly enlarged in people who require red blood cell transfusions on a continuing basis, the spleen becomes heavily siderotic. When the body burden of iron is grossly enlarged in hereditary hemochromatosis, it does not; moreover, the iron in the spleen is not abnormal. Here again, the spleen provides a clue to the solution of a systemic abnormality. The practically iron-free spleen of hemochromatosis demonstrates an inability of the cordal macrophages to store iron even when the amount of ambient iron in the body is enormous. (Marrow macrophages in hemochromatosis do not store iron either.) This suggests, in turn, an abnormality of macrophage ferritin, its synthesis, or its stability. The sparing of the spleen in this storage disease has been recognized for as long as hemochromatosis has been known to be an abnormality of iron metabolism.

The last 40 years have witnessed much change as regards the status of the spleen in the clinic. House officers have learned to spell "splenectomy," although the nurses still prefer "spleenectomy." "Hypersplenism" became a fad, and the spleen became the surgeons' hockey puck, removed for "surgical convenience" or hematologic curiosity. Then, in 1952, overwhelming postsplenectomy infection was rediscovered (it was first described in 1929), and slowly the rush to removal eased. Nowadays it is sometimes difficult to find a surgeon and hematologist who can agree to commit splenectomy, even to save a life. Partial ablation and partial infarction have been developed as alternatives to splenectomy.

During the splenectomy era we observed that removal of the spleen resulted, sometimes, in the cure of diseases remote from the spleen itself: chronic leg ulcer, aplastic anemia, pulmonary siderosis, the vascular lesions of thrombotic thrombocytopenic purpura. How does one define hypersplenism to encompass these phenomena?

During the 40 years that I have collected spleen books, many have been published, each until now a disappointment. The first spleen book ever has remained the best. In 1854 Henry Gray published *On the Structure and Use of the Spleen*. It was a book out of its time, a marvellous encyclopedia of the history of the spleen from Erasistratis, the first anatomist, onward. Gray recorded his own extensive research on the anatomy of the spleen and comparative anatomy based on necropsies of the animals that died in the London Zoo. This spleen book was Gray's scholarly preparation for the writing of his *Anatomy, Descriptive and Surgical,* published in 1858, which has gone through 30 editions. A pity that Gray's spleen book has never been reprinted.

I am convinced that this present encyclopedic work, *Disorders of the Spleen*, is as definitive as any book can be in our time. In these past 40 years it is the first spleen book that is not a disappointment.

William H. Crosby, M.D.
Director of Hematology
Chapman Regional Cancer Center
Joplin, Missouri

Preface

Rapid progress has been made in our understanding of the anatomy, physiology, and pathophysiology of the spleen during the past 10 years. This progress has come mainly as a result of the development of techniques in electron microscopy as well as from advances in cytology, cell physiology, and cell culture. Elucidating the functions of the spleen, and the study and documentation of these functions, present a supreme challenge to modern technology and ingenuity. But science has successfully responded to the challenge. And the product of this research has resulted in great improvements in patient care and led to enlightened understanding of the pathophysiology of various diseases.

Giant strides have been made toward gaining knowledge of the physiology of the spleen and its role in hematopoiesis and in functions related to immunity. The spleen was once a neglected and obscure organ, shrouded in fantasy and mystery. But now the spleen has been illuminated and vitalized by the glow of new knowledge in the related basic and clinical sciences and by the development of new research technologies.

The purpose of this book is to review concisely the state of current knowledge and to document progress in the anatomy and physiology of the spleen. Its purpose is also to clarify the role of this important organ in the pathophysiology of various diseases. Although knowledge and understanding have been greatly improved, it is obvious that we can now see only the tip of the iceberg. Much progress has been made, yet we still often find ourselves in the position of having only fragmentary information of uncertain significance. Many burning questions still remain that demand continued innovative investigation and intensive study.

It is hoped that this book will serve as a useful reference for primary care physicians as well as a resource for scientists involved in research related to the spleen. Physicians to whom this book will be most useful include: pediatricians, specialists in pediatric hematology/oncology, internists, medical oncologists, and hematologists, as well as surgeons, pathologists, and radiologists. All physicians involved in patient care are confronted by clinical problems that may be directly or indirectly associated with disorders of the spleen.

This book contains new information on the anatomy and physiology of the spleen. This new information permits improved understanding of the complex interrelationships of the spleen with other organs and systems in both health and disease. There have also been long strides in understanding the role of the spleen in immunology and control of infections as well as in hematopoiesis. This progress enables us to deal more effectively with the spleen in various diseases involving immunocytopenias and autoimmune phenomena. There has also been considerable progress in the technology of imaging of the spleen, using the newer imaging modalities. This sophisticated imaging has resulted in a better understanding of the normal anatomy and physiology of the spleen as well as a more accurate assessment of the functional and anatomical changes that occur in disease.

The study of the spleen is multidisciplinary in scope. The needed technology and clinical and laboratory expertise extend far beyond the capabilities of any one clinician or scientist. Contributors of this book represent the various disciplines that are the essential components of this research. The members of this distinguished team have pooled their experience and scholarship, and among them they have concisely and authoritatively reviewed all of the major aspects of the anatomy, physiology, and pathophysiology of the spleen. The scientific merits of this book are due solely to them. We limited the scope of the book to information of clinical relevance to satisfy the informational needs of the busy clinician. The material is presented in concise form so that it may be quickly and easily understood.

Finally, we are honored that Dr. William Crosby, a distinguished pioneer in spleen research, was willing to write the Foreword for this book. Mable Pochedly provided vital assistance as liaison with authors and publishers, as well as in copyediting and proofreading. Elizabeth Cavanaugh skillfully typed final drafts of edited manuscripts. Paul Dolgert, Kerry Doyle, Elaine Grohman, Brian Black, and Natascha Franco of Marcel Dekker, Inc., were most helpful and supportive throughout all stages in the planning and production of this book.

Carl Pochedly
Richard H. Sills
Allen D. Schwartz

Contributors

Reneé V. Gardner* Department of Pediatrics, University of Florida College of Medicine, Gainesville, Florida

Mary V. Gresik Department of Pathology, Baylor College of Medicine, Houston, Texas

Deborah Hurst Department of Hematology and Oncology, Children's Hospital, Oakland, Oakland, California

John G. Kelton Department of Pathology, McMaster University Medical Center, Hamilton, Ontario, Canada

Karen L. Kotloff Department of Pediatrics, University of Maryland School of Medicine, Baltimore, Maryland

William G. Murphy† Department of Hematology, McMaster University Medical Center, Hamilton, Ontario, Canada

Margaret B. Rennels Department of Pediatrics, University of Maryland School of Medicine, Baltimore, Maryland

---

Current affiliations: *Genetics and Biochemistry Section, National Institutes of Health, Bethesda, Maryland
†Royal Infirmary, Edinburgh, Scotland

Allen D. Schwartz Department of Pediatrics and Oncology, University of Maryland School of Medicine, Baltimore, Maryland

Mark F. Seifert Department of Anatomy, University of South Dakota School of Medicine, Vermillion, South Dakota

Charles M. Severin Department of Anatomical Sciences, State University of New York at Buffalo, Buffalo, New York

Irene N. Sills* Diabetes Program, Children's Hospital of Buffalo, Buffalo, New York

Richard H. Sills Division of Pediatric Hematology/Oncology, Children's Hospital of New Jersey, and the Department of Pediatrics, University of Medicine and Dentistry–New Jersey Medical School, Newark, New Jersey

James A. Stockman III[†] Department of Pediatrics, Northwestern University Medical School, Chicago, Illinois

John R. Sty Children's Hospital of Wisconsin, Milwaukee, Wisconsin

Elliott P. Vichinsky Department of Hematology and Oncology, Children's Hospital, Oakland, Oakland, California

Leon Weiss Department of Animal Biology, School of Veterinary Medicine of the University of Pennsylvania, Philadelphia, Pennsylvania

Robert G. Wells Children's Hospital of Wisconsin, Milwaukee, Wisconsin

---

Current affiliations: *Department of Pediatric Endocrinology, Children's Hospital of New New Jersey, Newark, New Jersey
†Children's Memorial Hospital, Chicago, Illinois

Contents

Series Introduction (Kenneth M. Brinkhous)		iii
Foreword		v
Preface		ix
Contributors		xi

PART I: General Features

1 Anatomy of the Spleen 1

Charles M. Severin

Development of the Spleen	1
Relationships and Appearance of the Adult Spleen	4
Microscopic Organization of the Spleen	7
Summary	17
References	18

2 Spleen in Blood Cell Regulation and Hematopoiesis 21

Mark F. Seifert

Phylogenesis and Ontogenesis of Splenic Hematopoiesis	21
Splenic Hematopoiesis in Man	24
Splenic Hematopoiesis in Disease	25
Regulation of Splenic Hematopoiesis	27
Summary and Conclusions	29
References	30

3	**Pathology of the Spleen**	37
	Mary V. Gresik	
	Examination of the Spleen	37
	Structural Abnormalities and Circulatory Disturbances	42
	Red Blood Cell Abnormalities	46
	Infectious Diseases	50
	Storage Diseases	56
	Immune and Autoimmune Disorders	62
	Benign Tumors	72
	Malignancy and Myeloproliferative Disorders	73
	Summary	89
	References	90
	PART II: Pathophysiology of Spleen Disorders	
4	**Hyposplenism**	99
	Richard H. Sills	
	Methods to Evaluate Adequacy of Splenic Function	99
	Overview of Laboratory Techniques to Evaluate Hyposplenism	110
	Causes of Functional and Anatomic Hyposplenism	110
	Congenital Hyposplenism	113
	Summary and Conclusions	132
	References	133
5	**Physiology of the Spleen and Consequences of Hyposplenism**	145
	Allen D. Schwartz	
	Reservoir Function	146
	Blood Production	147
	Destruction of Blood	147
	The Pitting Function	148
	The Spleen and Infection	149
	Management of the Asplenic State	154
	Summary	157
	References	158
6	**Hypersplenism**	167
	Richard H. Sills	
	Pathophysiology of Hypersplenism	168
	Laboratory Evaluation of the Hypersplenic State	169

	Etiologies of Hypersplenism	170
	Inflammatory and Collagen-Vascular Disorders as Etiologies of Hypersplenism	173
	Congestive Splenomegaly	174
	Storage Diseases as Causes of Hypersplenism	175
	Hematologic Diseases as Causes of Hypersplenism	175
	Neoplastic Conditions Associated with Hypersplenism	179
	Miscellaneous Conditions Associated with Hypersplenism	179
	Treatment of Hypersplenism	180
	Summary and Conclusions	180
	References	181
7	**Role of the Spleen in Autoimmune Disorders**	**187**
	William G. Murphy and John G. Kelton	
	Overview of the Process of Antibody and Complement-Mediated Cell Clearance	187
	Anatomy of the Spleen and Its Role as an Immune Clearance Organ	192
	The Spleen in Immune Thrombocytopenic Purpura	194
	The Spleen in Autoimmune Hemolytic Anemia	198
	The Spleen in Autoimmune Neutropenia	201
	Summary	202
	References	204

PART III: Splenomegaly

8	**Splenomegaly: Diagnostic Overview**	**217**
	James A. Stockman III	
	Functions of the Spleen	218
	Definition of Splenomegaly	222
	Diagnostic Overview	227
	Summary	236
	References	237
9	**Splenomegaly: Infectious Etiologies**	**239**
	Karen L. Kotloff and Margaret B. Rennels	
	Normal Anatomy and Physiology	239
	Pathophysiology	240
	Infections that Cause Splenomegaly	240
	Diagnostic Approach to the Patient with Splenomegaly	259

	Summary	261
	References	262
10	**Splenomegaly: Neoplastic and Histiocytic Causes**	**265**
	Renée V. Gardner	
	Role of the Spleen in Anti-Tumor Immunity	266
	Clinical Presentation	268
	Diagnosis	270
	Leukemias	272
	Lymphomas: Hodgkin's Disease and Non-Hodgkin's Lymphoma	281
	Myelofibrosis	284
	Histiocytosis	287
	Angiosarcoma	300
	Miscellaneous	302
	Summary	304
	References	306
11	**Splenomegaly: Storage Disorders**	**319**
	Irene N. Sills	
	Disorders of Carbohydrate Metabolism	321
	Disorders of Lipoprotein Metabolism	323
	Disorders of Sphingolipid Metabolism	326
	Mucopolysaccharidoses	333
	Sulfatide Lipidosis	337
	Mucolipidosis: I-Cell Disease	339
	Disorders of Glycoprotein Degradation	342
	Neutral Lipid Storage Diseases	343
	Amyloidosis	345
	Cystinosis	346
	Hemachromatosis	346
	Summary	347
	References	348

PART IV: Imaging and Surgery

12	**Imaging the Spleen**	**355**
	John R. Sty and Robert G. Wells	
	Anatomy and Embryology	360
	Variations in Spleen Size	360
	Techniques for Imaging the Spleen	361

	Clinical Applications of Imaging in Diagnosing Splenic Abnormalities	371
	Summary	399
	References	400
13	**Splenectomy: Indications in Childhood**	**407**
	Deborah Hurst and Elliott Vichinsky	
	Splenectomy for Traumatic Rupture	407
	Hematologic Indications for Splenectomy: Red Cell Disorders	410
	Hematologic Indications for Splenectomy: Immune Cytopenias	417
	Hypersplenism	418
	Miscellaneous Conditions	420
	Malignancy	420
	Infection	421
	General Considerations	422
	References	423

PART V: Perspectives

14	**New Trends in Spleen Research: Reticuloendothelial Basis of the Clearance of Blood by the Spleen**	**431**
	Leon Weiss	
	The Intermediate Circulation of the Spleen	431
	Reticuloendothelial Character of the Spleen	439
	Macrophages	439
	The Endothelium of Vascular Sinuses	441
	Reticular Cells	442
	Inductive Capacities of Fibroblasts	443
	Hegemonies of the Reticuloendothelial System: Barrier-Forming Systems of Activated Reticular Cells	444
	Clearance of Blood by the Spleen	446
	Summary	450
	References	451

Index   *455*

Part I

General Features

1
Anatomy of the Spleen

CHARLES M. SEVERIN
State University of New York at Buffalo, Buffalo, New York

The spleen is the largest multifunctional lymphatic organ in the human body. Early in fetal life, it serves the purpose of myeloid hematopoiesis. Later, it removes and destroys foreign microbial pathogens in the blood and also provides for the selective monitoring and removal of aged and damaged erythrocytes, leukocytes, and platelets.

In immune reactions, the spleen provides for the same processes of antigen trapping, cellular collaboration, lymphocyte proliferation, and antibody production seen in peripheral lymph nodes. In general, the immune responses to antigens and pathogens invading the blood stream are concentrated within the spleen. Before discussing how the microscopic organization of the spleen achieves these functions, the development and location of the spleen will be described.

DEVELOPMENT OF THE SPLEEN

The spleen is derived from condensations of mesenchymal tissue in the dorsal mesogastrium of the embryo. These condensations are seen in human embryos at about the fifth week of development (1). These cellular aggregates fuse to form a lobulated structure in the left side of the dorsal mesogastrium, opposite the urogenital fold, and to the left of the pancreas at the level of the fundus of the stomach. Evidence for this early lobulation is indicated in the adult spleen by notches usually present along its superior margin.

The classical theory of splenic development states that these mesenchymal cells differentiate into the reticulum and into primitive free cells resembling lymphocytes. Other mesenchymal cells become myeloid in type and contain all the various stages of developing erythrocytes, granulocytes, and platelets. A more recent investigation (2) has suggested that hematopoietic precursors are ultimately derived from cells that migrate from the yolk sac to the liver and spleen. Regardless of the origin of these myeloid precursors, the formation of these cells normally ceases shortly after birth, in contrast to lymphocyte development, which continues throughout life. The spleen's phagocytic potential, which is expressed late in gestation, is similarly maintained (3).

In its early stages of development, the primordium of the spleen is supplied with a capillary plexus connecting the afferent and efferent vessels. After the development of the characteristic distribution of vessels, lymphocytes gradually become more compactly arranged around the arteries to form the beginning of the white pulp. The focal enlargements of the white pulp that form definite splenic corpuscles are not found until the end of fetal development. The characteristic adult structure of the red pulp is not attained until after birth, when the myeloid characteristics of the tissue are lost as the development of erythrocytes and granulocytes ceases.

The development of the spleen is influenced to some degree by its close proximity to the stomach. The pressure of the rotating stomach upon the spleen forces the spleen to project from the left surface of the dorsal mesogastrium into the general peritoneal cavity (Figure 1). By this action the dorsal mesogastrium can be subdivided into a portion between the posterior abdominal wall and the

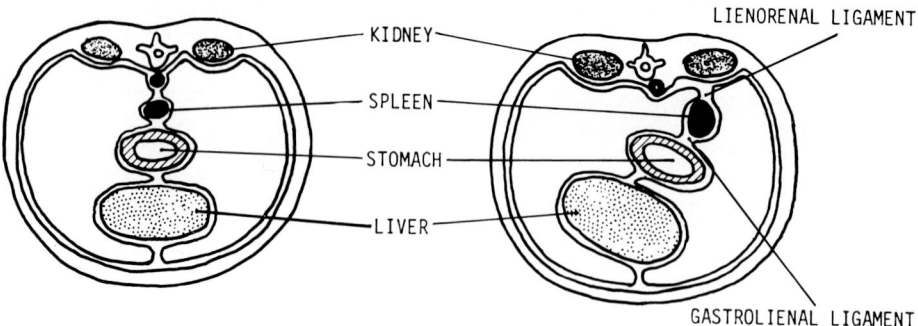

Figure 1 Transverse sections through the liver, stomach, spleen, and kidneys at the end of the fifth week of development. Note that with development and rotation of the stomach, the spleen is displaced to the left and, subsequently, the gastrolienal and lienorenal ligaments are formed.

ANATOMY OF THE SPLEEN

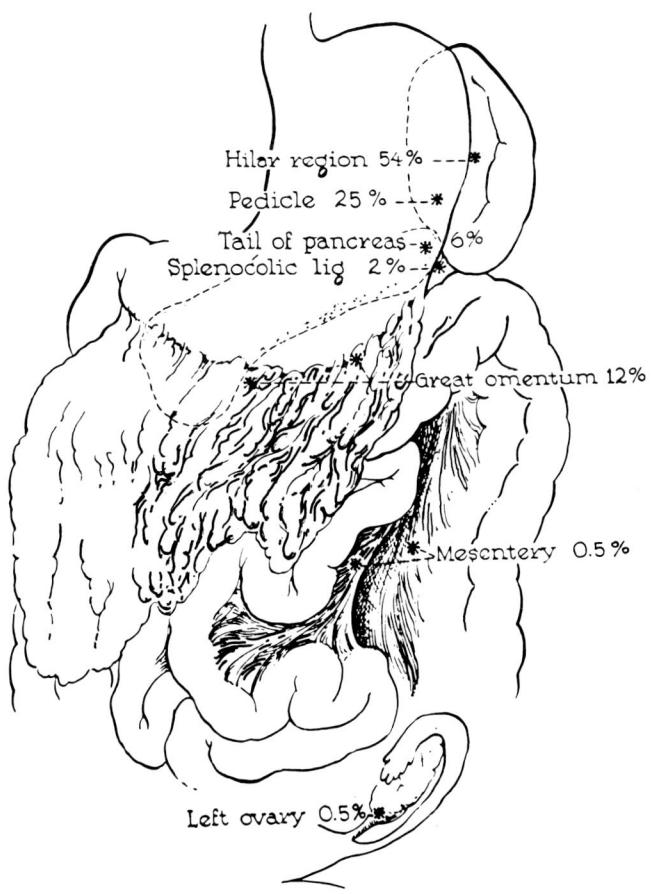

Figure 2 Diagram showing the location and frequency of ectopic spleens. (From Curtis and Movitz (5).)

spleen, and a segment between the spleen and greater curvature of the stomach. Another part of the dorsal mesogastrium fuses with the peritoneum of the posterior abdominal wall ventral to the developing left kidney. The connections between the stomach and the spleen form the gastrolienal ligament, and connections between the spleen and kidney form the lienorenal ligament.

Many structures that are asymmetrical in the human body are either of midline origin (such as the stomach) or, while originally bilateral (such as the aortic arches and the venae cavae), persist after the suppression of the component of one side. The spleen is an exception, since it is neither midline nor bilateral in origin. Some investigators feel that a splenic primordium does originate on the right side but fails to develop. In spite of a single report of paired symmetrical spleens (4), there is no further evidence of normally bilateral splenic primordia.

Absence of the spleen is unusual and may be clinically important. It may be accompanied by anomalies in the cardiovascular system. One of the more frequently encountered developmental aberrations of the body is the presence of accessory spleens. In most cases, this condition is asymptomatic and is first identified at surgery or autopsy. While only one or two accessory spleens are usually observed, as many as 10 have been reported (5). Accessory spleens most commonly (in about 80% of cases) occur near the hilum of the spleen. An accessory spleen may be embedded partly or wholly in the tail of the pancreas, or it may be embedded within the gastrolienal ligament. These supernumary organs result from a failure in fusion of the original individual splenic masses and are sometimes carried to ectopic sites by splenic ligaments. Ectopic splenic tissue is also encountered in splenogonadal fusion, where splenic tissue is found in the left side of the scrotum or adjacent to the left ovary. This abnormality originates due to an adherence of splenic primordia to the left gonadal ridge. An accessory spleen may be connected to the spleen proper by a thin cord of splenic or trabecular tissue. At times the accessory spleen is almost as large as the spleen itself, a condition known as duplicate spleen (6).

Ectopic spleens usually occur in patients with abdominal malformations, as in situs inversus. Thus, the demonstration of ectopic spleens should give rise to suspicion of the presence of other malformations. The locations and percentages of ectopic spleens are shown in Figure 2.

RELATIONSHIPS AND APPEARANCE OF THE ADULT SPLEEN

The spleen is a freely moveable dark purplish organ found principally in the left hypochondriac region of the abdomen, although its posterior edge may extend into the epigastric region. It is situated in the greater peritoneal sac between the diaphragm and stomach, and is sheltered entirely by the ribs. Because it is under the rib cage, the normal spleen cannot be palpated. However, if it becomes significantly enlarged, the lower end of the spleen may extend downward and forward toward the umbilicus and may be readily palpated below the costal margin. The spleen may enlarge due to increased blood pressure, or for a few hours after a meal. It diminishes in size after exercise, and with advancing age.

The normal length of the spleen varies from 10 to 14 cm, its width varies from 6 to 10 cm, and its thickness is 3 to 4 cm. The weight of the spleen varies from 80 to 300 g or more. It has a rather smooth, convex diaphragmatic surface that faces posterolaterally, and a more irregular concave visceral surface that faces the abdominal cavity. The superior border of the spleen may be notched as compared with its inferior border. The posterolateral surface of the spleen is related through the diaphragm to the base of the left lung, the costodiaphrag-

ANATOMY OF THE SPLEEN

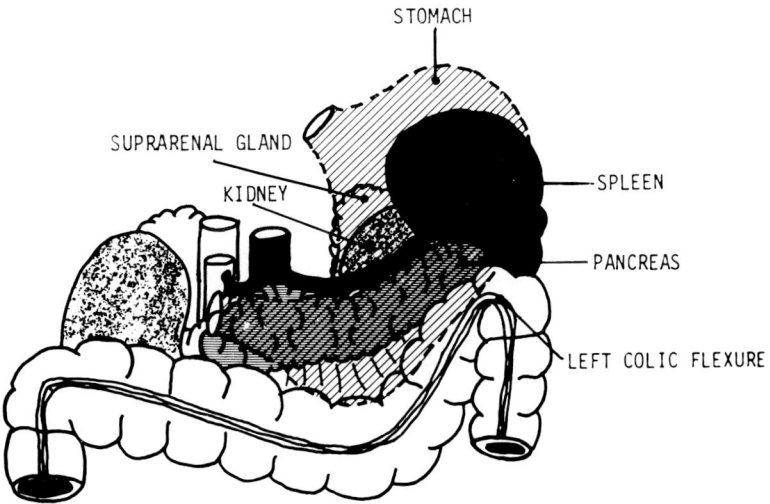

Figure 3 Relationship of spleen to other organs.

matic recess of the left pleura, and the ninth, tenth, and eleventh ribs. In the recumbent position, the longitudinal axis of the spleen lies along the tenth rib. In the adult the spleen is in contact with the stomach, pancreas, left kidney, and the splenic flexure of the colon. In a child, the spleen also contacts the left suprarenal gland (Figure 3).

As stated previously, the spleen develops in the dorsal mesogastrium, so that except for its hilum, it is completely invested with peritoneum. The peritoneum fuses to the fibrous capsule of the spleen. The hilum is a longitudinal fissure on the visceral surface of the spleen which admits the vessels, nerves, and lymphatics conveyed to the spleen in the lienorenal ligament. This ligament is attached to the posterior lip of the hilum, and generally contains the tail of the pancreas, making it the only organ that directly contacts the spleen. The gastrolienal ligament, attached to the anterior lip of the hilum, conveys branches of the splenic vessels to the stomach. A peritoneal reflection may run from the lower pole to the greater omentum. A tearing of this reflection during surgical retraction of the stomach to the right may result in severe bleeding.

The arterial supply of the spleen originates from the splenic artery, which is a branch of the celiac trunk (Figure 4). Upon emerging from the celiac trunk, the splenic artery courses along or within the superior margin of the pancreas toward the spleen. Near the hilus, and within the lienorenal ligament, the artery divides into numerous branches. The most important branches are the superior polar, left gastroepiploic, and superior and inferior terminal arteries. The su-

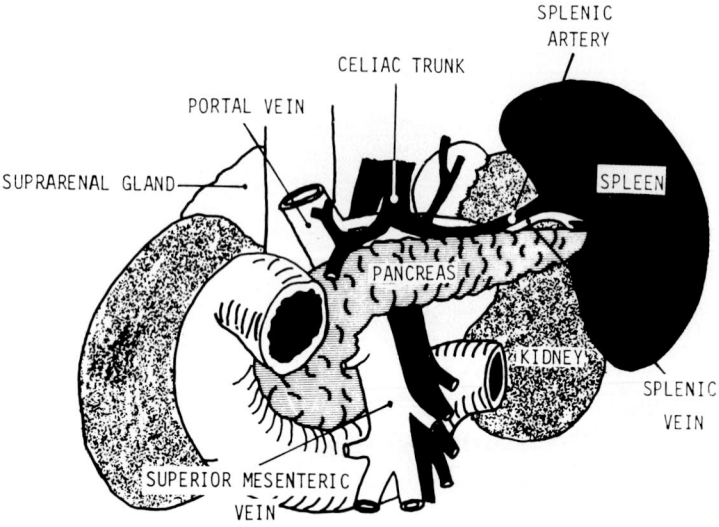

Figure 4 Vascular supply of the spleen.

perior polar artery arises some distance from the hilus and, before entering the spleen, distributes short gastric arteries to the stomach. The left gastroepiploic artery passes along the inferior pole of the spleen to supply a part of the greater curvature of the stomach and the greater omentum. The superior and inferior terminal arteries divide into secondary branches, which penetrate the splenic parenchyma at the hilus. These give rise to end arteries supplying a wedge-shaped area of the spleen. If these terminal arteries are blocked, a splenic infarct may result.

The notches on the surface of the spleen delineate zones of venous drainage. Most authors describe three zones, although others define between two and six regions of venous drainage. Regardless of the pattern of drainage, all splenic zones eventually drain into the splenic vein. This vein begins as several large branches leaving the hilum of the spleen (Figure 4). It runs dorsal to the splenic artery and pancreas, joining with the superior mesenteric vein to form the portal vein. Shortly before joining the superior mesenteric vein, the inferior mesenteric vein may empty into the splenic vein. Lymphatics within the spleen are confined to its capsule and to large trabeculae within the parenchyma.

Nerve fibers from the median and anterior parts of the celiac plexus as well as fibers directly from the splanchnic nerves form a dense network along the splenic artery. This splenic plexus is composed mainly of nonmyelinated fibers.

ANATOMY OF THE SPLEEN

Recent studies (7,8) suggest that these fibers influence not only the vasculature of the spleen but they also influence the immune reactions elicited by the parenchyma.

MICROSCOPIC ORGANIZATION OF THE SPLEEN

Capsule and Trabeculae

The spleen is surrounded by a dense fibrous capsule a few millimeters thick. From the internal capsular surface, a network of trabeculae project inward toward the splenic parenchyma or pulp, subdividing it into numerous communicating compartments (Figure 5). These septae contain the blood vessels and nerves that supply the splenic pulp. The presence of lymphatics within these trabeculae has been debated for many years. Lymphatics can be found in the adventitia of arteries, but it is not certain whether they penetrate to any extent into the pulp. Goldberg's findings suggest that lymphatics do indeed extend deeply into the parenchyma (9).

The connective tissue of the capsule and the trabeculae contains numerous elastic fibers and some smooth muscle cells. In humans, these cells are not numerous. In certain other mammals (such as the dog and cat) these cells are quite abundant and their contraction causes the expulsion of accumulated blood from the spleen. The paucity of smooth muscle cells in the splenic capsule and trabeculae in humans, however, does not support this concept for the release of blood from the spleen. Nonetheless, because of the abundance of elastic tissue, and because of the arrangement of fibrous connective tissue in wavy bundles, the spleen is distensible and capable of considerable change in volume.

Splenic Pulp

The splenic pulp may be subdivided into red and white pulp. These contain an extensive network of reticular fibers that support the cellular elements of the spleen (Figure 6). Fixed cellular elements of the splenic pulp consist of the reticular cells. The relationship between the reticular cells and reticular fibers has not been fully explained. Electron photomicrographs show that the reticular fibers may be encased in extensions of reticular cells (Figure 6).

Owing to the presence of numerous erythrocytes, most of the splenic pulp is red, the red pulp occupying 76-79% by volume. Another prominent cell within the red pulp is the platelet. The normal spleen can sequester about 45% of the platelets released from the bone marrow. In cases of splenomegaly the spleen can sequester over 90% of the body's platelets. The red pulp contains the venous sinuses (or sinusoids) and splenic cords (cords of Billroth) (Figure 7, *A* and *B*). The venous sinuses are vascular channels lined by endothelial cells (stave cells) and hoop-like arrangements of basement membrane.

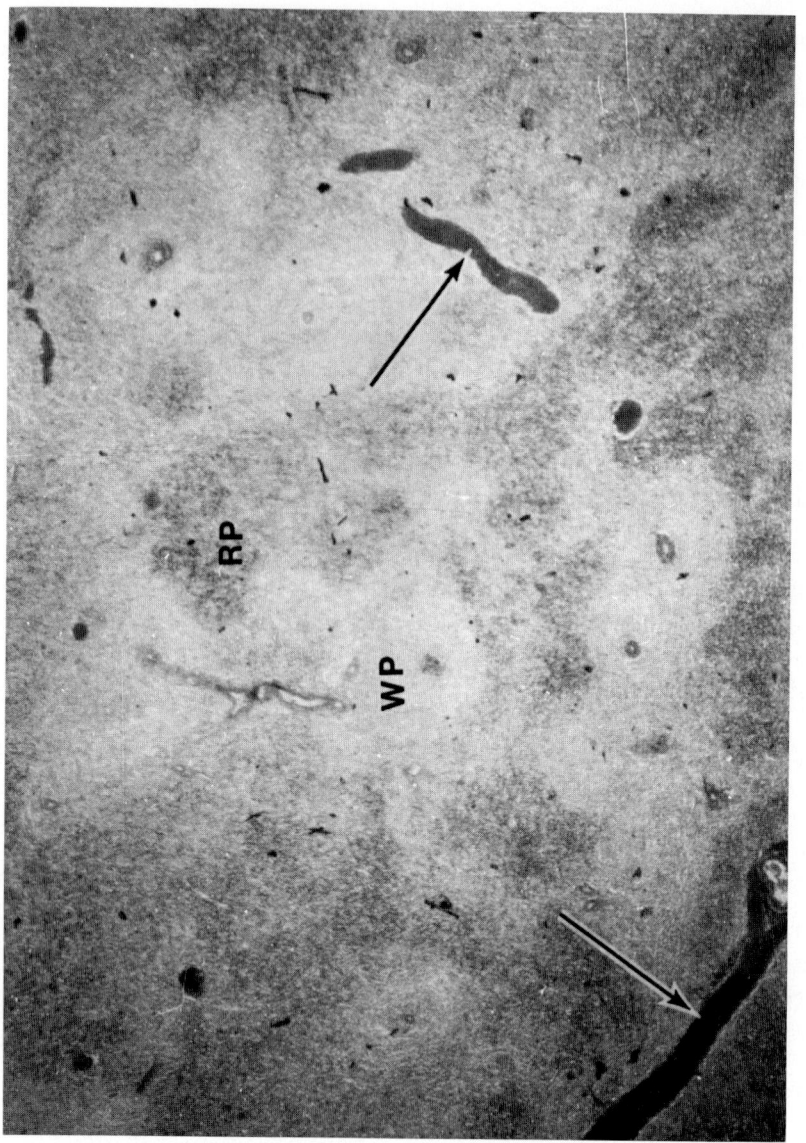

Figure 5 Photomicrograph of adult spleen showing areas of white pulp (WP) and red pulp (RP). Note the vessels within the trabeculae (arrows). (Gomori stain, × 104)

ANATOMY OF THE SPLEEN

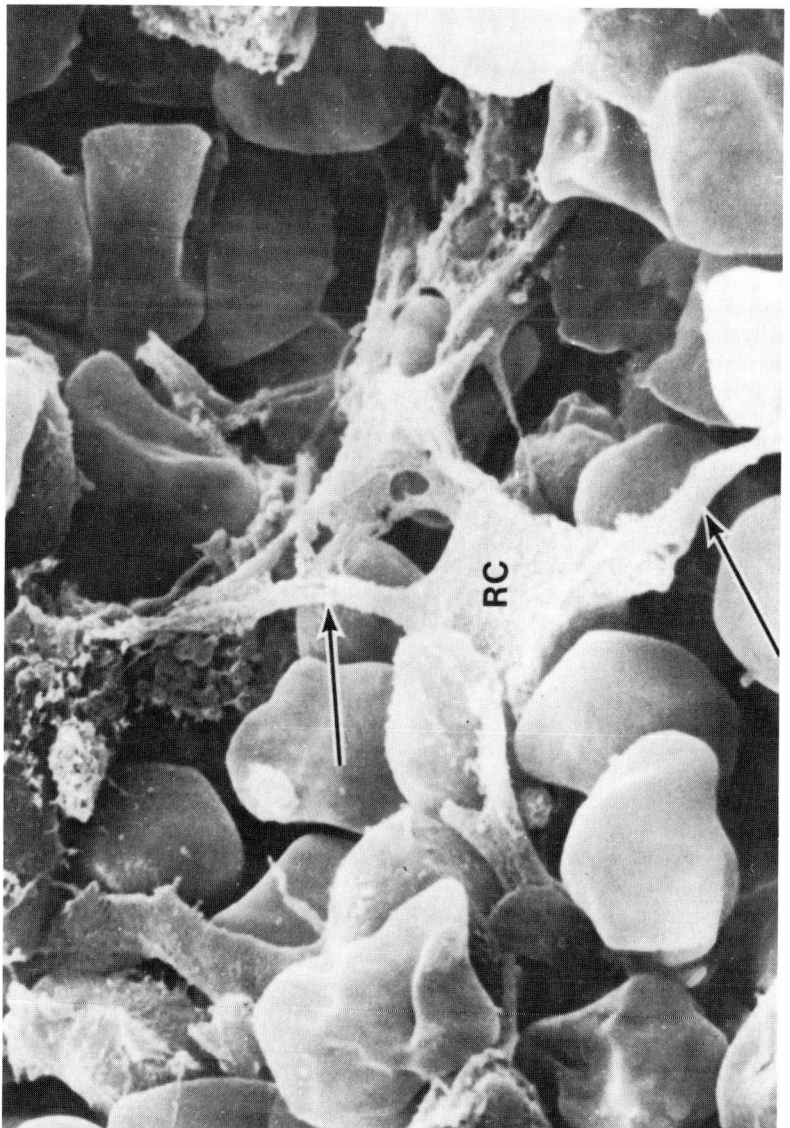

Figure 6 Scanning electron micrograph of a reticular cell (RC) and its processes (arrows) within the red pulp. (× 800)

Figure 7A

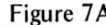

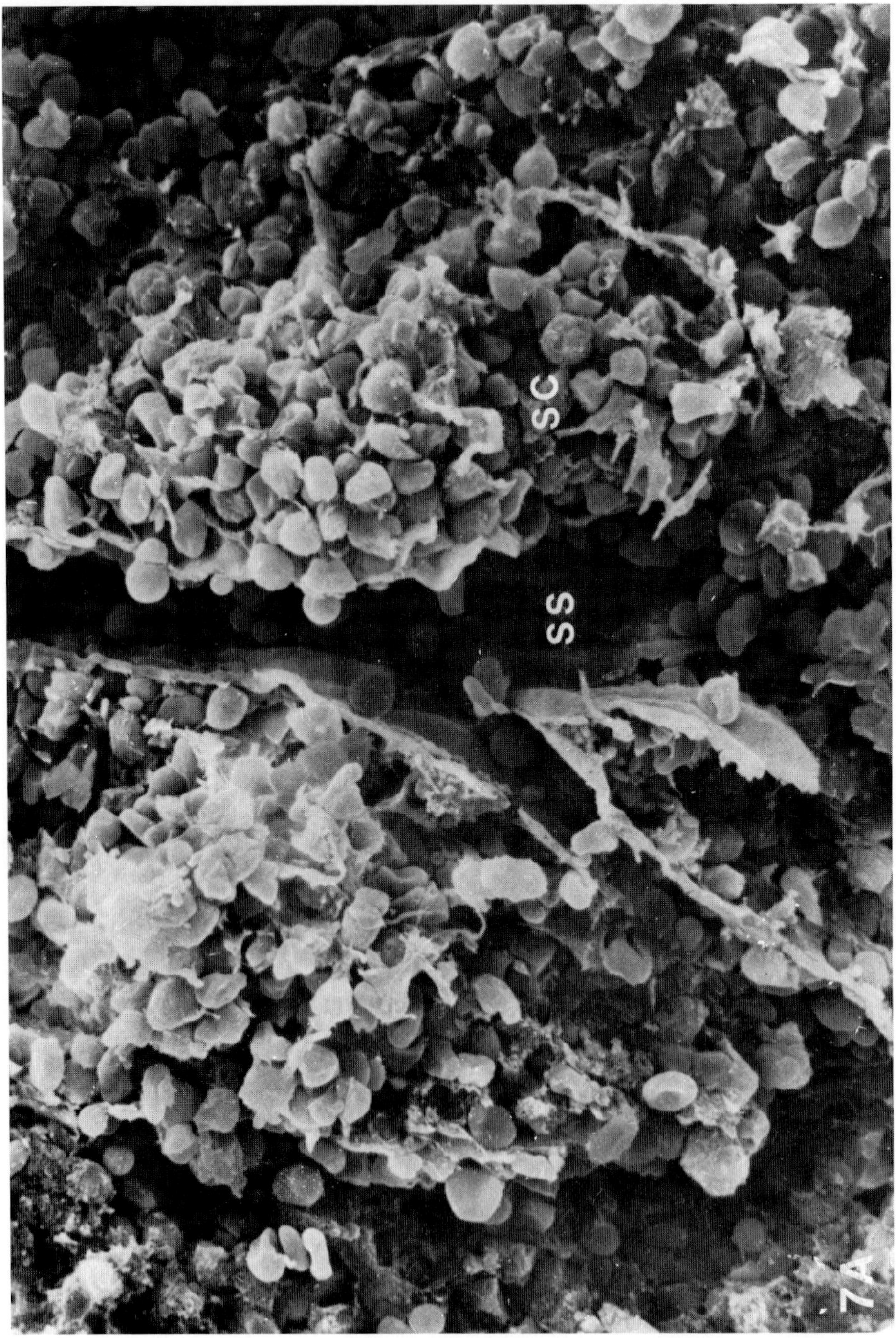

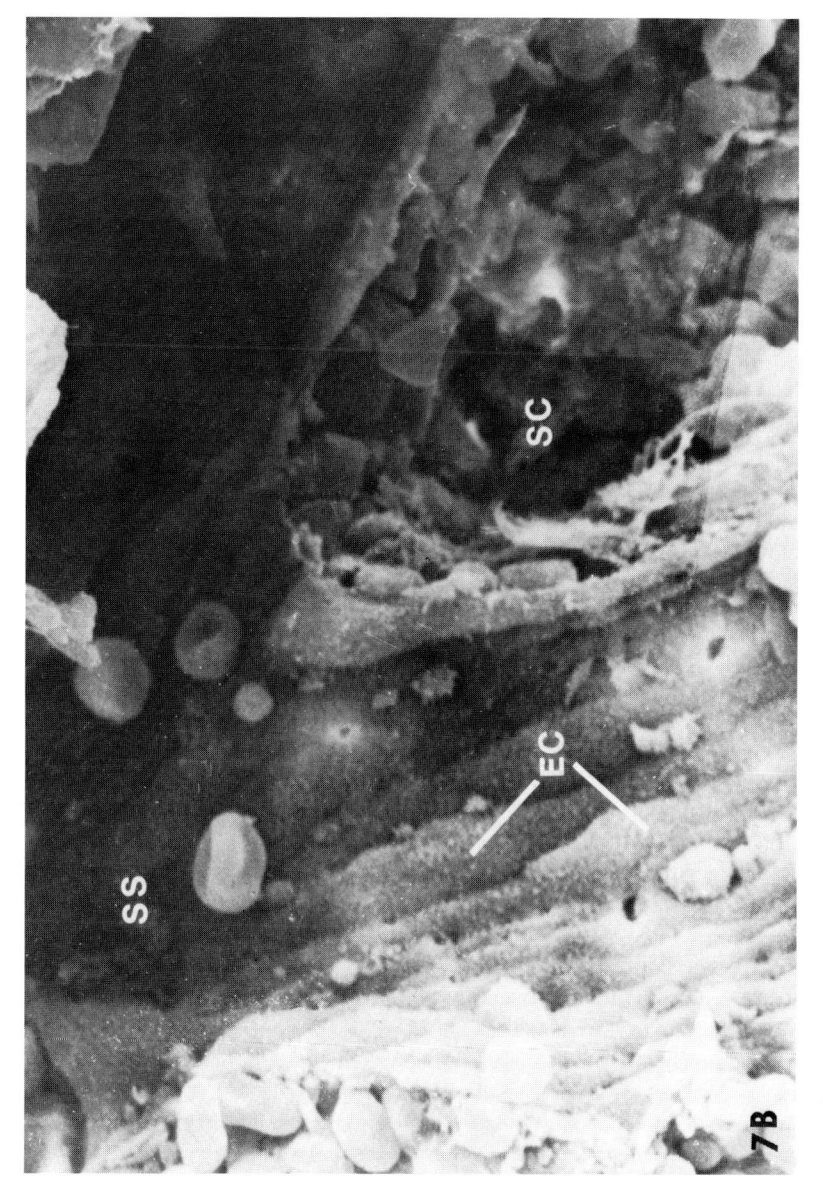

Figure 7 (A) Scanning electron micrograph of a splenic sinus (SS) surrounded by a splenic cord (SC). (X 780) (B) Scanning electron micrograph of a splenic sinus (SS) and adjacent splenic cord. Note the endothelial cells (EC) forming the sinus. (X 1300)

The endothelial cells measure more than 50 μm in length and are arranged in a manner such that there are numerous slits or openings between the cells. The sinus has been compared to a barrel made of green wood and allowed to dry in the sun. The lining cells represent the staves of the barrel and the ring fibers represent the hoops (10). Within the limits of its surface area and volume, the erythrocyte can be deformed to pass through pores as small as 1 μm in diameter. The size of the slits or pores between the endothelial cells are large enough to allow an erythrocyte easy passage between the cord and the sinus. It is of further interest that the sinus endothelium is characterized by numerous pinocytotic vesicles. These vesicles may be the means or route for the incorporation of hemoglobin that escapes into the splenic sinus by pinocytotic activity, rather than the hemoglobin being incorporated by the mechanism of phagocytosis characteristic of macrophages.

The splenic cords, on the other hand, are continuous partitions of tissue between the venous sinuses. The cords contain erythrocytes, lymphocytes, macrophages, granulocytes, and numerous antibody-secreting plasma cells. Erythrocytes liberated into the splenic cords must squeeze through slits between the endothelial cells of the sinus to enter its lumen (Figure 8). The spleen monitors abnormal erythrocytes by this mechanical sieving, and cells that have lost their plasticity are destroyed as they pass from cord to sinus (11). Sequestration of abnormal red cells in the cordal compartment of the spleen is due to decreased plasticity (or increased rigidity), which prevents their easy passage through the walls of the sinuses. Sequestration may also be due to other membrane abnormalities that make the red cells vulnerable to phagocytic digestion.

Another mechanism for the removal and subsequent destruction of cells or cellular elements involves the arterioles and their surrounding reticulum. Shortly before they terminate, arterioles within the red pulp may be modified by passing through a periarterial macrophagic sheath (12). Erythrocytes, granulocytes, and other blood cells may be present in the sheath. These sheaths may represent a site for a major population of macrophages in the spleen. Well-developed sheaths possess an extraordinary phagocytic capacity and can be a major site of clearance of blood-borne particles in the red pulp.

The white pulp is composed of compact lymphatic tissue arranged around branches of the trabecular arteries (Figure 9). Lymphocytes infiltrate the adventitia of these arteries and subsequently surround or ensheath them, forming a lymphatic periarterial sheath (**PALS**). These lymphocytes are predominantly T cells of the recirculating pool. Along the course of these arteries, the periarterial or lymphatic sheath periodically expands to help form a number of spherical or ovoid lymphatic nodules. These lymphatic nodules are sometimes referred to as splenic nodules or Malpighian corpuscles. The nodules lie within the periarterial lymphatic sheath and contain high concentrations of B cells. Although in each of

ANATOMY OF THE SPLEEN

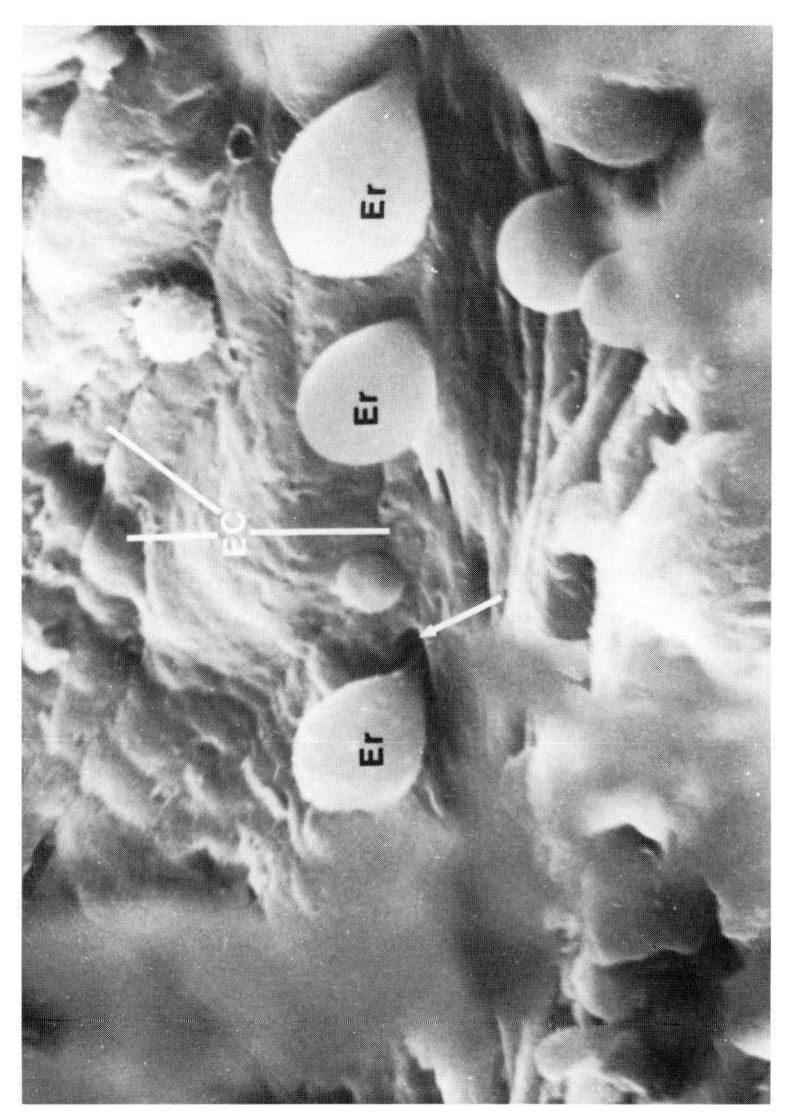

Figure 8 Scanning electron micrograph within a splenic sinus. Notice the erythrocytes (Er) entering the lumen of the sinus through pores or slits (arrows) between endothelial cells. (× 4000)

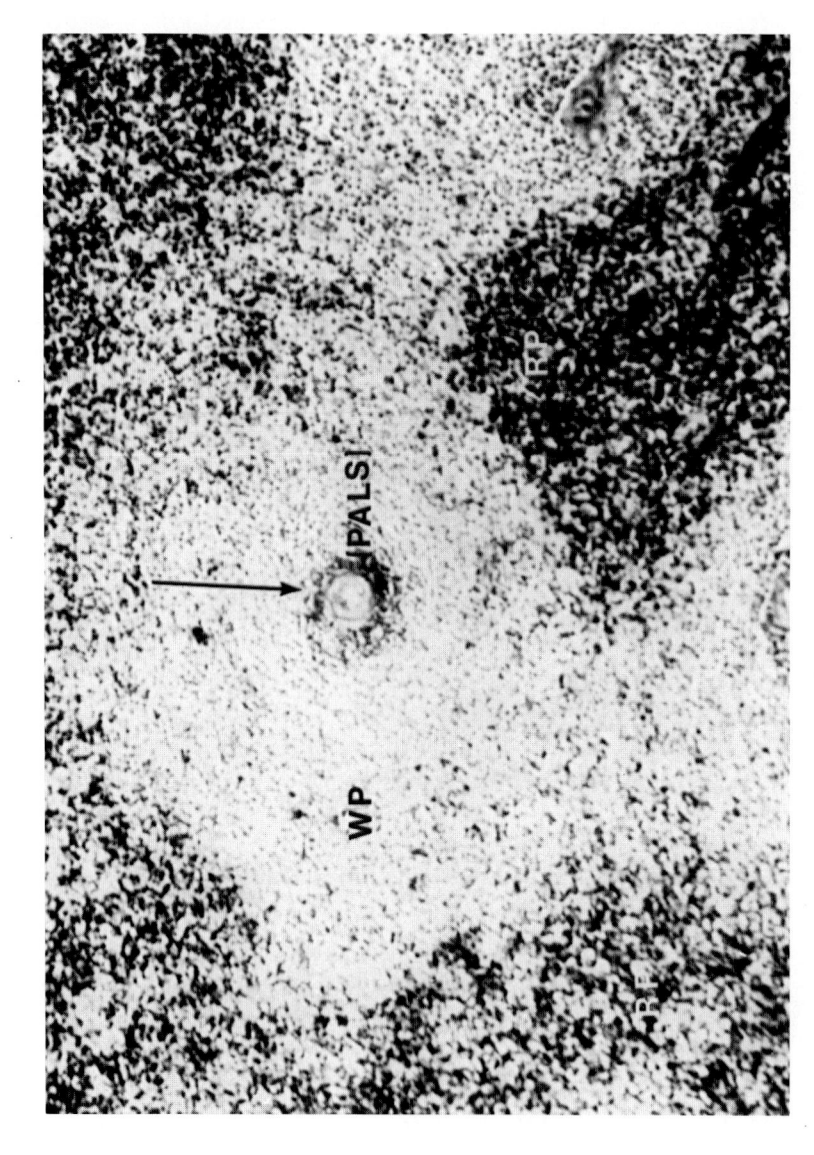

Figure 9 Photomicrograph of an adult spleen showing white pulp (WP) and red pulp (RP). Note the periarterial lymphatic sheath (PALS) surrounding a central artery (arrow). (Gomori stain, X 256)

ANATOMY OF THE SPLEEN

these nodules an artery usually occupies an eccentric position, this artery is called a central artery. Except for their larger blood vessels, the lymphatic nodules of the spleen are very similar in structure to lymphatic nodules found in lymph nodes and, like the latter, may contain germinal centers. In children, a germinal center is usually found in each nodule or follicle, but in the adult spleen the germinal centers are less numerous. Disease also influences the state of the germinal centers. In lymphocytic leukemia, the white pulp hypertrophies and the red pulp atrophies; while in myeloid leukemia the red pulp expands and the white pulp shrinks.

The cells of the white pulp of the spleen are similar to those in lymph nodes; the white pulp consists of lymphocytes, macrophages, and other cells of the reticulum. Large, medium, and small lymphocytes are numerous and compactly arranged. Large and medium lymphocytes are especially numerous in the germinal centers. Both free and attached macrophages are found throughout the white pulp. These macrophages may contain foreign particles, degenerating granulocytes, and fragmented or whole erythrocytes. Frequently, the macrophages of white pulp contain reddish or brownish pigment granules (hemosiderin) derived from the hemoglobin of phagocytosed erythrocytes.

Monocytes and plasma cells are also fairly numerous in the white pulp of the spleen. Monocytes enter the spleen via the circulating blood. They have phagocytic properties and, when very active, may enlarge to become macrophages. The plasma cells are similar to those observed in the red pulp in that they are also involved in the production of antibodies. Although megakaryocytes similar to those in bone marrow have been observed in splenic pulp in the fetal spleen, they are absent in the adult.

Between the red and white pulp is an area termed the marginal zone. In this region a great deal of the processing and filtration of blood occurs. Its matrix consists of many sinuses and a reticular meshwork interspersed with a few lymphocytes but with many macrophages showing active phagocytosis. The marginal zone retains large amounts of blood antigens and thus plays a major role in the immunologic activity of the spleen. Many of the pulp arterioles, derived from the central artery, extend out and away from the white pulp, but then they turn back and empty into the moatlike sinuses of the marginal zone that encircles the nodules. As a consequence of this drainage, this area plays a significant role in filtering the blood and initiating the immune response. A large number of macrophages trap antigens and then present them to immunologically competent cells. T and B lymphocytes are also removed from the blood in the marginal zone. As these lymphocytes leave the systemic circulation to penetrate the white pulp, they pass macrophages presenting exposed antigen. If the appropriate B cells, T cells, and antigen are present, an immune response will be initiated.

Splenic Vasculature

The spleen is supplied by the splenic artery and vein, which pass through the hilus and subsequently branch to pass into the trabeculae. The trabecular arteries are relatively thick-walled and are especially rich in elastic fibers. As the arteries pass through the trabeculae they narrow and eventually leave the trabeculae at a diameter of 150-250 μm to enter the white pulp. The smaller-sized trabeculae contain only veins. As the arteries enter the pulp, they are surrounded by a sheath of lymphatic tissue, called the periarteriolar lymphatic sheath. These vessels, termed central arteries, travel through the sheath and enter the red pulp (Figure 9). Walls of the central arteries are composed of the layers characteristic of an artery, namely, an endothelium with prominent nuclei, an internal elastic lamina, a smooth muscle media, and an adventitia. Splenic arteries are noted for their tall endothelium (13).

As the central artery courses through the lymphatic sheath, it sends out many branches, termed arterioles, that supply the lymphatic nodules. These arterioles branch at large angles approaching 90°. This branching of arteries favors plasma skimming, since the cellular elements flow in the middle of the vessel while the plasma is at the periphery. This mechanism may be a way in which the arterial system contributes to hemoconcentration in the spleen (14). In the human spleen most branches travel to the periphery of the sheath and terminate in the marginal zone.

Within the sheath these arterioles contribute to the vascular bed of the nodule by encircling it, similar to a hand grasping a ball. Before the arterioles finally lose their sheaths of lymphatic tissue and enter the surrounding marginal zone, they divide into a number of straight vessels termed penicilli. After passing through the marginal zone, each of these vessels develops a slight thickening of its coat known as the sheath of Schweigger-Seidel. These sheaths are formed by an aggregation of macrophages, lymphocytes, and reticular cells. They are well-developed in some mammals, such as the cat and dog, but are small and inconspicuous in man. The sheaths are elongated tubular structures in man and dog, but are spherical or ellipsoid in the cat.

Many different functions have been ascribed to these arterial sheaths. Early investigators felt they were vasomotor centers, regulating blood pressure between the arterial system and the pulp. Others thought they were nervous centers, receiving terminations of the splenic nerves. Studies by Solnitzky (15), and by French, Wilkinson, and White (16) showed that these sheaths serve as phagocytic sites, which sequester particulate matter soon after its entry into the spleen and also serve as important structures involved in the fixation of antigen.

In the red pulp and in the marginal zone, blood flows through cords and enters splenic sinuses (Figure 8). The splenic sinuses penetrate the entire red pulp and are especially numerous outside the marginal zone surrounding the white pulp. These vessels are called sinuses because they have a wide (12-40 µm) irregular lumen, the size of which varies with the amount of blood in the organ.

The venous sinuses empty into the veins of the pulp. The walls of these veins consist of endothelium supported externally by a condensed stroma of the red pulp and a few elastic fibers. The pulp veins coalesce to form the veins of the trabeculae. Walls of these vessels consist only of endothelium supported by the connective tissue of the trabeculae. The trabecular veins form the splenic vein, which leaves the organ at the hilus and empties into the portal vein.

Open Versus Closed Circulation

The exact manner in which arterial capillaries terminate within the spleen has been debated for many years. Is the circulation open or closed? Do the arterial vessels connect directly to venous vessels, with endothelial continuity (closed circulation)? Or, do the arterial vessels terminate and empty into the cords or pulp spaces, with the blood flowing through these spaces and then through the walls of venous vessels (open circulation)? Alternatively, is the circulation through the red pulp partly open and partly closed?

Although some investigations have suggested that the circulation through the red pulp of the spleen is closed (17), most of the evidence suggests that the vascular channel through the red pulp, whether of the sinusal or nonsinusal type, is open (12,18). Arterial terminations can be seen by light and electron microscopy to open into the cords or pulp spaces that contain large accumulations of blood. Blood cells, moreover, may regularly be observed crossing the wall of vascular sinuses through interendothelial slits or pores (Figure 8). There is no convincing evidence of continuity of endothelium between arterial capillaries and venous sinuses or pulp veins. Thus, it appears that the circulation of the spleen is open. Blood may pass from the arterial endings through the reticular meshwork of the marginal zone and thence to the venous sinuses or veins.

SUMMARY

The spleen is derived from condenstations of mesenchymal tissue in the left side of the dorsal mesogastrium. Upon development, it is found in the left hypochondriac region adjacent to ribs nine, ten, and eleven. In the adult, the spleen contacts the stomach, pancreas, left kidney, and splenic flexure of the colon. In a child, the spleen also contacts the left suprarenal gland.

The spleen is surrounded by a dense connective tissue capsule, which sends trabeculae into the parenchyma. These trabeculae contain vessels, nerves, and lymphatics. The parenchyma is composed of lymphatic nodules (white pulp) and areas rich in blood cells (red pulp). Cells contained in the white pulp include lymphocytes, macrophages, monocytes, and plasma cells. The red pulp consists of a network of open sinusoids and a reticular meshwork between them. The intersinusoidal area contains numerous erythrocytes and platelets. Due to its open pattern of circulation, the adult spleen functions to remove and destroy microbial pathogens as well as monitor and remove aged and damaged erythrocytes, leukocytes, and platelets.

ACKNOWLEDGMENTS

The author is grateful to Drs. Harold Brody and Chester Glomski and Dr. Judith Tamburlin for reviewing this manuscript, to Dr. Ted Szczesny for technical assitance in electron microscopy, and to Mrs. Shirley Travers for typing the text.

REFERENCES

1. Ono K: Untersuchungen ueber die Entwicklung der menschlichen Milz. *Ztschr f Zellforsch u mikr Anat* 1930; 10:573.
2. Moore MAS, Metcalf D. Ontogeny of the haemopoietic system: Yolk sac origin of in vivo and in vitro colony forming cells in the developing mouse embryo. *Br J Haematol* 1970;18:279.
3. Suzuki HK: Development of phagocytic activity in the reticuloendothelial system of the albino rat; a comparison of prenatal, neonatal, juvenile and adult periods. *Yale J Biol Med* 1957; 29:504.
4. Gurich HG: Doppelmilz bei partiellem situs inversus du Bauchorgane. *Acta Hepatosplen* 1968; 15:43-48.
5. Curtis GM, Movitz D: The surgical significance of the accessory spleen. *Ann Surg* 1946; 123:276-298.
6. Cremer J, Schleiblinger W: *Klinik der Milzkrankheiten*. Ferdinand Enke Verlag, Stuttgart, 1967.
7. Williams JM, Peterson RG, Shea PA, Schmedtje JF, Bauer DC, Felten DL: Sympathetic innervation of murine thymus and spleen: evidence for a functional link between the nervous and immune systems. *Brain Res Bull* 1980; 6:83-94.
8. Felten DL, Felten SY, Carlson SL, Olschowka JA, Liunat S: Noradrenergic and peptidergic innervation of lymphoid tissue. *J Immunol* 1985; 135:755-765.
9. Goldberg GM, Ungar H: The lymphatics of the spleen in leukaemia. *Lab Invest* 1958; 7:146.
10. Wennberg E, Weiss L: The structure of the spleen and hemolysis. *Ann Rev Med* 1969; 20:29-40.
11. Chen LT, Weiss L: The role of the sinus wall in the passage of erythrocytes through the spleen. *Blood* 1973; 41:529-537.
12. Blue J, Weiss L: Vascular pathways in non-sinusal red pulp; an electron microscope study of cap spleen. *Am J Anat* 1981; 161:135.

13. Hummel KP: The structure and development of the lymphatic tissue in the intestine of the Albino rat. *Am J Anat* 1935; 57:351.
14. Weiss L: The structure of the intermediate vascular pathways in the spleen of rabbits. *Am J Anat* 1962; 113:51-91.
15. Solnitzky O: The Schweigger-Seidel sheath (ellipsoid) of the spleen. *Anat Rec* 1937; 69:55.
16. Frenci VI, Wilkinson PC, White RG: Localization by immunofluorescence of 19S and 7S immunoglobulin in the lymphoid tissue of the chicken and its relation to specific antibody production. In Fiore-Donata L, Hanna MG (eds): *Lymphatic Tissue and Germinal Genters in Immune Response,* Plenum Press, New York, 1969, p. 211.
17. Knisely MH: Spleen studies; microscopic observations on the circulatory systems of living unstimulated mammalian spleens. *Anat Rec* 1936; 65:23.
18. McCuskey RS, McCuskey PA: In vivo microscopy of the spleen. *Bibl Anat* 1977; 16:121.

2
Spleen in Blood Cell Regulation and Hematopoiesis

MARK F. SEIFERT
University of South Dakota School of Medicine, Vermillion, South Dakota

The adult spleen is a large lymphoid organ situated in the bloodstream and performs multiple functions. Principal among these functions are (1) filtration, (2) phagocytosis and removal of senescent or damaged blood cells, (3) antigen uptake and antibody formation, (4) lymphocyte production, and (5) storage of platelets and certain blood cells for release under conditions of stress (1). During the second trimester of fetal development the spleen is also active in hematopoiesis (2,3). This hematopoietic function gradually decreases after the fifth month of gestation as the bone marrow becomes the predominant blood cell forming site.

The purpose of this chapter is to review the role of the spleen as a hematopoietic organ during its ontogenesis in man, and to discuss its potential capacity for hematopoiesis postnatally in health and disease.

PHYLOGENESIS AND ONTOGENESIS OF SPLENIC HEMATOPOIESIS

Study of the evolutionary history of splenic structure and function reveals this organ to be very complex (4). Research during the past few decades has done much to increase our understanding of this organ. But the spleen continues to be of special interest to physicians and investigators who are concerned with diseases of the blood and blood forming organs.

In all vertebrates the hematopoietic system originates with the appearance of pluripotent hematopoietic stem cells in blood islands of the yolk sac. During embryonic development in lower vertebrates blood cell formation is exclusively extramedullary, occurring in various sites, such as in the intestinal wall, gonads, kidney, liver, lymph nodes, and spleen (5). It is in the cartilagenous and bony fishes that the spleen first develops in the dorsal mesentery of the stomach and becomes an essential and primary blood-producing organ (6).

With the appearance of hollow bones beginning in anuran amphibians, conditions became favorable for a shift in erythropoietic activity from the spleen to bone marrow (7). In reptiles, birds and certain mammals, erythropoiesis, granulopoiesis and, somewhat later in evolution, thrombopoiesis, was transferred entirely from the spleen to the bone marrow in adult animals. Lymphocyte production, though retained in adults, also became partially transferred to lymph nodes and bone marrow. In adult spleens of higher mammals, the primary cell-forming functions are the formation of lymphocytes and monocytes, which are central to the animal's surveillance and immune functions.

The evolutionary advantage of this transfer of hematopoietic function from spleen to bone marrow and lymph nodes is unknown. Two possibilities, however, have been proposed (1). The first possible advantage is that the transfer of hematopoietic function from spleen to bone marrow results in decentralization of blood cell production. Bone marrow cavities present a more favorable and efficient environment for hematopoiesis. Locating hematopoiesis in the various bones of the body also decreases the vulnerability of an organism to injury or disease, as might occur when the blood forming organ is centralized.

The second proposed advantage of transfer of hematopoietic function from the spleen to bone marrow and lymph nodes is that the development of lymph nodes and lymphocyte production in peripheral parts of an organism also provides an evolutionary advantage. Such peripheral placement of lymph nodes and lymphocyte production places cells responsible for identifying foreign antigens invading the individual in a better position to respond to these antigens and to neutralize them.

Embryonic development of the hematopoietic system in higher vertebrates essentially recapitulates the phylogenesis of this system (8,9). That is, there is a sequential movement of hematopoietic centers from the yolk sac to the body mesenchyme (meninges, mesentery, and gonads), to the kidneys, to the liver, to the spleen, and lymph nodes, and to the bone marrow (5,8,9) (Figure 1).

In certain mammals, notably the mouse and rat, the spleen is a significant organ of hematopoietic activity (10-13). Immediately after birth, the spleen and liver in these animals are the principal hematopoietic centers (10,14,15). At this time, the bone marrow contains few if any erythroid elements, which only first appear about 12 hours after birth (16). In rats there is a decline in splenic

YOLK SAC
↓
BODY MESENCHYME
↓
KIDNEYS
↓
LIVER
↓
SPLEEN AND LYMPH NODES
↓
BONE MARROW

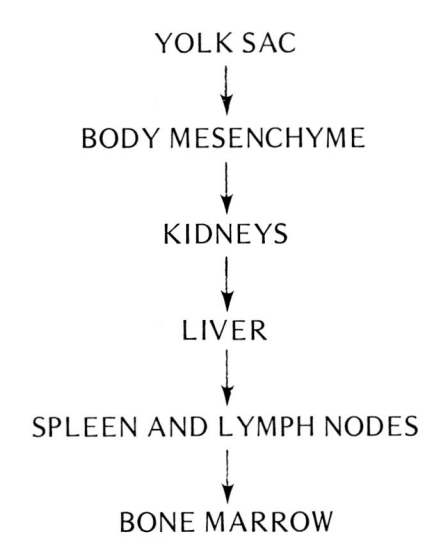

Figure 1 Sequential movement of centers of hematopoiesis during embryologic development of higher vertebrates. There is sequential movement of hematopoietic centers from the yolk sac, to the body mesenchyme, to the kidneys, to the liver, to the spleen and lymph nodes, and then to the bone marrow. This scheme recapitulates the phylogenesis of the hematopoietic system.

hematopoietic activity between the fifth and tenth days of life (17). This decline in splenic hematopoiesis is coincident with the transition from the presence in the spleen of an actively proliferating stem cell pool to a more resting stem cell pool. In the adult rat, less than 5% of erythropoiesis occurs in the spleen (18).

In contrast, the mouse demonstrates an explosive growth of the spleen during the first 2 weeks of postnatal life. As a result, by the fourteenth day of life the amount of erythropoiesis in the spleen is almost twice that of the bone marrow (10). This hematopoietic activity in the murine spleen subsequently wanes as the bone marrow assumes this function. But the transfer of hematopoietic activity is incomplete, with the spleen retaining a considerable amount of erythropoietic activity for the whole life of the animal (13,19). Thus, the degree of erythropoietic development in the newborn mouse corresponds to that found in the fifth or sixth month of gestation in humans (15). The mechanisms underlying the postnatal transition of erythropoietic activity in rodents from the spleen to the bone marrow are unclear. However, these transition mechanisms most likely involve developmental changes in the hematopoietic microenvironment of the spleen.

SPLENIC HEMATOPOIESIS IN MAN

Hematopoiesis in the spleen of the human fetus begins early in the second trimester and reaches a peak on about the thirteenth week of gestation. The splenic hematopoiesis gradually declines during the fifth month when intramedullary hematopoiesis begins (2,3,20). However, the contribution of the spleen to blood cell formation in the developing fetus is small, as compared to the liver, which is the principal extramedullary blood forming organ in the fetus.

Extremely high numbers of hematopoietic progenitor cells circulate in the blood of the human fetus at as early as 12 weeks of gestation (21,22). On the basis of this finding, it is hypothesized that developing fetal tissues are colonized by these circulating progenitor cells (23). Intense hematopoietic activity, primarily erythroblastic, in the liver is maintained until the bone marrow becomes an effective blood forming center. The reason for the predominance of the liver as a hematopoietic center in the developing fetus is unknown. However, intensive blood cell formation in the liver may relate to the presence of a more favorable hematopoietic microenvironment in this organ, or it may be related to the fact that during fetal development the liver is a major producer of erythropoietin (24,25). Immature forms of granulocytes and megakaryocytes which are intimately associated with cytoplasmic processes of reticular cells have been observed in the liver (26), but not in the spleen (27). Normally, by the end of pregnancy almost all erythropoiesis is taking place in the bone marrow, while liver and splenic hematopoiesis cease shortly before birth (28).

Much of our earlier knowledge of hematopoiesis in the fetal spleen has been derived from studies using nonhuman species (8,29,30) or from studies of human fetuses using conventional morphological techniques (31-33). However, recent studies challenge earlier concepts regarding hematopoiesis in the spleen and suggest that the spleen is not a significant organ of hematopoiesis in the human fetus.

In an ultrastructural study of human fetal spleens, Ishikawa (27) could not detect progenitor cells of the erythrocytic, granulocytic and megakaryocytic series. This finding implies that the differentiation of pluripotent hematopoietic stem cells into cells of these lineages (erythrocytes, granulocytes, and platelets) does not take place. In addition, there was no observable association between reticular cells and immature granulocytes or megakaryocytes. This lack of association suggests that the reticular cells in the human fetal spleen are unable to regulate the differentiation of pluripotential stem cells. Reticular cells of the spleen are also unable to provide a suitable hematopoietic inductive microenvironment (34) for support and differentiation of immature blood forms. In support of this concept, ultrastructural studies of human fetal spleens were unable to confirm a high degree of hematopoiesis (35).

Studies examining hematopoiesis in the fetal human yolk sac and liver failed to mention the presence of blood cell formation in the spleen (36,37). Furthermore, the use of immunohistological and cytochemical techniques to identify erythroid and granulocytic precursors more primitive than those recognizable by routine microscopy alone failed to demonstrate early progeny in any of the 3 myeloid cell lines from spleens of fetuses 12 to 40 weeks of gestation (38). From this study it was concluded that the spleen of the human fetus is not a significant organ of hematopoiesis.

These morphological and immunohistochemical findings, however, conflict with the in vitro studies of Hann et al. (21). Using mixed colony assay techniques, this group was the first to delineate the development of hematopoiesis in the mid-trimester human fetus. Their data clearly show that pluripotent (CFU-GEMM) and unipotent (BFU-E, CFU-GM) stem cells populate the liver throughout weeks 12 to 23 of gestation. They also showed that the bone marrow becomes populated at weeks 15 and 16 and that the spleen becomes populated only later, at 18 to 19 weeks. This demonstration of the presence of hematopoietic stem cells in fetal spleens beginning at 18 to 19 weeks runs counter to the studies cited, which failed to detect these cells and their progeny in fetuses ranging from 12 to 40 weeks of gestation.

Phagocytosis of hematopoietic cells has been observed in fetal spleens at as early as 12 weeks of gestation (38). This observation has been interpreted to mean that the presence of these precursor cells resulted from their entrapment and filtration by the spleen. This phagocytic activity may explain why pluripotent stem cells were not observed in significant numbers until 18 to 19 weeks of gestation (21). Also, presence of hematopoietic cells at this time may be explained by the high circulating levels of these cells which overcomes the phagocytic capacity of this organ. These conflicting views as to the role of the spleen in the human fetus may relate to the different techniques used in the various studies.

Thus, it appears in man that the principal hematopoietic organs, and the sequence in the development of hematopoiesis, are: the yolk sac, liver, (spleen), bone marrow and/or (spleen) (2,3,21). The relative contribution and onset of function of the spleen in this developmental process is unresolved and requires more study. The simultaneous application of cell culture, plus morphological and immunocytochemical techniques, to this question should resolve some of these previously conflicting observations.

SPLENIC HEMATOPOIESIS IN DISEASE

From this phylogenetic history of hematopoietic development, it is presumed that there remains in adult animals and in man the potential for recovery of hematopoietic activity in sites of embryonic hematopoiesis. This reversion to extramedullary hematopoiesis occurs when the bone marrow is diseased, when it is damaged by irradiation or chemotherapy, or fails to develop (8,39).

Clinical features of the myeloproliferative diseases include marrow fibrosis, splenomegaly or hepatosplenomegaly, and extramedullary hematopoiesis (8,40, 41). These disorders, including myelofibrosis with myeloid metaplasia (MMM), chronic lymphocytic leukemia (CLL), chronic myelogenous leukemia (CML), polycythemia vera (PV), and idiopathic thrombocythemia (IT) are clonal hemopathies (42). Each of these disorders is thought to arise from some defect in pluripotent hematopoietic stem cells, which respond abnormally to regulatory factors. This abnormal response of the stem cells results in proliferation of myeloid and stromal cell lines in the bone marrow and in extramedullary sites (8, 40,43). The mechanisms underlying this response are unknown.

How does the adult spleen revert to an embryonic hematopoietic function? Are resident hematopoietic stem cells reactivated by some myelostimulatory factor, as is postulated by many (8,43,44)? Or, are the increased numbers of hematopoietic progenitor cells in such spleens the result of migratory influx of these cells to the spleen from other body sites? Is there de-repression of the splenic hematopoietic inductive microenvironment to support renewed blood cell formation?

A body of literature holds that the adult spleen and other previous hematopoietic centers are indeed capable of reversion to their earlier embryonic function, (8,43-46) however, this concept has been challenged recently by Wolf and Nieman (47,48). They cite studies (38) (noted above) of the lack of significant hematopoiesis in fetal spleens. Also, they were unable to demonstrate splenic hematopoiesis in patients with myelofibrosis and polycythemia vera (47,48), as evidence against reversion of hematopoiesis to embryonic sites. They suggest that the altered stromal microenvironment of the bone marrow allows access of immature hematopoietic cells to the circulation. These hematopoietic cells are then trapped and filtered out by the spleen, and their continued accumulation explains the progressive splenomegaly in this disease.

Extramedullary hematopoiesis is also a clinical feature of infantile malignant osteopetrosis. This is a congenital bone disease characterized by a generalized systemic sclerosis of the skeleton (49). As a result of the severe reduction of bone resorptive capacity in this disease, bone marrow cavities do not develop. Affected infants demonstrate pancytopenia and hepatosplenomegaly, and they are often anemic and show increased susceptibility to infections (50,51). Histologically, spleens from patients with osteopetrosis show extensive hematopoietic activity (51,52). Also, high concentrations of hematopoietic progenitor cells are found both in the spleen and peripheral blood of these individuals (52). The presence of pancytopenia and related hematologic abnormalities suggest that splenic and hepatic hematopoiesis is limited. The presence of pancytopenia also indicates that the continued hematologic requirements of the growing individual cannot be met by these sources of blood cell production.

Extramedullary hematopoiesis in osteopetrosis presumably occurs as a result of persistence of the embryonic function of the spleen and liver. Support for this comes from a study in which pregnant mice were injected with the bone-seeking (myelotoxic) radioisotope Strontium-89 in an effort to prevent fetal bone marrow development. The injection of Strontium-89 resulted in compensatory splenic hematopoiesis for several weeks after birth (53).

Other studies (39,54) have recently provided histological and immunohistological evidence of extramedullary hematopoiesis in spleens of patients undergoing bone marrow transplantation for aplastic anemia, acute leukemia or chronic myelogenous leukemia. They suggested that the conditioning regimen administered prior to transplantation may have damaged the marrow microenvironment, thus promoting a reactivation of the splenic hematopoietic microenvironment and repopulation by hematopoietic progenitors.

Thus, these studies indicate that there is hematopoietic activity in spleens of osteopetrotic infants and in patients undergoing bone marrow transplantation. These observations support the concept that the spleen is indeed a potentially significant organ of fetal, neonatal and adult hematopoiesis when bone marrow development or the hematopoietic microenvironment of the marrow is severely compromised.

REGULATION OF SPLENIC HEMATOPOIESIS

Hematopoiesis constitutes a process by which pluripotent stem cells give rise to committed progenitor cells that proliferate and differentiate to form all the cellular elements of the blood. This process normally occurs in the microenvironment of the bone marrow, liver or spleen (55) and is sustained by hormonal growth factors and differentiation substances (56–58). Proliferation of progenitor cells and differentiated function of these cells are dependent on a family of glycoproteins known as colony-stimulating factors (CSFs) (58). These factors were discovered when it was recognized that hematopoietic precursors could not survive or proliferate in vitro unless specifically stimulated (59,60).

Thus far, 5 murine and human hematopoietic growth factors have been identified that stimulate precursor cells to form colonies of specific progeny cells (57,61). Granulocyte-macrophage colony-stimulating factor (GM-CSF) stimulates the production of both granulocytes and macrophages. Granulocyte-CSF (G-CSF) and macrophage-CSF (M-CSF) preferentially stimulate the formation of granulocytes and macrophages, respectively. Erythropoietin (EP) stimulates the formation of erythroid cells. Finally, multi-CSF has the capacity to stimulate granulocyte and macrophage formation in addition to stimulating the proliferation of erythroid cells, megakaryocytes, eosinophils, mast cells, stem cells, and pluripotential cells. In addition, distinct membrane receptors for each factor have been identified on undifferentiated and maturing cells of the parent cell lineages (57,61). Production of colony-stimulating factors have been documented for fibroblasts (62,63), monocytes (64,65), T lymphocytes (66,67), endothelial cells (68,69), splenocytes (70) and, recently, for bone cells (71).

Another important class of hematopoietic interactions occurs between proliferating hematopoietic cells and stromal cells in bone marrow and extramedullary sites, including the spleen (72). Studies in animals and humans have shown that splenic tissue is capable of supporting hematopoiesis by providing necessary microenvironmental and humoral influences (34,70,73,74). In an elegant study of the inductive effects of a stromal microenvironment on stem cell differentiation, it was demonstrated that the splenic stroma preferentially supports erythropoiesis while the stromal microenvironment in the bone marrow primarily supports granulopoiesis (73). In irradiated mice receiving hematopoietic stem cells, the erythrocyte:granulocyte (E:G) colony ratio in spleen was 3 or more. On the other hand, the E:G colony ratio in bone marrow stroma was less than 1, regardless of whether the marrow stroma was in situ or implanted as plugs into spleens. Interestingly, when spleens receiving these plugs were examined histologically, colonies formed in the marrow implants were almost completely granulocytic, while those developing in adjacent splenic tissue were erythrocytic.

Further evidence indicating a determining effect of hematopoietic organ stroma on pluripotent stem cells derives from studies using the anemic mouse mutations Sl/Sl^d and W/W^v. Sl/Sl^d mice possess normal numbers of hematopoietic stem cells and their macrocytic anemia is due to a congenital defect in the hematopoietic microenvironment (75,76). W/W^v mice, on the other hand, have a congenital deficiency in hematopoietic stem cells, but they have a functioning stromal microenvironment as evidenced by the fact that irradiated W/W^v mice are cured of their anemia following transplantation of normal stem cells from Sl/Sl^d mice (75,77). The anemic condition in Sl/Sl^d mice is not reversed by transplantation of stem cells from normal animals (77). However, the anemia is improved when competent stroma (normal +/+ or W/W^v spleens or femora) are implanted into Sl/Sl^d recipients to receive and support proliferation and differentiation of transplanted stem cells (76,77).

The long term bone marrow culture technique described by Dexter et al. (78), has proved to be a powerful tool for exploring stromal cell/hematopoietic stem cell interactions during hematopoiesis. In this system, the proliferation, differentiation and maturation of hematopoietic cells is dependent on the development of an adherent cell population composed of endothelial cells, macrophages, fibroblasts, adipocytes and reticular cells (79,80). This population provides an in vitro microenvironment which supports stem cell renewal and differentiation.

Application of this technique to the $S1/S1^d$ and W/W^v mouse mutations demonstrated that the hematological defects in these animals could be reproduced in vitro (81). Bone marrow adherent cells from $S1/S1^d$ mice were defective in their capacity to support hematopoietic stem cell proliferation, and deficiencies in numbers of W/W^v stem cells resulted in a rapid and considerable reduction in the formation of progenitor cells. These respective defects could be overcome when W/W^v marrow, used to form the adherent stromal microenvironment, was co-cultured with $S1/S1^d$ marrow. This combination resulted in a sustained high level of hematopoiesis and demonstrated a "cure," similar to that achieved by reciprocal transplantation in vivo (75,77).

This culture technique has also provided the opportunity to examine the role of macromolecules in the extracellular matrix in supporting hematopoiesis. Adherent stromal cells have been shown to secrete fibronectin, type IV collagen, laminin and proteoglycans (80,82). Extensive deposition of these macromolecules by stromal cells was shown to precede the onset of active hematopoiesis, and was required for maintenance of this activity (80).

How these extracellular proteins function to support hematopoiesis is poorly understood. It is suggested that fibronectin, for example, provides an essential substrate for development and differentiation of erythroid progenitors (83,84). These progenitors preferentially bind to stromal cells or fibronectin-coated substrates and this binding can be blocked by anti-fibronectin antibodies. Binding is also blocked by a monoclonal antibody to the cell-binding domain of fibronectin (84).

SUMMARY AND CONCLUSIONS

The spleen has contributed significantly throughout its evolutionary history to blood cell formation in vertebrates. Despite its important hematopoietic function in higher vertebrates, the significance of the spleen during normal human development is not yet satisfactorily agreed upon. Similarly, the capacity of the adult spleen to revert to an embryonic hematopoietic function as a result of disease or due to treatment-related suppression of the bone marrow continues to be argued. Relevant aspects as to the phylogenetic and ontogenetic development of this organ, coupled with the examples of disease states where extramedullary hematopoiesis occurs have been presented. This evidence supports the concept that the spleen is indeed a potentially significant organ of fetal, neonatal and adult hematopoiesis.

Our level of understanding of splenic hematopoiesis and the mechanisms involved in its regulation pales in comparison to what is known about this process in the bone marrow. What we know regarding the cellular and molecular biology of the hematopoietic microenvironment and the requisite interactions for supporting and maintaining hematopoiesis has derived principally from studies using bone marrow cultures. Because of this, one is largely forced to assume that similar, though not necessarily the same, elements are central to this process in splenic tissue during normal human fetal development.

The opportunity exists for the simultaneous application of several techniques, presently being used to study marrow hematopoiesis, to fetal splenic tissue. These techniques may be applied at various ages in development to definitively establish the significance of the spleen as a blood cell forming organ in man. Furthermore, these techniques will provide the means to examine cellular and molecular mechanisms underlying the cessation of splenic hematopoiesis before birth and the transfer of this function to the bone marrow. In addition, similar methods could also be applied to diseased spleens active in extramedullary hematopoiesis, to examine the processes contributing to reversion of this tissue to its embryonic function. These studies will provide valuable new information and will enhance our understanding of the role of the spleen as a hematopoietic organ during development, as well as in health and disease.

REFERENCES

1. Videbaek A, Christensen BE, Jonsson V: *The Spleen in Health and Disease.* Year Book Medical Publishers, Inc., Chicago, 1982; pp. 11-33.
2. Custer RP: A*n Atlas of the Blood and Bone Marrow.* W.B. Saunders Company, Philadelphia, 1974; pp. 9-25.
3. Kelemen E, Calvo W, Fliedner TM: *Atlas of Human Hematopoietic Development.* Springer Verlag, New York, 1979; pp. 156-171.
4. Tischendorf F: On the evolution of the spleen. *Experientia* 1985; 41:145-152.
5. Jordan HE: Extramedullary blood production. *Physiol Rev* 1942;22:375-384.
6. Weidenreich F: Hämolytischer Gewebe. In, Bolk L, Goppert E, Lallius E, Lobosch W (eds): *Handbuch der Vergleichenden Anatomie der Wirbeltiere.* Urban and Schwarzenberg Verlag, Berlin, 1933; pp. 420-450.
7. Jordan HE: The evolution of blood-forming tissues. *Q Rev Biol* 1933;8: 58-76.
8. Ward HP, Block MH: The natural history of agnogenic myeloid metaplasia (AMM) and a critical evaluation of its relationship with the myeloproliferative syndrome. *Medicine* 1971;50:357-420.
9. Seifert MF, Marks SC Jr: The regulation of hemopoiesis in the spleen. *Experientia* 1985;41:192-199.

10. Aggio MC, Guisto N, Brizzo MT, Montano M: The participation of spleen and bone marrow in mice erythropoiesis as a function of age. *Acta Physiol Latinoam* 1972;22:1-5.
11. Boggs DR, Geist A, Chervenick PA: Contribution of the mouse spleen to post-hemorrhagic erythropoiesis. *Life Sci* 1969;8:587-599.
12. Grouls V, Helpap B: The development of the red pulp in the rat spleen. *Adv Anat Embryol Cell Biol* 1982;75:1-71.
13. Bozzini CE, Rendo MEB, Devoto FCH, Epper CE: Studies on medullary and extramedullary erythropoiesis in the adult mouse. *Am J Physiol* 1970;219:724-728.
14. Grouls V, Helpap B: The granulocytopoiesis in the spleen of newborn rats. *Res Exp Med* 1980;177:237-243.
15. Lucarelli G, Porcellini A, Carnevali C, et al: Fetal and neonatal erythropoiesis. *Ann N Y Acad Sci* 1968;149:544-559.
16. Haas RJ, Stehle H, Fliedner TM: Autoradiographic studies on rapidly and slowly proliferating cell systems in neonatal bone marrow. *Helv Med Acta* 1967;34:54-66.
17. Lord BI: Haemopoietic changes in the rat during continuous gamma irradiation of the adult animal. *Br J Haematol* 1965;11:525-536.
18. Garcia JF: Radioiron time-distribution studies at various ages in the normal male rat. *Am J Physiol* 1957;190:31-36.
19. Fruhman GJ: Blood formation in the pregnant mouse. *Blood* 1968;31:242-248.
20. Weiss L: *Histology-Cell and Tissue Biology*, 5th Ed, Elsevier Biomedical Publishers, New York, 1983; pp. 544-568.
21. Hann IM, Bodger MP, Hoffbrand AV: Development of pluripotent hematopoietic progenitor cells in the human fetus. *Blood* 1983;62:118-123.
22. Linch DC, Knott LJ, Rodeck CH, Huehns ER: Studies of circulating hemopoietic progenitor cells in human fetal blood. *Blood* 1982;59:976-979.
23. Barnes DWH, Ford CE, Loutit JF: Haemopoietic stem cells. *Lancet* 1964;1:1395-1396.
24. Fried W: The liver as a source of extrarenal erythropoietin production. *Blood* 1972;40:671-677.
25. Zanjani ED, Peterson EN, Gordon AS, Wasserman LR: Erythropoietin production in the fetus; the role of the kidney and maternal anaemia. *J Lab Clin Med* 1974;83:281-287.
26. Emura I, Sekiya M, Ohnishi Y: Ultrastructural identification of the hematopoietic inductive microenvironment in the human embryonic liver. *Arch Histol Jap* 1984;47:95-112.
27. Ishikawa H: Differentiation of red pulp and evaluation of hemopoietic role of human prenatal spleen. *Arch Histol Jap* 1985;48:183-197.
28. Wood WG: Haemoglobin synthesis during human fetal development. *Br Med Bull* 1976;32:282-287.
29. Djaldetti M, Bessler H, Rifkind RA: Hematopoiesis in the embryonic mouse

30. Block M: Studies on the blood and blood-forming tissues of the newborn spleen; an electron microscopic study. *Blood* 1972;39:826-841. opossum. I. Normal development. *Ergebnisse der Anatomie und Entwicklungs Geschichte* 1974;37:237-248.
31. Gilmour JR: Normal haemopoiesis in intra-uterine and neonatal life. *J Pathol* 1941;52:25-55.
32. Zamboni L, Westin B: The ultrastructure of the human fetal spleen. I. One type of mesenchymal cell in the early stages of development of the spleen. *J Ultrastruct Res* 1964;11:469-491.
33. Djaldetti MA: Hemopoietic events in human embryonic spleens at early gestational stages. *Biol Neonate* 1979;36:133-144.
34. Trentin JJ: Influence of hematopoietic organ stroma (hemopoietic inductive microenvironments) on stem cell differentiation. In, Gordon AS (ed): *Regulation of Hemopoiesis*. Appleton-Century-Crofts, New York, 1970, pp. 161-186.
35. Vellguth S, von Gaudecker B, Muller-Hermelink H-K: The development of the human spleen. Ultrastructural studies in fetuses from the 14th to 24th week of gestation. *Cell Tissue Res* 1985;242:579-592.
36. Fukuda T: Fetal hemopoiesis. I. Electron microscopic studies on human yolk sac hemopoiesis. *Virchows Arch B* 1973;14:197-213.
37. Fukuda T: Fetal hemopoiesis. II. Electron microscopic studies on human hepatic hemopoiesis. *Virchows Arch B* 1974;16:249-270.
38. Wolf BC, Leuvano E, Neiman RS: Evidence to suggest that the human fetal spleen is not a hematopoietic organ. *Am J Clin Pathol* 1983;80:140-144.
39. Arnold R, Calvo W, Heymer B, et al: Extramedullary haemopoiesis after bone marrow transplantation. *Scand J Haematol* 1985;34:9-12.
40. Tavassoli M, Weiss L: An electron microscopic study of spleen in myelofibrosis with myeloid metaplasia. *Blood* 1973;42:267-279.
41. Underwood JCE, Dangerfield WJM: Immunohistochemical identification of adult and fetal haemopoiesis in the spleen in lymphoma, leukemia and myeloproliferative disease. *J Path* 1981;134:71-80.
42. McCulloch EA, Till JE: Stem cells in normal early haemopoiesis and certain clonal haemopathies. In, Hoffbrand AV, Brian MC, Hirsch T (eds): *Recent Advances in Haematology*. Churchill Livingstone, New York, 1977; pp. 85-110.
43. Laszlo J: Myelofibrosis, myelosclerosis, extramedullary hematopoiesis, undifferentiated MPD, and hemorrhagic thrombocythemia. *Semin Hemat* 1975;12:409-432.
44. Dameshek W: Some speculations of the myeloproliferative syndromes. *Blood* 1952;6:372-375.
45. Gilbert HS: The spectrums of myeloproliferative disorders. *Med Clin N Am* 1973;57:355-393.
46. Glew RH, Haese WH, McIntyre PA: Myeloid metaplasia with myelofibrosis. The clinical spectrum of extramedullary hematopoiesis and tumor forma-

tion. *Johns Hopkins Med J* 1973;132:253-271.
47. Wolf BC, Neiman RS: Myelofibrosis with myeloid metaplasia; pathophysiologic implications of the correlation between bone marrow changes and progression of splenomegaly. *Blood* 1985;65:803-809.
48. Wolf BC, Neiman RS: The pathology of the spleen in polycythemia vera. *Lab Invest* 1985;48:95A.
49. Marks SC Jr: Congenital osteopetrotic mutations as probes of the origin, structure and function of osteoclasts. *Clin Orthop Rel Res* 1984;189:239-263.
50. Reeves JD, Huffer WE, August CS, et al: The hematopoietic effects of prednisone therapy in four infants with osteopetrosis. *J Pediatr* 1979;94:210-214.
51. Solcia E, Rondini G, Capella C: Clinical and pathological observation on a case of newborn osteopetrosis. *Helv Paed Acta* 1968;6:650-658.
52. Freedman MH, Saunders EF: Hematopoiesis in the human spleen. *Am J Hematol* 1981;11:271-275.
53. Kincaide PW, Moore MAS, Schlegel RA, Pye J: B-lymphocyte differentiation from fetal liver stem cells in ^{89}Sr-treated mice. *J Immunol* 1975;115:1217-1222.
54. Antin JH, Weinberg DS, Rappeport JM: Evidence that pluripotential stem cells form splenic colonies in humans after marrow transplantation. *Transplantation* 1985;39:102-105.
55. Wolf NS: The haematopoietic microenvironment. *Clin Haematol* 1979;8:460-500.
56. Quesenberry PJ, McNiece IK, Robinson BE, et al: Stromal cell regulation of lymphoid and myeloid differentiation. *Blood Cells* 1987;13:137-146.
57. Nathan DG, Sieff CA: The biological activities and uses of recombinant granulocyte-macrophage and multi-colony stimulating factors. *Progr Hematol* 1987;15:1-18.
58. Metcalf D: The Hematopoietic Colony Stimulating Factors. Amsterdam, Elsevier, 1984.
59. Bradley TR, Metcalf D: The growth of mouse bone marrow cells in vitro. *Aust J Exp Biol Med Sci* 1966;44:287-299.
60. Ichikawa Y, Pluznik DH, Sachs L: In vitro control of the development of macrophage and granulocyte colonies. *Proc Natl Acad Sci USA* 1966;56:488-495.
61. Metcalf D: The molecular biology and functions of the granulocyte-macrophage colony-stimulating factors. *Blood* 1986;67:257-267.
62. Bagby GC, McCall E, Layman DL: Regulation of colony stimulating activity production. Interactions of fibroblasts, mononuclear phagocytes and lactoferrin. *J Clin Invest* 1983;71:340-344.
63. Tsai S, Emerson SG, Sieff CA, Nathan DG: Isolation of a human stromal cell secreting hemopoietic growth factors. *J Cell Physiol* 1986;127:137-145.
64. Chervenick PA, LoBuglio AF: Human blood monocytes; stimulation of

granulocyte and mononuclear colony formation in vitro. *Science* 1972;178: 164-166.
65. Golde DW, Cline MJ: Identification of colony-stimulating cells in human peripheral blood. *J Clin Invest* 1972;51:2981-2983.
66. Cline MJ, Golde DW: Production of colony stimulating activity by human lymphocytes. *Nature* 1974;248:703-704.
67. Nathan DG, Chess L, Hillman DG, et al: Human erythroid burst-forming units; T-cell requirement for proliferation in vitro. *J Exp Med* 1978;147: 324-339.
68. Quesenberry PJ, Gimbrone MA: Vascular endothelium as a regulator of granulopoiesis; production and colony stimulating activity by cultured human endothelial cells. *Blood* 1980;56:1060-1067.
69. Bagby GC, Rigas VD, Bennett RM, et al: Interaction of lactoferrin, monocytes, and T-lymphocyte subsets in the regulation of steady-state granulopoiesis in vitro. *J Clin Invest* 1981;68:56-63.
70. Fabian I, Dover D, Levitt L, et al: Human spleen cell generation of factors stimulating human pluripotent stem cell, erythroid, and myeloid progenitor cell growth. *Blood* 1985;65:990-996.
71. Felix R, Elford PR, Stoerckle C, et al: Production of hemopoietic growth factors by bone tissue and bone cells in culture. *J Bone Min Res* 1988;3: 27-36.
72. Cline MJ, Golde DW: Cellular interactions in haematopoiesis. *Nature* 1979; 277:177-181.
73. Wolf N, Trentin J: Hemopoietic colony studies. V. Effect of hemopoietic organ stroma on differentiation of pluripotent stem cells. *J Exp Med* 1968; 127:205-214.
74. Metcalf D, Johnson G: Production by spleen and lymph node cells of conditioned medium with erythroid and other hemopoietic colony stimulating activity. *J Cell Physiol* 1978;96:31-42.
75. McCulloch EA, Siminovitch L, Till JF, et al: The cellular basis of the genetically determined hemopoietic defect in anemic mice of genotype S1/S1^d. *Blood* 1964;26:399-410.
76. Fried W, Chamberlin W, Knospe WH, et al: Studies on the defective haematopoietic microenvironment of S1/S1^d mice. *Br J Haematol* 1973;24: 643-650.
77. Bernstein SE: Tissue transplantation as an analytic and therapeutic tool in hereditary anemias. *Am J Surg* 1970;119:448-451.
78. Dexter TM, Allen TD, Lajtha LG: Conditions controlling the proliferation of haemopoietic stem cells in vitro. *J Cell Physiol* 1977;91:335-344.
79. Allen TD, Dexter TM: Cellular interrelationships during in vitro granulopoiesis. *Differentiation* 1976;6:191-194.
80. Zuckerman KS, Wicha MS: Extracellular matrix production by the adherent cells of long-term murine bone marrow cultures. *Blood* 1983;61:650-547.
81. Dexter TM, Moore MAS: In vitro duplication and 'cure' of haemopoietic defects in genetically anaemic mice. *Nature* 1977;269:412-414.

82. Gallagher JJ, Spooncer E, Dexter TM: Role of the cellular matrix in haemopoiesis. I. Synthesis of glycosaminoglycans by mouse bone marrow cell cultures. *J Cell Sci* 1983;632:155-171.
83. Patel VP, Lodish HF: Loss of adhesion of murine erythroleukemia cells to fibronectin during erythroid differentiation. *Science* 1984;224:996-998.
84. Tsai S, Patel V, Beaumont E, et al: Differential binding of erythroid and myeloid progenitors to fibroblasts and fibronectin. *Blood* 1987;69:1587-1594.

3
Pathology of the Spleen

MARY V. GRESIK
Baylor College of Medicine, Texas Children's Hospital, Houston, Texas

EXAMINATION OF THE SPLEEN

The spleen is regarded as a difficult organ to evaluate by most pathologists. The white pulp presents a series of confusing morphologic manifestations in lymphomas and Hodgkin's disease, and nonspecific changes are seen in most reactive processes. The red pulp is filled with erythrocytes, which dominate the histologic appearance and make specific alterations difficult to appreciate. Many of these problems in histopathologic diagnosis can be solved by careful handling of the specimen and communication between pathologist and surgeon. For example, if the surgeon ligates the splenic artery before ligation of the splenic vein, much of the red pulp congestion will be reduced. Cutting the ligature on the splenic vein before sectioning can drain more blood from the spleen. Inspection of the capsular surface may provide valuable information about the underlying disease process. The spleen normally has a finely wrinkled capsule. This may be stretched and smooth in expansive lesions of the red pulp. Other conditions such as infarcts, granulomas or nodules of Hodgkin's disease may be grossly visible on external examination.

The spleen should be sliced bread-loaf fashion into slices 3-4 mm thick and the surfaces carefully inspected. While most disease processes of the red pulp involve the spleen diffusely, many diseases are focal and must be identified grossly to insure adequate sampling. Fixation with Zenker's solution or B5 fixative provides good cytologic detail for many conditions involving the spleen.

Table 1 Anatomic Localization of Splenic Diseases

Red pulp	White pulp

Congestion
  hemolytic anemias
  passive congestion
	Reactive Hyperplasia
	  immune thrombocytopenic purpura
	  infections
	  autoimmune disorders
	  chronic antigenic stimulation

Infection
  infectious mononucleosis
  granulomas
	Lymphomas (including chronic lympho-
	    cytic leukemia)

Histiocytic diseases
  storage diseases
  Langerhan's Cell
    histiocytosis
  malignant histiocytosis
  infection-associated
    hemophagocytic syndrome
  familial hemophagocytic
    lymphohistiocytosis
	Hodgkin's disease

Leukemia/myeloproliferative
  diseases
  acute leukemia
  hairy cell leukemia
  chronic myelogenous
    leukemia
  myelofibrosis with myeloid
    metaplasia	

Tumors
  cysts
  hamartomas
  vascular neoplasms
  metastatic neoplasms	

Small thin sections must be taken from the initial spleen slices since there is limited penetration by these fixtures. Touch preparations and snap-frozen specimens are desirable for those disorders that may require monoclonal antibody studies.

The periodic acid-Schiff (PAS) stain is a valuable adjunct to the routine hematoxylin-eosin stained section; PAS stains the ring fibers (basement membranes),

Table 2 Indications for Splenectomy: Experience at Texas Children's Hospital (1954-1985)

Indication for splenectomy	Number
Trauma	62
Hemolytic anemia, (non-spherocytic)	47
Immune thrombocytopenic purpura	42
Hereditary spherocytosis	35
Hodgkin's disease for staging	25
Splenomegaly/hypersplenism	16
Portal hypertension	15
Lymphoma or leukemia	13
Sickle cell disease or thalassemia major	12
Gaucher's disease	7
Chronic renal failure	4
Incidental to other surgical procedures	4
Miscellaneous	26
Total	308

clearly separating sinuses from cords. The PAS stain does not stain red blood cells and, therefore, unmasks the other cellular components of the red pulp. Similar staining of the basement membrane is seen with the reticulin stain (Figure 1). Other stains may be useful in certain conditions. The Prussian blue stain for iron may help to differentiate various hemolytic anemias. The naphthyl-ASD chloroacetate esterase stain is useful in identifying granulocytes and mast cells in myeloid leukemias and in myeloproliferative disorders.

In examining the spleen both grossly and microscopically, it is helpful to categorize the diseases into those principally affecting the red pulp and those that affect the white pulp (Table 1). Red pulp expansion is responsible for the largest spleens, such as in Gaucher's disease and chronic myelogenous leukemia in the United States, and in patients with malaria and leishmaniasis in other parts of the world. Spleens in patients with these diseases may weigh as much as 100 times the normal weight. Many of the diseases involving the spleen show similar histologic changes; thus, complete clinical information is necessary for adequate interpretation. Conversely, some disorders have similar clinical presentations, such as malignant histiocytosis and the infection-associated hemophagocytic syndrome. In these cases, distinction is based on cytologic features.

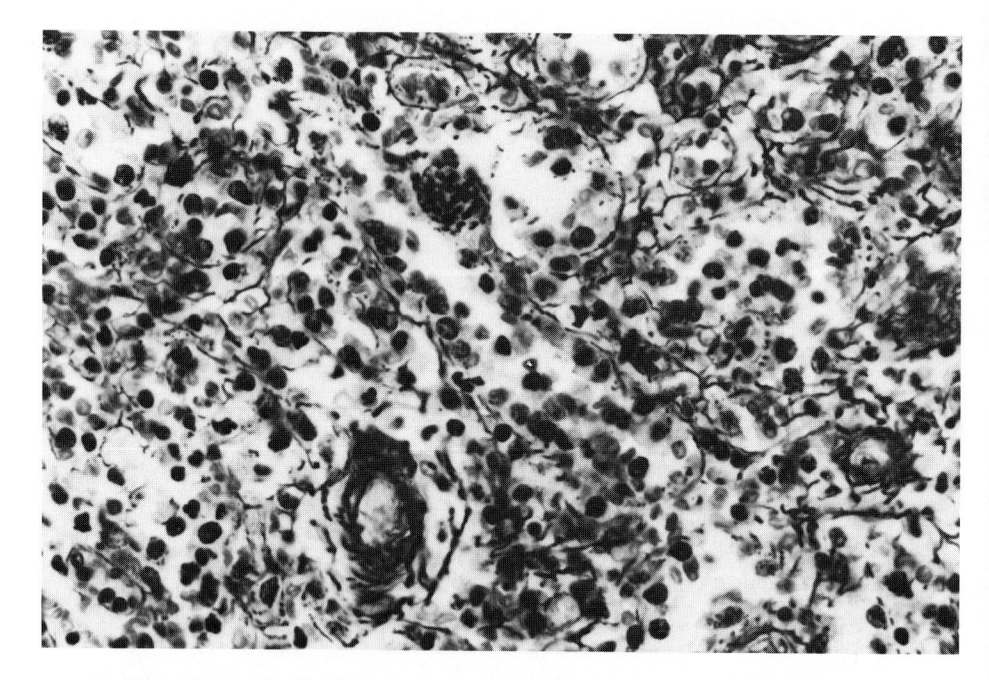

Figure 1 Normal splenic red pulp. The reticulin stain outlines the basement membrane demarcating sinuses from cords. (Wilder's reticulin stain × 400)

Although the spleen may have specific diagnostic features in many diseases, it is rarely removed solely for diagnosis. In evaluating the various causes of splenomegaly the diagnosis can usually be made by laboratory tests or from tissue obtained from other biopsy sites such as from lymph node, bone marrow or liver. Therefore, splenectomy is generally performed for therapeutic indications or for staging rather than for diagnosis. Table 2 lists the reasons for splenectomy at Texas Children's Hospital over a 30-year period. Similar figures would be obtained from a general hospital, with the addition of cases of hairy cell leukemia and chronic myelogenous leukemia.

While the spleen is not essential for life, its removal is not without consequence, especially in young children. The risk of overwhelming bacterial septicemia after splenectomy is well recognized (1,2) and is discussed in detail in Chapter 4. The age at splenectomy and the underlying disease are both important in determining the incidence of post-splenectomy sepsis. Singer (2) reviewed the incidence of sepsis and how it is affected by disease category, age and infecting organism.

The incidence of fulminant sepsis was greater in infants and young children than in older children and adults. The incidence of fatal post-splenectomy sepsis ranged from 0.58% for patients who had traumatic rupture of the spleen to 11% for patients who had splenectomy because of thalassemia. In his review of the literature, Singer found a 4.25% incidence of sepsis of which half were fatal. The most frequently recovered organisms were *Streptococcus pneumoniae, Neisseria meningitidis, Escherichia coli* and *Hemophilus influenzae.*

The spleen's unique combination of functions as a phagocytic organ and a major component of the immune system accounts for the increased susceptibility to infection in the asplenic patient. The infant's inexperienced immune system is severely compromised by the loss of a major antibody-producing organ, whereas the older individual with fully programmed lymphocytes may fare better. The spleen is the major site for removal of encapsulated organisms because of the large number of phagocytic cells in the red pulp and the production of tuftsin which facilitates the phagocytosis of microorganisms.

With the undesirable consequences of splenectomy, it would seem that splenic biopsy might be an attractive alternative for diagnostic evaluation of the spleen. Although the splenic biopsy is performed in other countries with apparent safety (3,4), it is rarely done in the United States. Fear of hemorrhage may be a major reason for this lack of enthusiasm, although the focal nature of many of the diseases is also a factor against doing splenic biopsy. In some centers hemisplenectomy has been attempted in children with Hodgkin's disease (5), in order to increase the sample size and still maintain some degree of splenic function to protect against overwhelming sepsis. However, if the spleen is included in the radiation field during radiotherapy, it may offer little protection against overwhelming sepsis due to the diffuse fibrosis in the red pulp and the significant lymphoid depletion.

Schellong et al. (6), correlated the presence of enlarged lymph nodes at the splenic hilus or in the tail of the pancreas with splenic involvement by Hodgkin's disease. If either of these two findings (enlarged lymph nodes or nodules on the surface of the spleen) was present at laparotomy a splenectomy was performed. Using this strategy, splenectomy was avoided in 64% of patients. This method was only used in patients who would receive chemotherapy, since approximately 10% of the nonsplenectomized patients may have minor splenic involvement. Recently, partial splenectomies have been performed on patients with Gaucher's disease (7). While some authors report no recurrence of hypersplenism or splenomegaly in these patients, this has not been the experience of others (8).

STRUCTURAL ABNORMALITIES AND CIRCULATORY DISTURBANCES

Isolated congenital absence of the spleen is rare and is associated with an increased risk of infection. More commonly, asplenia is associated with congenital heart disease (CHD), abnormal visceral situs (situs inversus) and bilateral right (tri-lobed) lungs (the Ivemark syndrome) (9). These patients demonstrate laboratory evidence of splenic hypofunction, including peripheral blood smear findings of Howell-Jolly bodies and the presence of erythrocyte "pits" using direct interference contrast microscopy (10-12).

Other splenic syndromes occur in association with congenital heart disease. The polysplenia syndrome consists of multiple small spleens of equal size (Figure 2) with bilateral left (bilobed) lungs, abnormal situs and congenital heart disease (13). Anisosplenia is the occurrence of one main spleen and one or more accessory spleens. There are two forms of anisosplenia (14). M-anisosplenia occurs in males with bilateral right lungs, and F-anisosplenia occurs in females with bilateral left lungs. Congenital heart disease and variably abnormal situs are found in both groups.

Accessory spleens are common and are found in 10 to 30% of autopsy series (15,16). The accessory spleen is generally found at the hilum of the spleen or in

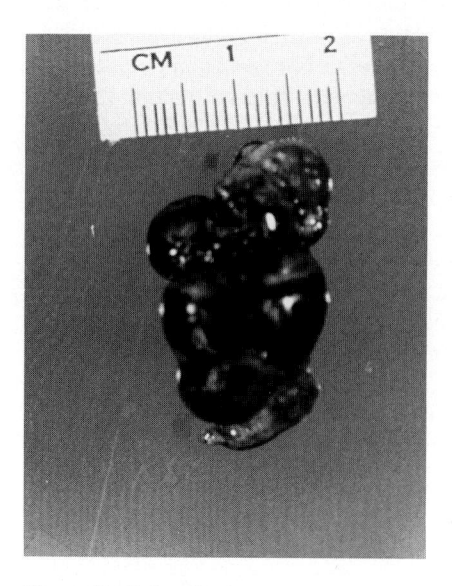

Figure 2 Polysplenia. There are multiple small splenic nodules all of approximately equal size.

the tail of the pancreas. Splenic tissue embedded in the tail of the pancreas is a common feature in trisomy 13 and trisomy 18 syndromes (17,18). Although accessory spleens are generally asymptomatic, they should be looked for when splenectomy is performed for a hemolytic anemia, immune thrombocytopenia, or hypersplenism. Failure to remove accessory splenic tissue may negate the therapeutic effects of splenectomy in these cases.

Splenosis is the autotransplantation of splenic tissue after traumatic rupture. This condition is generally confined to the abdomen, but in trauma associated with diaphragmatic tears splenic implants may be seen in the thoracic cavity (19,20). Although splenosis is generally asymptomatic, it may be the cause of unexplained recurrence of hemolysis or cytopenias after a therapeutic splenectomy, or rarely it may be a cause of abdominal pain.

Splenic-gonadal fusion is an uncommon anomaly. Two types are described (21,22). In the continuous form a cord of splenic or fibrous tissue connects the spleen and left gonad. In the discontinuous form an accessory spleen is present in or near the gonad, separate from the main spleen. Most cases of splenic gonadal fusion occur in males and are frequently seen with an ectopic or undescended testis and inguinal hernia. Bony defects of various types are also seen in association with this lesion. In one case hepatosplenic fusion was an incidental autopsy finding (23).

Peliosis of the spleen is a rare condition consisting of blood-filled cystic spaces in the spleen. While this condition is frequently associated with peliosis hepatis, it may also occur independently (24-26). The lesion in the spleen, like that in the liver, is of uncertain etiology. However, peliosis of the spleen has been seen in association with the use of androgenic anabolic steroids, glucocorticoids, birth control pills, and in chronic debilitating infectious disease or malignancies. The spleen is generally not enlarged and blood-filled cysts are grossly visible on cut section. Microscopically these cavities are unlined and most commonly involve the parafollicular regions (Figure 3). They are similar in appearance to the somewhat smaller blood lakes seen in hairy cell leukemia. Endothelial injury with resultant hemorrhage into the surrounding parenchyma is a possible explanation. These cysts may rupture into the abdominal cavity causing massive hemoperitoneum and shock (27).

Vascular congestion causing splenomegaly and hypersplenism is a common occurrence. Obstruction to portal blood flow by cirrhosis, obstruction by other liver pathology or portal-splenic vein thrombosis leads to chronic congestion, fibrosis and splenomegaly. There is expansion of the red pulp with thickened fibrous cords and congestion in the sinuses. Focal hemorrhages occur in the red pulp. These foci heal by scarring and with deposition of iron and calcium, creating Gamna-Gandy bodies (28) (Figure 4). The white pulp appears decreased in volume in congestive splenomegaly. In long-standing congestive heart failure

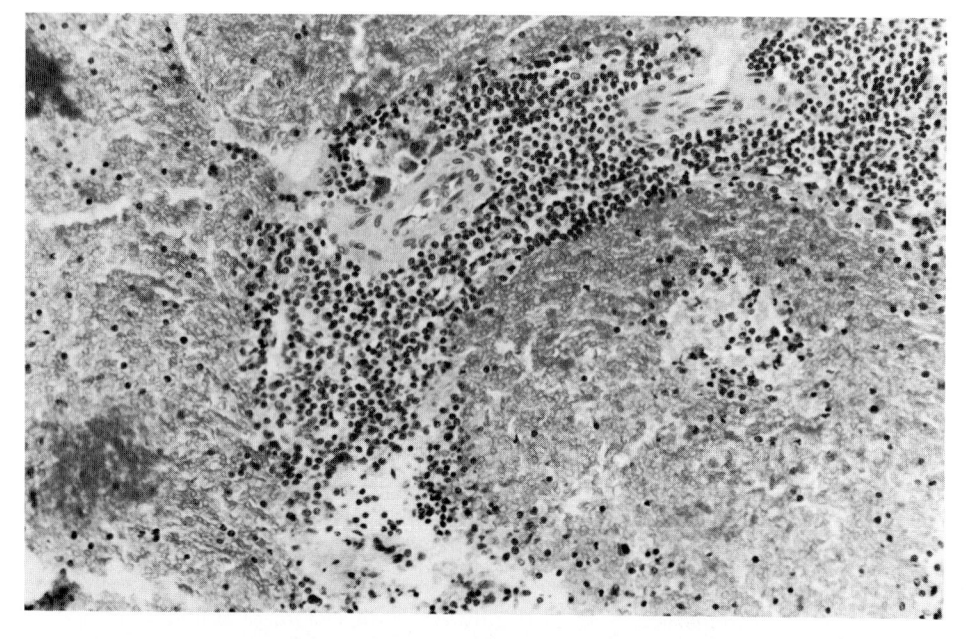

Figure 3 Peliosis of the spleen. Large unlined blood-filled spaces are present in the red pulp. (Hematoxylin-eosin stain × 400)

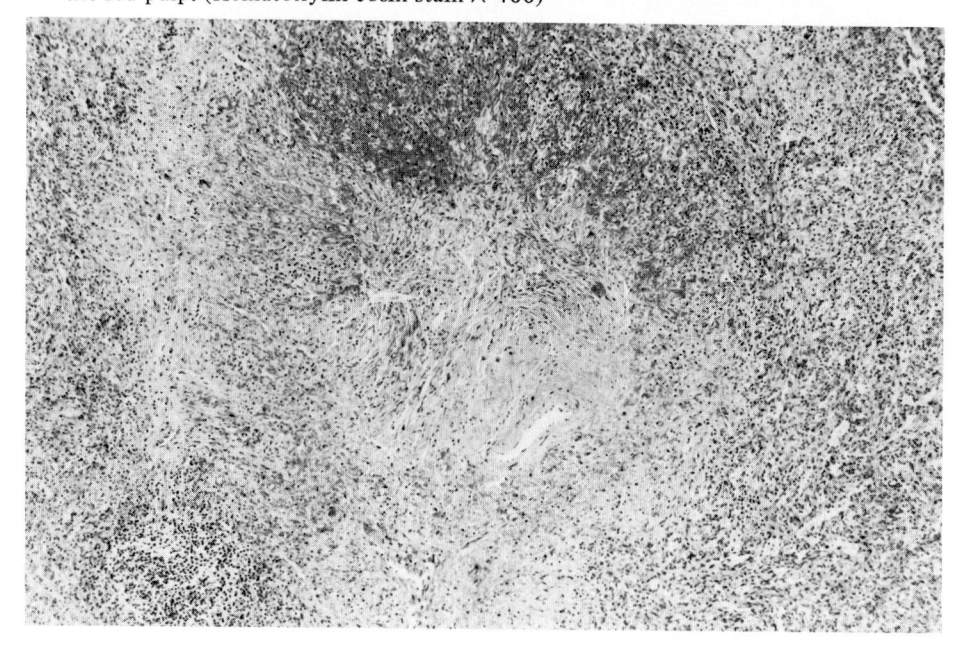

Figure 4 Sickle cell disease. A Gamma-Gandy body (fibrotic nodule encrusted with iron and calcium) is present in the center. This fibrous nodule was encrusted with iron. (Hematoxylin-eosin stain × 100)

PATHOLOGY OF THE SPLEEN

there is also an increase in fibrous connective tissue in the red pulp of the spleen; however, splenomegaly is minimal. The degree of hemosiderosis is much less in the congested spleen in congestive heart failure than in congestive splenomegaly due to portal hypertension.

Splenic infarcts are the result of occlusion of the splenic artery and its branches. Causes of these infarcts include thrombosis, sludging of abnormal red blood cells, infiltration of the vessel by leukemic cells, vasculitis and emboli from endocardial vegetations. Clinically, splenic infarcts may be asymptomatic or may be manifested by left upper quadrant abdominal pain. Infarcts vary in size. They may be single or multiple and are generally wedge-shaped (Figure 5). Depending on their age, these infarcts are either hemorrhagic or pale and scarred.

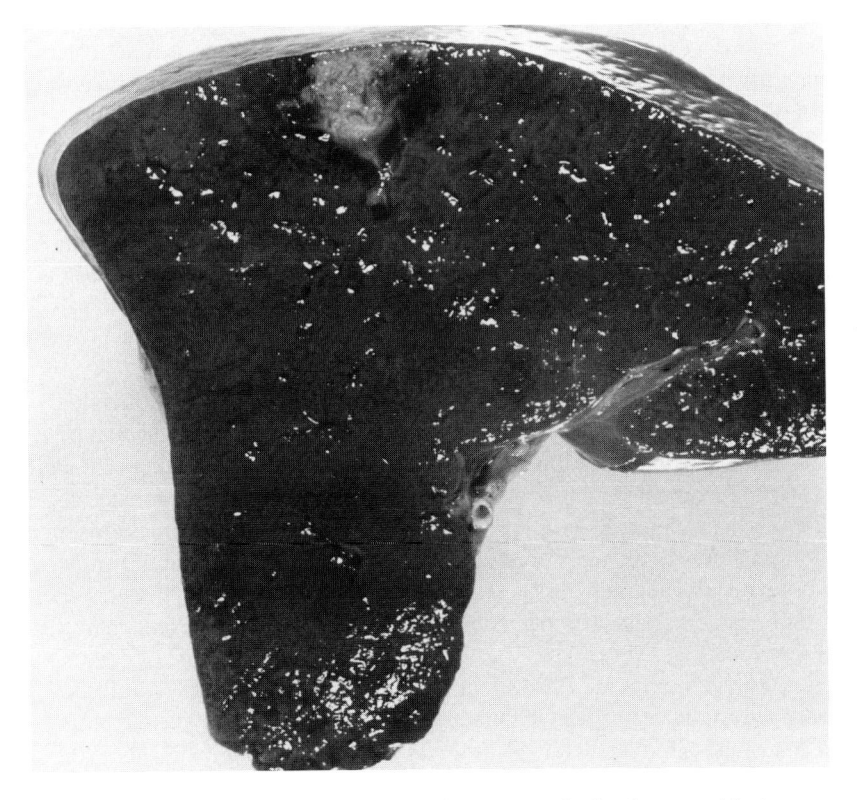

Figure 5 Splenic infarct. There is a well-circumscribed pale central lesion surrounded by a hemorrhagic border.

Repeated infarction may result in decreased splenic parenchyma as seen in sickle cell disease.

Splenic rupture is generally the result of blunt trauma, but it may occur in association with infection, tumor or leukemia. In the absence of a history of trauma, a pathologic process such as infection, malignancy or a structural defect should be searched for.

RED BLOOD CELL ABNORMALITIES

Hereditary spherocytosis (HS) is an inherited hemolytic anemia which is invariably associated with splenomegaly. The predominant mode of inheritance is autosomal dominant, although rare autosomal recessive cases are reported (29). Recently, a chromosomal translocation involving chromosomes 3, 8, and 12 was observed (30,31). These translocations, t(8; 12) (p11; p13) and t(3; 8) (p21; p11), suggest that the gene for heredity spherocytosis is located on the short arm of chromosome 8.

Although the exact molecular defect in hereditary spherocytosis is not clear, a variety of abnormalities have been described. These abnormalities are mainly related to the protein constitutent of the plasma membrane, spectrin, which may be reduced in quantity or have abnormal relationships to other constituents. The lack of deformability allows spherocytes to be trapped in the red pulp cords where they are subject to phagocytosis. The macroscopic appearance is that of a large spleen with inconspicuous white pulp and an expanded red pulp (Figure 6A). The histologic hallmark of hereditary spherocytosis in the spleen is congested red pulp cords with empty sinuses (Figure 6B). There is some hyperplasia of the lining cells of the splenic sinuses and a small amount of iron is present in the macrophages and endothelial cells.

In ultrastructural studies, Rappaport showed that the sinuses are not truly empty but filled with ghost erythrocytes (32). Other red blood cell membrane abnormalities, including hereditary elliptocytosis, hereditary stomatocytosis and acanthocytosis, may result in splenomegaly and a histologic picture similar to herediary spherocytosis. Splenectomy is curative in hereditary spherocytosis. In hereditary elliptocytosis and stomatocytosis, splenectomy may modify the disease, but cure is not certain. Splenectomy may be dangerous if it is performed for acanthocytosis secondary to liver disease as opposed to an inherited membrane abnormality (33).

The spleen in autoimmune hemolytic anemia is generally enlarged, but it is not enlarged to the degree seen in hereditary spherocytosis (34). The red pulp cords and sinuses are filled with erythrocytes to varying degrees. Patients with more spherocytes will have more red blood cells in the cords and fewer cells in the sinuses. Erythrophagocytosis may be prominent and it is easier to see in the

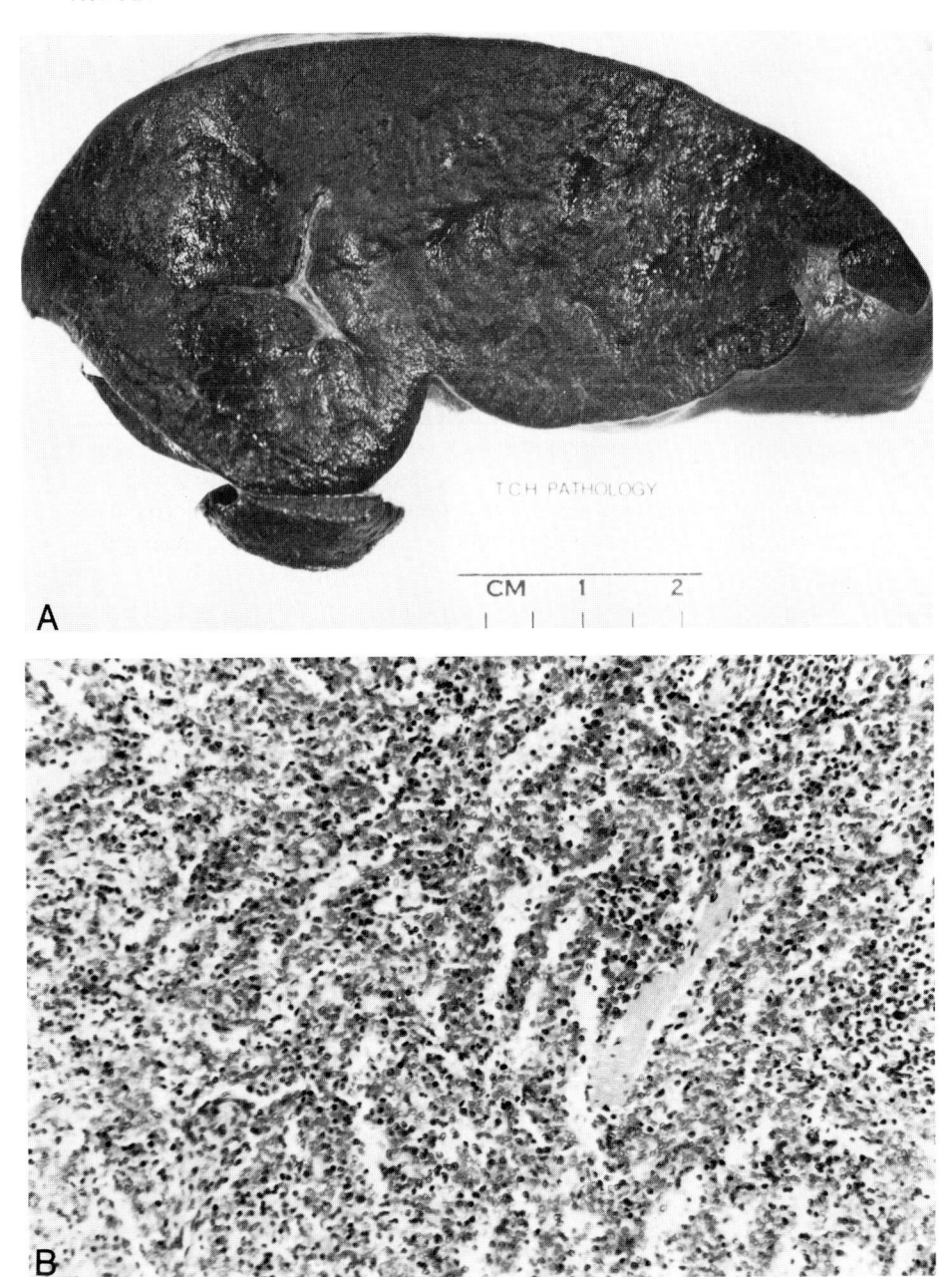

Figure 6 Hereditary spherocytosis. A. The spleen is enlarged, weighing 550 grams (normal for age is 73 grams). There is inconspicuous white pulp and expanded red pulp. B. The red pulp cords are filled with red blood cells and the sinuses are relatively empty. (Hematoxylin-eosin stain × 100)

sinuses than in the congested cords. Extramedullary hematopoiesis and prominence of the sinusoidal lining cells may be apparent. Stainable iron is more abundant in autoimmune hemolytic anemia than in hereditary spherocytosis. The white pulp usually is reactive in appearance and may be conspicuous on gross examination.

The spleen in sickle cell disease may have a variety of appearances depending on the age of the patient and status of the disease. Several poorly understood functional syndromes involving the spleen occur in patients with sickle cell disease. Acute splenic sequestration tends to occur in young children. The spleen enlarges rapidly with pooling of a large volume of blood, which may cause circulatory collapse and death. Acute splenic sequestration may occur repeatedly and can be fatal. Blood transfusions are needed immediately. In sickle cell disease, as in any condition requiring chronic transfusions, the use of phenotypically matched red blood cells is desirable. The development of multiple antibodies in response to multiple transfusions makes compatible blood difficult to obtain. Splenectomy may be of benefit (35) if the attacks of acute splenic sequestration are recurrent.

Functional asplenia may be seen in young children with splenomegaly (36). In these children, Howell-Jolly bodies and nucleated red cells are seen on the peripheral blood smear and the spleen is not visualized on radionucleotide scans. A possible mechanism for functional asplenia is reticuloendothelial blockade by red blood cell stroma. This condition may be reversed by blood transfusion, which increases the percentage of hemoglobin A. Chronic hypersplenism is a rare complication in patients with sickle cell disease (37).

The most common finding in older children and adults with sickle cell disease is autosplenectomy (37). Repeated episodes of vascular congestion and occlusion by sickled cells leads to progressive splenic infarction and siderofibrosis. The spleen removed for treatment of splenic sequestration is enlarged and markedly congested. The cords and sinuses are filled with sickled cells (Figure 7). Sickled forms are more readily appreciated in formalin-fixed specimens which allow reduction and encourage sickling than in specimens fixed in Zenker's solution or in B-5 fixative, which are oxidants and prevent sickling. In older patients who have some degree of autosplenectomy, there are large areas of infarction and variable degrees of fibrosis along with marked hemosiderin deposition within the irregularly shaped scars. These lesions are called siderotic nodules or Gamna-Gandy bodies. Little extramedullary hematopoiesis is seen in the spleen from patients with sickle cell disease.

Patients with the more severe forms of thalassemia have splenomegaly, which may contribute to their anemia. The spleen is enlarged with prominence of the

PATHOLOGY OF THE SPLEEN 49

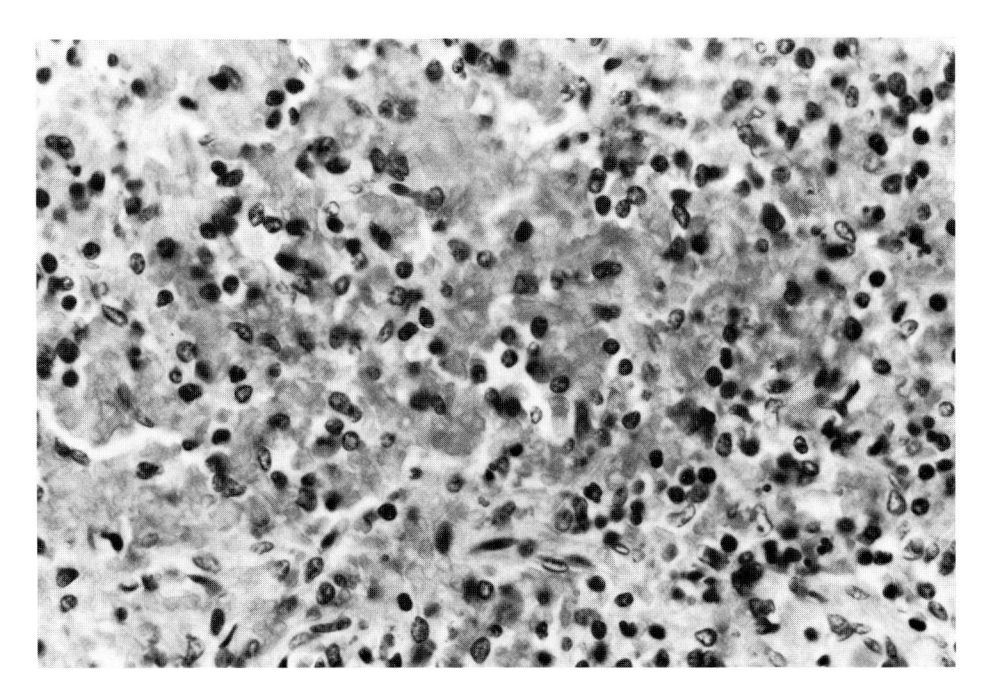

Figure 7 Sickle cell disease. The red pulp cords are massively congested with red blood cells and the sinuses are compressed. Sickled red cells are not well seen in this Zenker's fixed specimen. (Hematoxylin-eosin stain × 400)

red pulp. Infarcts are frequently present. Microscopically, there is congestion of the red pulp, extramedullary hematopoiesis, prominence of the cordal macrophages and lining cells, and hemosiderin deposition. Clusters of large histiocytes or Gaucher-like cells may be seen in the red pulp. Staining characteristics of these cells are similar to true Gaucher's cells. However, the Gaucher-like cells show presence of filamentous lysosomal material on ultrastructural examination, in contrast to the 30 to 60 nm tubules typical of Gaucher's disease (38) (see below). It has been postulated that the material in these storage cells represents incompletely digested breakdown products of the red blood cell membrane. This type of cell may also be seen in *chronic myelogenous leukemia* (CML), in *immune thrombocytopenic purpura* (ITP), in hyperlipoproteinemia, and occasionally in sickle cell disease.

INFECTIOUS DISEASES

The spleen acts as a blood filter and is generally involved in blood-borne infections. In adults and older children, the classic appearance of a "septic" spleen consists of reactive germinal centers associated with central necrosis and large numbers of neutrophils in the red pulp. This classic histologic picture is not seen in children less than 4–6 months of age. In a review of spleens of 131 children who died with bacterial sepsis between the ages of 24 weeks gestation and four and one-half years, we found that germinal center formation was rarely seen before 3 months of age. Polymorphonuclear leukocytes as well as other granulocytic and erythroid cells were seen in the red pulp, especially in premature in-

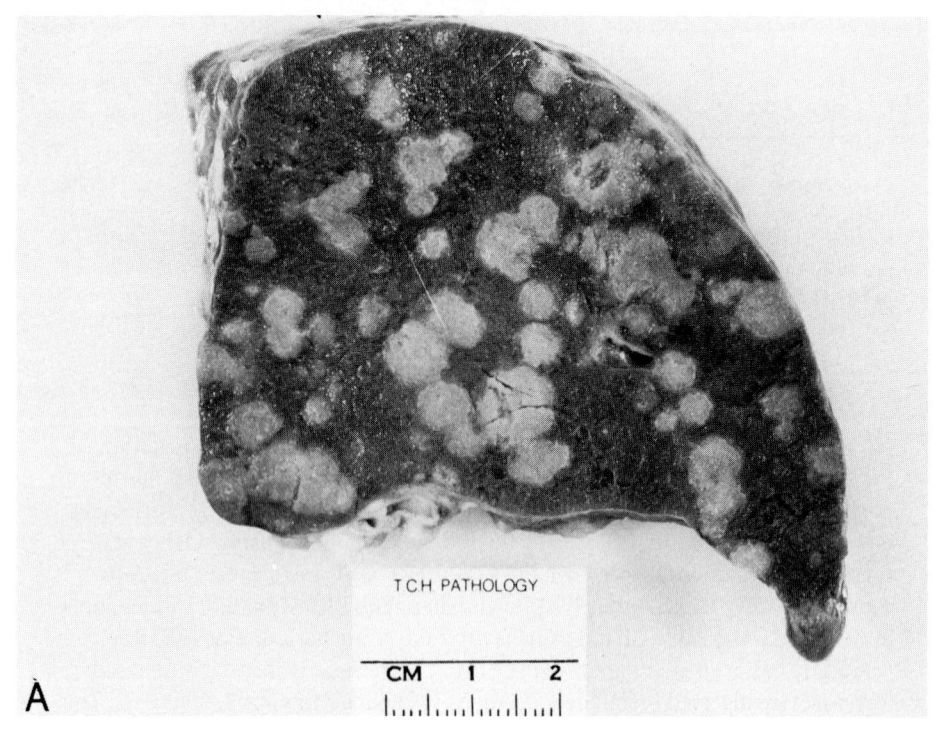

Figure 8 Systemic candidiasis. A. The cut surface is studded with dry, tan confluent nodules. B. A necrotizing granuloma is seen on the left. (Hematoxylin-eosin stain X 400) C. A sliver stain shows yeast and pseudohyphae in the granulomas. (Methenamine silver stain X 1000)

PATHOLOGY OF THE SPLEEN

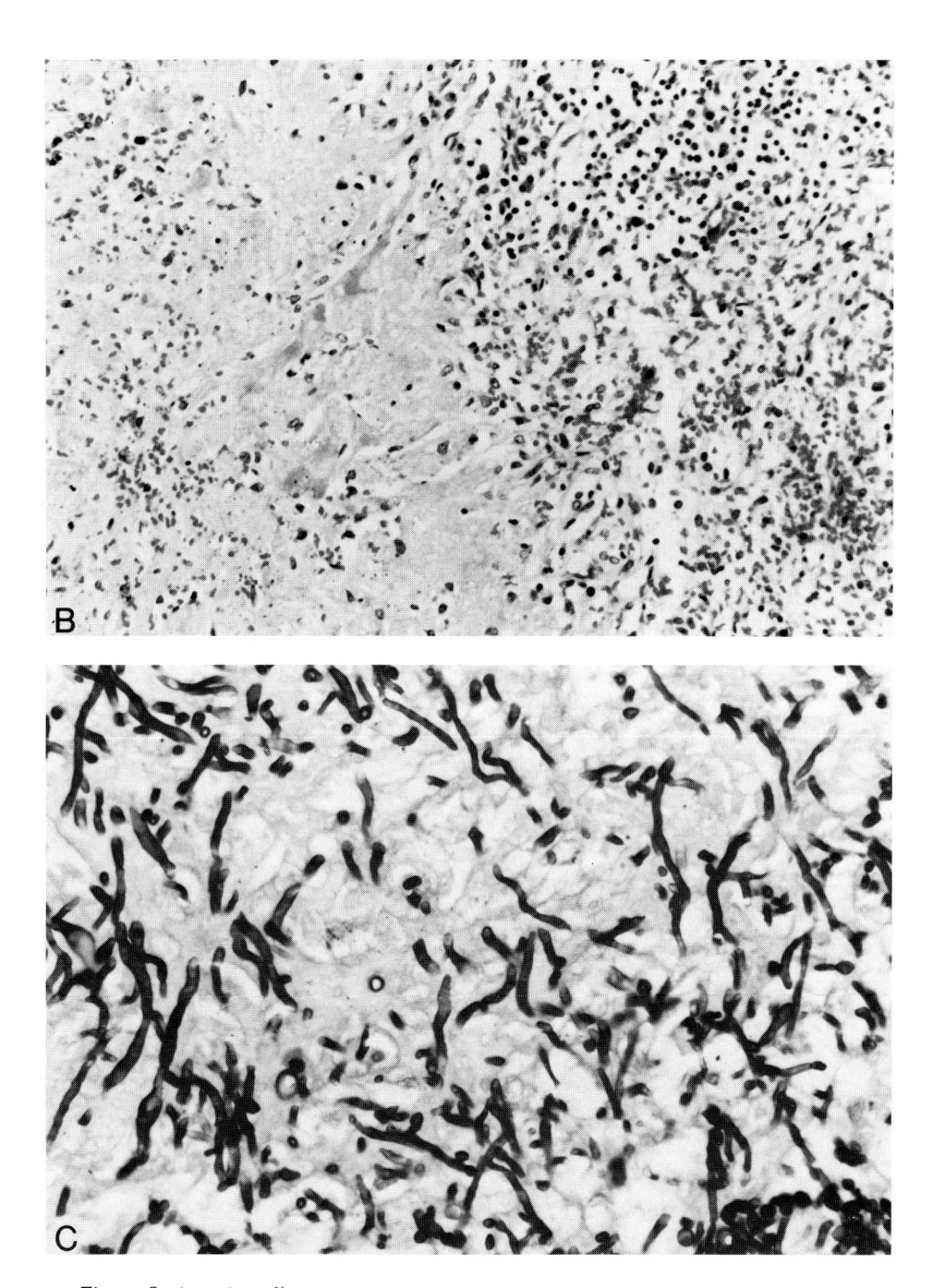

Figure 8 (continued)

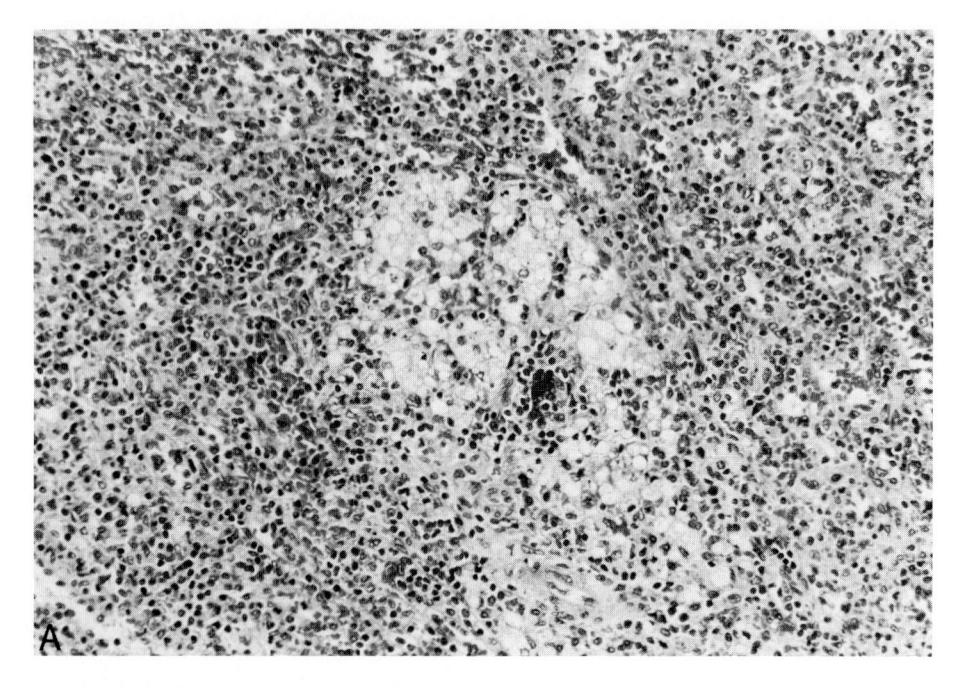

Figure 9 Leprosy. A. A granuloma containing bubbly histiocytes is present in the red pulp. (Hematoxylin-eosin stain × 100) B. The Fite stain shows large numbers of acid-fast bacilli. (Fite stain × 1000)

fants, as an expression of extramedullary hematopoiesis. The extent or severity of the reaction in the red pulp was not related to the type of microorganism cultured. Although young infants may be capable of an antibody response even in utero, their lymphoid organs do not display the expected histologic alterations associated with immune reactivity.

A large number of infectious diseases may involve the spleen and many cause significant splenomegaly. In most infections the pathologic changes in the spleen are similar to those seen in other organs, for example, there is granulomatous inflammation in mycobacterial and fungal diseases (Figures 8 and 9). Massive splenomegaly is seen in malaria and leishmaniasis. The parasites may be identified in the red pulp in macrophages and in endothelial cells. In malaria hematin pigment is present in macrophages, giving a dark brown color to the spleen.

B

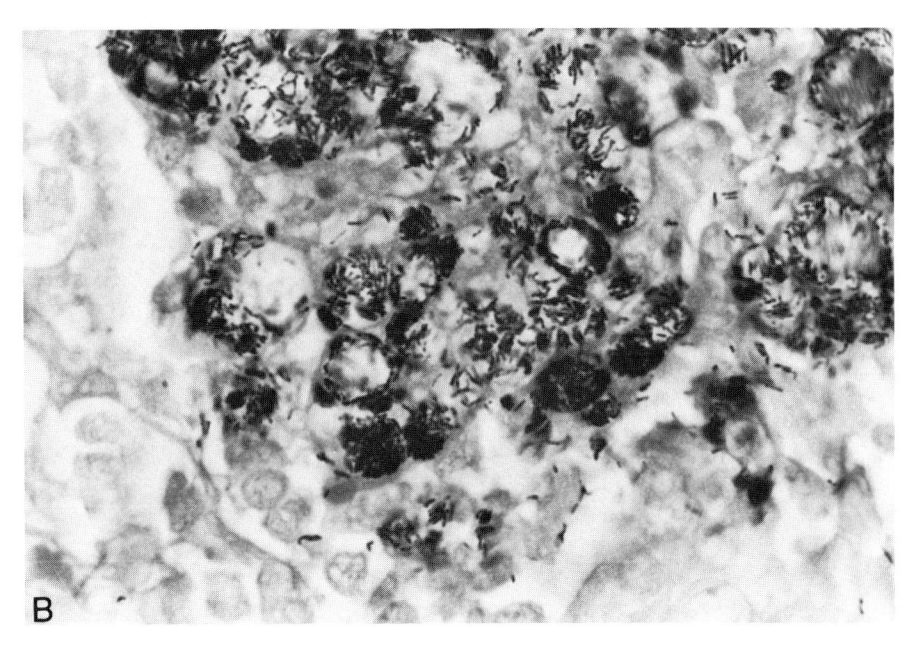

Figure 9 (continued)

Two entities deserve special mention because of their characteristic histologic features. These are *infectious mononucleosis* (IM) and the *infection-associated hemophagocytic syndrome* (IAHS). Infectious mononucleosis is generally a self-limited systemic infection and is caused by the Epstein-Barr virus. The spleen is generally enlarged but despite the fact that there is significant B and T lymphocytic activity, the white pulp is not enlarged or reactive in appearance. The red pulp is expanded and infiltrated by lymphocytes and immunoblasts of varying sizes (Figure 10). These cells infiltrate the capsule, trabeculae and walls of blood vessels. This infiltration of the connective tissue framework may lead to formation of hematomas or the occurrence of splenic rupture (39). As are observed in lymph nodes, large binucleated cells resembling *Reed-Sternberg cells* (RSC) may be seen in the spleen in infectious mononucleosis. Despite the presence of these cells, there should be no difficulty in differentiating infectious mononucleosis from Hodgkin's disease, either by gross inspection or by microscopic examination. On gross examination the spleen in Hodgkin's disease shows irregular nodules of white pulp, while in infectious mononucleosis the white pulp is not prominent and there is red pulp expansion. Microscopically the Reed-

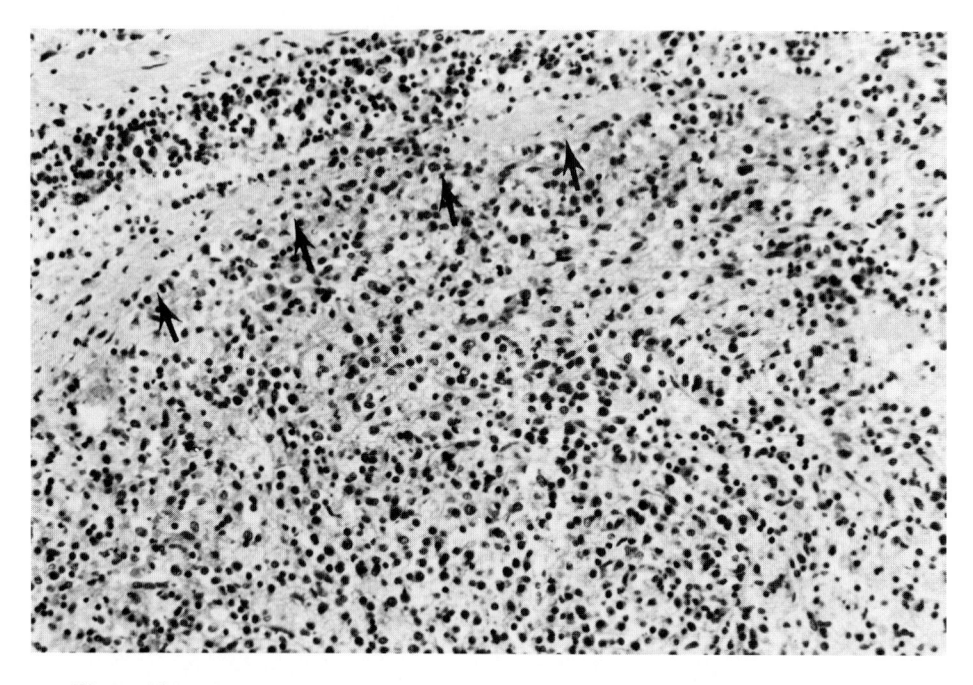

Figure 10 Infectious mononucleosis. The red pulp is diffusely infiltrated by lymphocytes and immunoblasts. A trabecula (arrows) has been almost completely destroyed, weakening the connective tissue framework. (Hematoxylin-eosin stain × 100)

Sternberg cells of Hodgkin's disease are present in a mixed background of small lymphocytes, eosinophils, plasma cells, histiocytes and connective tissue, while in infectious mononucleosis there is a relatively homogeneous proliferation of immunoblasts.

A more difficult differential diagnosis involves infectious mononucleosis and large cell lymphoma. While age, clinical presentation and serologic information may aid in the diagnosis, an occasional case may require the use of immunologic markers and evidence of a monoclonal proliferation to make this distinction. Involvement of the spleen by acute leukemia may also mimic infectious mononucleosis both grossly and microscopically. In both acute leukemia and infectious mononucleosis there are red pulp infiltrations with inconspicuous white pulp. In both diseases there is expansion of the red pulp by a homogeneous proliferation of large mononuclear cells. While the cytologic features of the blasts in acute leukemia may not be appreciated in tissue sections, they may be readily seen on touch preparations or by examination of the bone marrow and peripheral blood.

The virus-associated hemophagocytic syndrome was first described in 1979 (40). Since then a variety of etiologic agents, frequently viruses but also bacteria and protozoa, have been associated with this disorder. This finding makes the term *infection-associated hemophagocytic syndrome* (IAHS) a more appropriate name for the disorder. This condition presents with fever, constitutional symptoms, pancytopenia, coagulopathy, hepatosplenomegaly and lymphadenopathy. While a number of these patients died of overwhelming infection or hemorrhagic complications, a significant number had a self-limited disease which responded to supportive therapy. The spleen is enlarged; the white pulp is inconspicuous and the red pulp is congested. On microscopic examination, the red pulp is infiltrated by benign-appearing histiocytes which exhibit marked hemophagocytosis (Figure 11). The degree of phagocytosis of blood cells is greater than that seen in malignant histiocytosis and no atypical or malignant histiocytes are

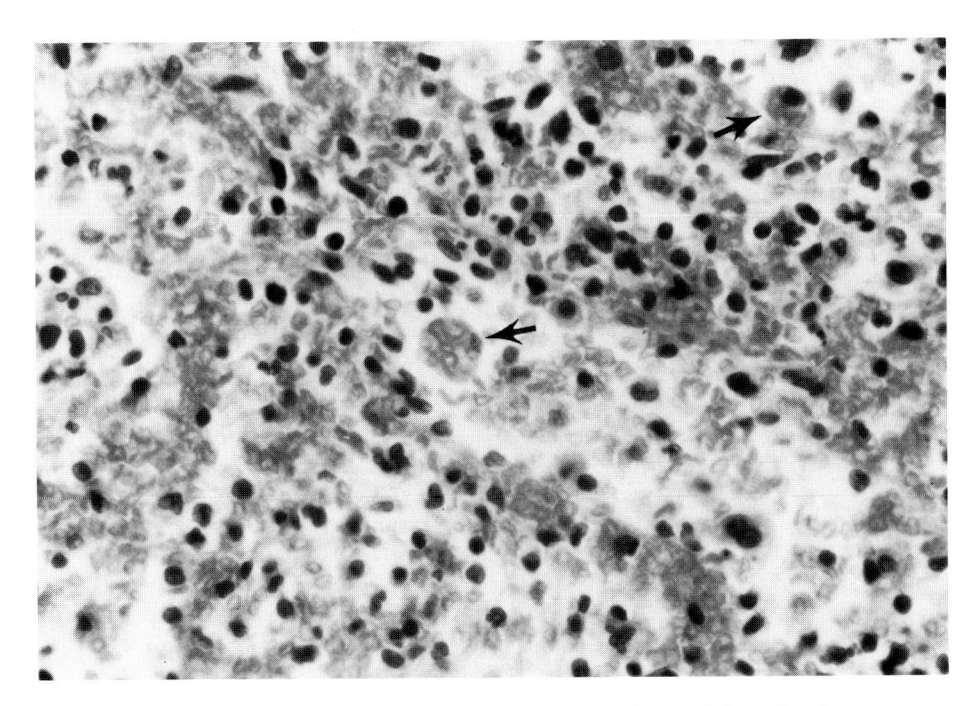

Figure 11 Infection-associated hemophagocytic syndrome. The red pulp contains a lymphohistiocytic infiltrate. Cytologically benign histiocytes exhibit marked erythrophagocytosis (arrows). (Hematoxylin-eosin stain × 400)

seen (41,42). Mononuclear cell infiltration of vessel walls and connective tissue as well as focal necrosis may be prominent (43). A similar histologic picture is seen in familial hemophagocytic lymphohistiocytosis and in the terminal or accelerated phase of Chediak-Higashi disease (44).

STORAGE DISEASES

A variety of inherited metabolic diseases result in storage of lipid or mucopolysaccharide compounds within histiocytes in the spleen. In Gaucher's disease there is accumulation of glucocerebroside in histiocytes in the spleen, liver, lymph nodes, and bone marrow. In some forms of Gaucher's disease these ac-

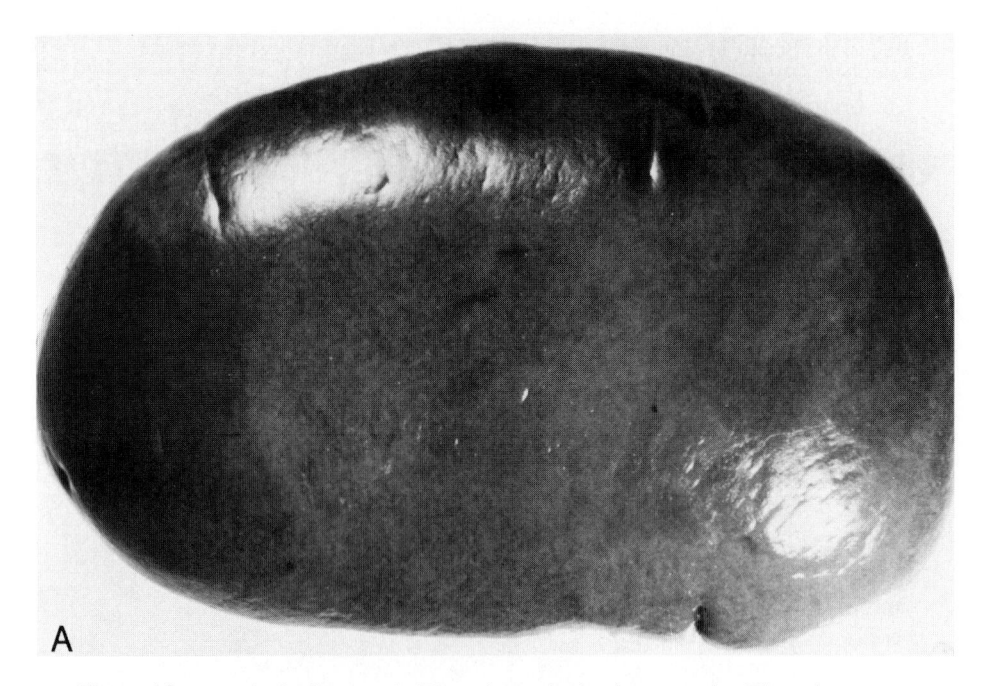

Figure 12 Gaucher's disease. A. There is marked splenomegaly. The spleen weighed 540 grams, normal for age 39 grams. B. A close-up view of the cut surface of the spleen shows red pulp expansion with a mottled red-yellow appearance. C. The red pulp sinuses are filled with collections of histiocytes. (Hematoxylin-eosin stain × 100) D. Spleen imprint. The Gaucher cells have eccentric nuclei and striated cytoplasm. (Wright-Giemsa stain × 1000) E. Electron micrograph of the Gaucher cell shows cytoplasmic microtubules. (Electron micrograph × 9000)

PATHOLOGY OF THE SPLEEN

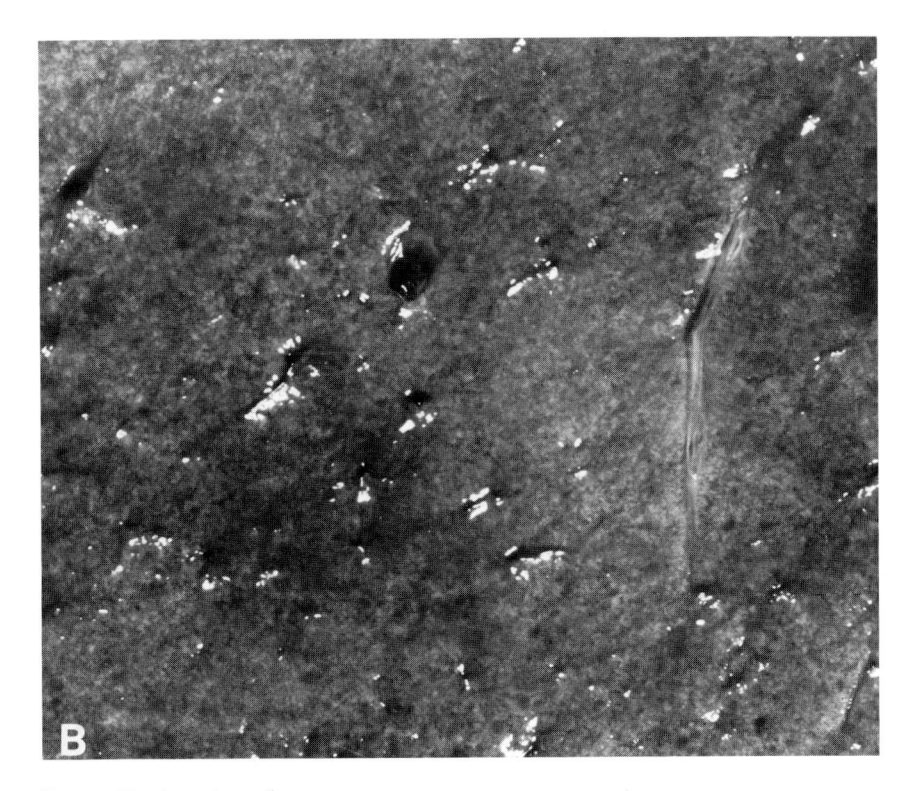

Figure 12 (continued)

cumulations are also present in the central nervous system. Massive splenomegaly is present. On gross examination of the spleen there is expansion of the red pulp and inconspicuous white pulp (Figure 12A, B). Microscopically, there is infiltration of the red pulp, especially the sinuses, with Gaucher cells (Figure 12C). These cells are large (20 to 100 μm) and have a single small hyperchromatic nucleus. The cytoplasm contains irregular striations resembling crumpled tissue paper or wrinkled silk (Figure 12D). Gaucher cells stain with PAS, Prussian blue for iron, acid phosphatase, and periodic acid-methenamine silver. Ultrastructurally, the cytoplasm contains membrane-bound tubules 30 to 60 nm in diameter (45) (Figure 12E). Gaucher-like cells have been observed in the spleen and other organs in a number of conditions characterized by increased cell turnover, such as thalassemia, chronic myeloid leukemia and *immune thrombocytopenic purpura* (ITP) (38).

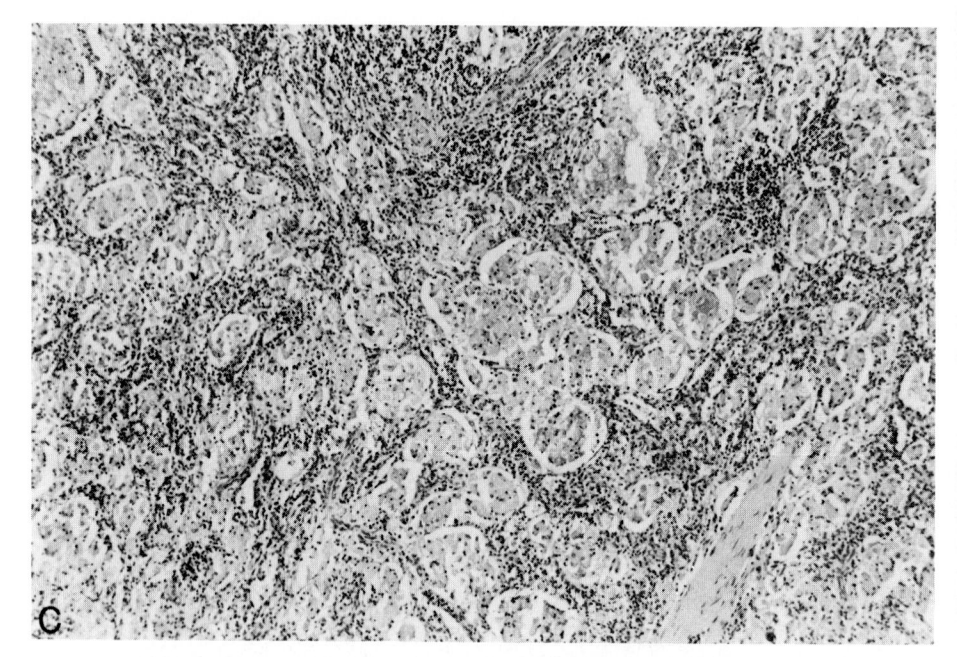

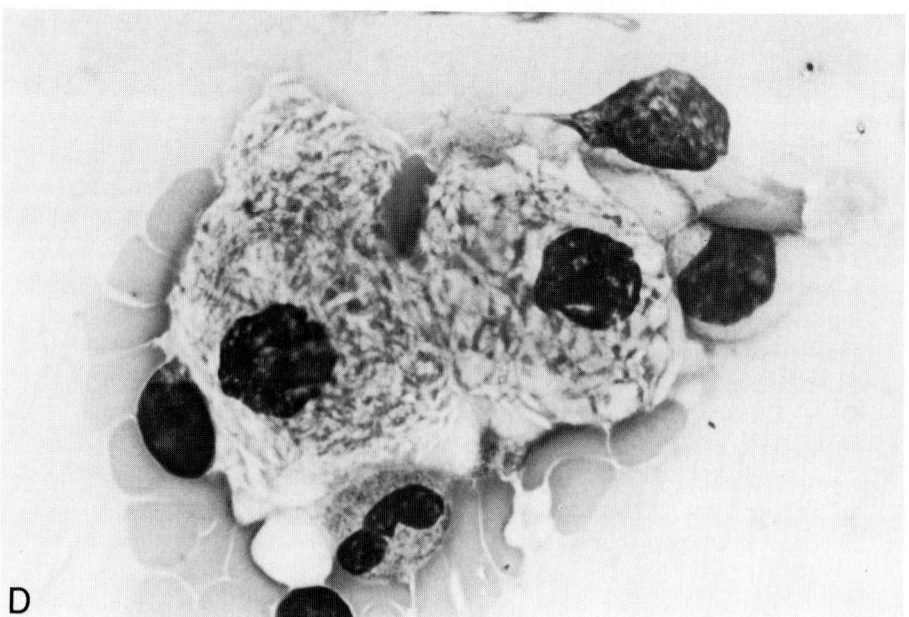

Figure 12 (continued)

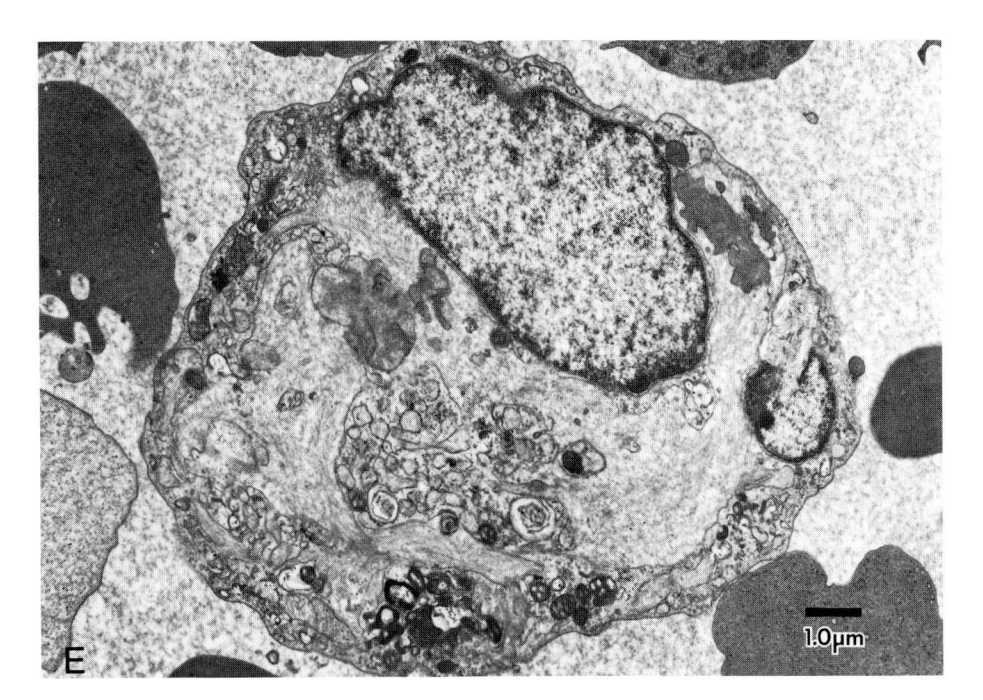

Figure 12 (continued)

The multiple clinical forms of Niemann-Pick disease have similar pathologic findings in the spleen. The storage of sphingomyelin in histiocytes of the cords result in red pulp expansion (Figure 13A). Variable degrees of vacuolization of sinusoidal lining cells are present. The histiocytes in Niemann-Pick disease are large (20 to 90 μm) and the cytoplasm has a bubbly or foamy appearance (Figure 13B), rather than the linear streaks of the Gaucher cell. The Niemann-Pick cell stains variably with PAS and is positive with a variety of lipid stains, including oil red-O, Sudan black, nile blue sulfate, and the Schultz stain for cholesterol. On electron microscopic examination the Niemann-Pick cells contain myelin figures within the cytoplasm (Figure 13C).

In addition to the classic Niemann-Pick cells, sea-blue histiocytes may be seen with the Giemsa stain in the spleen and other organs. Although sea-blue histiocytes were originally thought to be a marker for a specific syndrome (46,47), it is now believed that this disorder represents one of the adult types of Niemann-Pick disease (48,49). Sea-blue histiocytes may also be seen in a variety of other

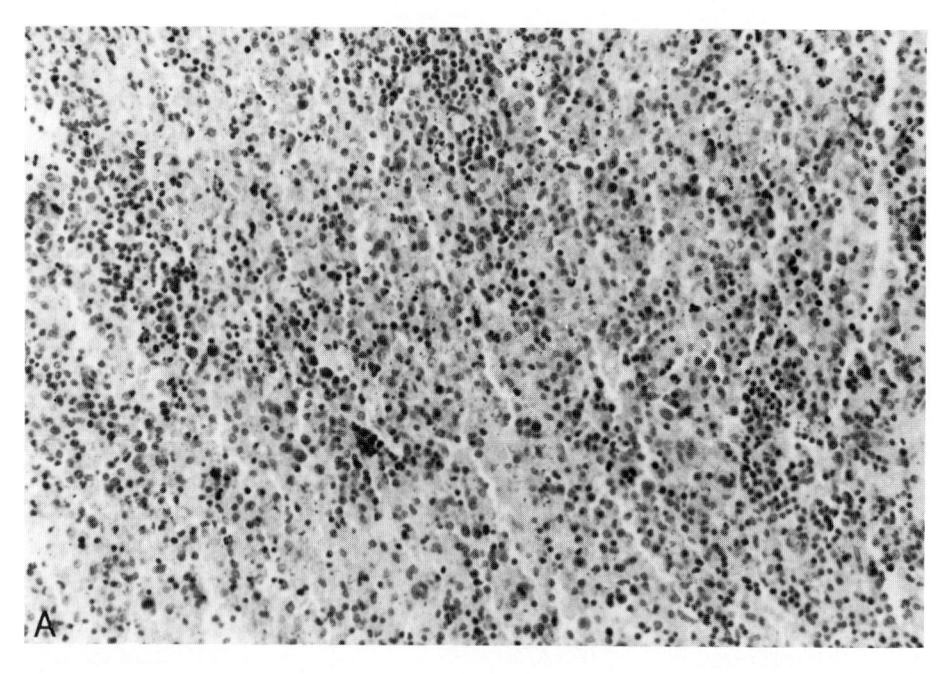

Figure 13 Nieman-Pick disease. A. The red pulp is diffusely infiltrated by histiocytes. (Hematoxylin-eosin stain × 100) B. Spleen imprint. The Nieman-Pick cell has a small eccentric nucleus and foamy cytoplasm. (Wright-Giemsa stain × 1000) C. Electron micrograph of the Nieman-Pick cell shows numerous cytoplasmic myelin figures. (Electron micrograph × 9000)

conditions including hyperlipidemias, chronic myeloid leukemia and ITP. Many other inherited storage disorders have splenic involvement and their storage histiocytes closely resemble those seen in Niemann-Pick disease. In Wolman's disease and cholesterol ester storage disease, cholesterol crystals may be seen in the histiocytes with polarizing lenses. Variable staining patterns for these disorders have been observed depending on the type of tissue examined, such as, touch preparations, frozen sections or fixed sections. Since many of these stored materials will be dissolved during tissue processing, the most reliable staining results are obtained using air-dried touch preparations or frozen sections.

A rare cause of splenomegaly and lipid storage disease is iatrogenic lipidosis following the intravenous administration of fat emulsions for hyperalimentation (50,51). This complication of hyperalimentation causes a variably enlarged salmon pink spleen. The splenic red pulp is filled with foamy macrophages contain-

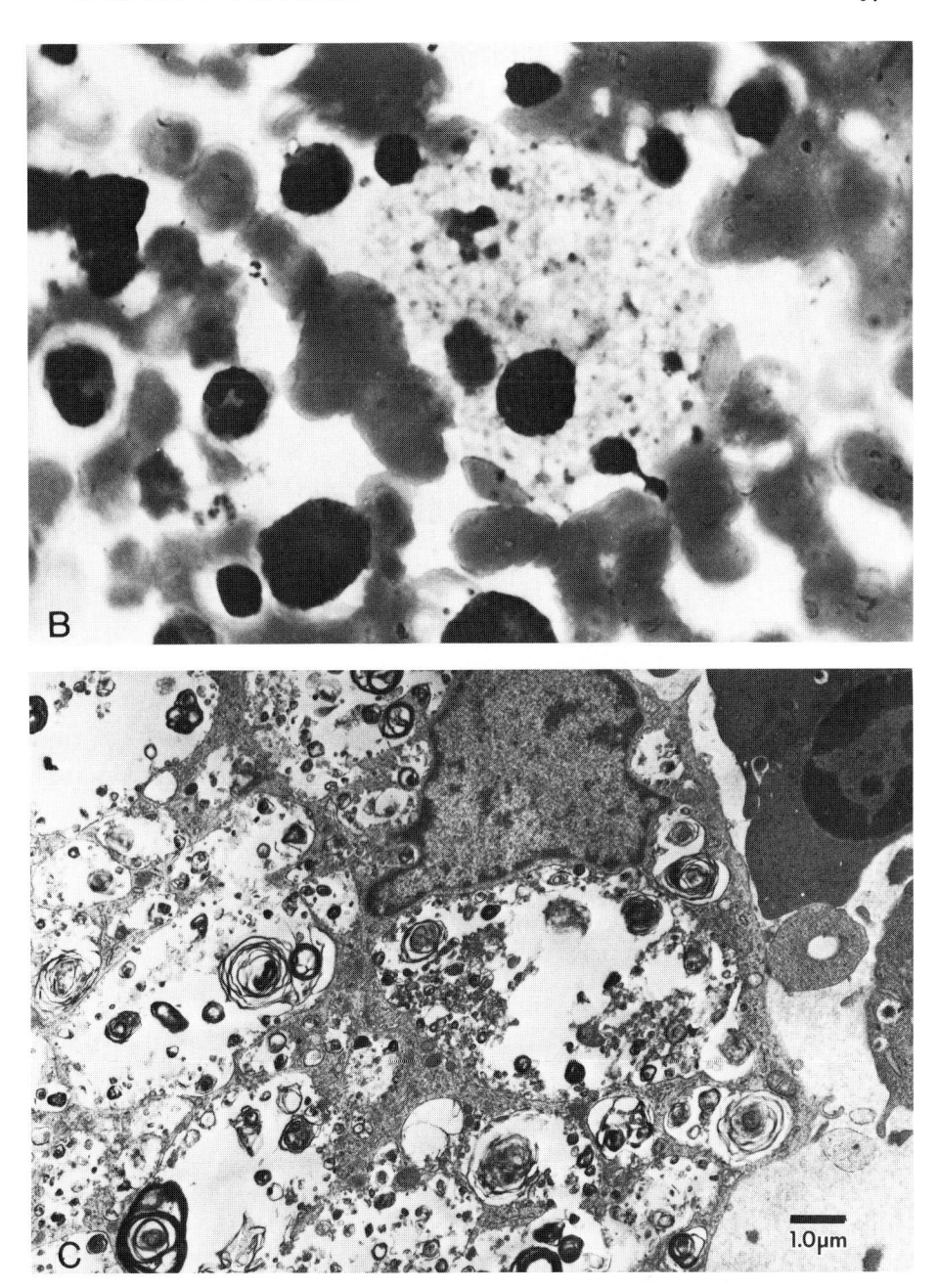

Figure 13 (continued)

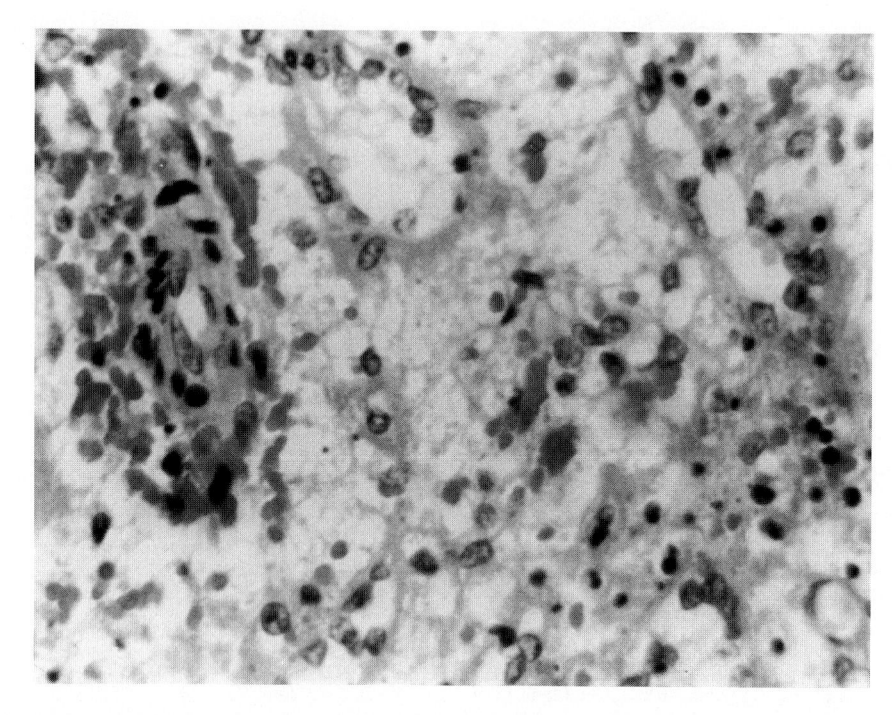

Figure 14 Hyperlipidosis. The red pulp is filled with foamy macrophages containing lipid.

ing lipid (Figure 14). These cells may also be seen in the kidney, liver, lungs, and blood vessels.

IMMUNE AND AUTOIMMUNE DISORDERS

The spleen is a major site of lymphoid tissue. Therefore it is not surprising that a variety of immune, autoimmune or immunodeficiency states involve the spleen. Immune thrombocytopenic purpura is a disorder associated with thrombocytopenia, shortened platelet survival, and compensatory megakaryocytic hyperplasia. Antiplatelet antibodies can be identified in most cases. This syndrome may be a postinfectious phenomenon, or it may be a harbinger of a collagen-vascular disease such as systemic lupus erythematosis. Although ITP frequently responds to steroid therapy, some cases are refractory to steroids and require splenectomy. Splenectomy is effective in most cases since it removes the major site of antibody formation (white pulp) as well as the major site of platelet se-

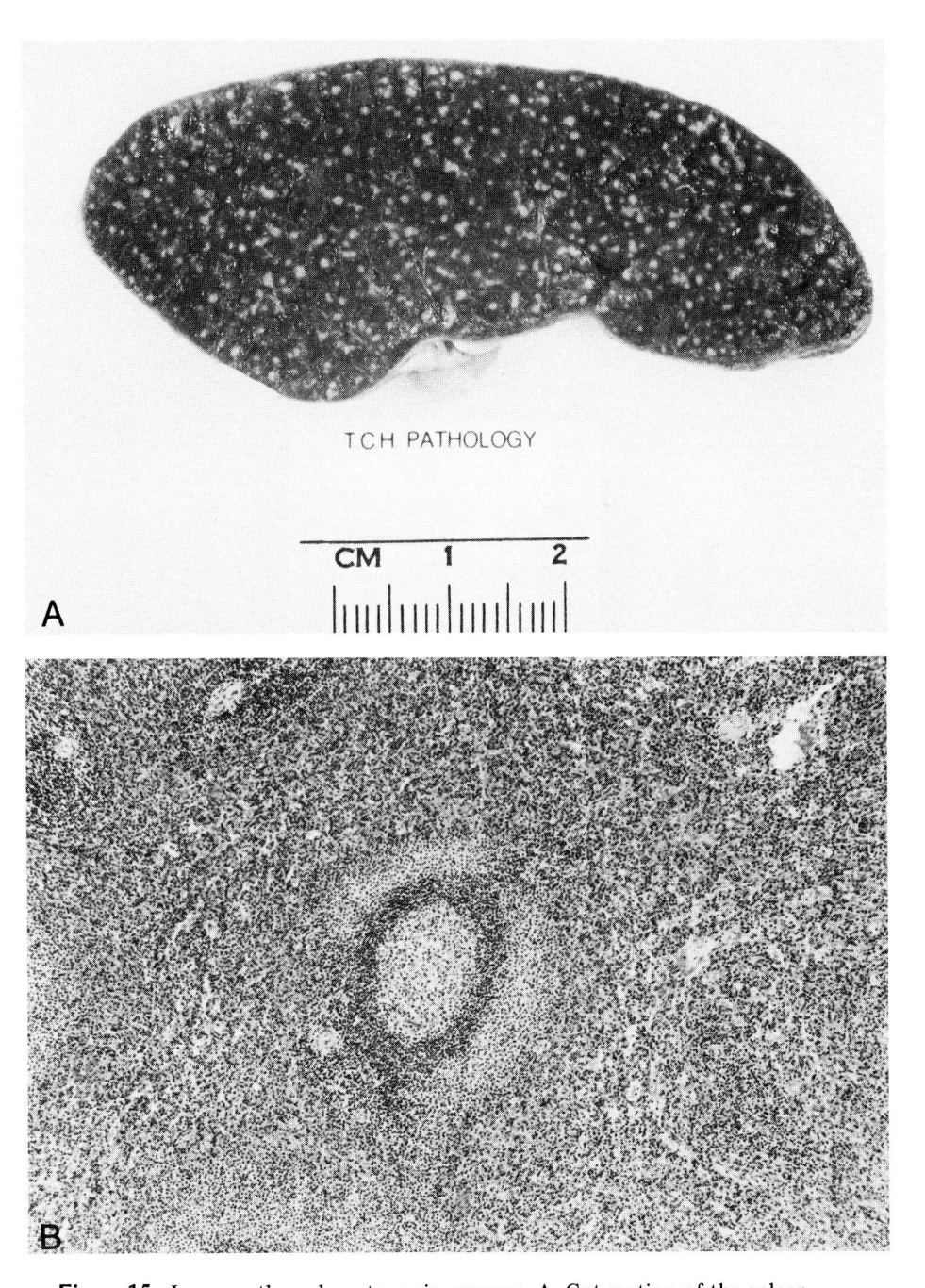

Figure 15 Immune thrombocytopenic purpura. A. Cut section of the spleen shows prominent white pulp nodules. The spleen weight was normal for age. B. There is reactive follicular hyperplasia with a prominent marginal zone. The red pulp is normal in appearance. (Hematoxylin-eosin stain × 100)

questration and destruction (red pulp). The spleen in ITP is generally not enlarged. On cut section the white pulp is prominent (Figure 15A). Microscopically, the white pulp is reactive with numerous germinal centers and prominent widened marginal zones (Figure 15B). Plasma cells may be numerous especially around vessels in the marginal zone (52). Macrophages in the cords contain phagocytized platelets, which are not discernable on routine stains but may be demonstrated immunohistochemically. Foamy histiocytes or Gaucher-like cells may be seen in the red pulp (53).

The classic appearance of the splenic white pulp in ITP may be altered by the use of corticosteroids prior to splenectomy (54). In these cases phagocytized platelets may still be demonstrated in the cords by the use of touch preparations or immunohistochemistry. Periarteriolar fibrosis or "onion skinning" of the blood vessels in the spleen is often seen in ITP. Some authors believe this finding may relate to underlying systemic lupus erythematosis in these patients (55).

A small percentage of patients with a long history of rheumatoid arthritis have splenomegaly and granulocytopenia (Felty's syndrome). These patients may have persistent or recurrent infections and respond well to splenectomy. This syndrome is occasionally seen in children with juvenile rheumatoid arthritis (56). The spleen does not have pathognomonic features in rheumatoid arthritis but shows reactive follicles with plasma cells and immunoblasts around vessels. The red pulp is expanded but granulocytes are not increased in numbers and little leukophagocytosis is seen. In systemic lupus erythematosis the characteristic "onion skin" lesion around arterioles is present, and in *thrombotic thrombocytopenic purpura* (TTP) the typical hyaline thrombi may be seen in vessels. Prominent hemophagocytosis by splenic macrophages has also been described in TTP (57). Amyloidosis may involve the spleen with nodules of amyloid deposition in the walls of the vessels in the white pulp also known as sago spleen (Figure 16A and B) or with diffuse red pulp deposition.

Immune deficiency states will show decreased white pulp with loss of B cell or T cell areas or both (Figure 17). Opportunistic infections are common in these patients and may involve the spleen as well as other organs. In the *acquired immunodeficiency syndrome* (AIDS), the lymphocyte depletion and possible infectious disease of the spleen may be accompanied by a malignant process, such as Kaposi's sarcoma or malignant lymphoma (58).

With the increasing use of organ transplantation as a therapeutic modality, the pathologist is seeing more evidence of *graft-vs.-host disease* (GVHD). The spleen in graft-vs.-host disease shows lymphoid depletion as a result of immunosuppressive therapy. There is frequently hemorrhage and hemosiderin deposition in the red pulp. A lymphohistiocytic infiltrate is present similar to that seen in other organs (59). If the patient has received whole body irradiation in preparation for bone marrow transplantation, in addition to lymphoid depletion there may be fibrosis in the red pulp and myointimal proliferation in the arteries (60).

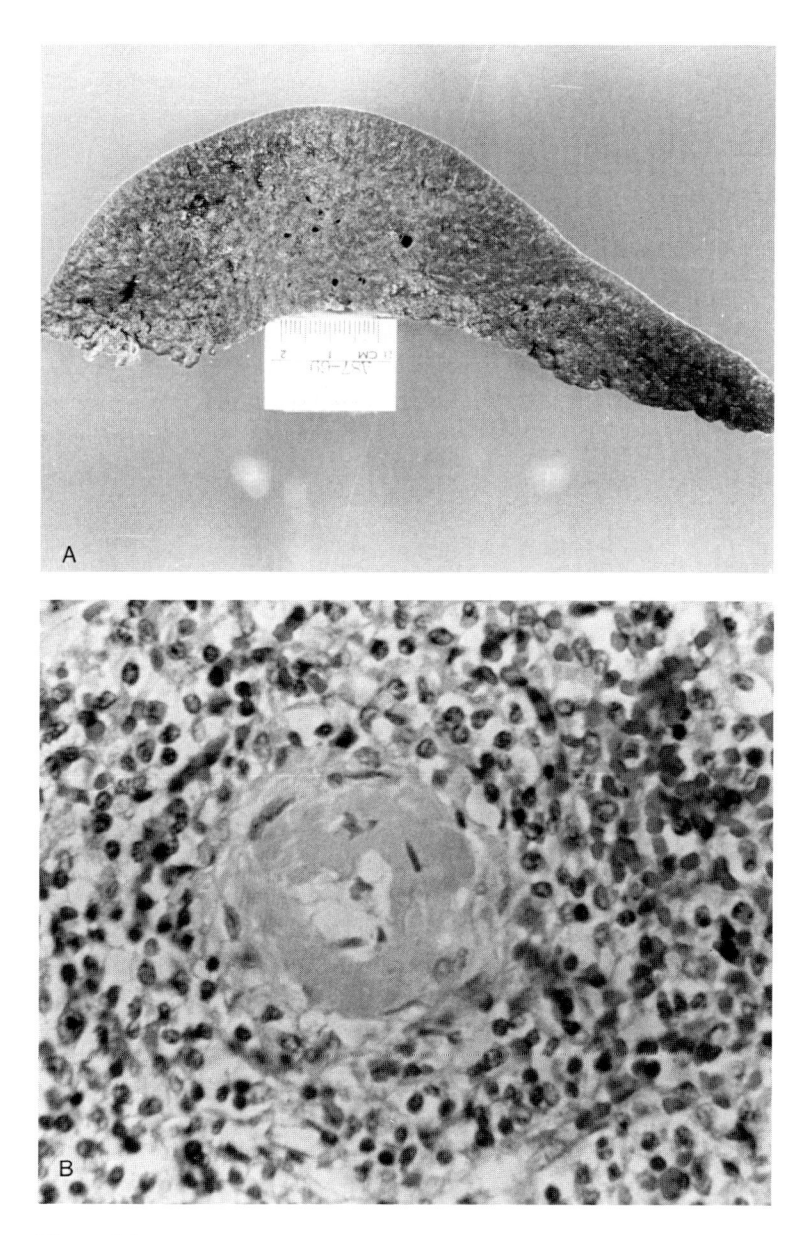

Figure 16 A. Amyloidosis. Cut section of the enlarged spleen has a firm texture and a pale waxy appearance. B. Amyloidosis: The vessels are thickened by a homogeneous eosinophilic material that stains positively for amyloid with congo red. (Hemotoxylin-eosin × 100)

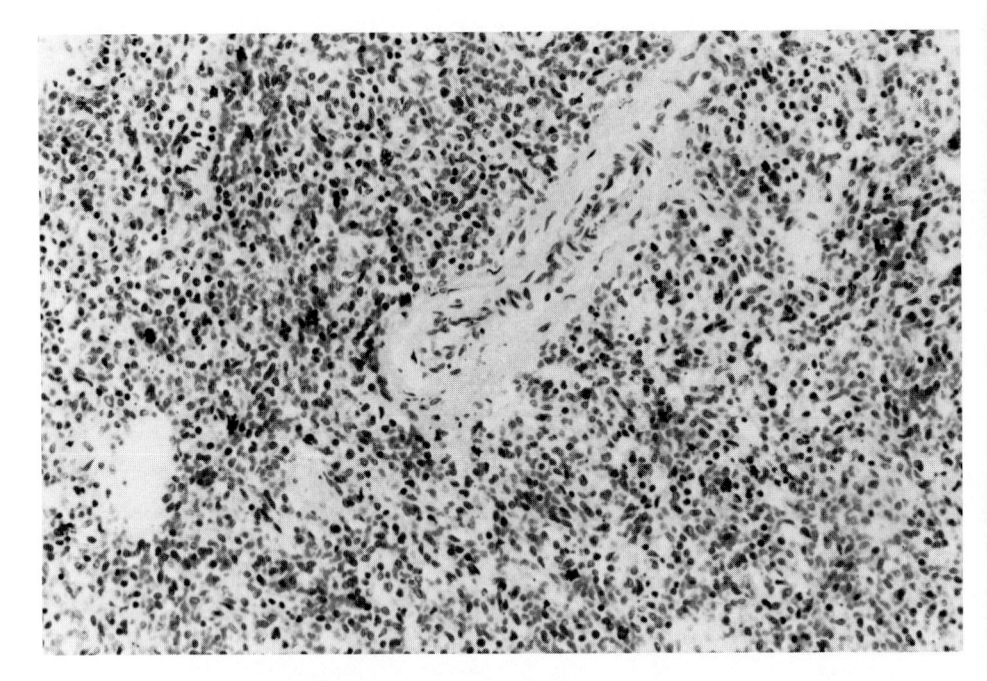

Figure 17 Severe combined immune deficiency. There is absence of the periarteriolar sheath (T cells) as well as germinal centers (B cells). The red pulp is normal in appearance. (Hematoxylin-eosin stain × 100)

Histiocytosis X (Langerhans cell histiocytosis) is a disorder with variable clinical manifestations, characterized by a proliferation of Langerhans cells, which are histiocytes of the dendritic cell family. At present this disease is believed to be a disorder of immune regulation rather than a malignancy (61). In Langerhans cell histiocytosis the splenic architecture may not be greatly disturbed. Granuloma-like collection of Langerhans cells are present in the red pulp and the marginal zone of the white pulp (Figure 18A). The Langerhans cells have a characteristic appearance with abundant eosinophilic cytoplasm and an oval or bean-shaped nucleus (Figure 18B). These cells are characterized ultrastructurally by the presence of the Birbeck granule (Figure 18C) and immunohistochemically by positive staining for S100 protein, OKT6, OKT4, HLA-DR (Ia), αD mannosidase and a specific staining pattern with peanut agglutinin (61).

Several other disorders are associated with abnormalities of splenic function. Most of these involve impaired splenic function and are discussed in detail in Chapter 4 on hyposplenism (62,63).

PATHOLOGY OF THE SPLEEN

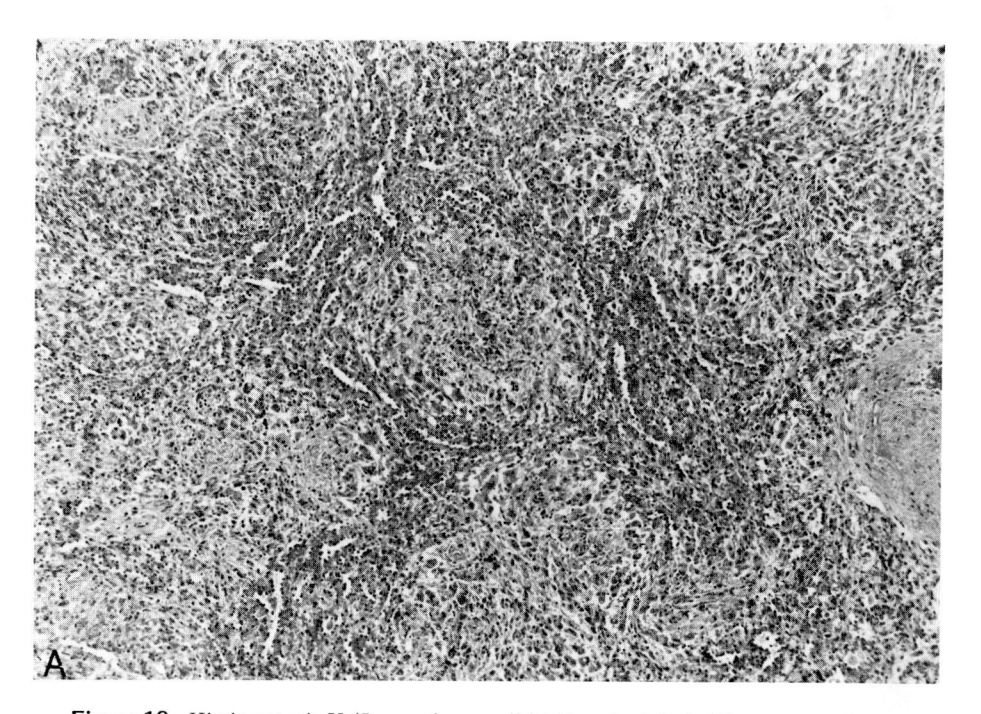

Figure 18 Histiocytosis X (Langerhans cell histiocytosis). A. There are multiple granuloma-like aggregates of histiocytes in the red pulp. (Hematoxylin-eosin stain X 100) B. There is a proliferation of Langerhans cells in the red pulp. The Langerhans cell has an eccentric oval to bean-shaped nucleus and ample eosinophilic cytoplasm (arrow). C. Electron micrographs shows Birbeck granules (the rod- or racket-shaped pentalaminar structures) in the cytoplasm of a Langerhans cell. (Electron micrograph X 67,000)

In patients with chronic renal failure on hemodialysis, a hypersplenic state may be present (64,65). Splenectomy generally relieves this situation. Microscopically, there is prominent reactive white pulp with germinal centers and expanded marginal zones (Figure 19). Plasma cells are often present. There is congestion in the red pulp and increased numbers of mast cells. It is postulated that the patient with renal failure on dialysis has numerous sources of chronic antigenic stimulation, including sepsis, multiple transfusions and repeated exposure to hepatitis as well as contamination of the dialysis fluid. This results in lymphoid hyperplasia, splenomegaly and hypersplenism.

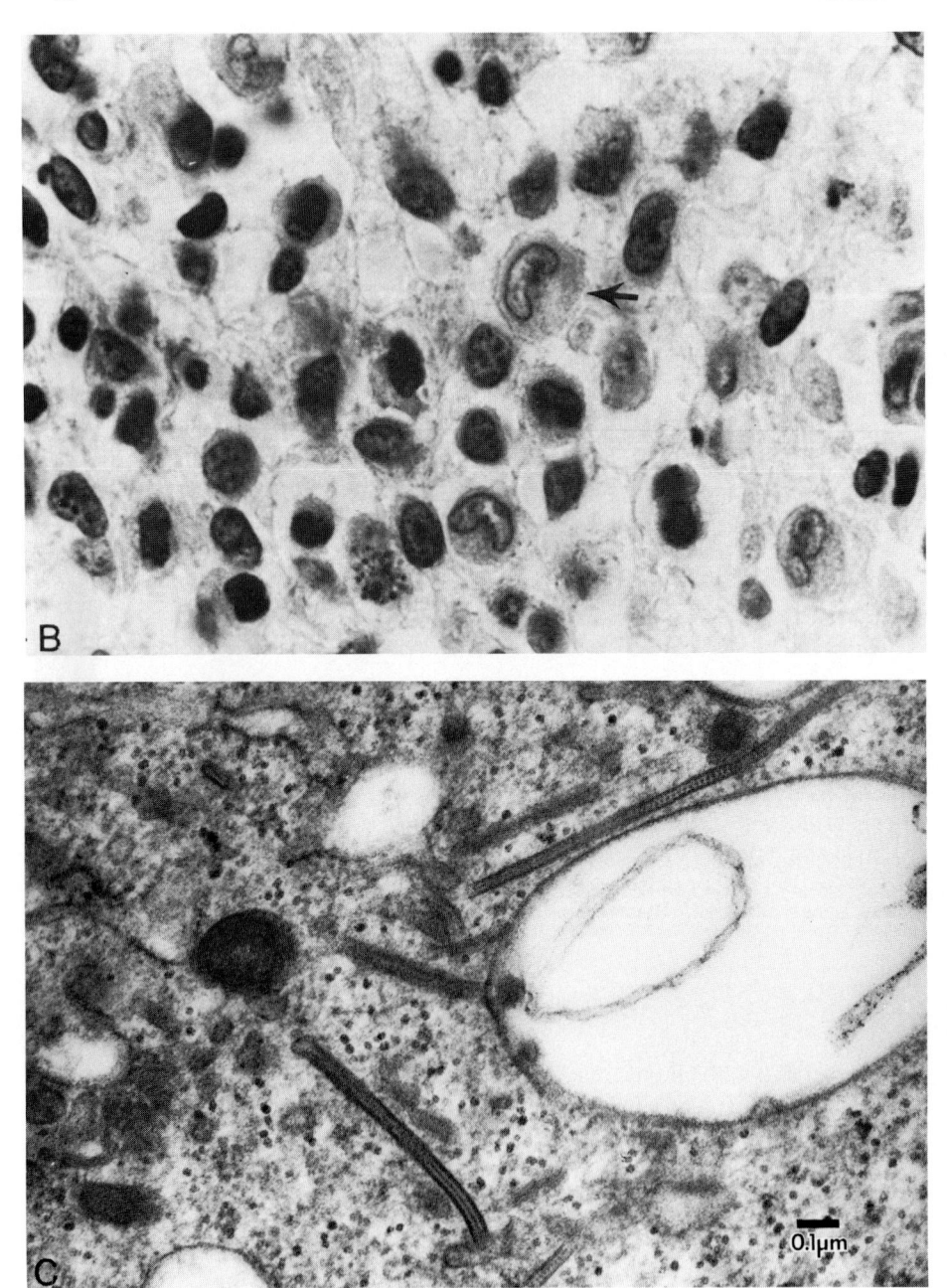

Figure 18 (continued)

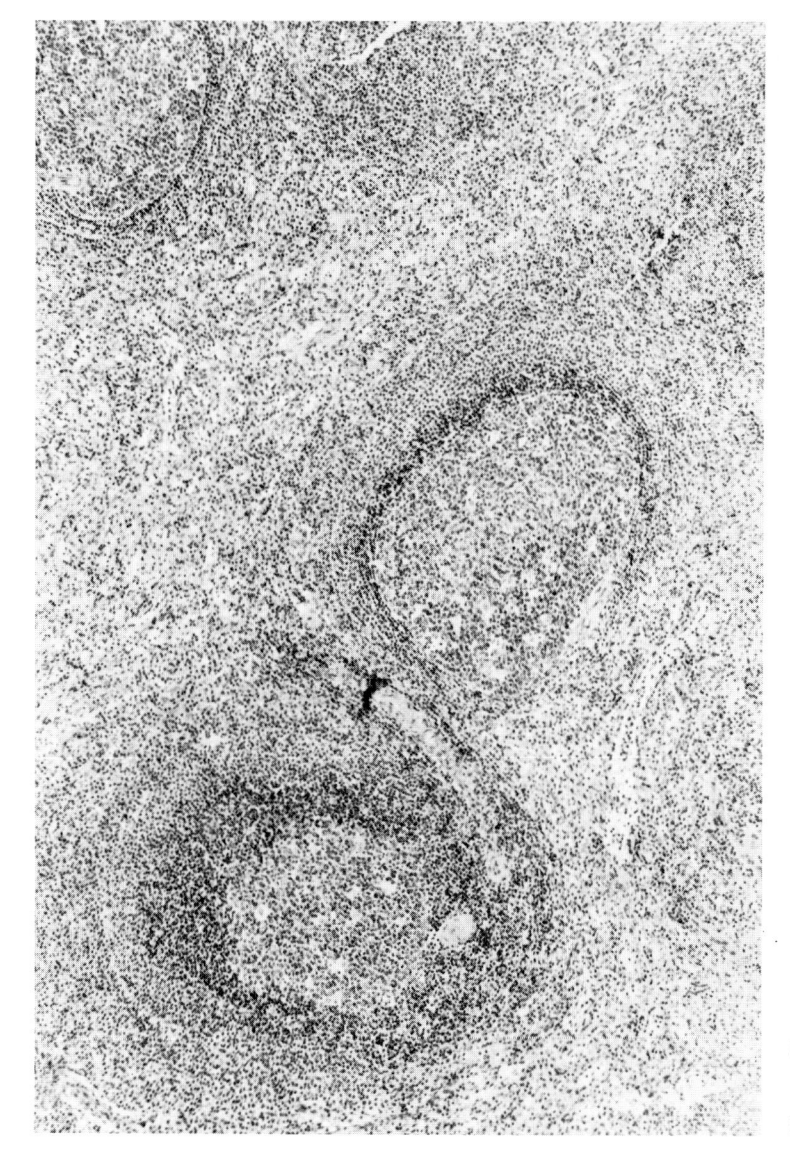

Figure 19 Chronic renal failure in a patient treated with hemodialysis. Reactive follicular hyperplasia is present with normal appearing red pulp.

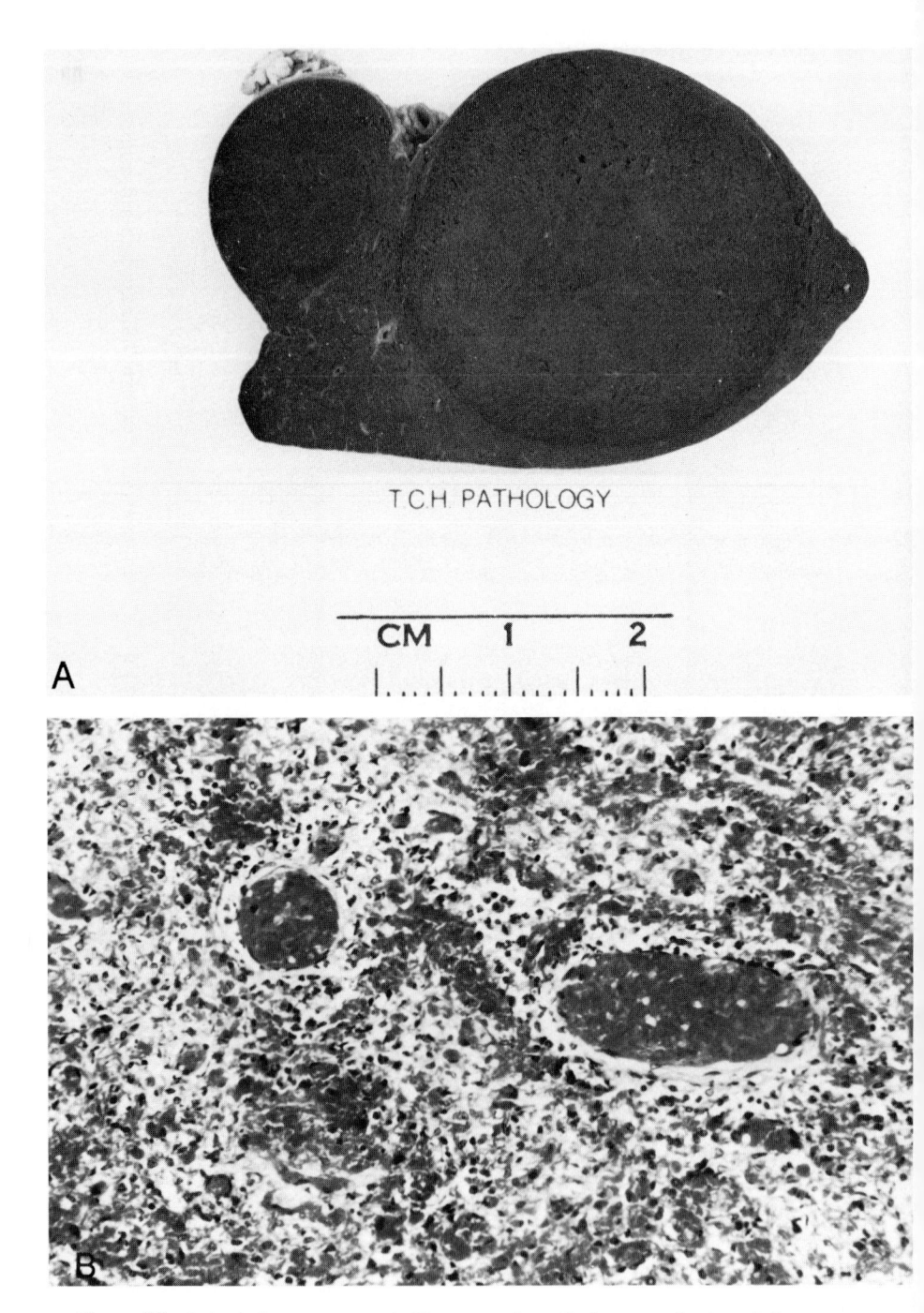

Figure 20 Splenic hamartoma. A. Two round, well-circumscribed nodules are present. They are similar in appearance with the uninvolved spleen. B. Sections from the nodules show congested red pulp without any white pulp present. (Hematoxylin-eosin stain × 400)

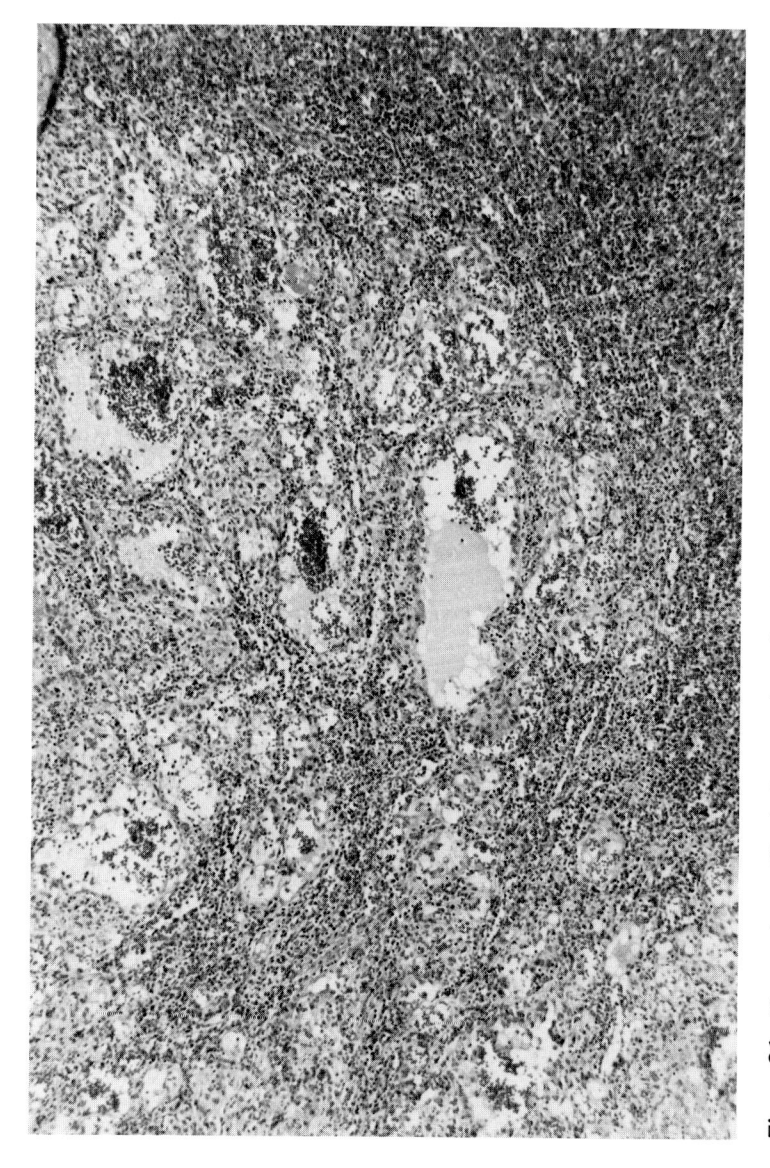

Figure 21 Hemangioma. The lesion consists of multiple blood-filled spaces lined by endothelial cells. The adjacent red pulp is compressed. (Hematoxylin-eosin stain × 100)

BENIGN TUMORS

Benign splenic tumors include hamartomas, hemangiomas, lymphangiomas and cysts. These lesions may present as an abdominal mass or abdominal pain, or may be incidental findings at autopsy or laparotomy. Splenic hamartomas, also called splenomas or nodular hyperplasia of the spleen, are well demarcated nodules compressing the normal parenchyma (66) (Figure 20A). The microscopic appearance of these tumors consists of splenic red pulp without trabeculae or white pulp (Figure 20B). Hamartomas are generally incidental findings and are asymptomatic. Hemangiomas in the spleen may be single or multiple and present as blood-filled spongy spaces in the spleen. These hemagiomas may be capillary or cavernous in type and are lined by flat endothelial cells without atypia (Figure 21). An associated coagulopathy may be present.

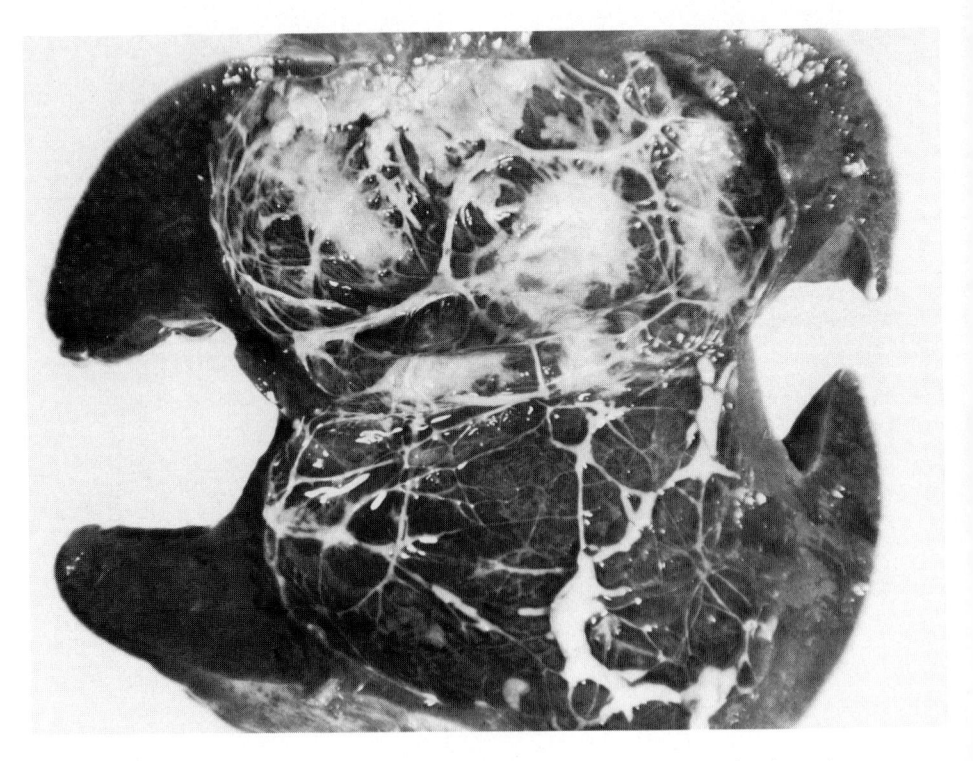

Figure 22 Primary nonparasitic cyst of the spleen. The bisected spleen shows a large central cyst with a pale trabeculated lining.

Lymphangiomas are similar in appearance but contain proteinaceous fluid rather than blood and typically occur beneath the capsule and around large trabeculae. Splenic cysts are of two types: true or primary cysts and secondary or false cysts (67,68) (Figure 22). True cysts have a cellular lining and are parasitic (echinococcal) or nonparasitic (squamous lined). The secondary cysts are more common and generally are associated with trauma. Cysts produce symptoms only if they are large enough. Most cysts contain bloody fluid.

MALIGNANCY AND MYELOPROLIFERATIVE DISORDERS

Malignant lymphoma in the spleen is generally part of a widely disseminated process, but 1 to 2% of lymphomas may present as primary splenic disease (69-72). Lymphomas involve the white pulp, which is present as scattered nodules throughout the spleen. Thus, the terms nodular or diffuse are not meaningful, since initially all lymphomas will have a nodular pattern. A lymphoma with uniform involvement of all the Malpighian bodies may not be distinguishable grossly from exuberant reactive hyperplasia. The cell type of the lymphoma determines the gross appearance of the spleen. Lymphomas of small cells show a fairly uniform distribution of nodules. Large cell lymphomas present with larger irregular masses which represent coalescence of a number of expanded white pulp foci.

Lymphoma of small lymphocytes (such as in well differentiated lymphocytic lymphoma or chronic lymphocytic leukemia) expands the Malpighian bodies and may extend into the red pulp (Figure 23A). There also may be subendothelial infiltration of the trabecular veins (73). The cells are round and regular with scant cytoplasm and condensed, clumped nuclear chromatin (Figure 23B). Lymphoma of small cleaved cells (poorly differentiated lymphocytic lymphoma) as well as other follicular center cell lymphomas tend to involve the central portions of the Malpighian bodies. The lesions are surrounded by a paler marginal zone of small round lymphocytes (74) (Figure 24A). At low power magnification these nodules may appear normal. However, at higher power the central regions are composed exclusively of small angulated, cleaved lymphocytes (Figure 24B), rather than the heterogeneous population of reactive germinal centers. Large numbers of epitheloid histiocytes may be seen in association with small cell lymphomas and these cells may be so numerous as to obscure the diagnosis (75).

Large cell lymphomas involve the spleen in a nonuniform manner with varying sized, grossly visible nodules (Figure 25A). The cells are large (20 to 30 μm) in diameter and have abundant cytoplasm, vesicular nuclear chromatin and prominent nucleoli (Figure 25B). Mycosis fungoides and other lymphomas of T

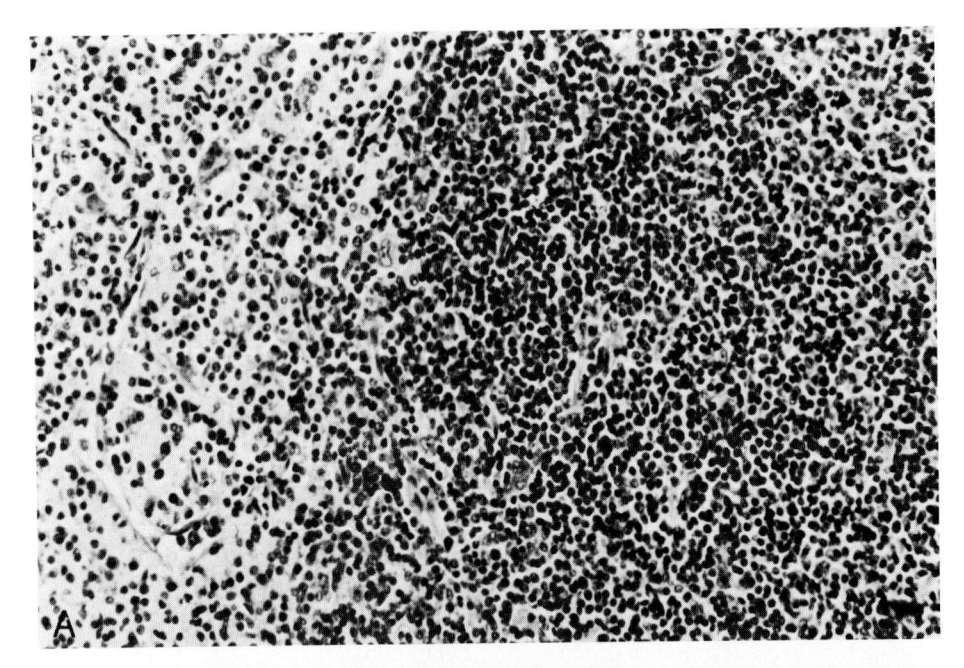

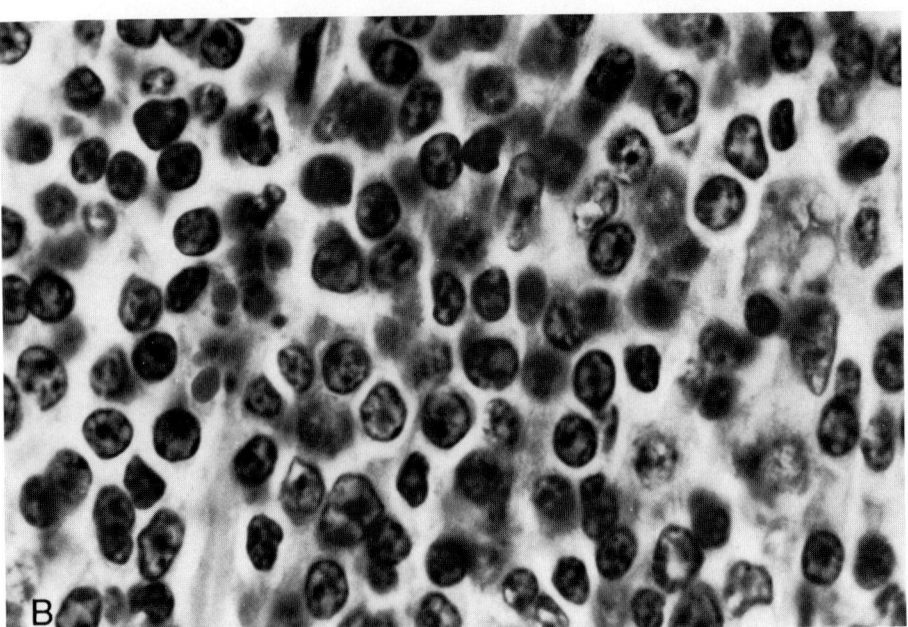

Figure 23 Malignant lymphoma, small lymphocytic type. A. A white pulp nodule (right) is expanded with extension of small lymphocytes into the surrounding red pulp. (Hematoxylin-eosin stain × 400) B. The white pulp is expanded by a homogeneous population of small round lymphocytes. (Hematoxylin-eosin stain × 1000)

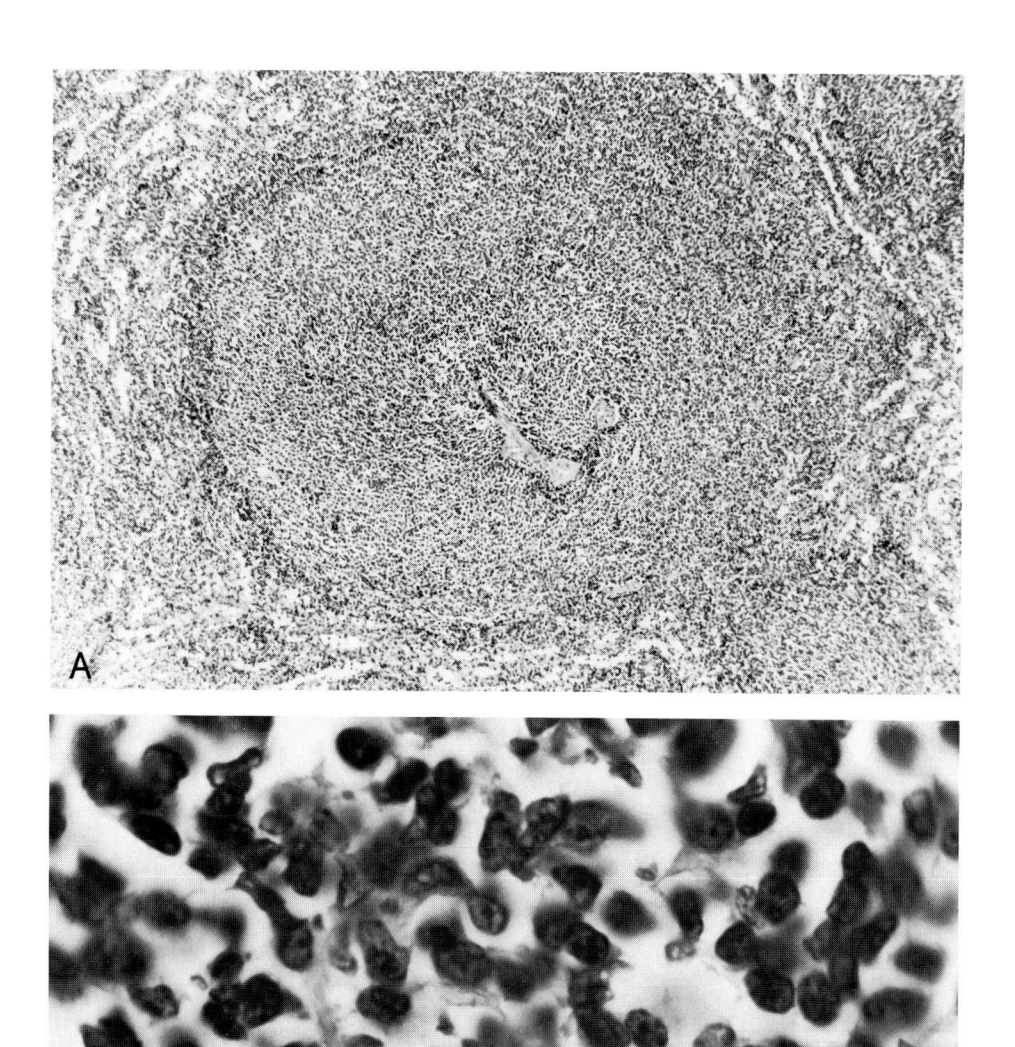

Figure 24 Malignant lymphoma, small cleaved lymphocytic type. A. The white pulp is expanded and partially surrounded by a denser mantle zone. B. The white pulp is expanded by small angulated cleaved lymphocytes. (Hematoxylin-eosin stain × 1000)

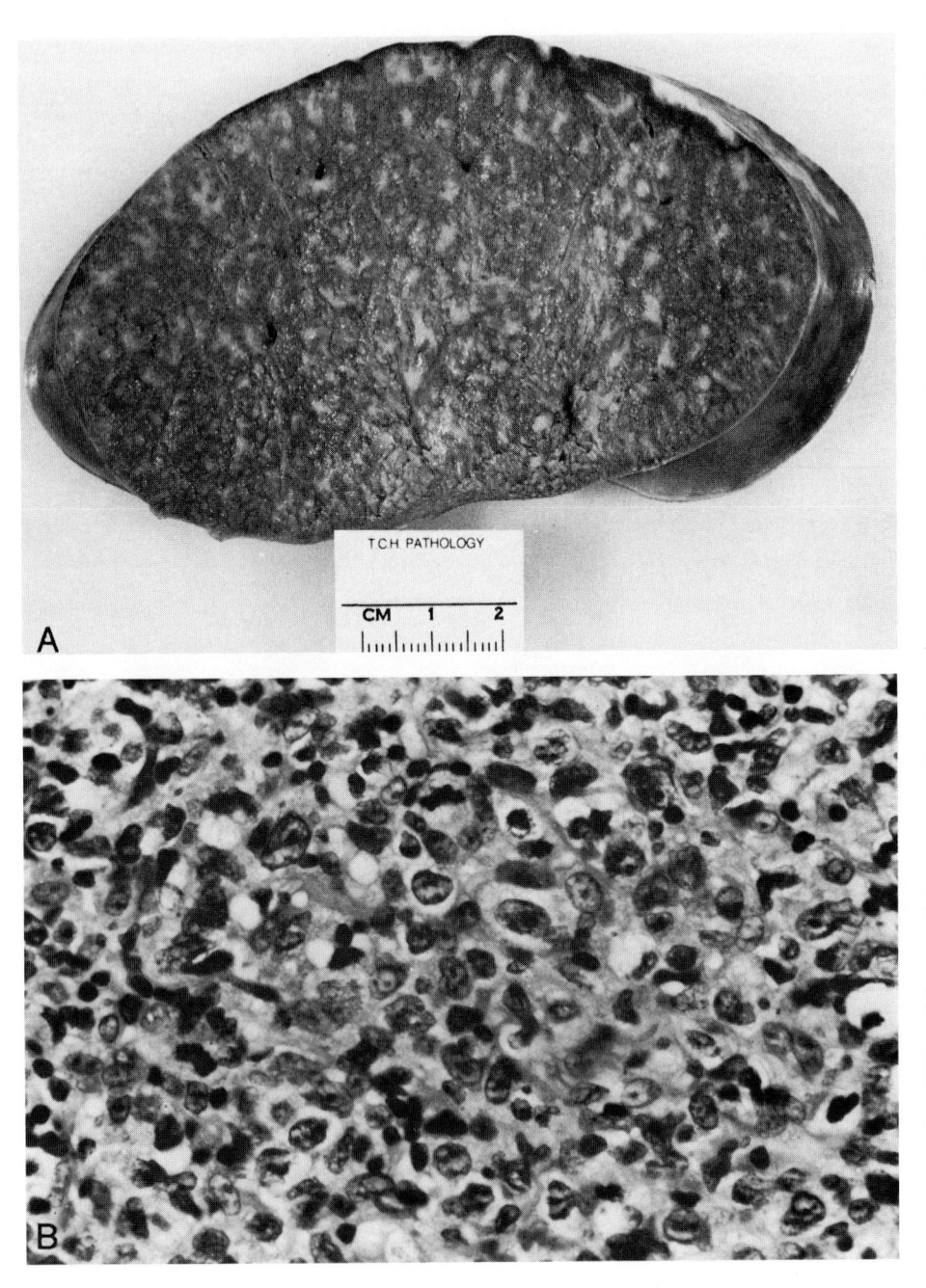

Figure 25 Large cell lymphoma. A. The spleen is enlarged. It weighed 690 grams, normal for age being 120 grams, and is diffusely studded by poorly defined pale tan nodules. B. The grossly-visible nodules are composed of large lymphocytes with oval to irregularly shaped nuclei, and ample cytoplasm. (Hematoxylin-eosin stain × 400)

cell origin may show early involvement of the spleen, with formation of nodules of white pulp along the periarteriolar sheath. With progression, patchy involvement of the red pulp is present. Small to medium-sized lymphocytes with highly convoluted nuclei are seen in mycosis fungoides. On occasion, localized follicular hyperplasia may present with grossly visible nodules that simulate lymphoma (76). Microscopically, these nodules have the appearance of reactive lymphoid tissue rather than lymphoma or Hodgkin's disease.

Involvement of the spleen by Hodgkin's disease ranges from microscopic foci to grossly visible tumors formed by confluence of smaller nodules (Figure 26). Microscopic involvement is uncommon in the absence of gross lesions, if the spleen is adequately sectioned. Once a diagnosis of Hodgkin's disease has been established in a lymph node, the criteria for involvement of the spleen and other

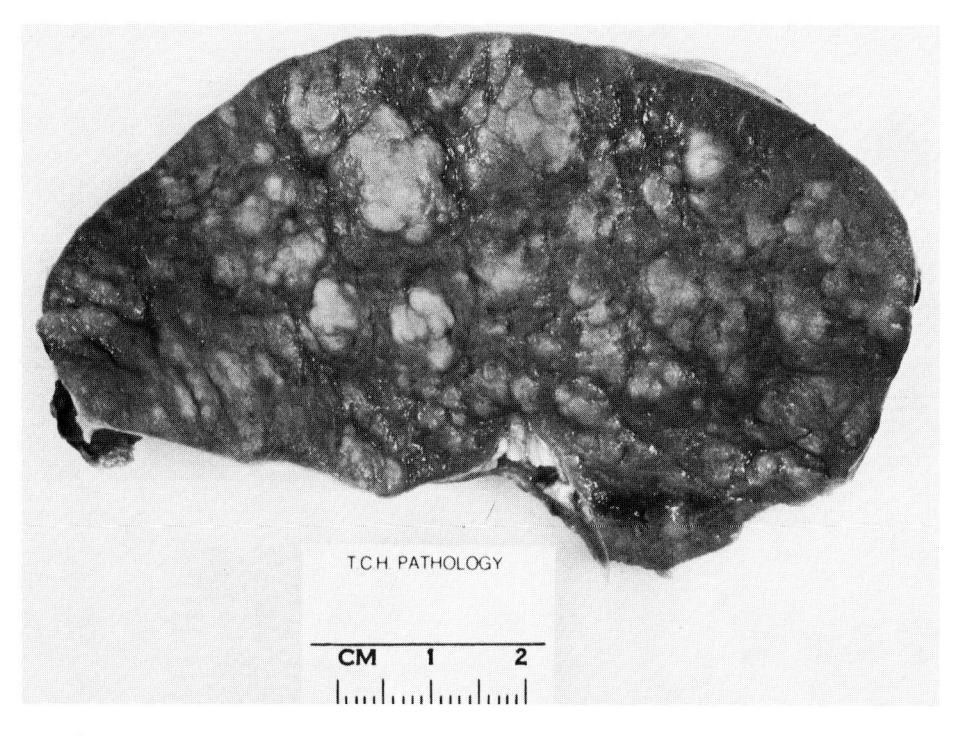

Figure 26 Hodgkin's disease. Cut section of the spleen shows confluent mulberry-like tan nodules. The spleen was enlarged. It weighed 370 grams, normal for age being 120 grams.

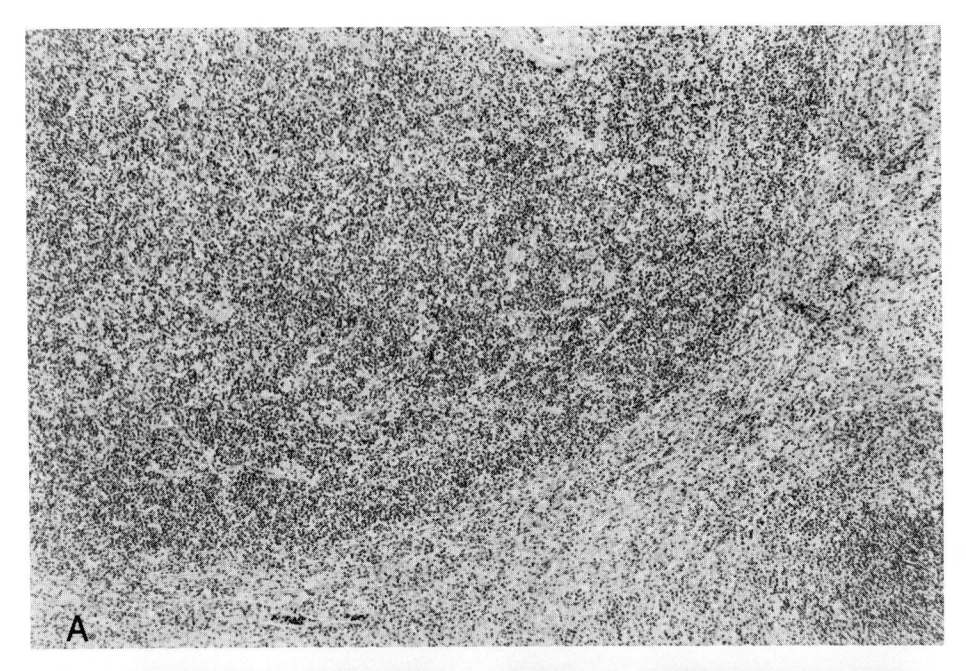

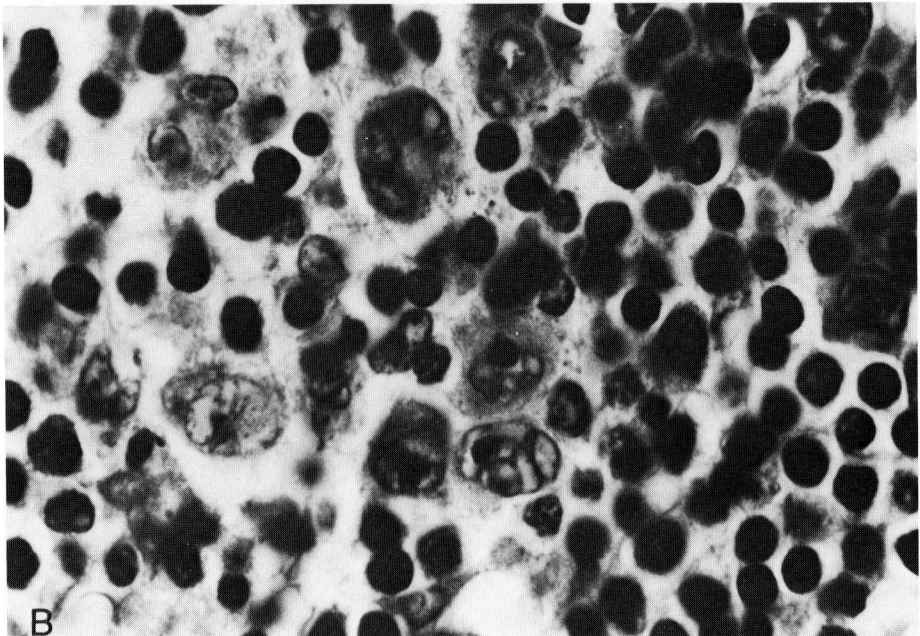

Figure 27 Hodgkin's disease. A. A fairly well circumscribed nodule is present in the upper left portion of the field. It is composed of histiocytes, lymphocytes, plasma cells and eosinophils. (Hematoxylin-eosin stain × 100) B. A cluster of Reed-Sternberg cell variants is seen within the nodule. (Hematoxylin-eosin stain × 1000)

extranodal sites are less stringent (77). The presence of Reed-Sternberg cell variants in an appropriate cellular background is sufficient to document involvement, even if acceptable classic Reed-Sternberg cells are not found (Figure 27A and B). Subtyping of Hodgkin's disease is generally not based on the splenic morphology since it is often not possible to distinguish the mixed cellularity type from nodular sclerosis types (78). Granulomas formed by discrete aggregates of epitheloid histiocytes may be seen in the spleen and other organs in patients with Hodgkin's disease (79-81) (Figure 28). While some of these lesions may be lipid granulomas in patients who have had lymphangiograms, lipid may not be present in many of the granulomas. Some patients who have these granulomas have not had lymphangiograms or other procedures using lipid-containing

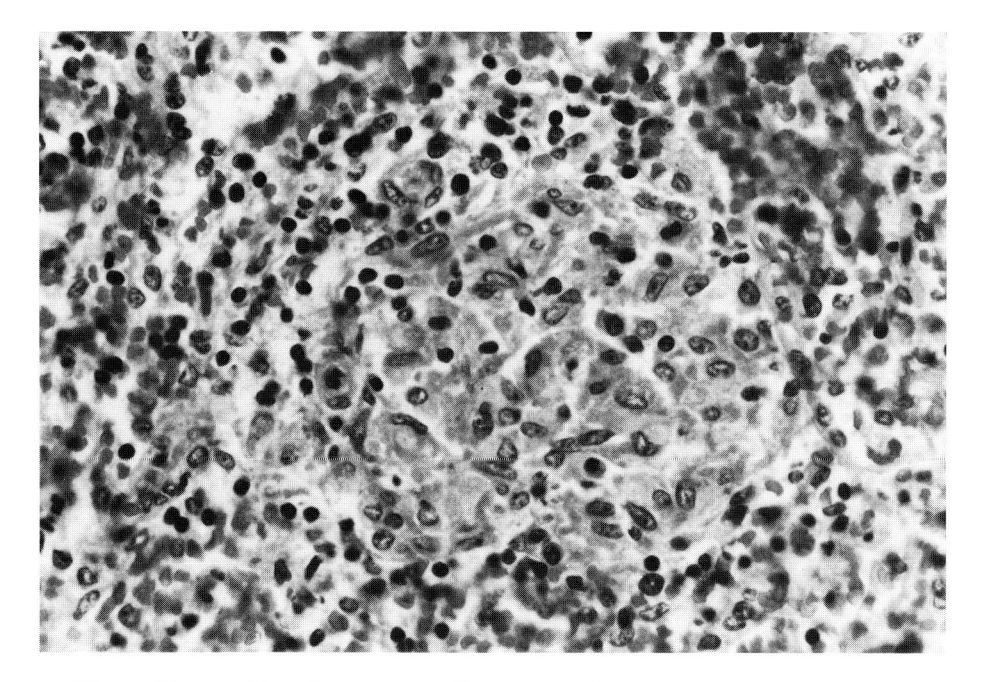

Figure 28 Hodgkin's disease. A small granuloma formed by epitheloid histiocytes is present in the red pulp. This, by itself, does not indicate involvement by Hodgkin's disease. (Hematoxylin-eosin stain × 400)

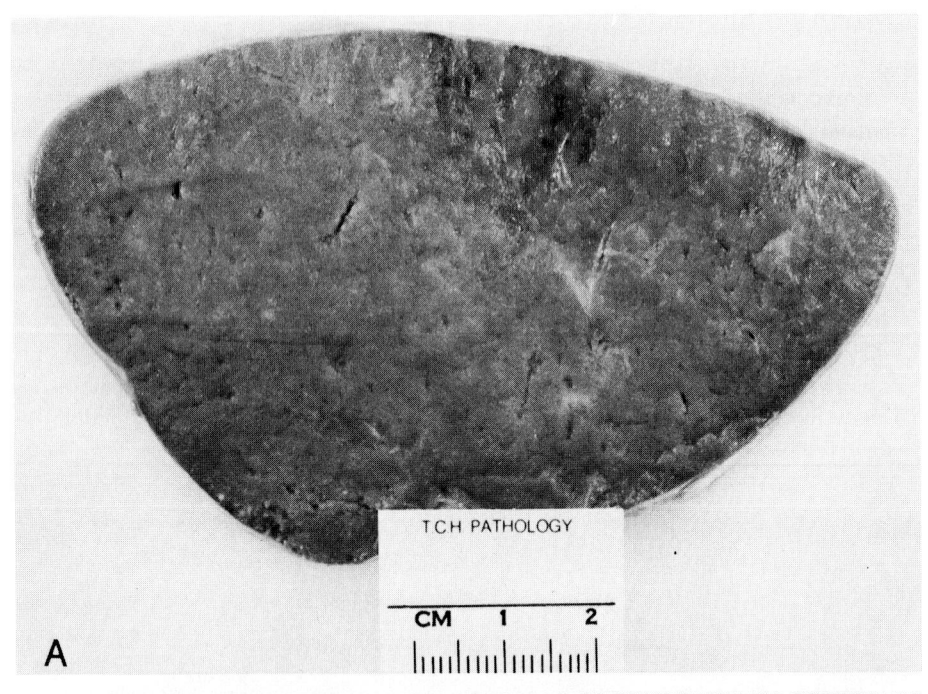

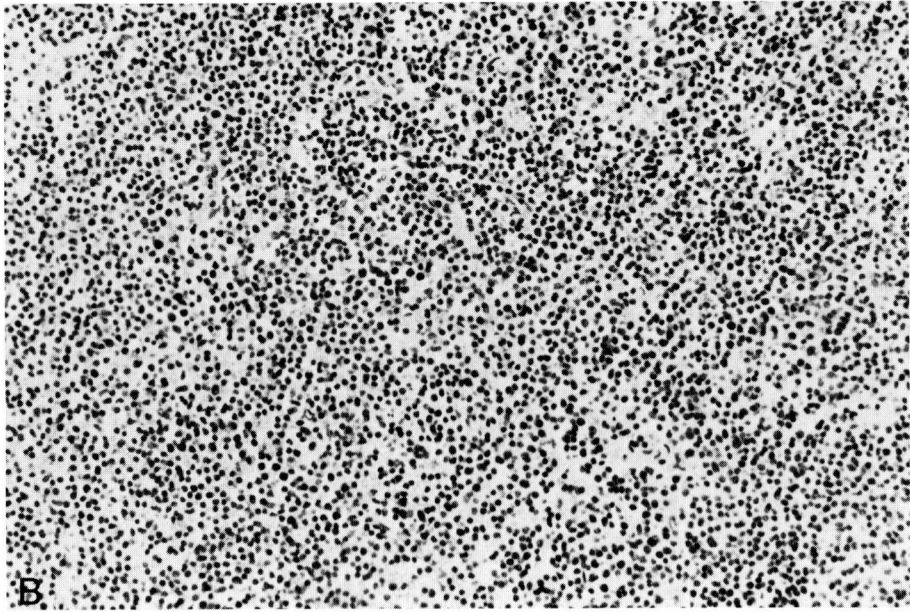

Figure 29 Acute lymphoblastic leukemia. A. The spleen is enlarged. It weighed 1500 grams, normal for age being 50 grams. The white pulp is inconspicuous. B. There is diffuse infiltration of the red pulp by a homogeneous population of blasts. The cytologic features of these cells cannot be well appreciated in tissue sections. (Hematoxylin-stain × 100)

contrast material. These granulomas are seen in approximately 10% of patients with Hodgkin's disease and do not imply splenic involvement by this disease.

Acute leukemias, regardless of the cell type, show diffuse red pulp infiltration (Figure 29A). The cords and sinuses are filled with blasts (Figure 29B). The distinction between lymphoid and myeloid blasts may be impossible on tissue sections. However, cytochemical or immunohistochemical stains may be done on touch preparations or frozen sections to make this distinction if the primary diagnosis is not known.

Typical *chronic lymphocytic leukemia* (CLL) is the circulating form of small lymphocytic lymphoma and is generally a B cell disorder. In the spleen, it involves the white pulp as shown by a homogeneous infiltrate of small round lymphocytes. A small number of cases of chronic lymphoid leukemia are of T cell origin. These cases have prominent involvement of the spleen and skin. The few reports of the splenic morphology describe white pulp expansion with leukemic cells surrounding the larger trabecular vessels, and large numbers of small lymphocytes in the red pulp sinuses (82). In tissue sections, these small lymphocytes resemble their B cell counterparts, but in smears the leukemic T cells have more abundant cytoplasm and may contain granules. Phenotypically, these cells have been shown to be of helper, suppressor or natural killer cell types by various authors (82,83).

Prolymphocytic leukemia, another variant of chronic lymphoid leukemia, may have prominent splenic involvement (84). There may be focal or diffuse infiltration of the red pulp, with or without white pulp involvement. In appearance, the cells or prolymphocytic leukemia may present a spectrum from small round lymphocytes to large "blast-like" forms. Both B cell and T cell types of prolymphocytic leukemia have been observed (85). A translocation between chromosomes 6 and 12 (t(6; 12) (q15; p13)) has been reported in 5 cases of B cell prolymphocytic leukemia (86).

Hairy cell leukemia, originally described as leukemic reticuloendotheliosis, presents with splenomegaly and pancytopenia (87). On gross examination, the spleen shows expanded, meaty red pulp with inconspicuous white pulp. Scattered infarcts may be present. Microscopically, there is diffuse infiltration of the cords and sinuses by hairy cells (Figure 30A). The hairy cell is a medium sized cell (10-20 μ in diameter) with abundant pale cytoplasm and oval-bean shaped nucleus (Figure 30B). The cells are quite monotonous and bland in appearance. A characteristic microscopic feature of hairy cell leukemia is the blood lake or pseudosinus (88). These are vessel-like structures filled with red blood cells whose walls have been infiltrated by hairy cells, replacing the endothelial lining cells (Figure 30C). Touch preparations from the cut surface of the spleen or frozen sections may be used to demonstrate the *tartrate-resistant acid phosphatase* (TRAP) staining reaction which is characteristic of hairy cells. While the

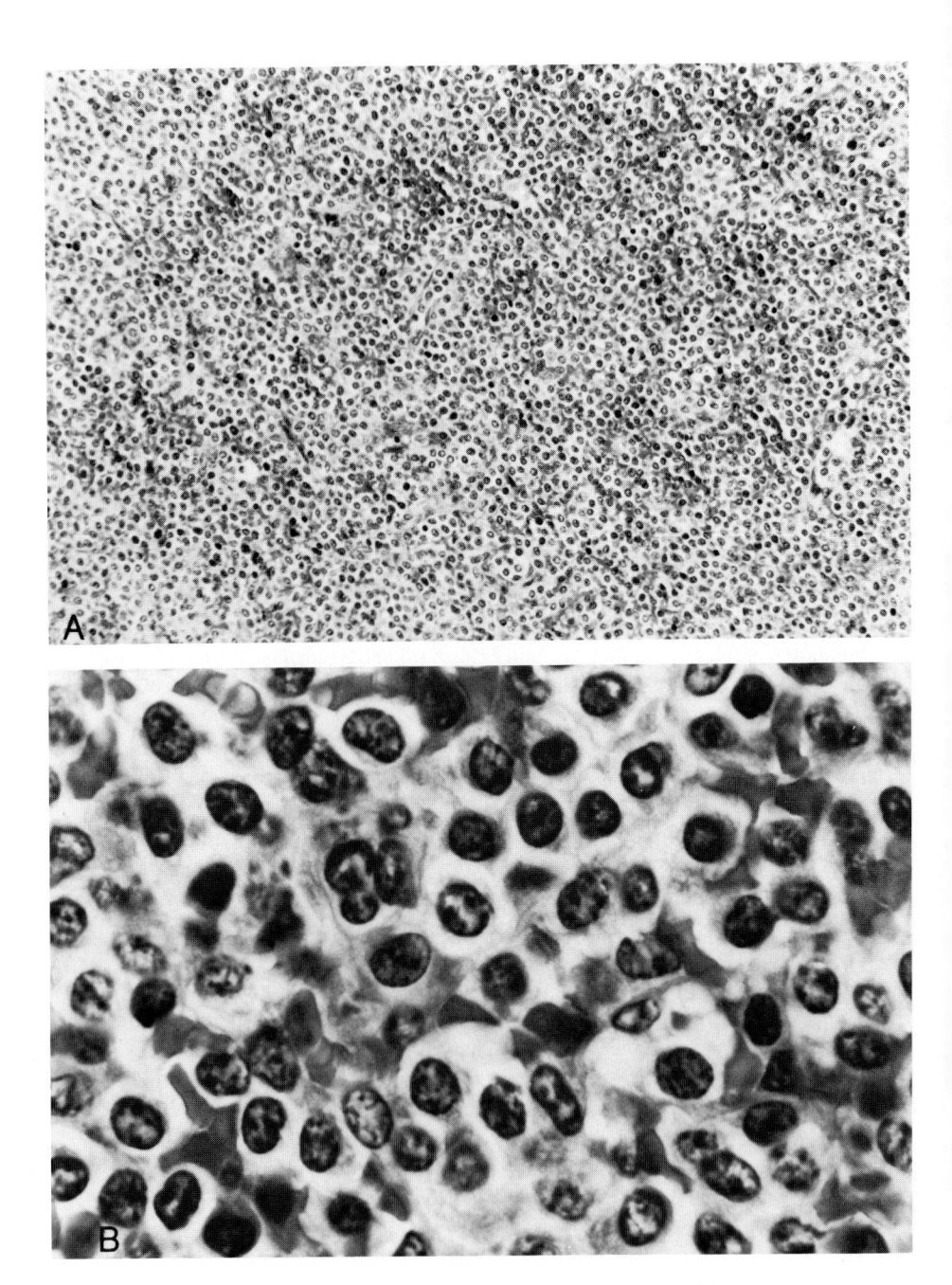

Figure 30 Hairy cell leukemia. A. There is diffuse red pulp infiltration by a monotonous population of cells producing a mosaic pattern. (Hematoxylin-eosin stain × 100) B. The hairy cells have round, regular nuclei with small nucleoli and abundant pale cytoplasm. (Hematoxylin-eosin stain × 1000) C. A blood lake is present in the center of the field. No endothelial lining is seen in this structure.

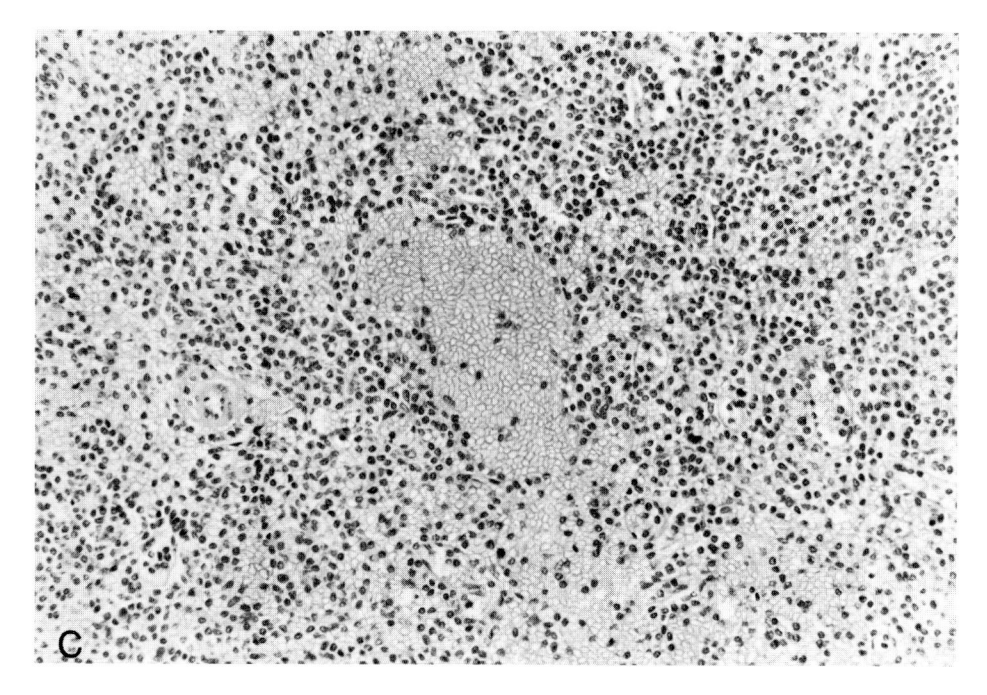

Figure 30 (continued)

typical cytoplasmic processes of hairy cells are not apparent in light microscopic sections of the spleen, these processes may be demonstrated by ultrastructural examination to be intertwining with neighborning cells (89). The origin of the hairy cells has been debated for many years, but they are now thought to be of B cell origin (90,91) on the basis of surface and cytoplasmic immunoglobulin.

Malignant histiocytosis is a systemic disease presenting with fever, wasting, generalized lymphadenopathy, and hepatosplenomegaly. Frequently there is jaundice and pancytopenia (92,93). On rare occasions malignant histiocytosis may present as splenomegaly without systemic symptoms (94). The neoplastic proliferation in the spleen primarily involves the red pulp, with secondary extension into the white pulp (Figure 31A). In contrast to large cell lymphoma, grossly visible nodules are not present. A mixture of cell types is seen in the infiltrate, including large atypical cells with hyperchromatic nuclei or prominent nucleoli (Figure 31B), intermediate cells called prohistiocytes (Figure 31B), and bening-appearing histiocytes which may exhibit hemophagocytosis (Figure 31C). These cells may infiltrate the walls of the trabecular veins. The histiocytic nature of these cells is shown by immunohistochemical techniques. Chromosomal

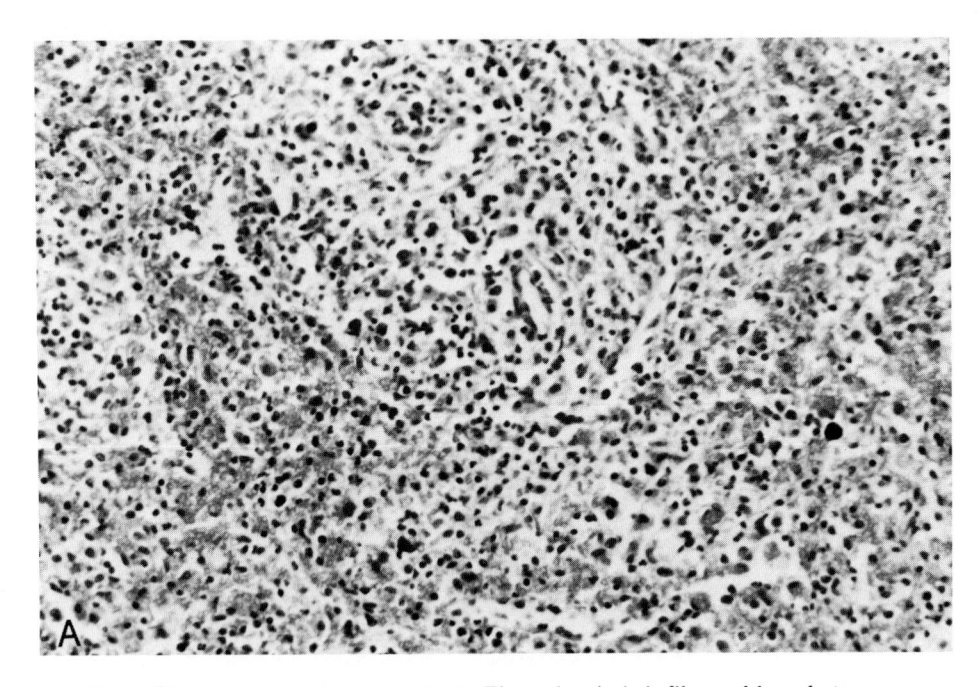

Figure 31 Malignant histiocytosis. A. The red pulp is infiltrated by a heterogeneous population of histiocytic cells, some with large hyperchromatic nuclei, others showing erythrophagocytosis. (Hematoxylin-eosin stain × 100) B. Large, bizarre hyperchromatic cells are present (black arrows) as well as prohistiocytes (white arrow). (Hematoxylin-eosin stain × 1000) C. A benign-appearing histiocyte showing erythrophagocytosis (arrow) is also present in the red pulp infiltrate. (Hematoxylin-eosin stain × 1000)

translocations with a constant breakpoint (5q 35) have been observed in cases of malignant histiocytosis (95). This location on the chromosome is just distal to the reported site of the c-fms oncogene. It is possible that translocations in the region of this oncogene may have a role in causing malignant histiocytosis.

Primary nonhematologic malignancies of the spleen are rare. The most commonly reported malignancy is the angiosarcoma (96-98). These patients present with splenomegaly and left-sided abdominal pain and may show a microangiopathic anemia or coagulopathy. On gross examination, the spleen is enlarged and has multilobulated nodules containing prominent hemorrhage and necrosis. Microscopically, the tumor is composed of vascular spaces lined by plump poly-

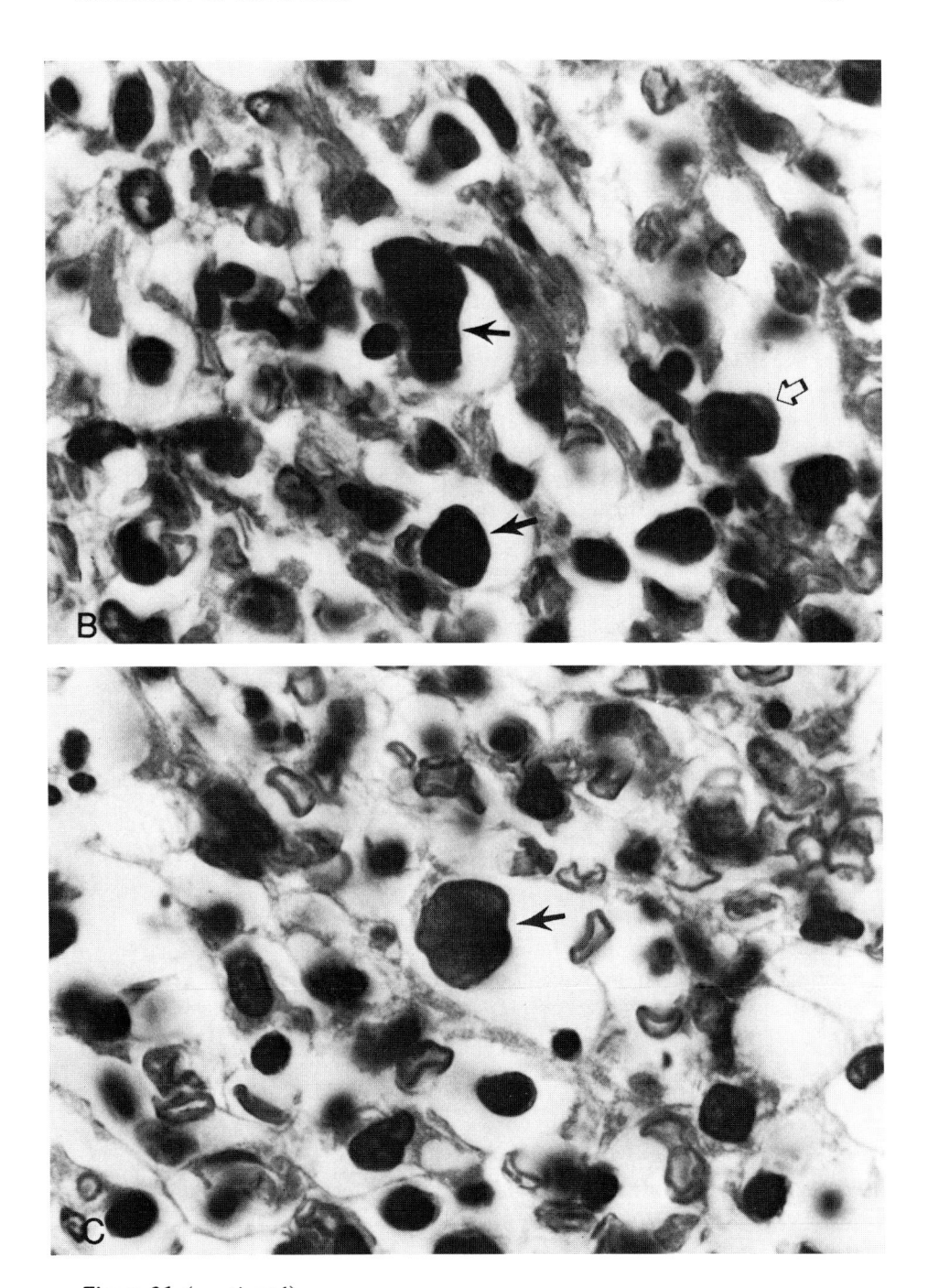

Figure 31 (continued)

gonal or oval hyperchromatic cells which may "pile up" projecting into the vascular lumen. Hemosiderin deposits are common. On ultrastructural examination, the cells show pinocytotic vessels and Weibel-Palade bodies (rod-shaped microtubulated bodies, specific for endothelial cells). Anti-factor VIII and the plant lectin Ulex Europaeus are immunohistochemical markers for endothelial cells. Tumors of vascular origin show positive staining with these markers. Metastasis of angiosarcomas may occur early, with spread to liver, lung, lymph node and bone. Patients with this tumor may initially present with splenic rupture, but there seems to be no relationship of the size of tumor with incidence of rupture (98). Splenic rupture following chemotherapy for a follicular lymphoma has been reported (99).

Other primary splenic malignancies include malignant fibrous histiocytoma and fibrosarcoma. The spleen is also occasionally the site of metastatic tumor, the most common primary sites of the primary malignancy being the lung and breast (100).

The spleen is generally involved in myeloproliferative disorders, in which splenomegaly is a significant clinical finding. In adult *chronic myeloid leukemia* (CML) the spleen may be massively enlarged (Figure 32A). In juvenile chronic myeloid leukemia, splenomegaly is present, but not to the degree seen in adult CML. Extramedullary hematopoiesis predominantly of the granulocytic series is seen in the red pulp (Figure 32B). Granulocytes at all stages of differentiation are present, including eosinophils and basophils. The chloroacetate esterase (specific esterase) stain may be helpful in identifying the full extent of red pulp involvement. Early blastic transformation of chronic myeloid leukemia may be seen as nodules of myeloblasts in the splenic red pulp (101). Gaucher-like cells may be seen in the spleen.

Virtually all patients with myelofibrosis have splenomegaly and myeloid metaplasia. On gross examination of the spleen there is expansion of the red pulp with the white pulp being inconspicuous. All hematopoietic cell lines are present in the cords and sinusoids (Figure 33). Red cell precursors may have megaloblastoid features and are found predominantly in the sinuses. Megakaryocytes involve the sinuses and occasionally the cords, while myeloid precursors are principally located in the cords (102). The marked degree of splenomegaly

Figure 32 Chronic myelogenous leukemia. A. Marked splenomegaly is present. The spleen weighed 330 grams, normal for age being 20 grams. The red pulp is expanded and the white pulp is inconspicuous. B. The red pulp contains large numbers of granulocytes at various stages of maturation. (Hematoxylin-eosin stain X 400)

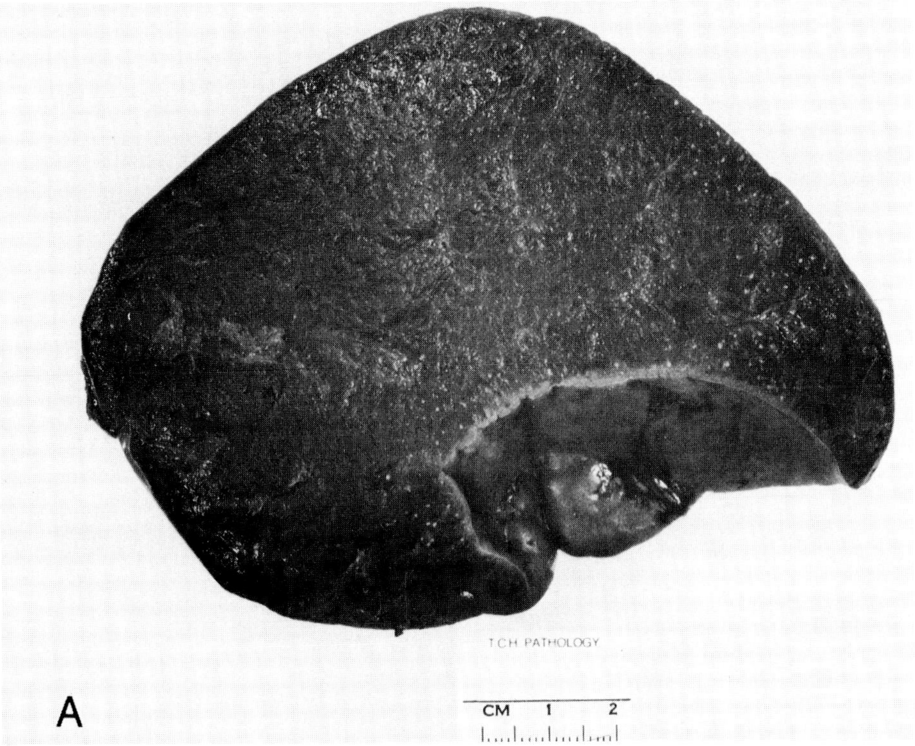
T.C.H. PATHOLOGY
CM 1 2
A

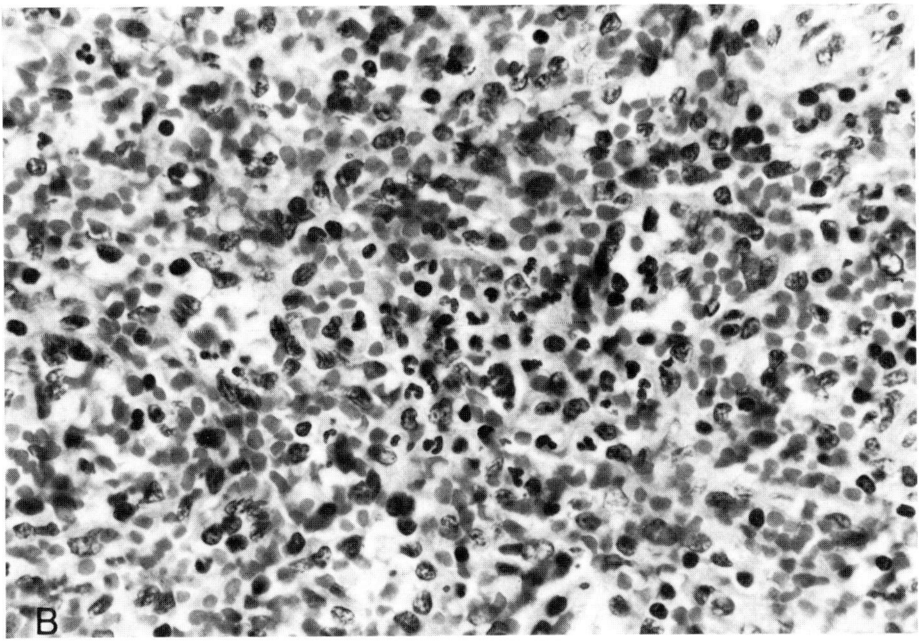
B

Table 3 Differential Features of Splenic Abnormalities Found in Various Lympho/Hematologic Malignancies

	Hodgkin's Disease	WDLL[a] CLL[b]	PDLL[c]	Large cell lymphoma	Malignant histiocytosis	Hairy cell leukemia	CML[d]	Acute leukemia
Location	white pulp marginal zone	white pulp	white pulp	white pulp	red pulp	red pulp	red pulp	red pulp
Gross Appearance	irregular nodules	nodules	uniform nodules	irregular large nodules	expanded red pulp decreased white pulp	expanded red pulp decreased white pulp	expanded red pulp decreased white pulp	expanded red pulp decreased white pulp
Cellular Pleomorphism	present	absent	absent	may be present	present	absent	present	absent
Nuclei	vary with cell type	small round	small cleaved	large vesicular	large vesicular	round-oval bean-shaped	variety of granulocytes	large, round-convoluted fine chromatin
Nucleoli	prominent in RSC[e]	0	0	prominent	prominent in atypical cells	0	0	prominent in ANLL[f]
Cytoplasm	abundant in RSC	scant	scant	abundant	abundant	moderate	moderate	scant
Immunologic Markers/ Cytochemistry	LEU M1+ in RSC	B cell	B cell	B,T or histiocytic markers	Histiocytic or dendritic cell markers	TRAP +[g]	Specific esterase +	myeloid or lymphoid markers
Other Features	± sarcoid-like granulomas	infiltration vein walls	may have intact marginal zone	frequent mitoses	erythrophago-cytosis	pseudosinuses or blood lakes	eosinophils ± megakaryocytes ± Gaucher-like cells	frequent mitoses blastic crisis of CML may present as nodules in red pulp

[a]WDLL = well differentiated lymphocytic lymphoma
[b]CLL = chronic lymphocytic leukemia
[c]PDLL = poorly differentiated lymphocytic lymphoma
[d]CML = chronic myelogenous leukemia
[e]RSC = Reed-Sternberg cell
[f]ANLL = acute non-lymphoid leukemia
[g]TRAP = Tartrate-resistant acid phosphatase

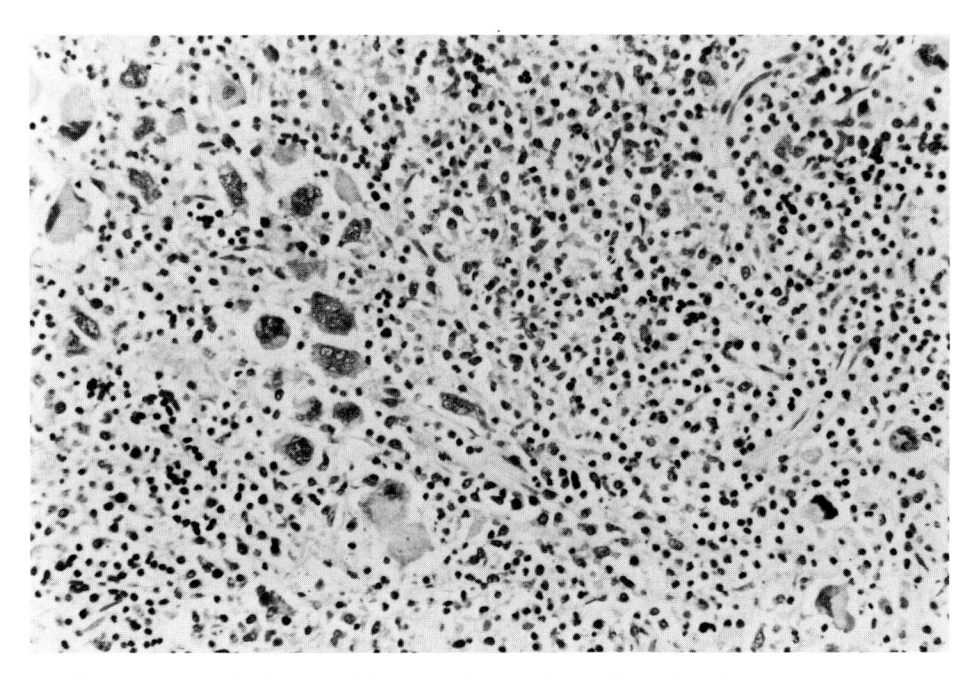

Figure 33 Myelofibrosis with myeloid metaplasia. The red pulp contains erythroid, granulocytic and megakaryocytic cells. The megakaryocytes are clustered and somewhat dysplastic in appearance. (Hematoxylin-eosin stain × 100)

with resultant hypersplenism may result in anemia and thrombocytopenia. Thus, splenectomy may be of benefit in patients with myelofibrosis.

Splenomegaly is present in 75% of patients with polycythemia vera at diagnosis. The enlargement of the spleen may not be due to myeloid metaplasia as previously thought but may be a result of red cell sequestration. Splenectomy is not beneficial in polycythemia vera. In fact, it may be contraindicated due to the resultant thrombocytosis and hypercoagulable state that occurs following splenectomy.

Differential features of malignancies involving the spleen are given in Table 3.

SUMMARY

The spleen, regarded as a difficult organ to evaluate by pathologists, is involved in a variety of benign and malignant diseases. Although the spleen is generally removed for therapeutic rather than diagnostic reasons, the pathologist has the opportunity to study splenic pathology in many clinical settings. It was the widespread use of therapeutic splenectomy that led to the discovery of "post splenectomy sepsis" and gave valuable information concerning the vital role of the spleen in the normal immune system.

Congenital abnormalities of size, position or number of spleens are frequently associated with other anomalies, especially congenital heart disease. Circulatory disturbances secondary to liver disease, congestive heart disease or abdominal vascular disease are frequent causes of splenomegaly. In its role of removing abnormal erythrocytes from the circulation the spleen plays an important role in the symptomatology of red blood cell membrane abnormalities and hemoglobinopathies. While most systemic infections involve the spleen, few have a characteristic histologic appearance. Inherited enzyme deficiencies with the resultant proliferation of storage histiocytes generally exhibit prominent splenomegaly and may have characteristic histologic or ultrastructural findings. Because of its role in the immune system, the spleen is involved in many immune and autoimmune disorders such as ITP and Felty's syndrome. Benign tumors of the spleen are uncommon but splenic involvement in lymphoproliferative and hematologic malignancies is a frequent finding.

Although examination of the spleen is perceived as a difficult task, it may be a valuable diagnostic tool. In addition to routine microscopic studies, newer techniques such as immunohistochemistry, flow cytometry, DNA analysis, and in situ hybridization may aid in the diagnosis as well as giving information about the basic biology of the disease process.

REFERENCES

1. King H, Shumacker HB: Splenic Studies: I. Susceptibility to infection after splenectomy performed in infancy. *Ann Surg* 1952;136:239-242.
2. Singer DB: Postsplenectomy Sepsis. In: Rosenberg HS, Bolande RP: *Perspectives in Pediatric Pathology*; Chicago, Yearbook Medical Publishers, Inc. 1973;285-311.
3. Lambert IA: Splenectomy as a diagnostic technique. *Clin Haematol* 1983; 12:535-563.
4. Suzuki T, Shibuya H, Yoshimatsu S, Suzuki S. Ultrasonically guided staging splenic tissue core biopsy in patients with non-Hodgkin's lymphoma. *Cancer* 1987;60:879-882.
5. Boles ET, Haase GM, Hamoudi AB: Partial splenectomy in staging laparotomy for Hodgkin's disease: An alternative approach. *J Pediatr Surg* 1978; 13:581-586.
6. Schellong G, Waubke-Landwehr A, Langermann JH, et al: Prediction of splenic involvement in children with Hodgkin's disease. *Cancer* 1986;57: 2049-2056.

7. Bar-Maor JA, Govrin-Yehudain J: Partial splenectomy in children with Gaucher's disease. *Pediatrics* 1985;76:398-401.
8. Stellin GP, Lilly JR, Githens JH: On partial splenectomy in Gaucher's disease. *Pediatrics* 1986;77:618-619.
9. Ivemark BI: Implications of agenesis of the spleen on the pathogenesis of cono-truncus abnormalities in childhood. An analysis of the heart malformations in the splenic agenesis syndrome, with fourteen new cases. *Acta Pediatr* 1955;44:Suppl 104:1-110.
10. Holroyde CP, Oski FA, Gardner FH: The "pocked" erythrocyte. Red-cell surface alterations in reticuloendothelial immaturity of the neonate. *N Engl J Med* 1969;281:516-519.
11. Casper JT, Koethe S, Rodey GE, Thatcher LG: A new method for studying splenic reticuloendothelial dysfunction in sickle cell disease patients and its clinical application: A brief report. *Blood* 1976;47:183-188.
12. Bates HM: Evaluating splenic function. *Laboratory Management* 1981;19:9-12.
13. Arnold GL, Bixler D, Girod D: Probable autosomal recessive inheritance of polysplenia, situs inversus and cardiac defects in an Amish family. *Am J Med Genet* 1983;16:35-42.
14. Landing BH, Lawrence TYK, Payne VC, Wells TR: Bronchial anatomy in syndromes with abnormal visceral situs, abnormal spleen and congenital heart disease. *Am J Cardiology* 1971;28:456-462.
15. Halpert B, Gyorkey F: Lesions observed in accessory spleens of 311 patients. *Am J Clin Path* 1959;32:165-168.
16. Das Gupta TK, Busch RC: Accessory splenic tissue producing indentation of the gastric fundus resembling gastric neoplasm. *N Engl J Med* 1960;263:1360-1361.
17. Hashida Y, Jaffe R, Ynis EJ: Pancreatic pathology in trisomy 13: Specificity of the morphologic lesion. *Pediatric Pathology* 1983;1:169-178.
18. Smith DW: Chromosomal abnormality syndromes. In: *Recognizable Patterns of Human Malformation. Genetic, Embryologic and Clinical Aspects*; Philadelphia, W.B. Saunders Co., 1970;38-45.
19. Dalton ML, Strange WH, Downs EA: Intrathoracic splenosis. *Am Rev Resp Dis* 1971;103:827-830.
20. Fleming CR, Dickson ER, Harrison EG: Splenosis: Autotransplantation of splenic tissue. *Am J Med* 1976;61:414-419.
21. Putschar WGJ, Manion WC: Splenic-gonadal fusion. *Am J Path* 1956;32:15-34.
22. Watson RJ: Splenogonadal fusion. *Surgery* 1986;63:853-858.
23. Cotelingam JD, Saito R: Hepatolienal fusion; case report of an unusual lesion. *Hum Pathol* 1978;9:234-236.
24. Warfel KA, Ellis GH: Peliosis of the spleen. *Arch Pathol Lab Med* 1982;106:99-100.
25. Tada T, Wakabayashi T, Kishimoto H: Peliosis of the spleen. *Am J Clin Pathol* 1983;79:708-713.

26. Bleiweiss IJ, Thung SN, Goodman JD. Peliosis of the spleen in a patient with cirrhosis of the liver. *Arch Pathol Lab Med* 1986;110:669–671.
27. Diebold J, Audovin J: Peliosis of the spleen. *Am J Surg Pathol* 1983;197–204.
28. Rywlin AM: Hematopoietic system. In: Kissane JM, ed. *Anderson's Pathology* ed 8; St Louis Missouri, C.V. Mosby Co., 1985;1257–1351.
29. Becker PS, Lux SE: Hereditary spherocytosis and related disorders. *Clin. Haematol* 1985;14:15–43.
30. Kimberling WJ, Taylor RA, Chapman RG, Lubs HA: Linkage and gene localization of hereditary spherocytosis. *Blood* 1978;52:859–867.
31. Bass EB, Smith SW, Stevenson RE, Rosse WF: Further evidence for location of the spherocytosis gene on chromosome 8. *Ann Intern Med* 1983;99:192–193.
32. Molnar Z, Rappaport H: Fine structure of the red pulp of the spleen in hereditary spherocytosis. *Blood* 1972;39:81–97.
33. Ferrant A: The role of the spleen in haemolysis. *Clin Haematol* 1983; 12:489–504.
34. Rappaport H, Crosby WH: Auto-immune hemolytic anemia. II Morphologic observations and clinicopathologic correlations. *Am J Pathol* 1957;33:429–458.
35. Emond AM, Collis R, Darvil D, et al: Acute splenic sequestration in homozygous sickle cell disease: Natural history and management. *J Pediatr* 1985; 107:201–206.
36. Pearson HA, Spencer RP, Cornelius EA: Functional asplenia in sickle cell anemia. *N Engl J Med* 1969;281:923–926.
37. Milner PF: The sickling disorders. *Clin Haematol* 1974;3:289–331.
38. Beltrami CA, Bearzi I, Fabirs G: Storage cells of spleen and bone marrow in thalassemia: An ultrastructural study. *Blood* 1973;41:901–902.
39. Gowing NFC: Infectious mononucleosis: Histopathologic aspects. In: Sommers SC, Rosen PP, eds; *Path Annual*; New York, Appleton-Century-Crofts, 1971;1–20.
40. Risdall RJ, McKenna RW, Nesbit ME, et al: Virus-associated hemophagocytic syndrome. *Cancer* 1979;44:993–1002.
41. Wieczorek R, Greco MA, McCarthy K, et al: Familial erythrophagocytic lymphohistiocytosis. *Hum Pathol* 1986;17:55–63.
42. Spritz RA: The familial histiocytoses. *Pediatric Pathology* 1985;3:43–47.
43. Riesmann RP, Greco MA: Virus-associated hemophagocytic syndrome due to Epstein-Barr virus. *Hum Pathol* 1984;15:290–293.
44. Rubin CM, Burke BA, McKenna RW, et al: The accelerated phase of Chediak-Higashi syndrome; an expression of the virus-associated hemophagocytic syndrome. *Cancer* 1985;56:524–530.
45. Ghadially FN: Lysosomes in Gaucher's cells, Gaucher-like cells and sea-blue histiocytes. In: *Ultrastructural Pathology of the Cell and Matrix* ed 2; London, Butterworths, 1982;526–533.

46. Sawitsky A, Rosner F, Chodsky S: The sea-blue histiocyte syndrome, a review: Genetic and biochemical studies. *Semin Haematol* 1972;9:285-297.
47. Silverstein MN, Ellefson RD: The syndrome of the sea-blue histiocyte. *Seminol Hematol* 1972;9:299-307.
48. Dawson PJ, Dawson G: Adult Nieman-Pick disease with sea-blue histiocytes in the spleen. *Hum Pathol* 1982;13:1115-1120.
49. Landas S, Foucar K, Sando GN, et al: Adult Niemann-Pick disease masquerading as sea-blue histiocyte syndrome: Report of a case confirmed by lipid analysis and enzyme assays. *Am J Hematol* 1985;20:391-400.
50. Freund J, Krausz Y, Levij IS, Eliakim M. Iatrogenic lipidosis following prolonged intravenous hyperalimentation. *Am J Clin Nutr* 1975;28:1156-1160.
51. Forbes GB. Splenic lipidosis after administration of intravenous fat emulsions. *J Clin Path* 1978;31:765-771.
52. Tavassoli M, McMillan R: Structure of the spleen in idiopathid thrombocytopenic purpura. *Am J Clin Pathol* 1975;64:180-191.
53. Cohn J, Tygstrup I: Foamy histiocytes of the spleen in patients with chronic thrombocytopenia. *Scand J Haematol* 1976;16:33-37.
54. Hassan NMR, Nieman RS. The pathology of the spleen in steroid-treated immune thrombocytopenic purpura. *Am J Clin Pathol* 1985;84:433-438.
55. Berendt HL, Mant MJ, Jewell LD. Periarterial fibrosis in the spleen in idiopathic thrombocytopenic purpura. *Arch Pathol Lab Med* 1986;110:1152-1154.
56. Toomey K, Hepburn B: Felty syndrome in juvenile arthritis. *J Pediatr* 1985;106:254-255.
57. Kadri A, Moinuddin M, deLeeuw NKM: Phagocytosis of blood cells by splenic macrophages in thrombotic thrombocytopenic purpura. *Ann Intern Med* 1975;82:799-802.
58. Welch K, Finkbeiner W, Alpers CE, et al: Autopsy findings in the acquired immune deficiency syndrome. *JAMA* 1984;252:1152-1159.
59. Kruger GRF, Berard CW, DeLellis RA, et al: Graft-versus-host disease. *Am J Pathol* 1971;63:179-196.
60. O'Dailey MD, Coleman CN, Fajardo LF: Splenic injury caused by therapeutic irradiation. *Am J Surg Pathol* 1981;5:325-331.
61. Favara BE, McCarthy RC, Mierau GW: Histiocytosis X. In: Finegold MJ, ed. *Pathology of Neoplasia in Children and Adolescents*; Philadelphia, W. B. Saunders Co., 1986; 126-144.
62. Corazza GR, Gasbarrini G: Defective splenic function and its relation to bowel disease. *Clin in Gastroenterology* 1983;12:651-668.
63. O'Grady JG, Stevens FM, Harding B, et al: Hyposplenism and gluten-sensitive enteropathy. *Gastroenterology* 1984;87:1326-1331.
64. Nieman RS, Bischel MD, Lukes RJ: Hypersplenism in the uremic hemodialyzed patient: Pathology and proposed pathophysiologic mechanisms. *Am J Clin Pathol* 1973;60:502-511.

65. Berne TV, Bischel MD, Payne JE, Barbour BH: Selective splenectomy in chronic renal failure. *Am J Surg* 1973;126:271-276.
66. Silverman ML, Livolsi VA: Splenic hamartoma. *Am J Clin Pathol* 1978;70:224-229.
67. Garvin DF, King FM: Cysts and nonlymphomatous tumors of the spleen. In: Sommers SC, ed; *Path Annual* part 1; New York, Appleton-Century-Croft, 1981;61-80.
68. Tsakraklides V, Hadley TW: Epidermoid cysts of the spleen. *Arch Pathol* 1973;96:251-254.
69. Harris NL, Aisenberg AC, Meyer JE, et al: Diffuse large cell (histiocytic) lymphoma of the spleen. *Cancer* 1984;54:2460-2467.
70. Kraemer BB, Osborne BM, Butler JJ: Primary splenic presentation of malignant lymphoma and related disorders. *Cancer* 1984;54:1606-1619.
71. Narang S, Wolf BC, Neiman RS: Malignant lymphoma presenting with prominent splenomegaly. *Cancer* 1985;55:1948-1957.
72. Spier CM, Kjeidsberg CR, Eyre HJ, Behm FG: Malignant lymphoma with primary presentation in the spleen. *Arch Pathol Lab Med* 1985;109:1076-1080.
73. Rosai J: Spleen. In: Rosai J, ed. *Archerman's Surgical Pathology* ed 6; St Louis, Missouri, C.V. Mosby Co., 1981;1229-1250.
74. Butler JJ: Pathology of the spleen in benign and malignant conditions. *Histopathology* 1983;7:453-474.
75. Braylan RC, Long JC, Jaffe ES, et al: Malignant lymphoma obscured by concomitant extensive epitheloid granulomas. *Cancer* 1977;39:1146-1155.
76. Burke JS, Osborne BM: Localized reactive lymphoid hyperplasia of the spleen simulating malignant lymphoma. A report of seven cases. *Am J Surg Pathol* 1983;7:373-380.
77. Lukes RJ: Criteria for involvement of lymph node, bone marrow, spleen, and liver in Hodgkin's disease. *Cancer Res* 1971;31:1755-1767.
78. Burke JS: Surgical pathology of the spleen: An approach to the differential diagnosis of splenic lymphomas and leukemias. Part 1. Diseases of the white pulp. *Am J Surg Pathol* 1981;5:551-563.
79. Kadin ME, Donaldson SS, Dorfman RF: Isolated granulomas in Hodgkin's disease. *N Engl J Med* 1970;283:859-861.
80. O'Connell MJ, Schimpff SC, Kirschner RH, et al: Epitheloid granulomas in Hodgkin's disease. *JAMA* 1975;233:886-889.
81. Pak HY, Friedman NB: Pseudosarcoid granulomas in Hodgkin's disease. *Hum Pathol* 1981;12:832-837.
82. Palutke M, Eisenberg L, Kaplan J, et al: Natural killer and suppressor T-cell chronic lymphocytic leukemia. *Blood* 1983;62:627-634.
83. Feller AC, Parwaresch MR, Lennert K: Subtyping of chronic lymphocytic leukemia of T-type by dipeptidylaminopeptidase IV (DAP IV), Monoclonal antibodies, and Fc-receptors. *Cancer* 1983;52:1609-1612.
84. Galton DAG, Goldman JM, Wiltshaw E, et al: Prolymphocytic leukaemia. *Brit J Haematol* 1974;27:7-23.

85. Tsai LMC, Tsai CC, Hyde TP, et al: T-cell prolymphocytic leukemia with helper-cell phenotype and a review of the literature. *Cancer* 1984;54:463-470.
86. Sadamori N, Han T, Minowada J, et al: Possible specific chromosome change in prolymphocytic leukemia. *Blood* 1983;62:729-736.
87. Burke JS, Byrne GE, Rappaport H: Hairy cell leukemia (Leukemic reticuloendotheliosis) 1. A clinical pathologic study of 21 patients. *Cancer* 1974;33:1399-1410.
88. Nanba K, Soban EJ, Bowling MC, Berard CW: Splenic pseudosinuses and hepatic angiomatous lesions. *Am J Clin Pathol* 1977;67:415-426.
89. Burke JS, Mackay B, Rappaport H: Hairy cell leukemia (Leukemic reticuloendotheliosis) II. Ultrastructure of the spleen. *Cancer* 1976;37:2267-2274.
90. Meijer CJLM, Albeda F, Van Der Valk P, et al: Immunohistochemical studies of the spleen in hairy-cell leukemia. *Am J Pathol* 1984;115:266-274.
91. Mori N, Tsunoda R, Kojima M, et al: Ultrastructural localization of immunoglobulins in hairy cell leukemia. *Hum Pathol* 1984;15:1042-1047.
92. Byrne GE, Rappaport H: Malignant histiocytosis. In: Akazaki K, ed. *Malignant Diseases of the Hemotopoietic System* Gann Monograph on Cancer Research, Vol 15; Tokyo, University of Tokyo Press, 1973;145-162.
93. Warnke RA, Kim H, Dorfman RF: Malignant histiocytosis (histiocytic medullary reticulosis). *Cancer* 1975;35:215-230.
94. Vardiman JW, Byrne GE, Rappaport H: Malignant histiocytosis with massive splenomegaly in asymptomatic patients. *Cancer* 1975;36:419-427.
95. Morgan R, Hecht BK, Sandberg AA, Hecht F: Chromosome 5q 35 breakpoint in malignant histiocytosis. *N Engl J Med* 1986;314:1222.
96. Wick MR, Scheithauer BW, Smith SL, Beart RW: Primary nonlymphoreticular malignant neoplasms of the spleen. *Am J Surg Pathol* 1982;6:229-242.
97. Wilkinson HA, Lucas JC, Foote FW: Primary splenic angiosarcoma. *Arch Path* 1968;85:213-218.
98. Smith VC, Eisenberg BL, McDonald EC: Primary splenic angiosarcoma case report and literature review. *Cancer* 1985;55:1625-1627.
99. Zwi LJ, Evans DJ, Wechsler AL, Catovsky D: Splenic angiosarcoma following chemotherapy for follicular lymphoma. *Hum Pathol* 1986;17:528-530.
100. Marymont JH, Gross S: Patterns of metastatic cancer in the spleen. *Am J Clin Pathol* 1963;40:58-66.
101. Inoshita T, Lee CY, Tabor DC: Localized blast crisis in the spleen in a patient with chronic myelocytic leukemia. *Arch Pathol Lab Med* 1984;108:609-610.
102. Soderstrom N, Bandmann U, Lundh B: Patho-anatomical features of the spleen and liver. *Clin Haematol* 1975;4:309-329.

Part II

Pathophysiology of Spleen Disorders

4
Hyposplenism

RICHARD H. SILLS
Children's Hospital of New Jersey, and University of Medicine and Dentistry-New Jersey Medical School, Newark, New Jersey

The spleen, as the largest lymphoid organ in the body, plays a critical role in host defense. A variety of clinical disorders have adverse effects upon splenic function. Some conditions decrease splenic function while others result in excessive splenic activity. The recognition of the post-splenectomy sepsis syndrome as an entity has led to an increased awareness of the consequences of impaired splenic function.

While surgical splenectomy remains the most common cause of asplenia, a variety of disorders have been associated with impairment of splenic function in the last 10 to 15 years. In many instances there is only partial, as opposed to total, functional impairment. On this basis, the terms hyposplenism or hyposplenia seem more appropriate and less restrictive than the more traditionally used term, asplenia.

METHODS TO EVALUATE ADEQUACY OF SPLENIC FUNCTION

A variety of laboratory studies have been used to evaluate or to assess splenic function (Table 1). Many clinical findings, such as thrombocytosis and normoblastemia, are suggestive of hyposplenia but are also nonspecific. Even the more specific studies, such as radionuclide scans and enumeration of erythrocyte pits, have limitations. These laboratory studies will be reviewed below, but it is important to recognize a limitation common to all of them. The crucial function to

Table 1 Laboratory Studies Which Detect Findings Associated with Hyposplenism

A. Radiologic
  1. Routine radiographs **
  2. Ultrasonography **
  3. Computerized axial tomography **
  4. Nuclear magnetic resonance **
  5. Radionuclide scans
    a. Chromium-51 heat-damaged erythrocyte clearance ****
    b. Technetium-99m sulfur colloid scanning ****
    c. IgG-sensitized, chromium-51 labelled autologous erythrocyte clearance ****
B. Hematologic
  1. Enumeration of erythrocyte pits ****
  2. Howell-Jolly bodies ****
  3. Normoblastemia ***
  4. Target cells, siderocytes, basophilic stippling *
  5. Leucocytosis *
  6. Thrombocytosis *

**** = very useful in identifying hyposplenism.
*** = a useful finding suggestive of hyposplenism but nonspecific.
** = provides anatomic but not functional information concerning the spleen.
* = a finding consistent with hyposplenism but too nonspecific to be clinically useful.

measure is clearance of nonantibody coated, encapsulated bacteria, since this reflects the true clinical risk of septicemia. Unfortunately, it is not known how our various methods of evaluating the spleen relate to this one crucial function.

When impairment of splenic function is severe, all aspects of splenic function are probably impaired, so any functional study is likely to reflect this. When the impairment is less severe, the degree of impairment of different splenic functions may vary. In these instances, our present techniques for measuring splenic function may not correlate with the specific and vital function of bacterial clearance. More research is needed to identify techniques which will accurately reflect this particular splenic function.

Radiologic Studies

Radiography, ultrasound and computerized tomography provide anatomic, but not functional information about the spleen. A splenic shadow may be seen on routine radiographs, but this finding is unreliable. Ultrasound examination can demonstrate the presence of a spleen, and provide measurement of splenic size

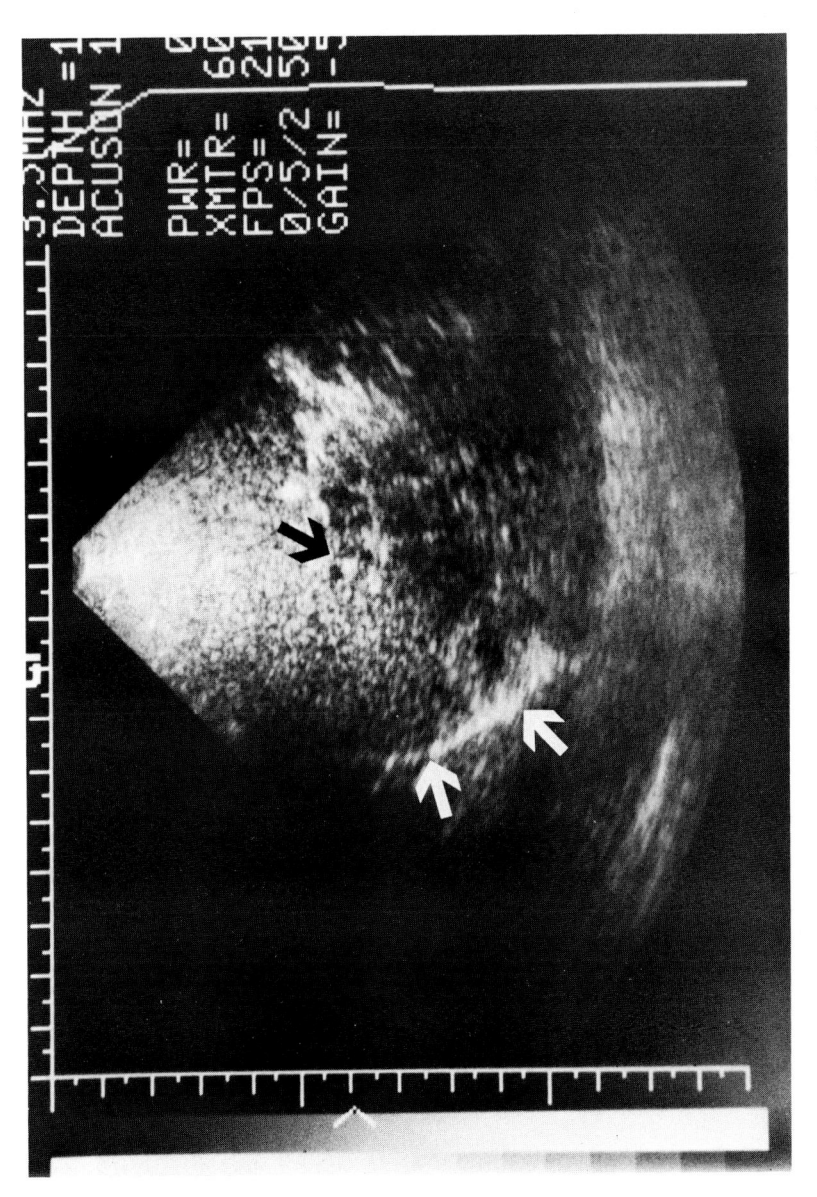

Figure 1 Ultrasound image of a normal spleen. The white arrows delineate the diaphragm. The black arrow points to the splenic hilum. Splenic tissue lies between these arrows.

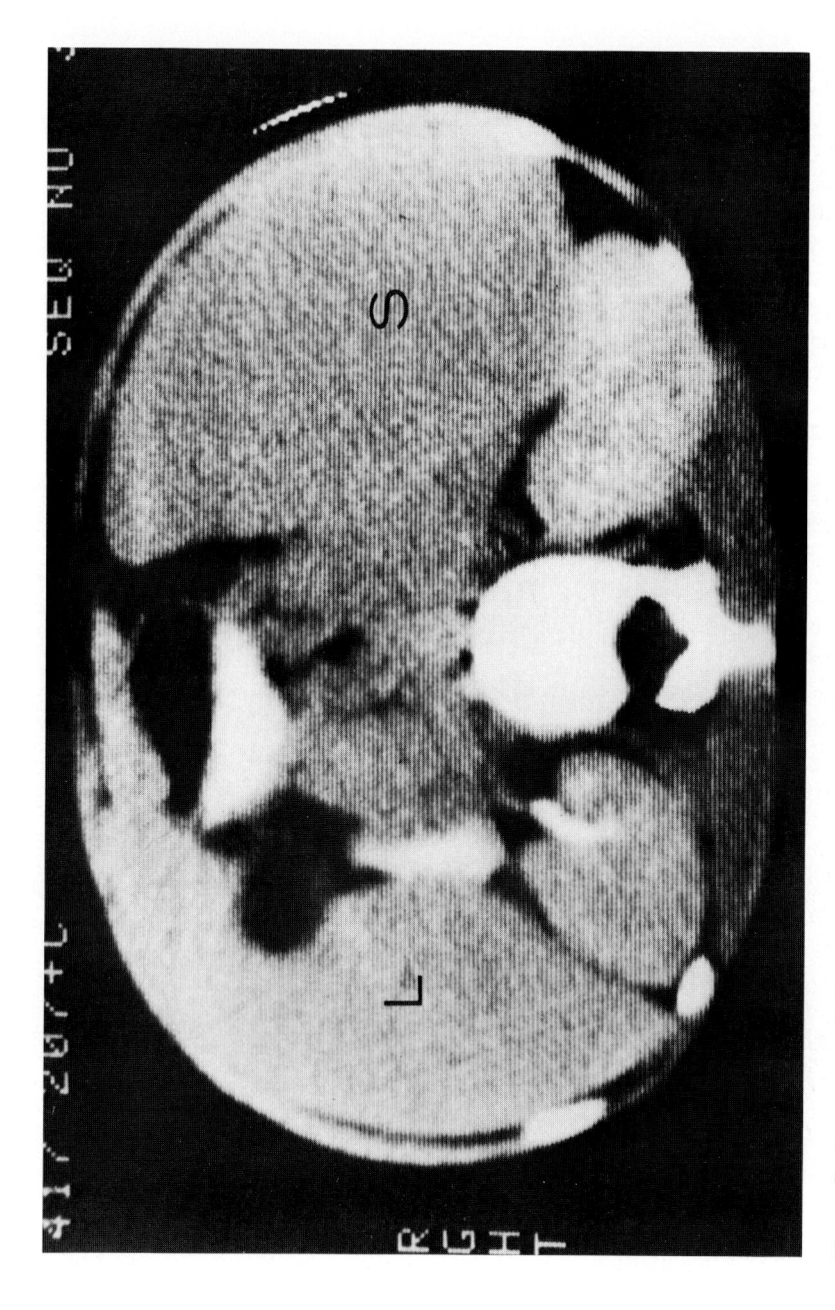

Figure 2 Computerized tomography image of the spleen. The spleen (S) is massively enlarged. The liver (L) is of normal size.

(1-3) (Figure 1). Computerized tomography can document both the anatomic presence of the spleen and the presence of intrasplenic defects (4-6); it can also identify splenosis (7,8) and estimate splenic volume (6) (Figure 2). Studies are in progress to identify specific emulsions or liposomes for use with computerized tomography to act as contrast materials with specificity for the liver and spleen (9,10). Until such specific contrast media are developed, computerized tomography will remain a tool primarily for anatomic but not for functional assessment of the spleen. Nuclear magnetic resonance can visualize the spleen and its blood supply, but experience with this imaging technique is limited (11).

Radionuclide scanning can provide both functional and anatomic information, depending on the radioactive label used. The two most commonly used methods involve chromium-51-labelled, heat-damaged red cells or technetium-99m sulfur colloid.

The clearance of chromium-51 heat-damaged red cells examines both splenic anatomy and function. Since the spleen is both sensitive and efficient at recognizing and removing abnormal erythrocytes, the clearance of heat-treated red cells provides an excellent measurement of the spleen's ability to cull red cells. The scanning procedure involves damaging autologous red cells in vitro by heating them to 50 degrees C for 20 min and then labelling the cells with chromium-51. In another technique that is utilized less often, red cell damage can also be produced chemically with compounds such as 1-mercury-2-hydroxypropane (12). The damaged red cells are infused back into the patient and are rapidly cleared from the circulation. As many as 90% of these cells are removed from the circulation by the spleen (13). Calculating the clearance of the damaged cells from the circulation provides a measure of splenic function. Scintillation scans are done to locate the anatomic sites of splenic sequestration.

The heat-treated red cell technique can be more sensitive than sulfur-colloid scanning. While approximately 90% of heat-damaged red cells are trapped in the spleen, only 10% of cells labeled with sulfur-colloid are localized to this organ. When only 10% of normal splenic function remains, the 9% of heat-damaged red cells that are trapped in the spleen will be easily identified. The equivalent 1% of sulfur-colloid will likely be missed because of the limits of sensitivity of the technique (12). The use of heat-damaged red cells is also likely to be superior to sulfur-colloid when the left lobe of the liver is overlying the spleen, since there is much less hepatic uptake (14).

However, the heat-damaged red cell technique does present a number of technical problems. These include (1) false indications of hyposplenia because of insufficient heat-induced red cell damage, (2) inadequate red cell uptake of chromium, and (3) difficulties in comparing erythrocyte destruction at various reticuloendothelial sites (15). These technical difficulties can be critical. Experience and very careful technique are necessary to obtain useful results (12). The study

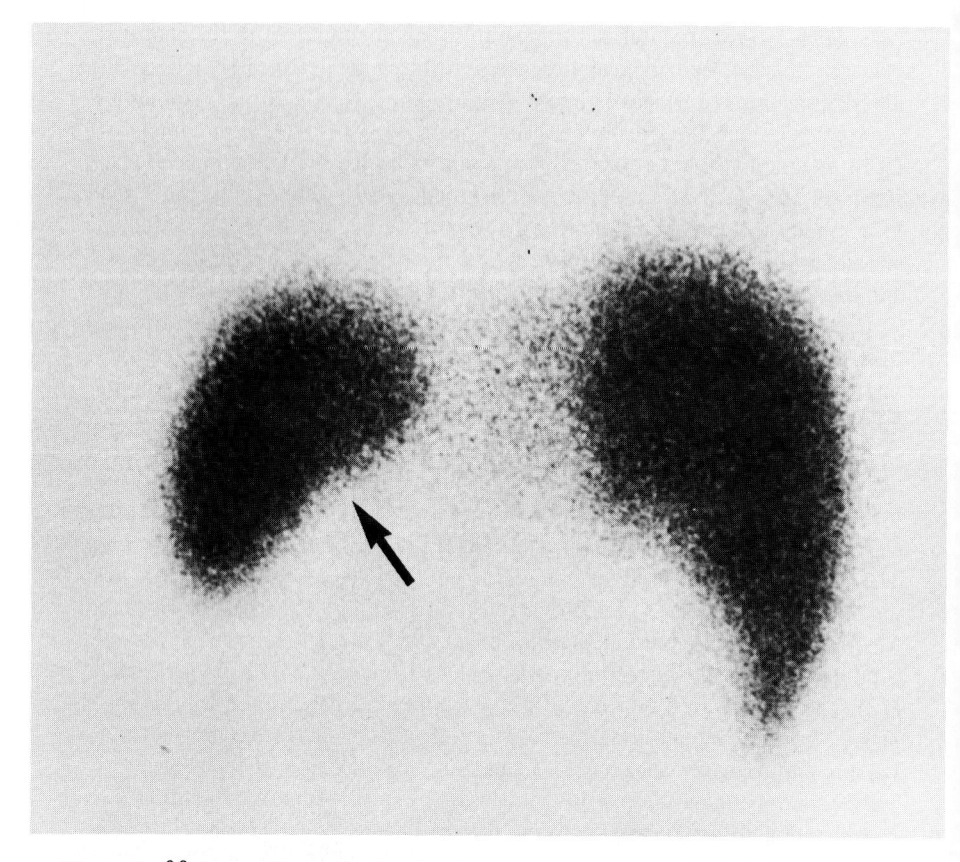

Figure 3 $^{99}Tc_m$-sulfur colloid scan of a normal subject. The arrow points to the uptake of sulfur colloid by the spleen. The distinctly larger mass of uptake (right) represents the liver.

using heat-damaged red cells may also be inadequate if the patient has an underlying erythrocyte defect (16). In general, the complex preparations which this test requires have led to its replacement with technetium-99m sulfur-colloid scanning for routine clinical studies.

Technetium-99m sulfur-colloid scanning is now the most commonly used method of splenic scanning. It measures the functional capacity of the spleen to clear particulate matter. Sulfur-colloid particles 1.0 micron in diameter are used, 10% of which are normally phagocytized by the spleen (Figure 3). In functional asplenia, sulfur-colloid is not trapped in the spleen in spite of evidence of the anatomic presence of splenic tissue (17). The neonatal spleen does trap this colloid, so this study is useful for assessing neonatal splenic function (1,18). The sensitivity of the study may be increased by comparing it with a HIDA (N-(2,2-dimethyl phenylcarbamoylmethyl iminodiacetic acid) or a PIPDA (technetium-99m-acetanilido-iminodiacetic acid) scan which should not identify the spleen (19). Whether the benefit of doing these two studies outweighs the risk of the excess potential side effects and increased cost remains to be determined. The presence of ascites or a large left lobe of the liver hampers interpretation of these imaging studies (16).

Technetium sulfur-colloid scanning and the clearance of heat-treated erythrocytes specifically measure the ability of the spleen to remove (or sequester) particulate matter. They do not provide any measurement of the spleen's ability to clear immunologically active material from the circulation, which is mediated by specific Fc receptor sites. Function of the Fc receptor sites is measured by the ability to clear chromium-51-labelled Rh(D) positive erythrocytes sensitized with anti-D. Since anti-D antibody does not fix complement, the clearance of these Rh positive red cells is dependent upon attachment to the Fc receptor sites of splenic macrophages (20-22). These Fc-receptor sites are the same ones involved in the clearance of antibody-antigen complexes. At least 5 times as many Rh-sensitized cells are removed in the spleen, as opposed to the liver. This is in spite of the fact that hepatic blood flow is 10 times greater than that of the spleen (13). A limitation of the technique utilizing Rh (D) positive erythrocytes is that the patient must be Rh(D) positive to avoid sensitization to the Rh antigen. Clearance of IgG sensitized red cells therefore provides an important tool to measure specific immunologic function of the spleen.

Hematologic Changes

There are a number of hematologic changes in the asplenic state which may be helpful in recognizing anatomic or functional asplenia.

Erythroid alterations associated with asplenia include (1) non-specific hematologic changes, (2) Howell-Jolly bodies and (3) erythrocyte pits. Asplenia is also associated with certain leukocyte and platelet abnormalities.

Red cell survival and hemoglobin levels are unchanged in otherwise normal asplenic individuals. The reticulocyte count can increase, but it usually remains normal (23,24). The mean corpuscular volume remains normal but cell surface area increases, causing red cells to appear thinner and target cells to form in smears of peripheral blood. Acanthocytes and fragmented red cells may also be seen (24). None of these changes are specific for the asplenic state.

Basophilic stippling and siderocytes are non-specific changes commonly found in asplenic patients. Normoblastemia, the presence of nucleated erythrocytes in peripheral blood, is an abnormal finding that is a more specific indication of hyposplenism (25). Normoblasts that escape from the marrow are normally

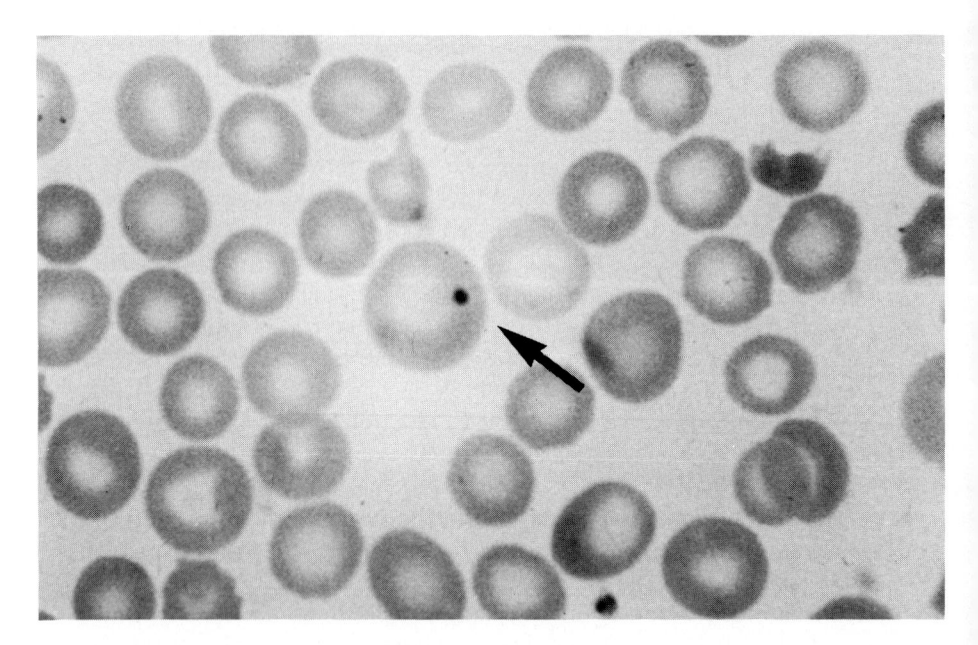

Figure 4 Photomicrograph of a Howell-Jolly body on a routine peripheral blood smear. The dark inclusion in the cell marked by the arrow is the Howell-Jolly body. (Wright's stain, X 1200)

cleared rapidly by the spleen. The presence of normoblasts in the peripheral blood therefore suggests a hyposplenic state. However, marrow stress and release of excessive numbers of normoblasts can overcome the ability of a normal spleen to clear them from the circulation. This situation can occur with hypoxia, hemolytic anemia (or during recovery from anemia), megaloblastic anemia, ineffective erythropoiesis, as well as infections, collagen-vascular disorders, malignancies, and during therapy with vinca alkaloids (vincristine or vinblastine) (26).

The most useful peripheral blood smear abnormality in diagnosing asplenia is the *Howell-Jolly body* (Figure 4). These nuclear fragments are removed from circulating erythrocytes by the spleen and are not normally seen in peripheral blood. In asplenic states, Howell-Jolly bodies are almost always present (23,27). They may be found as frequently as in 1 out of 100 (28) or as rarely as in 1 out of 10,000 red cells (92). Therefore, a careful and prolonged search of the peripheral blood smear is essential.

Howell-Jolly bodies are a sensitive indicator of splenic function. In a comparative study, Howell-Jolly bodies were noted when the T 1/2 (half-survival

HYPOSPLENISM

time) of heat-treated red cells was only mildly prolonged (30,31). One study of functional asplenia in adults suggested that Howell-Jolly bodies are a more sensitive indicator of splenic function than sulfur-colloid scanning (32). However, other workers found radionuclide sulfur-colloid and heat-treated red cell studies to be more sensitive (33,34). Unfortunately, Howell-Jolly bodies are also found in patients with hemolytic and megaloblastic anemias, so they are not specific for splenic dysfunction.

In general, these inclusions represent an inexpensive, readily available indicator of splenic dysfunction and their presence should suggest hyposplenism. However, it must be recognized that significant false positive and false negative results occur when the finding of Howell-Jolly bodies alone is used in assessing splenic function.

The most useful morphologic feature in diagnosing anatomic or functional asplenia is the appearance of red cell surface "pits" or "pocks." Their visualization requires examining wet preparations of red cells under a special optical system, called direct interference contrast microscopy. Routine microscopy cannot be used (Figure 5). These apparent surface pits are actually an illusion inherent to the optical system. Under electron microscopy, they are seen to be submembranous vacuoles unattached to the cell membrane (35-37).

Post-splenectomy, patients demonstrate pits in from 10 to 50% of their red cells, and many cells have multiple pits as well as pits larger than 0.5 microns in diameter (33,38-40). In contrast, normal individuals with normal spleens have pits in no more than 2% of their red cells; multiply pitted red cells and individual pits larger than 0.5 microns in diameter are very rarely seen. Erythrocytes from asplenic individuals lose their pits when injected into a normal host, while normal erythrocytes acquire pits when injected into an asplenic host (35). Presumably the spleen's normal "pitting" function removes these surface pits, leaving the remainder of the cell unharmed. Hyposplenic subjects are unable to remove the pits, so the number of pitted erythrocytes increases. The percentage of red cells containing pits, the "pit count," is useful in identifying functional hyposplenism as well as anatomic asplenia (33,38-43).

Two studies were done comparing the number of red cell pits with the findings of heat-damaged erythrocyte scanning of the spleen. These studies showed a significant inverse correlation between the number (or percentage) of pitted red cells and the calculated splenic size derived from the scan (44,45). Thus, as the size of the spleen increased the numbers of pitted red cells decreased. In the first study, all patients with normal red cell clearances (half-survival time) had pit counts of less than 4%, while all patients with a calculated splenic volume of less than 158 cm^3 had pit counts of more than 4%. Only 1 out of 16 patients with a prolonged red cell clearance had a pit count of less than 4% (44). In the second study (108) all post-traumatic surgically asplenic patients with less than 16.2%

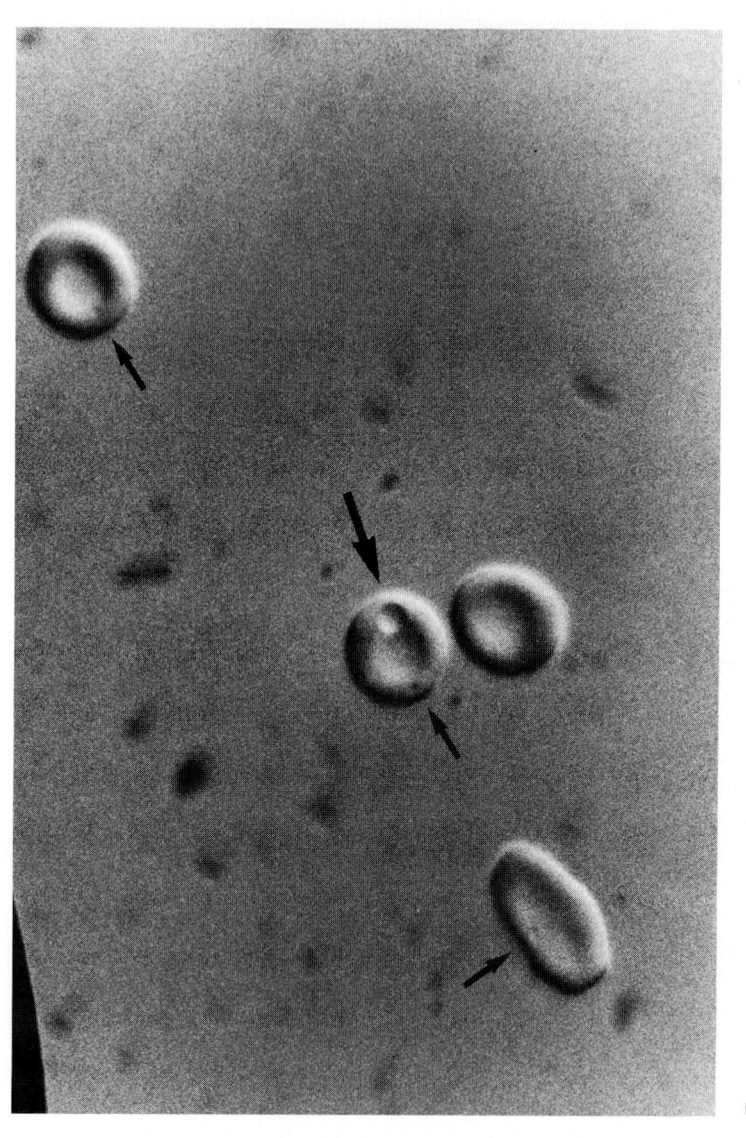

Figure 5 Photomicrograph of erythrocytes using direct interference-contrast microscopy. The blood sample is from an asplenic donor. Small erythrocyte pits are indicated by the small arrows. The single pit is noted by the larger arrow. The pits are much more distinct under direct visualization with the microscope because of the limitations of photomicroscopy and the ability to easily vary the direction of the light source to best outline individual pits. In taking this particular photograph, the light was adjusted to delineate the outline of the large pit at the expense of the smaller ones. (× 1000)

pitted erythrocytes demonstrated splenosis. It was calculated that, in adults, the pit count would theoretically reach 0% at a splenic volume of 180 cm^3.

A large cooperative study has assessed splenic function in more than 2,000 patients with sickle cell anemia. Normal sulfur-colloid splenic scans correlated closely with the finding of less than 3.5% pitted red cells, while abnormal scans correlated with the presence of 3.5% or more pitted red cells. The predictive value of these correlations was 95% (46). An earlier report on this population of patients with sickle cell disease demonstrated a high percentage of pitted erythrocytes in all 14 children who developed severe bacterial infections (47). This preliminary study is extremely important because it suggests that by measuring red cell pitting one is able to identify hyposplenic patients at risk for septicemia.

It has been reported that patients with hereditary spherocytosis have lower pit counts than expected following splenectomy (40). It was assumed that this reflected a specific membrane defect in spherocytosis which impairs pit formation. However, subsequent studies have failed to confirm this finding (40a).

The quantitation of red cell surface pits is a very sensitive and specific measurement of splenic function. The single drop of blood required for the study can be obtained by fingerstick. The sample can be accurately restudied years later if it has been appropriately fixed in glutaraldehyde. The technique is reproducible and quantitative, and it is ideal for use in longitudinal studies. Proper adjustment of the microscope, experience, and counting adequate numbers of red cells is crucial. One should examine 500 to 2,000 red cells, with the larger number preferable if the percentage of pitted erythrocytes is low. The only drawbacks of this technique are (1) the equipment is not widely available, (2) technical consistency is important, and (3), as with other studies of splenic function, it is not clear how accurately it reflects the spleen's ability to clear encapsulated bacteria in the absence of type-specific antibody.

A transient leucocytosis usually follows splenectomy, although this is persistent in only a minority of patients (23,48). The leucocytosis consists primarily of a lymphocytosis and monocytosis. Eosinophilia may be noted and a transient neutrophilia may occur. Immature white cells are not generally seen (23,27). None of these findings are specific enough to be of significant use in evaluating splenic function.

One-third to one-half of patients will demonstrate a thrombocytosis after splenectomy, which can persist for several months to a year or more (24,27,49). Animal studies suggest that the initial thrombocytosis is due to general perioperative stress, but persistence of the elevated platelet count appears to be related to alteration of megakaryocyte ploidy in the bone marrow (50). This thrombocytosis is too non-specific to be an aid in specific diagnosis.

Other non-specific changes in platelets associated with asplenia include the appearance of giant platelets (34) and a possible increase in platelet adhesion (24).

Certain other hematologic changes are also associated with asplenia. Thus, asplenic individuals demonstrate decreased saline osmotic fragility of red cells (24) and elevated transferrin levels (51). These findings are of no specific diagnostic assistance in identifying the asplenic state.

OVERVIEW OF LABORATORY TECHNIQUES TO EVALUATE HYPOSPLENISM

Splenic radionuclide scanning has been the accepted, traditional means to measure splenic function. These scanning procedures are accurate and widely available. Other studies, however, can be very useful. The presence of Howell-Jolly bodies, although nonspecific, can be critical in identifying hyposplenism especially when it is not otherwise suspected. The quantitation of red cell pits appears to be as accurate as radionuclide scanning. The test is simpler to perform, less expensive, and superior for longitudinal studies. However, availability of this technique is more limited because of the specific optical system it requires. Further research is needed to identify techniques that more accurately reflect the spleen's ability to clear bacteria.

CAUSES OF FUNCTIONAL AND ANATOMIC HYPOSPLENISM

Many clinical conditions and diseases are associated with hyposplenism (Table 2). The true incidence of hyposplenism in these disorders is often difficult to determine because of bias in case reporting and the various methodologies used to measure splenic function. Potential causes of hyposplenism, based on experimental data in animals, are briefly mentioned. In some hyposplenic disorders, the spleen is physically absent and the hyposplenia is thereby anatomic. In many other instances, splenic tissue is present but function is impaired. This latter form of hyposplenism is considered to be functional. No attempt is made to separately classify the anatomic and functional forms of hyposplenism since the two forms often exist in a continuum.

The consequences of hyposplenism and their treatment will be discussed in Chapter 4, "Physiology of the Spleen and Consequences of Hyposplenism."

Hyposplenism in the Neonate

The normal neonate demonstrates several findings suggestive of impaired splenic function. These findings include occasional Howell-Jolly bodies and normoblasts (23,52), Heinz bodies (53), siderocytes, and a small percentage of distorted red cells (23). Clearance of transfused erythrocytes containing Heinz bodies is very prolonged in premature infants as well as asplenic adults, which supports the concept of neonatal hyposplenism. The additional finding of impaired clearance

Table 2 Causes of Anatomic and Functional Hyposplenism

A. The normal neonate
B. Congenital hyposplenism
    1. Isolated congenital hyposplenism
    2. Asplenia syndrome
    3. Polysplenia syndrome
    4. Fanconi's syndrome
    5. Syndrome of the refractory sideroblastic anemia and vacuolization of marrow precursors
    6. Congenital hypoplastic anemia **
    7. Teratogenic effect of warfarin **
C. Hyposplenism of old age *
D. Hyposplenism due to in situ splenic congestion
    1. Sickle hemoglobinopathies
    2. Myeloproliferative disorders
        a. Essential thrombocytosis *
        b. Myelofibrosis **
    3. Hemolytic anemias ***
    4. Malaria ***
E. Hyposplenism due to impaired vascular supply to the spleen *
F. Immunologic or autoimmune disorders
    1. Glomerulonephritis *
    2. Systemic lupus erythematosis
    3. Rheumatoid arthritis
    4. Other forms of vasculitis *
    5. Graft-vs.-host disease
    6. Sarcoidosis *
    7. Hyperthyroidism or thyroiditis *
    8. IgA Deficiency **
    9. Combined immunodeficiency **
   10. Idiopathic thrombocytopenic purpura **
G. Gastrointestinal Disorders
    1. Celiac disease
    2. Dermatitis herpetiformis *
    3. Ulcerative Colitis *
    4. Regional enteritis
    5. Intestinal lymphangiectasia **
    6. Chronic aggressive hepatitis **
H. Malignancies
    1. Sezary syndrome *
    2. Multiple myeloma *
    3. Gastric carcinoma *
    4. Breast carcinoma *

Table 2 (Continued)

H. Malignancies (continued)
   5. Primary splenic angiosarcoma **
   6. Non-Hodgkin's lymphoma *
   7. Mild splenic hypoplasia in many childhood malignancies (may be due to therapy, primary disease or both)
   8. Splenic irradiation
   9. Thorotrast therapy *
I. Miscellaneous
   1. Systemic amyloidosis *
   2. Drug-induced
      a. Intravenous gamma globulin
      b. Methyldopa
      c. Corticosteroids **
   3. Nephrotic syndrome
   4. The "born-again" spleen syndrome
   5. Malignant mastocytosis **
   6. Fibronectin deficiency **
   7. Experimental etiologies of hyposplenism
      a. Viral infections **
      b. Folate deficiency ***
      c. Lipid Emulsions (palmitates) ***

* = Reported in adults but not in children or adolescents.
** = Based upon sparse clinical data.
*** = Experimental animal data but no evidence of an effect in humans.

of heat-damaged red cells in premature infants confirms the relationship of these findings to hyposplenism (53).

However, enumeration of erythrocyte pits has provided much more quantitative data. The first study of red cells of newborns using erythrocyte pit counts found the numbers of pitted cells to be similar to those found in asplenic adults. Full-term infants had a mean pit count of 24% with multiple pits in 40-70% of their red cells. The mean pit count in premature infants was 47%, with even higher counts in the smallest infants weighing less than 1500 grams. Asplenic adults, by comparison, had average pit counts of 50% (41). These findings were recently confirmed, although the pit counts were considerably lower (42). Both studies confirmed the existence of an inverse correlation between the pit count and increasing gestational age and birth weight, although the correlation with gestational age was more significant (41,42). Therefore, splenic maturity in the neonate is more dependent on maturational factors than birth weight. Postmature infants had higher counts suggesting that their exposure to fetal malnutrition and hypoxia impair splenic development (42). After birth, the percentage of red cell pits falls to normal levels by 2 months in the full term infant and somewhat later in the premature (41).

These pits may form in red cells of newborns for reasons other than hyposplenism. However, the presence of findings in peripheral blood smear consistent with hyposplenism, and impaired clearance of heat-treated red cells, support the presence of an impairment of splenic function in the neonate. Further experimental evidence is provided by a rat model. The spleen of the newborn rat is small in size and markedly impaired in its ability to take up technetium sulfurcolloid. However, adult weight and function of the spleen is rapidly attained by 2 weeks of age (54). The role of functional hyposplenism, if any, in predisposing newborns to bacterial infections is uncertain.

CONGENITAL HYPOSPLENISM

This includes isolated congenital asplenia, asplenia syndrome, polysplenia syndrome, Fanconi's anemia, the syndrome of refractory sideroblastic anemia and vacuolization of marrow precursors, congenital hypoplastic anemia, and congenital malformations dur to warfarin.

Isolated congenital asplenia is a very rare disorder (55-58). Although usually sporadic, familial involvement has been reported (59). These children do not demonstrate immunologic abnormalities other than asplenia, which has been documented by the presence of Howell-Jolly bodies and the absence of splenic tissue on radionuclide scanning. However, the presence of a rudimentary spleen at 10 months of age in one infant suggests that the spleen is not always absent (60). Bacterial meningitis, sepsis, or both, are frequent complications of isolated congenital asplenia (59).

Asplenia syndrome is a sporadic disorder which can be simply considered as bilateral right-sidedness. These patients usually demonstrate bilateral tri-lobed lungs, right-sided stomach, and severe conotruncal cardiac abnormalities in addition to asplenia (23,61,62). The occurrence of both asplenia and heart disease probably reflects the simultaneous formation of the splenic anlage and the arterio-venous cushions of the heart on the twenty-fifth day of embryonic life. The associated cardiac malformations include abnormalities of the venae cavae and pulmonary venous connections, transposition of the great arteries, pulmonary stenosis or atresia, truncus arteriosis, and absence of the coronary sinus. Rare patients have partial situs inversus without significant cardiovascular disease (19,58).

Although the spleen is usually absent anatomically in patients with the asplenia syndrome, functional (instead of true anatomical) asplenia was observed in 2 infants (59). In one infant the presence of splenic tissue was confirmed at autopsy. The second infant did not demonstrate splenic tissue on an initial sulfur-colloid scan, but a second scan following clinical improvement of his heart disease revealed the presence of a normal spleen. It is not clear if this functional asplenia represents a variant of the asplenia syndrome, or whether hypoxia in these infants exaggerates the "physiologic" hyposplenia of the neonate.

Septicemia is a common complication of the asplenia syndrome, occurring in 27% of 59 patients. Under the age of 6 months, *Escherichia coli* and *Klebsiella pneumoniae* are the common organisms. After 6 months, *Streptococcus pneumoniae* and *Hemophilus influenzae* predominate. Although the majority of children who develop septicemia do so in the first year of life, it has been reported to occur as late as 13 years of age (56). Follow-up of a small group of these children has suggested that prophylactic penicillin is beneficial (55).

Asplenia syndrome should always be considered in patients with severe congenital heart disease, especially in those with other signs of bilateral right-sidedness. The functional hyposplenism of normal neonates may make it difficult to establish this diagnosis early in life. Radiologic studies confirming the anatomic presence of a spleen are helpful, but it is important to remember that the asplenia may be functional. Sulfur-colloid scanning, which is reported to be normal in neonates, may be indicated in this situation (18). In infants with asplenia syndrome, longitudinal studies of erythrocyte pit counts should fail to show the expected attainment of adult values by age 2 months. Early diagnosis is crucial because of the high risk of septicemia.

Polysplenia, also a sporadic disorder, is basically bilateral left-sidedness. Polysplenia occurs more rarely than the asplenia syndrome (60). Common manifestations include bilateral bilobed lungs, isomerism of the liver, biliary atresia, and multiple right-sided stomachs (63,64,64a). Cardiac abnormalities tend to be simple and benign. One-quarter of patients have normal hearts. Two main spleens and multiple smaller ones are generally found (63,64,64a). Although splenic function is classically normal, two cases have showed persistent Howell-Jolly bodies (65,66), and one died of overwhelming pneumococcal sepsis accompanied by disseminated intravascular coagulation (66). These small, multiple spleens may not always provide adequate splenic function.

Small spleens, weighing less than 40 gm, have been reported in patients with Fanconi's anemia. Autopsy examination revealed very small, but structurally normal spleens in 9 out of 12 patients in one study. This finding suggests that a small spleen may be a common finding. The clinical significance of the finding of a very small spleen is unclear since there have been no studies of splenic function in this disorder. The overwhelming septicemia typical of asplenia has not been reported in cases of Fanconi's anemia. However, such an overwhelming infection might have been attributed to the neutropenia commonly seen in these patients, and the hyposplenism could easily have gone undetected (67).

Hyposplenism is also associated with the syndrome of refractory sideroblastic anemia and vacuolization of marrow precursors. Five patients have been reported with a syndrome consisting of severe, transfusion-dependent, macrocytic anemia, together with bone marrow findings of vacuolization of erythroid and myeloid precursors, hemosiderosis and ringed sideroblasts. Varying degrees of thrombocytopenia and neutropenia were also noted. Associated abnormalities included intestinal malabsorption with evidence of exocrine pancreatic dysfunction (68,69). Two of these 5 patients had splenic atrophy, documented by autopsy in one case and sulfur-colloid scanning in the other. One died of bacterial sepsis due to *E. Coli* (69). Although the syndrome of refractory sideroblastic anemia is very rare, reports may become more frequent now that it has been described.

Two patients with congenital hypoplastic anemia have been reported with hyposplenia (70,70a). Both had the typical findings of Blackfan-Diamond syndrome. The hyposplenia was confirmed in one child by radionuclide scanning as well as finding a small spleen during abdominal surgery (70a). The second patient died of *Streptococcus pneumoniae* septicemia and no spleen or splenic blood vessels were found at autopsy (70).

One infant exposed to warfarin early in gestation had multiple congenital malformations including asplenia. The other congenital defects included cyanotic congenital heart disease, hypoplastic nails and short, broad, distal phalanges. The child died of septicemia, and asplenia was noted on autopsy. Asplenia has not been noted in previously reported cases of warfarin-induced congenital malformations, which only included minor cardiac abnormalities (71). It is unclear whether congenital asplenia is part of the teratologic syndrome, or it is a rare, coincidental finding.

Hyposplenism Associated with Old Age

Splenic weight is known to decrease in old age. Erythrocyte pitting was studied in a group of elderly persons, together with a younger control population, to determine the effect of aging on splenic function. A group of otherwise normal, elderly subjects (mean age 74 years) had a mean red cell pit count of 4.2%. The control group of younger adults (mean age 27) had a mean red cell pit count of 1.4%. The elderly group showed impaired clearance of heat-damaged red cells and slower accumulation of these red cells in the spleen. It was concluded that the decreasing weight of the spleen in the elderly is associated with some impairment of splenic function (72). The mean red cell pit count of the elderly subjects is increased, but the risk of septicemia from this mild degree of splenic impairment may not be very great. The actual clinical significance of this impairment is unknown.

Hyposplenism Due to In Situ Splenic Congestion

This occurs in sickle hemoglobinopathies, in myeloproliferative disorders, hemolytic anemias, and malaria.

Hyposplenism is a well recognized complication of homozygous (hemoglobin SS) sickle cell anemia. The hypoxic, acidotic and hypoglycemic environment of the splenic cords induces sickling and causes these erythrocytes to be trapped within the spleen. As more sickle cells are trapped, the environment becomes even more adverse to red cell function and a vicious cycle of continued sickling ensues. The circulation of the spleen eventually becomes so congested by sickled red cells that normal splenic function is impaired. This vascular congestion may result in diversion of splenic blood flow through intrasplenic shunts which bypass the reticuloendothelial elements of the spleen. Initially, transfusion of normal blood is capable of restoring normal splenic function. Eventually, the splenic vascular changes become irreversible and even blood transfusion fails to restore splenic function (73,74).

The age of onset of this splenic dysfunction appears to be related to decreasing levels of hemoglobin F (38). Since the spleen is usually palpable at the time hyposplenism is first noted (75), the initial impairment of the spleen appears to be functional and not anatomic.

Functional hyposplenism in homozygous sickle cell disease has been documented using sulfur-colloid scans, enumeration of erythrocyte pits, and heat-damaged red cell survival studies (38,39,46,76-78). The most detailed information has been obtained from enumerating erythrocyte pits, because of the ease in studying large numbers of patients with this technique, even on a longitudinal basis. Red cell pit counts above the normal range in patients with sickle cell anemia are first noted as early as 5 months of age and at a mean age of 13 months. There is a gradual increase in pit counts until the age of 6 to 8 years. Thereafter, the pit counts reach the range of asplenic adults and tend to remain stable. Splenomegaly, which is usually evident by one year of age in patients with sickle cell disease, tends to disappear after the age of 8 years (38,39,79).

Before the age of 6 to 8 years, the hyposplenia can be reversed by blood transfusions adequate to attain a hemoglobin A levels of 50% (38,39,46,73,79). The increased level of hemoglobin A presumably reestablishes a functional circulation in the spleen, allowing clearance of the obstructing sickle red cells (38, 46,79). At 6 to 8 years of age, the spleen usually becomes nonpalpable because it is gradually infarcting. Transfusions will no longer reverse the hyposplenism. By the age of adolescence, the spleen is totally scarred and the asplenia becomes anatomic as well as functional. Only a small number of patients with homozygous sickle cell disease will maintain splenic function into adulthood (33,46). Interestingly, some children with sickle cell disease from Saudi Arabia manifest little or no splenic dysfunction. These children have high levels of hemoglobin F which appear to protect them from splenic infarction and resulting asplenia (80-82).

Patients with sickle cell anemia demonstrate a number of immunologic findings which are associated with asplenia. These include abnormalities of the alternate pathway of complement (83-85), decreased levels of tuftsin (86,87), and immunoglobulin abnormalities (88).

The hyposplenism associated with sickle cell disease is extremely important. Infection has been the leading cause of death from sickle cell anemia at all ages (89). The risk of overwhelming bacterial sepsis or meningitis in these patients has been estimated as being 300-600 times higher than that of the general population (90). As many as 15.2% of children with homozygous sickle cell anemia will develop pyogenic septicemia or meningitis. Up to 35% of those with sepsis and 10% of those with meningitis will die. Functional hyposplenism plays a critical role in causing this increased susceptability to serious infections (91).

Enumeration of erythrocyte pits may be helpful in predicting the future risk of infection for individual patients. Infants whose pit counts are increased before 12 months of age may have a higher risk of developing sepsis than those whose counts are normal. Since only 23% of these infants show increased pit counts at age one year, this may be an important finding (79). When pit counts were available, all patients who developed overwhelming bacterial septicemia had elevated pit counts prior to septicemia or at the time of the infection (46,92).

Although recent studies suggest that the morbidity and mortality due to infection has fallen significantly, it remains a major problem (93). Generally, children with homozygous sickle cell anemia who have fever over 38.5-39 degrees centigrade should routinely have blood cultures taken. Then they should immediately be given intravenous antibiotics which will provide adequate therapy directed against *Streptococcus pneumoniae* and *Hemophilus influenzae*. Such intensive antibiotic therapy is necessary because of our inability to initially differentiate overwhelming sepsis from acute illness due to viral infection as a cause of fever in these patients.

The paucity of controlled studies concerning the risk of septicemia in adults with sickle cell disease makes it difficult to establish firm recommendations for the management of fever in these patients. Until such information is available, the life-threatening nature of overwhelming sepsis must be emphasized. Thus, an aggressive approach to fever in these patients should be pursued. It must also be remembered that adolescents and even adults with sickle cell disease are still at risk for infection with *Hemophilus influenzae*.

All adults, as well as children of appropriate age, should receive pneumococcal vaccine. Penicillin prophylaxis is also of benefit in preventing septicemia. It can be given monthly as a long-acting penicillin intramuscularly (94), or orally twice-a-day (94a). Although this prophylaxis is usually given orally, compliance is a significant problem (94b). Prophylaxis should be instituted before 6 months of age and continued until at least 5 years of age. *Hemophilus influenzae* vaccine should be given to children with sickle cell disease. There have been no studies of this vaccine in adults with sickle cell anemia, but it may prove to be of benefit.

It is interesting that life-threatening, acute splenic sequestration crises of homozygous sickle cell disease still occur in patients who are functionally asplenic. This complication is discussed in the chapter on hypersplenism (Chapter 5).

The incidence of hyposplenism and the risk of serious infections in the sickle variants is less well defined. Hyposplenism is a common complication of hemoglobin SC disease, having been identified by sulfur-colloid scanning, heat-damaged erythrocyte survival studies, and enumeration of red cell pits (33,38, 39,47,95-99). Although there is some inconsistency among the various studies, it appears that hyposplenism occurs less frequently and is less severe in degree in hemoglobin SC disease than that seen with homozygous sickle cell anemia (47,95,97). There is disagreement as to whether there is (95) or is not (47,97) a relationship between age and hyposplenism. It may be that only certain patients with hemoglobin SC disease are likely to develop hyposplenism, unlike homozygous sickle cell anemia in which it develops in almost all patients. Acute splenic infarction, with classic symptoms including abdominal pain, is also seen in patients with hemoglobin SC disease (99).

Patients with hemoglobin SC disease do have an increased risk of serious bacterial infection, but the risk is not as high as in patients with homozygous sickle cell disease (95). Bacterial septicemia is usually associated with a recognized focus of primary infection, which is usually not found in the young patient with homozygous sickle cell anemia (95,100). The classic, fatal, overwhelming sepsis syndrome associated with asplenia has been noted in only 2 cases (66,96). It is not clear whether the small risk of septicemia in these patients justifies the aggressive antibiotic therapy of high fevers used in homozygous sickle cell anemia, but it must be recognized that overwhelming, fatal sepsis can occur.

Patients with sickle beta-thalassemia may also develop hyposplenism (33,39, 47,97). Patients with sickle beta^0-thalassemia develop splenic hypofunction of a degree comparable to that seen in homozygous sickle cell anemia. On the other hand, patients with sickle beta$^+$-thalassemia develop less severe splenic hypofunction which is comparable to that seen in patients with hemoglobin SC disease (47). Transient, functional asplenia was reported in one patient with hemoglobin SE disease (101). A patient with Hemoglobin SD—Los Angeles disease developed asplenia confirmed by liver-spleen scanning and complicated by pneumococcal septicemia (101a). Based on limited available studies (47), febrile episodes in beta^0-thalassemia should be treated in the same manner as those in homozygous sickle cell anemia. Less clinical data are available for patients with other hemoglobinopathies, so it is difficult to make firm recommendations concerning the management of their febrile episodes.

Essential thrombocysosis is a myeloproliferative disease which occurs predominately in adults (102). Splenic atrophy in patients with this disease was initially identified only at autopsy (103,104). In a study of 8 patients hyposplenism was detected in 3, based on the finding of prolonged clearance of heat-damaged red cells and failure to identify splenic tissue with scintillation scans (105). Splenic atrophy in these patients is probably the result of thrombosis secondary to the thrombocytosis and abnormal platelet function, which are typical of this disorder. Hyposplenism has not been described in children with essential thrombocytosis.

Another myeloproliferative syndrome has also been associated with hyposplenism. A single adult with myelofibrosis and hyposplenia has been reported (106).

There is no convincing evidence that hemolytic anemias, other than sickling disorders, can cause sufficient splenic congestion to result in hyposplenism. However, studies in rats have shown that phenylhydrazine-induced hemolysis can result in splenic congestion (107) and increased mortality from innoculated *Hemophilus influenzae* (108). It is not known if these findings have any significance in man.

Among 100 children with hereditary spherocytosis, 4 showed Howell-Jolly bodies and 24% normoblastemia on blood smears prior to splenectomy (109). These findings probably represent an "overload" syndrome. Thus, increased numbers of Howell-Jolly bodies produced by a hyperplastic marrow are delivered to a functionally normal spleen too rapidly to be cleared (110). However, a less likely explanation is that the spleen has been chronically overloaded and its function impaired.

In animals, infection with the parasites of malaria can cause diminished clearance of heat-treated red cells by the spleen during rising parasitemia (111). It is not known if this occurs in malaria in man.

Hyposplenism Due to Impaired Vascular Supply to the Spleen

Hyposplenism can result from impaired blood flow in the splenic artery or vein. Most cases of vascular impairment appear to result from atherosclerotic vascular disease of the splenic artery. Other cases are due to splenic vein thrombosis. The diagnosis of impaired vasculature is usually established by radionuclide splenic scanning performed because of acute left upper quadrant pain, the presence of Howell-Jolly bodies in the peripheral blood, or both. The youngest reported patient with impaired vascular supply to the spleen was 57 years old (29,112,113). Overwhelming septicemia has not been reported. Thromboembolism can also cause splenic infarction, but significant loss of splenic function has not been reported (113a).

Immunologic or Autoimmune Disorders Associated with Hyposplenism

Association of autoimmune disorders with hyposplenism is being recognized with increasing frequency. The pathophysiology is unknown, but in cases with fulminant nephritis or vasculitis, immune complexes may play a role (20).

Hyposplenism in association with autoimmune disorders has generally been reported in adults. This finding may merely be due to the fact that autoimmune disorders occur much more frequently in adults. It may also be that years of disease activity in cases of autoimmune disorders are required to develop this complication. However, the fact that exchange transfusion can cause rapid reversal of the manifestations of autoimmune-related hyposplenia in some cases would seem to make the latter possibility less likely (20).

Immunologic disorders associated with hyposplenism include glomerulonephritis, systemic lupus erythematosis, rheumatoid arthritis, other forms of vasculitis, graft-vs.-host disease, sarcoidosis, hyperthyroidism or thyroiditis, IgA deficiency, combined immunodeficiency, and idiopathic thrombocytopenic purpura.

Hyposplenism, as shown by decreased clearance of labelled antibody-coated and heat-treated erythrocytes, is a common finding in glomerulonephritis (20, 114-116). These impaired splenic clearances of red cells have been observed in mesangial IgA nephropathy, acute post-infectious glomerulonephritis, antiglomerular basement membrane disease, focal glomerulonephritis, minimal change glomerulonephritis (114), Goodpasture's syndrome, Wegener's granulomatosis (115,116), and idiopathic membranous nephropathy. Mesangio-capillary glomerulonephritis, however, is usually associated with normal or enhanced splenic function (115).

Hyposplenism was identified in the majority of patients in these studies, which only included adults. It is not clear whether the degree of hyposplenism is related to the severity of disease activity (20,114). The degree of hyposplenism was related to the level of circulating immune complexes in one study. However, some hyposplenic patients failed to demonstrate any immune complexes (20). Furthermore, a second study found no such correlation (114), and a third study failed to identify circulating immune complexes in any of the patients (115). The mechanism by which splenic function is impaired in glomerulonephritis remains undefined.

Treatment of 10 glomerulonephritis patients with plasma exchange resulted in improvement or, more commonly, complete reversal of the hyposplenism within 48 hours (20). This rapid improvement is consistent with an immune-complex dependent mechanism. Another potential mechanism is the lowering of the serum concentration of the IgG by the plasma exchange. Decreasing serum IgG levels may cause an "unblocking" of the reticuloendothelial system (117). Regardless of whether immune complexes are responsible for the impaired splenic function, the hyposplenism may exacerbate the immune complex disease by prolonging clearance of these complexes (115).

Therapy other than plasma exchange can also improve splenic function. Three of five patients treated with corticosteroids, either alone or in combination with cytotoxic drugs, had return of splenic function. However, the improvement in the hyposplenism was more gradual compared to that seen following plasma exchange (20).

It is not clear whether the hyposplenism is associated with an increased risk of infection. Confirmation of these findings using indicators of splenic function other than than erythrocyte clearances have not been reported, except for systemic lupus erythematosis (see below). Also, there have been no reports of overwhelming bacterial septicemia. However, cases of overwhelming bacterial septicemia may not have been identified as being associated with hyposplenism because of failure to recognize the hyposplenic state.

A number of reports have confirmed that hyposplenia is associated with systemic lupus erythmatosis (20,43,118-122). The impairment of splenic function has been confirmed using erythrocyte pitting, sulfur-colloid scans, labelled red cell clearance studies, computerized tomography and autopsy studies. The frequency of hyposplenism among 114 patients with lupus erythematosis in 2 studies was 6% (43,119). Both functional and anatomic hyposplenism occur in children as well as adults (119,120). Changes in splenic function do not appear to correlate with disease activity (43). Patients with untreated systemic lupus erythematosis show impaired clearance of IgG sensitized chromium-labelled red cells, suggesting abnormal clearance by Fc receptor sites. This impairment correlated with levels of immune complexes, suggesting that the splenic hypofunction associated with lupus may also be related to immune complex disease (22,121). Plasma exchange rapidly reversed the impaired clearance of labelled erythrocytes in two patients. Corticosteroid therapy, given either alone or in combination with cytotoxic drugs, improved splenic function more gradually in 2 out of 3 patients (20).

Septicemia may complicate the hyposplenism of systemic lupus erythematosis. Two patients with lupus have been reported who died of fulminant bacterial septicemia. Death in one patient was due to *Streptococcus pneumoniae* (119) and the other was due to *Salmonella typhimurium* (122). Splenic atrophy was noted at autopsy in one report (119).

Rheumatoid arthritis has also been associated with hyposplenism (123-126). Impaired splenic function in this disorder has been documented by heat-treated red cell clearances (116,124,126), by the presence of Howell-Jolly bodies, and by sulfur-colloid scanning (123). The frequency of hyposplenism among 33 patients with rheumatoid arthritis in 2 studies was approximately 50%. There is conflicting evidence as to whether the severity of hyposplenism is related to the clinical activity of the disease (124,125). Gold therapy, which is used in the treatment of this disease, also impaired clearance of heat-damaged red cells in normal controls as well as in a patient with rheumatoid arthritis (126).

Only a single case of asplenia has been reported in association with juvenile rheumatoid arthritis (126). Overwhelming bacterial septicemia as a complication of hyposplenism has not been reported in rheumatoid arthritis.

Hyposplenism has also been reported in association with a number of less common collagen-vascular disorders. They include Sjogren's syndrome, Wegener's granulomatosis, Goodpasture's syndrome, polyarteritis nodosa and cutaneous vasculitis (20,121). None of the reports specify whether hyposplenism is seen in children with this disease. Of 19 patients with Sjogren's syndrome, 12 had delayed clearance of IgG-sensitized erythrocytes. Almost all the patients with evidence of hyposplenism had either extraglandular disease or another collagen-vascular disease, in addition to the Sjogren's syndrome. Although many of these patients had increased circulating immune complexes, the levels of immune complexes did not correlate with the impaired splenic function as measured by erythrocyte clearance (121).

The hyposplenism in some patients with these collagen-vascular disorders improved rapidly following plasma exchange. Others responded to corticosteroid therapy, although more slowly (20). Overwhelming bacterial septicemia has not been recognized as a complication in patients with hyposplenism associated with these less common collagen-vascular diseases.

Functional hyposplenism is a complication of chronic graft-vs.-host disease following bone marrow transplantation (127,128). It has been identified by both radionuclide scans and erythrocyte pit counts in children and adults. There was no relationship between the development of hyposplenism and the pre-transplantation therapy (preparative regimen) or the time interval since the transplantation. Impaired splenic function was not noted in patients with acute graft-versus-host disease or in those who did not show evidence of graft-versus-host disease (127). The asplenia can reverse without evidence of graft failure or reactivation of the graft-vs.-host disease (128). The pathophysiology is not well defined.

Overwhelming sepsis has not been associated with hyposplenism in these bone marrow transplant patients. However, such an association might not have been made considering the great susceptibility of these patients to infection. Since infection is a major cause of death in these patients, all patients with chronic graft-vs.-host disease should have their splenic function evaluated.

Functional hyposplenism has been reported in adults with sarcoidosis, but not in children with this disease. Presence of hyposplenism has been documented at autopsy, by the presence of Howell-Jolly bodies and by sulfur-colloid scanning (129-131). One patient who was previously well died of overwhelming *Streptococcus pneumoniae* septicemia complicated by disseminated intravascular coagulation. The diagnosis of sarcoidosis, including the finding that splenic tissue was replaced by granuloma, was only established at autopsy (130). This suggests that the hyposplenism associated with sarcoidosis may be complicated by the development of overwhelming septicemia.

Three patients with thyrotoxicosis (132) and two with hypothyroidism secondary to thyroiditis (133) developed evidence of hyposplenism including presence of Howell-Jolly bodies and diminished uptake using sulfur-colloid scan or clearance of heat-damaged red cells. The mechanism by which hyposplenism develops is not known. All patients were adults and none developed bacterial sepsis.

Two patients with IgA deficiency were reported to have hyposplenism based upon abnormal radionuclide scans (133,134). One patient was 12 years old and had a history of recurrent septicemia and meningitis (134). Hyposplenism should be considered a potential complication of IgA deficiency.

Hyposplenism has also been noted to occur in cases of combined immunodeficiency. This association is mentioned briefly and without details in two reports (135,136). It is impossible to judge the significance of this finding without specific clinical data.

A single adult with idiopathic thrombocytopenic purpura (ITP) being treated with high doses of prednisone developed hyposplenism which was confirmed by peripheral blood findings, sulfur-colloid scan and heat-damaged red cell clearance. On the basis of this one case, it is impossible to judge whether the hyposplenism was related to the platelet disorder (ITP), to the prednisone therapy, or was due to an unrecognized, underlying collagen-vascular disorder (137).

Hyposplenism in Association with Gastrointestinal Disorders

Celiac disease, dermatitis herpetiformis, and inflammatory bowel disease (ulcerative colitis and regional enteritis), plus intestinal lymphangectasia and chronic active hepatitis are associated with hyposplenism. The pathophysiology of hyposplenism in these disorders remains undefined. All of these disorders may have an autoimmune basis which could provide a common link to the hyposplenism associated with autoimmune diseases. However, such an autoimmune etiology remains unproven.

Another possibility is a genetic predisposition. Celiac disease and dermatitis herpetiformis are associated with the presence of HLA alloantigens B8/DRw3. These alloantigens are also associated with impaired Fc-dependent splenic function (138). Further research is necessary to define the role of these and other potential pathophysiologic mechanisms as causes of hyposplenism.

Hyposplenism is a common finding in adults with celiac disease. The pathophysiology underlying this association is poorly understood, but studies of HLA haplotypes suggest a genetic predisposition. HLA types B8 and DRw3 are present in more than 80% of patients with celiac disease. These specific antigens are also associated with impairment of reticuloendothelial Fc-receptor function. The defect in reticuloendothelial function was identified by the prolonged clearance of IgG-sensitized red cells in otherwise normal subjects as well as patients with dermatitis herpertiformis (138). However, a statistically significant relationship between these haplotypes and hyposplenism in celiac disease could not be documented. This might be because the very high frequency of these HLA haplotypes make it difficult to confirm such a relationship.

However, another study casts some doubt upon the role of this mechanism. Family members of patients with celiac disease were examined. As many as 20% of siblings or children of patients with celiac disease demonstrated erythrocyte pit counts that were significantly higher than normal, but lower than pit counts seen in the celiac disease patients. There was considerable interfamily variation, but the pattern of splenic function tended to be consistent within a family. However, there appeared to be no relationship between the presence of hyposplenism and HLA-B8 positivity. It was suggested that other genetic factors, probably recessive in nature, influence splenic function and the inheritance of celiac disease (139). A direct relationship between HLA haplotypes and hyposplenism in celiac disease remains unproven.

Hyposplenism is found in at least 30-50% of adults with celiac disease (31, 112,140,141). It has been identified by typical findings on peripheral blood smears (31,34,133,142), by heat-treated red cell clearance or sulfur-colloid scans (31,44,142-146), and by erythrocyte pit counts (44,141,147). Hyposplenism has been the initial presenting finding in some patients with celiac disease (133,142).

There is some debate whether there is (44,140,141,148) or is not (112,144) a relationship between the duration, activity and therapy of celiac disease and the occurrence of hyposplenism. Several observations from the larger studies (44, 141) support the concept that hyposplenism is related to duration and activity of the disease. First, patients whose therapy was started later in life, and were therefore untreated longer, are more likely to be hyposplenic (44). Secondly, there is a direct relationship between the degree of hyposplenism as measured by erythrocyte pit counts and the severity of the celiac disease based on the extent of small bowel biopsy abnormalities. Thirdly, pit counts are significantly lower in patients less than 20 years of age compared to patients over 30, while the highest counts were found in patients aged 50-60 years. Finally, pit counts were significantly lower after 4 to 6 months of therapy than after one month of therapy. These data strongly support a relationship between hyposplenism and the duration and degree of activity of celiac disease (141).

Immune function has been evaluated in patients with celiac disease and hyposplenism to determine whether there is an etiologic relationship between these complications. Primary and secondary antibody responses were significantly impaired in one group of these patients with celiac disease and associated hyposplenism (148). Another study failed to demonstrate any impairment of T cell function (149). Further work is necessary to determine the etiologic relationship, if any, between immune abnormalities and hyposplenism.

Patients with celiac disease are at increased risk for the development of malignant lymphomas (133,145,150). One study suggested that those celiac disease patients with hyposplenism are at greater risk for developing lymphomas (133), but others did not confirm this finding (150).

The incidence of hyposplenism in children with celiac disease is considerably lower than that of adults. This is not surprising in view of the findings supporting a relationship between the development of hyposplenia and the duration of untreated disease (44,141). Children are more likely to have had a shorter duration of disease. Although two individual children with celiac disease have been reported to have impaired splenic function (151,152), three studies including a total of 41 children failed to identify any instance of hyposplenia (44,153,154). However, a recent, large survey of 177 patients studied using erythrocyte pit counts showed that hyposplenia is fairly common in children. Seven out of 25 patients less than 20 years of age had pit counts of more than 10%, which is well above normal. More than half of the patients had pit counts that were above the normal range (141).

There have been no reports of overwhelming sepsis in this population, although this might be explained in part by the development of hyposplenism at an older age when the risk of septicemia is decreased. The clinical significance of the hyposplenism associated with celiac disease remains unclear.

Dermatitis herpetiformis is a chronic, recurrent, cutaneous disease. It is complicated by a celiac-type gluten sensitive enteropathy in 60-70% of patients (155). As with celiac disease, hyposplenism is a common finding in dermatitis herpetiformis. At least one-third of patients have evidence of impaired splenic function on the basis of erythrocyte pit counts and heat-damaged red cell survival (44,156).

The role of HLA haplotypes in the pathogenesis of hyposplenia has also been examined in dermatitis herpetiformis. More than 90% of patients with dermatitis herpetiformis are HLA-B8/DRw3 positive. Patients with these haplotypes, both with and without dermatitis herpetiformis, have impaired function of the Fc-receptor, as demonstrated by impaired clearance of IgG-sensitized erythrocytes. Abnormalities of T cells bearing Fc receptors for IgG were also identified. It was concluded that these haplotypes are associated with a functional defect of the Fc-receptor in dermatitis herpetiformis (138). Confusion arises in comparing the association of HLA haplotypes and hyposplenism in both celiac disease and dermatitis herpetiformis. It seems logical that the mechanism of hyposplenism is similar in both disorders, yet studies of celiac disease fail to directly associate HLA haplotypes and splenic function. More research is necessary to clarify the role of specific HLA haplotypes, the specific impairment of Fc-receptor function associated with these haplotypes, and the broader aspects of hyposplenism which occur in both celiac disease and dermatitis herpetiformis.

A relationship between splenic dysfunction and disease activity or therapy has not been recognized in dermatitis herpetiformis (44,156). A larger study may identify such a relationship, since a similar finding was confirmed for celiac disease. The hyposplenia of dermatitis herpetiformis has not been recognized in children. Bacterial septicemia has not been reported as a complication of this disorder.

Hyposplenism is also common in ulcerative colitis. It has been identified in this disease using peripheral blood findings, heat-treated red cell clearance and scintigraphy, and erythrocyte pits (30,112,143,157-160). Approximately one-half of patients with ulcerative colitis show prolonged heat-treated red cell clearances consistent with impaired splenic function (32,143,160). All patients were normal at diagnosis, with hyposplenia developing later during periods of active disease (112). The location of disease activity is also important; hyposplenism is rare with distal ulcerative colitis, but common with total colonic disease (143, 159).

Hyposplenism has not been specifically reported in children with ulcerative colitis, although it was found in a number of patients between 20 and 30 years of age (157-159). Four adults with ulcerative colitis and hyposplenia developed early, sudden-onset post-colectomy sepsis, which was complicated by disseminated intravascular coagulation in two cases (30,161). *Streptococcus pneumoniae* was isolated in one instance, and gram negative bacteria in the others. This suggests that the hyposplenia associated with ulcerative colitis can result in septicemia.

Hyposplenism is also associated with regional enteritis, although it occurs less frequently than in ulcerative colitis (30,159). Approximately one-quarter of patients have either prolonged heat-treated red cell clearances or Howell-Jolly bodies (30,159,160). Patients with isolated ileal disease do not appear to develop this complication (159). Hyposplenism does occur in adolescents with regional enteritis (159,160). Overwhelming bacterial septicemia has not been reported in these patients.

Intestinal lymphangiectasia is characterized by dilated lymphatics, protein-losing enteropathy, hypoalbuminemia and edema. A patient with this disorder developed hyposplenia documented by the presence of Howell-Jolly bodies, increased numbers of red cell pits, and decreased splenic size on sulfur-colloid scan. Impaired splenic function was not present at the time of diagnosis but appeared later in the disease. Hyposplenism resolved as the lymphangiectasia improved clinically. It was proposed that lymphocyte loss into the gut may have resulted in hyposplenism. Further study of splenic function in intestinal lymphangiectasia is necessary to confirm this report (162).

In a case of chronic acitve hepatitis in an adult there was absence of the spleen on sulfur-colloid scanning. After treatment with high-dose steroids, splenic function returned (136). The mechanism involved in producing hyposplenism and the significance of this single case is unclear.

Malignancies

There have been many case reports of hyposplenism occurring in association with malignancies in adults. The malignancies involved have included Sezary syndrome (135), multiple myeloma (163), gastric carcinoma (164), breast carcinoma (165), primary splenic angiosarcoma (166,167), and immunoblastic as well as lymphoblastic lymphoma (168). The pathophysiology of the hyposplenia in these malignant diseases appears to involve direct splenic infiltration by malignant cells (165,168), or obstruction of either the splenic artery or the splenic vein (164).

Although none of these reported cases involved children, they do suggest that similar findings might be found in childhood malignancies. Using enumeration of erythrocyte pits, splenic function was studied in 181 children with cancer (169). Approximately one-third of the children demonstrated increased numbers of pitted erythrocytes; 13% of the patients had pit counts greater than 3.0%. The newly diagnosed, untreated patients did not demonstrate increases in red cell pits, while patients who had undergone therapy did show increased pit counts. However, there was no correlation between the percentage of pitted red cells and either the specific chemotherapy used or the activity of the disease. Increased numbers of red cell pits were seen in patients in remission, regardless of whether they were on or off therapy, as well as patients in relapse.

Children with acute lymphoblastic leukemia and Wilms' tumor were more likely to have increased red cell pitting, while those with neuroblastoma, non-Hodgkin's lymphoma and other solid tumors were less likely to have increased numbers of pitted erythrocytes. The significance of these findings is not clear. It seems unlikely that the finding of increased red cell pit counts is an isolated effect of therapy alone. However, the absence of this finding at diagnosis and its presence in patients in remission, in both those on and off therapy, certainly makes it unlikely that increased red cell pitting is primarily related to the malignancy itself. Further studies are necessary to better understand this finding.

Another question is whether this relatively mild degree of hyposplenism predisposes these patients to infection. Children with cancer do develop *Hemophilus influenzae* and *Streptococcus pneumoniae* infections which usually occur in remission and are unrelated to neutropenia (170,171). The small percentage of patients in this study with pit counts above 3% may have been at increased risk for septicemia. One of the 181 children did develop sepsis, but that is not conclusive (169). With such minor degrees of hyposplenism it may be difficult to prove conclusively whether there is such an increased risk of serious infection.

Splenic irradiation used as part of cancer therapy is associated with hyposplenism. Irradiation of the spleen in a dose of approximately 4,000 rad (40 G) will cause splenic atrophy (172). The average weight of the spleen of patients with Hodgkin's disease who received such irradiation was 75 grams compared to a weight of 210 grams in those patients who were not given splenic irradiation. On pathological examination, the irradiated spleens contained fibrosis, atrophy of the red pulp, intimal thickening of the vasculature, and loss of sinusoidal patterns (172,173).

Twenty-five patients with lymphomas who were treated with splenic irradiation were studied 5 to 16 years later with erythrocyte pit counts and sulfur-colloid scans. As many as 13 out of 14 patients with Hodgkin's disease and 5 out of 6 patients with non-Hodgkin's lymphomas had red cell pit counts above the normal range. The mean pit count for both groups was 13%, compared to 0.94% for the normal controls. Size of the spleen of patients treated with splenic irradiation, as measured by splenic diameter on sulfur-colloid scanning, was significantly smaller than that of controls. The onset of splenic hypofunction following irradiation appears to be a gradual process (174). Chemotherapy does not appear to play a role in its development (172). This hyposplenism has been observed in children and it has been clearly associated with increased risk of bacterial septicemia (174).

Thorotrast is a colloidal suspension which was used in the 1940's to treat liver tumors. It causes splenic and hepatic fibrosis, with resulting hyposplenia (175, 176). Overwhelming pneumococcal septicemia has been reported in patients who were treated with thorotrast (175).

Miscellaneous Conditions Associated with Hyposplenism

These include systemic amyloidosis, drug-induced hyposplenia, the "born again" spleen, malignant mastocytosis, fibronectin deficiency, and various experimentally-induced conditions.

Systemic amyloidosis is associated with hyposplenia (32,177-182). Howell-Jolly bodies and other peripheral blood findings characteristic of hyposplenism and abnormal sulfur-colloid scans were found in 24% of 91 patients. Interestingly, the sulfur-colloid scans were not always abnormal when Howell-Jolly bodies were seen (32). None of the patients reported were children.

Pathological examination of the spleen in patients with amyloidosis reveals amyloid replacement of the splenic cords. Presumably, this replacement of normal tissue by amyloid causes the hyposplenism (179). There may be a relationship between amyloid involvement of the spleen and the deficiency of factor X that occurs in amyloidosis. Amyloid fibrils in the liver and spleen may remove part of the factor X molecule from the circulation, causing its deficiency. Splenectomy may improve the factor X deficiency (181,182).

Patients with amyloidosis who have hyposplenism have poorer survival rates than those who have normal splenic function. It appears that this finding is primarily a reflection of the severity of the amyloidosis, with severe cases having hyposplenism, and is not due to a greater risk of infection (32). Overwhelming septicemia has not been reported in cases of amyloidosis.

Intravenous gamma globulin is the most important pharmacologic agent that induces hyposplenism. Further study is needed to completely elucidate its mechanism of action, which may be multifactorial. It seems clear, however, that intravenous gamma globulin blocks the clearance of IgG-sensitized red cells by way of competitive inhibition of Fc-receptors in the spleen and the reticuloendothelial system. Other mechanisms, including interference with immune regulation, may also be involved in causing hyposplenism (183,184). It is assumed that the primary effect of gamma globulin on the spleen is inhibition of imune function. It is not clear if other splenic functions, such as culling or clearance of particulate matter, are affected.

The hyposplenism induced by gamma globulin was initially used as therapy in autoimmune hematologic disorders to specifically block destruction of antibody-coated hematologic cells. It is now being used experimentally in a variety of other disorders which may have autoimmune etiologies (185). Further discussion of gamma globulin, a rapidly evolving therapeutic modality, is beyond the scope of this discussion.

Gold thiomolate (sodium aurothiomolate), which is used in the treatment of rheumatoid arthritis, can impair splenic function (126). Three out of 4 normal subjects given 100 mg of gold developed severe impairment of heat-treated red cell clearances by the spleen. This finding indicated that splenic hypofunction was due to gold therapy and not the underlying rheumatoid arthritis. The clinical significance of this impairment is unknown.

Methyldopa is another drug which can impair reticuloendothelial function (21). This drug was investigated in an attempt to understand why the 20% of patients who develop anti-erythrocyte antibodies while using this drug rarely develop hemolysis. Of 5 patients with anti-erythrocyte antibodies induced by methyldopa, 4 demonstrated impaired Fc-dependent receptor function as measured by impaired clearance of IgG-sensitized autologous erythrocytes. These 4 had no clinical evidence of hemolysis, while the one patient who demonstrated hemolysis had normal Fc-receptor function. Four other patients who were given methyldopa but who did not have anti-erythrocyte antibodies also had impaired Fc-receptor function. This finding suggests that hemolysis often fails to develop in patients given methyldopa who have anti-erythrocyte antibodies because the drug impairs the Fc-receptor mediated destruction of the antibody-coated red cells. Splenic function in these patients has not been assessed using other techniques.

Overwhelming septicemia has not been reported as a complication of methyldopa therapy. Given the usually uneventful or self limited clinical course of patients given methyldopa, the clinical significance of this finding is unclear.

It has been proposed that corticosteroids may induce hyposplenism. Corticosteroids do inhibit binding to Fc receptors in the reticuloendothelial system, but it is not clear whether this causes a significant impairment of splenic function. One study suggested that patients with well-controlled acute rheumatic fever on moderate to high doses of corticosteroids have impaired reticuloendothelial clearance of specific lipid emulsions. This was not true for patients with other disorders, such as systemic lupus erythematosis and polymyositis. But disease activity in these patients was poorly controlled in spite of steroid therapy (186). A single case report of functional asplenia in idiopathic thrombocytopenia purpura was also attributed in part to steroid therapy, but these changes in splenic function may have been related to the underlying autoimmune process (137). Neither report provides strong evidence that corticosteroids cause hyposplenism.

Minimal change nephrotic syndrome has also been associated with hyposplenia (186a). Three of seven patients with minimal change disease, as well as one with focal glomerulosclerosis, demonstrated prolonged clearance of heat-treated erythrocytes. Bacterial infections other than overwhelming sepsis appeared to be more common in the patients with hyposplenia. The mechanism is unclear. There is conflicting data whether HLA-B8 (and its association with hyposplenia) (138) is more common in patients with this disease. There are also several theories, as yet unsubstantiated, that this disorder may have an autoimmune basis.

The "born-again spleen" syndrome should be mentioned. Splenosis, or the development of autologous implants of splenic tissue, has long been recognized to occur following splenectomy for rupture of the spleen. It was thought to be a rare phenomenon, but the ease of doing red cell pit counts allowed surveys of surgically asplenic patients. In a study of 22 children undergoing splenectomy for splenic rupture, 13 had red cell pit counts well below the range expected in asplenia. Sulfur-colloid scans demonstrated multiple nodules capable of concentrating the colloid. This phenomenon was labelled the "born-again" spleen.

It was felt that the high incidence of splenosis in these patients might help to account for the lower incidence of septicemia in patients undergoing splenectomy for trauma as opposed to those undergoing splenectomy for other indications (187). A second study confirmed that splenectomized children do demonstrate evidence of splenosis, although the incidence was lower. However, there was no evidence of the born-again spleen among 17 adults, with the exception of one patient with an accessory spleen (188). It is not clear whether this is due to an increased likelihood of finding accessory spleens in children (189) or, more likely, due to a greater ability of the splenic cells of children to successfully form implants.

The functional capabilities of these implants in preventing post-splenectomy sepsis is unknown. Although these implants are capable of concentrating sulfur-colloid, red cell pit counts in these patients are often within the asplenic range or at least above the normal range. It is not known whether the born-again spleen is capable of adequate clearance of encapsulated bacteria in humans. Studies using animal models of splenosis have produced conflicting results (190, 191). Until better information is produced conflicting results (190,191). Until better information is available, the born-again spleen remains a potentially hyposplenic condition.

In recent years, the risk of post-splenectomy sepsis has resulted in the use of nonsurgical management of splenic rupture. In order to determine whether hyposplenism may result from nonsurgical management of splenic rupture, 22 patients treated in this fashion were evaluated after a minimum interval of 6 months. None demonstrated any Howell-Jolly bodies and all had normal red pit counts (192). Thus, nonsurgical management of splenic rupture does not appear to result in impairment of splenic function.

In one case of malignant mastocytosis in an adult, the spleen failed to demonstrate splenic uptake of technetium sulfur-colloid. Although there was no primary skin involvement, visceral organs including the spleen and bone marrow were heavily infiltrated with mast cells. The hyposplenia was presumably due to replacement of normal splenic tissue by mast cells (193). The significance of this single case is unclear.

Fibronectin, a major opsonin, may be important in the clearance of particulate debris. An adult patient with pneumococcal pneumonia and septicemia was found to have significant fibronectin consumption and reticuloendothelial blockade, with no splenic uptake of technetium sulfur-colloid. The clinical significance of this splenic hypofunction is unknown, but it is interesting to consider that such a blockade might be reversible by providing fibronectin with fresh frozen plasma (194,195).

Hyposplenism has been induced in a number of experimental models. The significance of these models for humans is unclear. Several viral infections are capable of causing splenic damage in animal models. Lymphoid depletion as well as necrosis of the spleen have been associated with experimental infections with cytomegalovirus, dengue virus, coxsackievirus B, and lymphocytic choriomeningitis virus (196-199). Lassa fever, a rare severe febrile viral illness indigenous to Africa, has been reported to cause splenic damage in humans. Although there was no premortem evidence of hyposplenism, autopsy findings included depletion of reticuloendothelial elements in the splenic pulp and marked splenic congestion (200). Disseminated varicella has been associated with splenic infarction and functional asplenia in a child with acute lymphoblastic leukemia. The child has disseminated intravascular coagulation and it is not clear whether the asplenia was related to the infection or the secondary coagulopathy (200a). It remains unclear whether viral infections can cause clinically significant hyposplenism, but the theoretical possibility needs to be considered.

Animal studies have suggested that asplenia may occur during folate deficiency (153,201). This finding has not been recognized in folate-deficient humans.

In other animal models, certain lipid emulsions containing ethyl palmitate and methyl palmitate can result in chemical splenectomy (202). These lipids have not been used in man, although the possibility of splenic blockade with newly developed lipid emulsions should be considered.

SUMMARY AND CONCLUSIONS

A wide variety of disorders can impaire splenic function. The pathophysiology appears to be clearly defined in some instances, such as in congenital asplenia and in disorders of splenic vascular obstruction or congestion of the spleen. In other situations, such as in the autoimmune and gastrointestinal disorders, the mechanism remains poorly defined.

Overwhelming bacterial septicemia has been reported to occur in some disorders that are associated with evidence of hyposplenism, but not in others. The absence of reported cases of septicemia in many of these hyposplenic disorders should not be interpreted to mean that it does not occur. There are several reasons why the occurrence of overwhelming septicemia could easily be missed. First, the lack of awareness of the association of hyposplenism with many of these disorders might easily cause such occurrences to go unrecognized and unreported. Secondly, the incidence of septicemia is very low. The risk of sepsis with surgical asplenia is only 1.5% (203), while the highest incidence rates with disorders such as sickle cell anemia are no higher than 10 to 15% (125). In disorders with partial impairment of splenic function, as opposed to total absence of splenic function, the incidence of septicemia could presumably be even less than the 1.5% incidence following splenectomy for trauma. Given these data, a very large number of patients would likely have to become asplenic before one would develop septicemia that would be recognized as being related to hyposplenism. An excellent case in point is the failure to recognize post-splenectomy sepsis syndrome as a complication of splenectomy until the 1950s. Finally, the age of the patients studied is important. The risk of septicemia is known to be considerably lower in adults than in children (203-205). Therefore, studies of adults may underestimate the incidence of septicemia in children.

Many of the disorders reported to cause hyposplenism in adults have not been noted to cause hyposplenism in children. In instances such as celiac disease, it may take many years for hyposplenism to develop, so that it is much less likely for a child to manifest this complication. In other instances, the primary disorder is so uncommon in pediatrics that not enough children have been studied to be confident that the hyposplenia and its associated risk of sepsis are not potential complications.

Hyposplenia-related bacterial septicemia is a catastrophic complication. If a patient develops a disorder that is potentially associated with impaired splenic function, the patient's peripheral blood should be observed for signs of hyposplenia. If the technique is available, enumeration of erythrocyte pits should be performed. If not, performing other studies of splenic function, such as radionuclide scans, should be considered depending on the incidence of hyposplenia in that particular disorder. If evidence of asplenia develops, pneumococcal (and depending on age) *Hemophilus influenzae* vaccines should be administered, penicillin prophylaxis should be given at least in younger children, and significant febrile episodes managed aggressively. Most importantly, the patient and family should be carefully educated about this complication. Most deaths from hyposplenia-related septicemia are preventable.

REFERENCES

1. Peters PE, Lorenz R, Fischer M: Splenic imaging. *Lymphology* 1983;16: 90-100.
2. Froelich JW, Simeone JF, McKusick KA et al: Radionucleotide imaging and ultrasound in liver-spleen trauma: a prospective comparison. *Radiology* 1982;145:457-461.
3. Koga T, Morikawa Y: Ultrasonographic determination of the splenic size and its clinical usefulness in various liver diseases. *Radiology* 1975;115:157-161.
4. Lutzker LG: Radionucleotide imaging of the injured spleen and liver. *Semin Nucl Med* 1983;13:184-198.
5. Kaufman RA: Liver-spleen computed tomography: a method tailored for infants and children. *CT* 1983;7:45-58.
6. Cools L, Osteaux M, Divano L et al: Prediction of splenic volume by a simple CT measurement; a statistical study. *J Comput Assist Tomogr* 1983; 7:426-430.
7. Mendelson DS, Cohen BA, Armos RR: CT appearance of splenosis; case report. *J Comput Assist Tomogr* 1982;6:1188-1190.
8. Gentry LR, Brown JM, Lindgren RD: Splenosis: CT demonstration of heterotopic autotransplantation of splenic tissue. *J Comput Assist Tomogr* 1982;6:1184-1187.
9. Vermess M, Lau DHM, Adams MD et al: Biodistribution study of ethiodized oil emulsion 13 for computed tomography of the liver and spleen. *J Comput Assist Tomogr* 1982;6:1115-1119.
10. Coride VJ, Sostman HD, Twickler J et al: Brominated radiopaque liposomes: Contrast agent for computed tomography of liver and spleen: A preliminary report. *Invest Radiol* 1982;17:381-385.
11. Higgins CB, Goldberg H, Hricak H et al: Nuclear magnetic reasonance of vasculature of abdominal viscera: normal and pathologic features. *AJR* 1983;1217-1225.

12. Armos RR: Splenic function and imaging studies. *Semin Nucl Med* 1985; 15:260-275.
13. Crome P, Mollison PL: Splenic distruction of Rh-sensitized, and of heated red cells. *Br J Haematol* 1964;10:137-154.
14. Ehrlich CP, Papavicolaou N, Treves S et al: Splenic scintigraphy using Tc-99-m-labelled heat-denatured red blood cells in pediatric patients: Concise communication. *J Nucl Med* 1982;23:209-213.
15. Rao BK, Shore RM, Leiberman LM et al: Dual radiopharmaceutical imaging in congenital asplenia syndrome. *Radiology* 1982;145:805-810.
16. McIntyre PA, Wagner HN Jr: Current procedures for scanning of the spleen. *Ann Intern Med* 1970;73:995-1001.
17. Sty Jr, Conwax JJ: The spleen: Development and functional evaluations. *Semin Nucl Med* 1985;15:276-298.
18. Spencer RP: Spleen scanning as a diagnostic tool. *JAMA* 1977;237:1473-1474.
19. Hauser GJ, Silberman C: Incidental discovery of asplenia syndrome, with situs inversus and a normal heart by radionuclide biliary imaging: A case report. *Clin Nucl Med* 1982;7:543-545.
20. Lockwood CM, Worlledge S, Nicholas A: Reversal of impaired splenic function in patients with nephritis or vasculitis (or both) by plasma exchange. *N Engl J Med* 1979;300:534-530.
21. Kelton JG: Impaired reticuloendothelial function in patients treated with methyldopa. *N Engl J Med* 1985;313:596-600.
22. Frank MM, Hamburger MI, Lawley TJ et al: Defective reticuloendothelial system Fc-receptor function in systemic lupus erythematosis. *N Engl J Med* 1979;300:518-523.
23. Crosby WH: Hyposplenism: An inquiry into normal functions of the spleen. *Annu Rev Med* 1963;14:349-370.
24. Wintrobe MM, Lee RG, Boggs DR et al: Clinical Hematology, Lea and Febriger, Philadelphia, PA, 1981, pp 259-270.
25. Polhemus DW, Schafer WB: Absent spleen syndrome: Hematologic findings as an aid to diagnosis. *Pediatrics* 1959;24:254-257.
26. Sills RH, Hadley RAR: The significance of nucleated red blood cells in the peripheral blood of children. *Am J Pediatr Hematol Oncol* 1983;5:174-177.
27. Lipson RL, Bayrd ED, Watkins CH: The postsplenectomy blood picture. *Am J Clin Path* 1949;32:526-532.
28. Singer K, Miller EB, Dameshek W: Hematologic changes following splenectomy in man with particular reference to target cells. *Am J Med Sci* 1941; 202:171-180.
29. Dhowan V, Spencer RP, Pearson HA et al: Functional asplenia in the absence of Howell-Jolly bodies. *Clin Nucl Med* 1977;2:395-396.
30. Ryan FP, Smart RC, Holdsworth CD, Preston FE: Hyposplenism in inflammatory bowel disease. *Gut* 1978;19:50-55.
31. Marsh GW, Stewart JS: Splenic function in adult coeliac disease. *Br J Haematol* 1970;19:445-457.

32. Gertz MA, Kyle RA, Greipp PR: Hyposplenism in primary systemic amyloidosis. *Ann Intern Med* 1983;98:475-477.
33. Casper JT, Koethe S, Rodey FE et al: A new method for studying splenic reticuloendothelial function in sickle cell disease and its clinical application. *Blood* 1976;47:183-191.
34. Robertson DAF, Bullen AW, Hall R et al: Blood film appearances in the hyposplenism of coeliac disease. *Br J Clin Pract* 1983;37:19-22.
35. Holrodye CP, Gardner FH: Acquisition of autophagic vacuoles by human erythrocytes; Physiologic role of the spleen. *Blood* 1970;36:566-575.
36. Schnitzer B, Rucknagel DL, Spencer HH: Erythrocytes: pits and vacuoles as seen with transmission and scanning electron microscopy. *Science* 1971; 173:251-252.
37. Kent G, Minick OT, Volini FT et al: Autophagic vacuoles in human red cells. *Am J Pathol* 1966;48:831-841.
38. Pearson HA, McIntosh S, Ritchey AK: Developmental aspects of splenic function in sickle cell anemia. *Blood* 1978;53:358-365.
39. Sills RH, Oski FA: RBC surface pits in the sickle hemoglobinopathies. *Am J Dis Child* 1979;133:526-527.
40. O'Grady JG, Harding B, Egan EL et al: "Pitted erythrocytes": Impaired formation in splenectomized subjects with congenital spherocytosis. *Br J Haematol* 1984;57:441-446.
40a. Buchanan GR, Holtkamp CA: Pocked erythrocyte counts in patients with hereditary spherocytosis before and after splenectomy. *Am J Hematol* 1987;25:253-257.
41. Holrodye CP, Oski FA, Gardner FH: The "pocked" erythrocyte. Red-cell surface alterations in reticuloendothelial immaturity of the neonate. *N Engl J Med* 1969;281:516-520.
42. Freedman RM, Johnston D, Mahoney MJ et al: Development of splenic reticuloendothelial function in neonates. *J Pediatr* 1980;96:466-468.
43. Neilan BA, Berney SN: Hyposplenism in systemic lupus erythematosis. *J Rheumatol* 1983;10:332-334.
44. Corazza GR, Bullen AW, Hall R et al: Simple method of assessing splenic function in coeliac disease. *Clin Sci* 1981;60:109-113.
45. Corazza GR, Tarozzi C, Vaira D et al: Return of splenic function after splenectomy: How much tissue is needed? *Br Med J* 1984;289:861-864.
46. Pearson HA, Chilcote R, Sullivan E et al: Splenic function in sickle cell disease in America and Saudi Arabia. *Pediatr Res* 1983;17:240A.
47. Pearson HA, Falleta J, Chilcote R et al: Splenic function in sickle cell disease. *Pediatr Res* 1982;16:211A.
48. McBride JA, Dacie JV, Shopley R: The effect of splenectomy on the leucocyte count. *Br J Haematol* 1968;14:225-231.
49. Ellison EC, Fabri PJ: Complications of splenectomy: Etiology, prevention and management. *Surg Clin North Am* 1983;63:1313-1330.
50. Tanum G, Sonstevold A, Jakobsen E: The effect of splenectomy on platelet formation and megakaryocyte DNA content in rats. *Blood* 1984;63:593-597.

51. Schumacher MJ: Serum immunoglobulin and transferrin levels after childhood splenectomy. *Arch Dis Child* 1970;45:114-117.
52. Padmanabhan J, Risemberg HM, Rome RD: Howell-Jolly bodies in the peripheral blood of full-term and premature neonates. *Johns Hopkins Med J* 1973;132:146-150.
53. Acevedo G, Mauer AM: The capacity for removal of eryrthrocytes containing Heinz bodies in premature infants and patients following splenectomy. *J Pediatr* 1963;63:61-64.
54. Ossoylu S, Hosein F, Mc Intyre PA: Functional development of phagocyte activity of the spleen. *J Pediatr* 1977;90:560-562.
55. Biggar WD, Ramirez RA, Rose V: Congenital asplenia: Immunologic assessment and a clinical review of eight surviving patients. *Pediatrics* 1981;67:548-551.
56. Waldman JD, Rosenthal A, Smith AL et al: Sepsis and congenital asplenia. *J Pediatr* 1977;90:555-559.
57. Muir CS: Splenic agenesis and multilobulate spleen. *Arch Dis Child* 1959;34:431-435.
58. Brivet F, Herer B, Fremaux A et al: Fatal post-splenectomy pneumococcal sepsis despite pneumococcal vaccine and penicillin prophylaxis (letter). *Lancet* 1984;2:356-357.
59. Kevy SV, Tefft M, Vawter GF et al: Hereditary splenic hypoplasia. *Pediatrics* 1968;42:752-757.
60. Muir CS: Splenic agenesis and multilobulate spleen. *Arch Dis Child* 1959;34:431-435.
61. Pearson HA: The spleen and disturbances of splenic function. In Nathan DG, Oski FA (eds): *Hematology of Infancy and Childhood*. WB Saunders, Philadelphia, PA, 1981, pp 887-907.
62. Putschar WGJ, Manion WC: Congenital absence of the spleen and associated anomalies. *Am J Clin Path* 1956;26:429-469.
63. Arnold GL, Bixlar D, Girod P: Probably autosomal recessive inheritance of polysplenia, situs inversus and cardiac defects in an Amish family. *Am J Med Genet* 1983;16:35-42.
64. Smith DW, Jones EL: *Recognizable Patterns of Human Malformation*. Philadelphia, PA, 1982, pp 458-459.
64a. Abramson SJ, Berdon WE, Altman RP, Amodio JB, Levy J: Biliary atresia and noncardiac polysplenic syndrome: US and surgical considerations. *Radiology* 1987;163:377-379.
65. Rodin AE1, Sloane JA, Nghiem QX: Polysplenia with severe congenital heart disease and Howell-Jolly bodies. *Am J Clin Pathol* 1972;58:127-134.
66. Sills RH, Deshpande GN, Humbert Jr: Unpublished observations.
67. Garriga S, Crobsy WH: The incidence of leukemia in families of patients with hypoplasia of the marrow. *Blood* 1959;14:1008-1014.
68. Stoddard RA, McCurnin DC, Shultenover SJ et al: Syndrome of refractory sideroblastic anemia with vacuolization of marrow precursors and exocrine pancreatic dysfunction presenting in the neonate. *J Pediatr* 1981;99:259-261.

69. Pearson HA, Lobel JS, Kochoshis SA et al: A new syndrome of refractory sideroblastic anemia with vacuolization of marrow precursors and exocrine pancreatic dysfunction. *J Pediatr* 1979;95:976-984.
70. Robinson RG, Adler R, Swanson VL et al: Congenital hypoplastic anemia (CHA) associated with congenital absence of the spleen. *Am J Pediatr Hematol Oncol* 1982;4:341-343.
70a. Lutz P, Seiller F, Desfossez J, et al: Erythroblastopenia chronique avec hyposplenic chez une filette de dix ans. *Ann Pediatr (Paris)* 1985;32:537-539.
71. Cox DR, Martin L, Hall BD: Asplenia syndrome after fetal exposure to warfarin. *Lancet* 1977;2:1134.
72. Zago MA, Figueiredo MS, Conas PT, Botturd C: Aspects of splenic hypofunction in old age. *Klin Wochenshcr* 1985;63:590-592.
73. Pearson HA, Cornelius EA, Schwartz AD, et al: Transfusion-reversible functional asplenia in sickle cell anemia. *N Engl J Med* 1970;283:334-337.
74. Serjeant GR: *Sickle Cell Disease*. Oxford University Press, Oxford, 1985, pp 115-123.
75. Vaidya S, Serjeant GR: Early splenomegaly in homozygous sickle-cell disease: an indicator of susceptibility to infection. *Lancet* 1978;2:963-965.
76. Pearson HA, Spencer RP, Cornelius EA: Functional asplenia in sickle-cell anemia. *N Engl J Med* 1969;281:923-926.
77. O'Brien RT, McIntosh LS, Aspnes GT et al: Prospective study of sickle cell anemia in infancy. *J Pediatr* 1976;89:205-210.
78. Zago MA, Bottura C: Splenic function in sickle-cell diseases. *Clin Sci* 1983; 65:297-302.
79. Rogers DW, Serjeant BE, Serjeant GR: Early rise in "pitted" red cell count as a guide to susceptibility to infection in childhood sickle cell anemia. *Arch Dis Child* 1982;5:338-342.
80. Al-Awamy B, Wilson WA, Pearson HA: Splenic function in sickle cell disease in the Eastern province of Saudi Arabia. *J Pediatr* 1984;104:714-717.
81. Babiker MA, El-Hazmi MAF, Al-Jobori AM, et al: Splenic function in children with sickle cell disease: Two different patterns in Saudi Arabia. *Scand J Haematol* 1985;35:191-193.
82. Mallouh A, Burke GM, Salamah M, et al: Splenic function in Saudi children with sickle cell disease. *Ann Trop Paediatr* 1984;4:87-91.
83. Johnston RB Jr, Newman SL, Struth AE: An abnormality of the alternate pathway of complement activation in sickle-cell disease. *N Engl J Med* 1973; 288:803-806.
84. Koethe SM, Casper JT, Rodney GE: Alternative complement pathway activity in sera from patients with sickle cell disease. *Clin Exp Immunol* 1976; 23:56-60.
85. Winkelstein JA, Drachman RH: Deficiency of pneumococcal serum opsonizing activity in sickle cell disease. *N Engl J Med* 1968;279:459-466.
86. Constantopoulous A, Najjar VT, Wish JB: Defective phagocytosis due to tuftsin deficiency in splenectomized subjects. *Am J Dis Child* 1973;125: 663-665.

87. Spirer Z, Weisman Y, Zakuth V: Decreased serum tuftsin concentrations in sickle cell disease. *Arch Dis Child* 1980;55:566–567.
88. Gavrilis P, Rothenburg SP, Guy DR: Correlation of low serum IgM levels with absence of functional splenic tissue in sickle cell disease syndromes. *Am J Med* 1974;57:542–545.
89. Wintrobe MM, Lee GR, Boggs DR, et al: *Hematology*, 8th edition. Lea and Febiger, Philadelphia, PA, 1981, p. 843.
90. Barrett-Connor E: Bacterial infection and sickle cell anemia. *Medicine* 1971; 50:97.
91. Overturf GD, Powars P, Baroff LJ: Bacterial meningitis and septicemia in sickle cell disease. *Am J Dis Child* 1977;131:784–787.
92. Brainbridge R, Higgs DR, Maude PH, Serjeant GR: Clinical presentation of homozygous sickle cell disease. *J Pediatr* 1985;106:881–885.
93. Powars D, Overturf G, Weiss J: Pneumococcal septicemia in children with sickle cell anemia. *JAMA* 1981;245:1839–1842.
94. Serjeant GR: Treatment of sickle cell disease in early childhood in Jamaica. *Am J Pediatr Hematol Oncol* 1985;7:235–239.
94a. Gaston MH, Vertes JI: Prophylaxis with oral penicillin in children with sickle cell anemia. *New Engl J Med* 1986;314:1593–1596.
94b. Buchanan GR, Siegel JD, Smith SJ, DePasse BM: Oral penicillin prophylaxis in children with impaired splenic function; a study of compliance. *Pediatrics* 1982;70:926–930.
95. Buchanan GR, Smith SJ, Holtkamp CA et al: Bacterial infection and splenic reticuloendothelial function in children with hemoglobin S-C disease. *Pediatrics* 1983;72:93–98.
96. Chilcote RR, Dampier C: Overwhelming pneumococcal septicemia in a patient with HbSC disease and splenic dysfunction. *J Pediatr* 1984;104:734–736.
97. Sills RH: Splenic function in children with hemoglobin SC disease and sickle Beta-thalassemia. *J Natl Med Assoc* 1983;75:991–994.
98. Ballas SK, Lewis CN, Noone AM, et al: Clinical, hematological and biochemical features of Hb SC disease. *Am J Hematol* 1982;13:37–51.
99. Sears DA, Udden MM: Splenic infarction, splenic sequestration and functional hyposplenism in hemoglobin S-C disease. *Am J Hematol* 1985;18: 261–268.
100. Topley JM, Cupidore L, Vaidya S, et al: Pneumococcal and other infections in children with sickle cell-hemoglobin C (SC) disease. *J Pediatr* 1982;101: 176–179.
101. Engelstad BL: Functional asplenia in hemoglobin SE disease. *Clin Nucl Med* 1982;7:100–102.
101a. Kelleher JF Jr, Park JOK: Life-threatening complications in a child with hemoglobin SD-Los Angeles Disease. *Hemoglobin* 1984;8:203–213.
102. Alter BP, Rappeport JM, Parkman R: The bone marrow failure syndromes. In, Nathan DG, Oski FA (eds): *Hematology of Infancy and Childhood*. W. B. Saunders, Philadelphia, PA, 1981, p. 225.

103. Hardisty RM, Wolff HH: Haemorrhagic thrombocythaemia: a clinical and laboratory study. *Brit J Haematol* 1955;1:390-405.
104. Gunz FW: Hemorrhagic thrombocythemia: a critical review. *Blood* 1960; 15:706-723.
105. Marsh GW, Lewis SM, Szur L: The use of 51 Cr-labelled heat damaged red cells to study splenic function. *Br J Haematol* 1966;12:167-172.
106. Polga JP, Holstein G, Spencer RP: Radiocolloid redistribution and multiple splenic infarcts in myelofibrosis. *Clin Nucl Med* 1983;8:335-336.
107. Chen LT: Intrasplenic microcirculation in rats with acute hemolytic anemia. *Blood* 1980;56:737-740.
108. Chen LT, Moxon ER: Effect of splenic congestion associated with hemolytic anemia on mortality of rats challenged with Haemophilus influenzae b. *Am J Hematol* 1983;15:117-121.
109. Krueger HC, Burgert EO Jr: Hereditary spherocytosis in 100 children. *Mayo Clin Proc* 1966;41:821-830.
110. Spencer RP, Pearson HA: Splenic radiocolloid uptake in the presence of circulating Howell-Jolly bodies. *J Nucl Med* 1974;15:294-295.
111. Wyler DJ, Quinn TC, Chen LT: Relationship of alterations in splenic clearance function and microcirculation to host defense in acute rodent malaria. *J Clin Invest* 1981;65:1400-1404.
112. Ferguson A: Hazards of splenectomy. *Br Med J* 1982;285:1375-1376.
113. Spencer RP, Sqiklas JJ, Turner JW: Functional obstruction of splenic blood vessels in adults: a radiocolloid study. *Int J Nucl Med Biol* 1982; 9:208-211.
113a. O'Keefe JH Jr, Holmes DR Jr, Schaff HV, Sheedy PT II, Edwards WD: Thromboembolic splenic infarction. *Mayo Clin Proc* 1986;61:967-972.
114. Lawrence SE, Pussell BA, Charlesworth JA: Splenic function in primary glomerulonephritis. *Adv Exp Med Biol* 1982;155:641-648.
115. McGinley E, Martin W, Henderson N, et al: Defective splenic reticuloendothelial function in idiopathic membranous nephropathy. *Clin Exp Immunol* 1984;56:295-301.
116. Frank MM, Jaffee CJ, Kimberly RP, et al: An immunospecific clearance defect in patients with systemic lupus erythematosis (SLE) related to levels of circulating immune complexes. *Clin Res* 1977;25:357A.
117. Kelton J, Singer J, Rodger C, et al: The concentration of IgG in the serum is a major determinant of Fc-dependent reticuloendothelial function. *Blood* 1985;66:495-498.
118. Pines A, Kaplinsky N, Olchonsky D, et al: Hyposplenism in systemic lupus erythematosis. *Br H Rheumatol* 1983;22:176-178.
119. Dillon AM, Stein HB, English RA: Splenic atrophy in systemic lupus erythematosis. *Ann Intern Med* 1982;96:40-43.
120. Dillon AM, Stein HB, Kassen BO et al: Hyposplenia in a patient with systemic lupus erythematosis. *J Rheumatol* 1980;7:196-198.
121. Lawley TJ: Immune complexes and reticuloendothelial system functions in human diseases. *J Invest Derm* 1980;74:339-343.

122. Foster PN, Hardy GJ, Losowsky MS: Fatal salmonella septicaemia in a patient with systemic lupus erythematosis and splenic atrophy. *Brit J Clin Proc* 1984;38:434–435.
123. Jarolim DR: Asplenia and rheumatoid arthritis (letter). *Ann Intern Med* 1982;97:616–617.
124. Williams BD, Pussell BA, Lockwood CM et al: Defective reticuloendothelial system function in rheumatoid arthritis. *Lancet* 1979;1:1311–1314.
125. Gordon PA, Davis P, Russell AS, et al: Splenic reticuloendothelial function in patients with active rheumatoid arthritis. *J Rheumatol* 1981;8:490–493.
126. Williams BD, Lockwood CM, Pussell BA: Inhibition of reticuloendothelial function by gold and its relation to past injection reactions. *Br Med J* 1979;2:235–238.
127. Al-Eid MA, Tutschka PJ, Wagner HN Jr: Functional asplenia in patients with chronic graft-versus-host disease: Concise communication. *J Nucl Med* 1983;24:1123–1126.
128. Demetrakopoulos GE, Tsokos GC, Levine AS: Recovery of splenic function after GVHD-associated functional asplenia. *Am J Hematol* 1982;12:77–80.
129. Lascari AD: *Hematologic Manifestations of Childhood Diseases*, Theime-Statton Inc., NY, 1984, p 280.
130. Guyton JR, Fumwalt RE: Pneumococcemia with sarcoid-infiltrated spleen (letter). *Ann Intern Med* 1975;82:847–848.
131. Stone RW, Mc Daniel WR, Armstrong EM et al: Acquired functional asplenia in sarcoidosis. *J Natl Med Assoc* 1985;77:930–936.
132. Brownlie BEW, Hamer JW, Cook HB, et al: Thyrotoxicosis associated with splenic atrophy (letter). *Lancet* 1975;2:1046–1047.
133. Bullen AW, Hall R, Gowland G et al: Hyposplenism, adult coeliac disease, and autoimmunity. *Gut* 1980;21:28–33.
134. Taylor CJ: Recurrent meningitis in a child with combined IgA deficiency and splenic hypoplasia (letter). *Arch Dis Child* 1981;56:486.
135. Hazenberg HJA, Hiddink HJM, Link EAM, et al: In-111 leucocyte scanning and partial functional asplenia in a patient with Sezary syndrome. *Clin Nucl Med* 1983;8:3–6.
136. Dhawan VM, Spencer RP, Szikles JJ: Reversible functional asplenia in chronic aggressive hepatitis. *J Nucl Med* 1979;20:34–36.
137. Dekker PT, Propp RP: Functional asplenia in idiopathic thrombocytopenic purpura. *NY State J Med* 1977;77:2282–2285.
138. Lawley TJ, Hall RP, Fauci AS, et al: Defective Fc-receptor functions associated with the HLA-B8/DR w3 haplotype: Studies in patients with dermatitis herpetiformis and normal subjects. *N Engl J Med* 1981;304:185–192.
139. O'Grady JG, Stevens FM, McCarthy CF: Genetic influences on splenic function in coeliac disease. *Gut* 1985;26:1004–1007.

140. Robinson PJ, Bullen AW, Hall R, et al: Splenic size and functions in adult coeliac disease. *Brit J Radiol* 1980;53:532-537.
141. O'Grady JG, Stevens FM, Harding B, et al: Hyposplenism and gluten-sensitive enteropathy. *Gastroenterology* 1984;87:1326-1331.
142. Ferguson A, Hutton MM, Maxwell JD: Adult coeliac disease in hyposplenic patients. *Lancet* 1970;1:163-164.
143. Palmer KR, Barber DC, Sherriff S: Reticuloendothelial function in coeliac disease and ulcerative colitis. *Gut* 1981;22:A419.
144. Trewby PN, Chipping PM, Palmer SJ: Splenic atrophy in adult coeliac disease: Is it reversible? *Gut* 1981;22:628-632.
145. O'Grady JG, Stevens FM, Mc Carthy CF: Celiac disease: Does hyposplenism predispose to the development of malignant disease? *Am J Gastroenterol* 1985;80:26-29.
146. Marsh GW, Stewart JS: Splenic function in adult Coeliac disease. *Br J Haematol* 1970;19:445-457.
147. Corazza GR, Frisoni M, Vaira D: Effect of gluten-free diet on splenic hypofunction of adult coeliac disease. *Gut* 1983;24:228-230.
148. Baker PG, Jones JV, Peacock DB: The immune response to OX 174 in man: III Evidence for an association between hyposplenism and immunodeficiency in patients with coeliac disease. *Gut* 1975;16:538-542.
149. Foster PN, Heatley RV, Losowsky MS: Hyposplenism and T lymphocyte subpopulations in coeliac disease and after splenectomy. *J Clin Lab Immunol* 1985;17:75-77.
150. Robertson DAF, Swinson CM, Hall R et al: Coeliac disease, splenic function and malignancy. *Gut* 1982;23:666-669.
151. Meyer A: Ueber Coeliakie. *Z Klin Med* 1932;119:665.
152. MacCrae O, Morris N: Metabolism studies in coeliac disease. *Arch Dis Child* 1931;6:75-83.
153. McCarthy CF, Fraser ID, Evans KT: Lymphoreticular dysfunction in idiopathic steatorrhea. *Gut* 1966;7:140-148.
154. Corazza GR, Lazzari R, Frisoni M: Splenic function in childhood coeliac disease. *Gut* 1982;23:415-416.
155. Hurwitz S: *Clinical Pediatric Dermatology*, WB Saunders Company, Philadelphia, PA, 1981, pp 331-332.
156. Pettit JE, Hoffbrand AV, Seah PP: Splenic atrophy in dermatitis herpetiformis. *Br Med J* 1972;2:438-440.
157. Ardeman S, Benan G: Hyposplenism and ulcerative colitis. (letter). *Lancet* 1974;2:588.
158. Ryan FP, Smart RC, Preston FE, et al: Hyposplenism in ulcerative colitis. *Lancet* 1974;2:318-320.
159. Palmer KR, Sherriff SB, Holdsworth CD, et al: Further experience of hyposplenism in inflammatory bowel disease. *Q J Med* 1981;50:463-471.
160. Jewell DP, Berney JJ, Pettit JE: Splenic phagocytic function in patients with inflammatory bowel disease. *Pathology* 1981;13:717-723.

161. Ryan FP, Limperley WR, Preston FF, et al: Cerebral involvement with disseminated intraveascular coagulation in intestinal disease. *J Clin Path* 1977;30:551-555.
162. Foster PN, Bullen AW, Robertson DAF, Chalmers DM, Losowsky MS: Development of impaired splenic function in intestinal lymphangiectasia. *Gut* 1985;26:861-864.
163. Spencer RP, Dhauvan V, Swesh K, et al: Causes and temporal sequence of onset of functional asplenia in adults. *Clin Nucl Med* 1978;3:17-18.
164. Spencer RP, Johnson PM, Sziklas JJ: Unusual scan presentations of splenic vasculative occlusion by tumor. *Clin Nucl Med* 1977;2:197-199.
165. Costello P, Gramm HF, Steinberg D: Simultaneous occurrence of functional asplenia and splenic accumulation of diphosphonate in metastatic breast carcinoma. *J Nucl Med* 1977;18:1237-1238.
166. Smith VC, Eisenberg BL, Mc Donald EC: Primary splenic angiosarcoma: Case report and literature review. *Cancer* 1985;55:1625-1627.
167. Mathews J, Szeklas JJ, Spencer RP: Functional asplenia and uptake of bone imaging agent in angiosarcoma of spleen. *Clin Nucl Med* 1985;10:527-528.
168. Gross DJ, Braverman AJ, Koren G: Functional asplenia in immunoblastic lymphoma. *Arch Intern Med* 1982;142:2213-2215.
169. Buchanan GR, Holtkamp CA: Splenic reticuloendothelial function in children with cancer. *J Pediatr* 1985;106:239-242.
170. Barlett Av, Fusman J, Daum RS: Unusual presentations of Haemophilus influenza infections in immunocomprised hosts. *J Pediatr* 1983;102:55-58.
171. Allen JB, Wierner LB: Pneumococcal sepsis in childhood leukemia and lymphoma. *Pediatrics* 1981;67:292-294.
172. Dailey MO, Coleman CN, Kaplan HS: Radiation-induced splenic atrophy in patients with Hodgkin's disease and non-Hodgkin's lymphoma. *N Engl J Med* 1980;302:215-217.
173. Daily MO, Coleman CN, Zajardo LF: Splenic irradiation caused by therapeutic irradiation. *Am J Surg Path* 1981;5:325-331.
174. Coleman CN, McDougall IR, Dailey MO: Functional hyposplenia after splenic irradiation for Hodgkin's disease. *Ann Intern Med* 1982;96:44-47.
175. Bensinger TA, Keller AR, Merrell LF: Thorotrast-induced reticuloendothelial blockade in man. *Am J Med* 1971;51:663-668.
176. Burroughs AK, Bass NM, Wood J: Absence of splenic uptake of radiocolloid due to thoroplast in a patient with thoroplast-induced cholangiocarcinoma. *Br J Radiol* 1982;55:598-600.
177. Wilson WA, Hughes GRV, Lochman PJ: Deficiency of factor B of the complement system in sickle cell anemia. *Br Med J (Clin Res)* 1976;1:367-369.
178. Hurd WM, Katholi RE: Acquired functional asplenia: Association with spontaneous rupture of the spleen and fatal rupture of the liver in amyloidosis. *Arch Intern Med* 1980;140:844-845.

179. Boyko WJ, Pratt R, Wass H: Functional hyposplenism, a diagnostic clue to amyloidosis. *Am J Clin Path* 1982;77:745-748.
180. Stone MJ, Trenkel EP: The clinical spectrum of light chain myeloma. *Am J Med* 1975;58:601-619.
181. Greipp RP, Kyle RA, Bowie EJW: Factor X deficiency in amyloidosis: a critical review. *Am J Hematol* 1981;11:443-450.
182. Greipp P, Kyle RA, Bowie EJW: Factor X deficiency in primary amyloidosis. *N Engl J Med* 1979;301:1050-1051.
183. Delfraissy JF, Lehernia G, Lawrian T, et al: Suppressor cell function after intravenous gammaglobulin treatment in chronic idiopathic thrombocytopenia purpura. *Br J Haematol* 1986;60:315-322.
184. Kimberly RP, Salmon JE, Bussel JB, et al: Modulation of mononuclear phagocyte function by intravenous gammaglobulin. *J Immunol* 1984;132:745-750.
185. Good RA: Intravenous immune globulin and the compromised host. *Am J Med* 1984;76:Supp 3A:1-209.
186. Salky NK, Mills D, Di Luzio N: Activity of the reticuloendothelial system in diseases of altered immunity. *J Lab Clin Med* 1965;66:952-960.
186a. McVicar MI, Chandra M, Margouleff D, Zanzi I: Splenic hypofunction in the nephrotic syndrome of childhood. *Am J Kidney Dis* 1986;5:395-401.
187. Pearson HA, Johnston D, Smith KA, et al: The born-again spleen. Return of splenic function after splenectomy for trauma. *N Engl J Med* 1978;298:1389-1392.
188. Neilan BA, Perry JF Jr: Persistence of vacuolated RBC's after splenectomy in adults. *JAMA* 1980;243:1741-1742.
189. Widmann WD, Laubscher FA: Splenosis: A disease or a beneficial condition. *Arch Surg* 1971;102:152-158.
190. Schwartz AD, Goldthorn JF, Winkelstein JA: Lack of protective effect of autotransplanted splenic tissue to pneumococcal challenge. *Blood* 1978;51:475-478.
191. Likhite VV: Protection against fulminant sepsis in splenectomized mice by implantation of autochthomous splenic tissue. *Exp Hematol* 1978;6:433-439.
192. Linne T, Erikson M, Lannergren K, et al: Splenic rupture after nonsurgical management of splenic rupture. *J Pediatr* 1984;105:263-265.
193. Roth J, Brudler O, Henze E: Functional asplenia in malignant mastocytosis. *J Nucl Med* 1985;26:1149-1152.
194. Boughton BJ, Simpon A, Chandler S: Functional hyposplenism during pneumococcal septicemia. *Lancet* 1983;1:121-122.
195. Scovill WA, Annest SJ, Soba TM: Cardiovascular hemodynamics after opsonic alpha-2-surface binding glycoprotein therapy in injured patients. *Surgery* 1979;86:285-293.
195a. Warrier I, Ravindranath Y: Splenic infarction and total functional asplenia in disseminated varicella. *J Pediatr* 1986;109:305-307.

196. Matteucci D, Toniolo A, Conaldi PG, et al: Systemic lymphoid atrophy in coxsackievirus B3-infected mice: Effects of virus and immunopotentiating agents. *J Infect Dis* 1985;151:1100–1108.
197. Bendinelli M, Matteuci D, Toniolo A, et al: Impairment of immunocompetent mouse spleen cell functions by infection with coxsackievirus B3. *J Infect Dis* 1982;146:797–805.
198. Tandon P, Chaturnedi VC, Mathur A: Differential depletion of T lymphocytes in the spleen of dengue virus-infected mice. *Immunology* 1979; 37:1–6.
199. Mims CA, Gould J: Splenic necrosis in mice infected with cytomegalovirus. *J Infect Dis* 1978;137:587–591.
200. Edington GM, White NA: The pathology of Lassa fever. *Trans R Soc Trop Med Hyg* 1972;66:381–389.
201. Asenjo CF: Pteroygtulamic acid requirement of the rat and a characteristic lesion observed in the spleen of the deficient animal. *J Nutr* 1948;36: 601–612.
202. Sebestik V, Brabec V: Experimental elimination of the splenic function by ethyl and methyl palmitate and significance of these substances from an immunological point of view. *Folia Haematol* (Lepiz) 1983;110:917–923.
203. Singer DB: Postsplenectomy sepsis. In, Rosenberg HS, Bolande RP (eds): *Perspectives in Pediatric Pathology*, Year Book Medical Publishers, Chicago, IL, 1973, vol 1, pp 285–311.
204. Walker W: Splenectomy in childhood: A review in England and Wales 1960-4. *Br J Surg* 1976;63:36–43.
205. Zarrabi MH, Rosner F: Serious infections in adults following splenectomy for trauma. *Arch Intern Med* 1984;144:1421–1424.

5
Physiology of the Spleen and the Consequences of Hyposplenism

ALLEN D. SCHWARTZ
University of Maryland School of Medicine, Baltimore, Maryland

A variety of functions have been attributed to the spleen since ancient times. Early Talmudic scholars thought that the spleen controlled our emotions and was the origin of laughter (1). The early Greek anatomist and physician, Erasistratus of Ceos, believed that its major purpose was to maintain the symmetry of the abdomen, thus acting as a balance to the liver. The organ itself, he believed, had no function at all. The spleen fascinated Galen. Despite the fact that he was considered to be the ultimate medical authority for over 14 centuries, he referred to the spleen as the *plenum mysterii organon*, or the organ full of mystery. Galen, however, fully accepted Aristotle's view that "Nature does nothing in vain" and sought to show that all parts of the body serve a function. He therefore created one for the spleen. Galen described a splenic canal into the stomach through which were excreted unsuitable humors (black bile), thus cleansing the body of "melancholy." Andreas Vesalius, the great Belgian anatomist of the sixteenth century, could find no such excretory duct connecting the spleen to the stomach in his careful dissection of cadavers, and finally ended 1400 years of Galenic dogma.

Greek and Roman athletes considered the spleen to be a hindrance to running, and older writings refer to certain beverages which, when taken by couriers, were supposed to reduce the size of their spleens (2). Such substances are unknown today and may have never existed, unless these references are to drugs with the properties of quinine, which may reduce the size of a spleen infected with malaria, a disease endemic to the Mediterranean area at the time. Pliny the Elder wrote that runners had a device to "burn and waste it" with a hot iron (3), but it is difficult to believe that such a method of splenectomy was actually used. Once the spleen was gone, however, its supposed ability to extract melancholic humors was also lost. Pliny wrote that "if it be man or woman that is thus cut for the spleen, he or she looseth their laughter," a conclusion not of great surprise, considering the method of removal to which he refers.

More recent studies have dispelled many of the antique mysteries of the spleen. In fact, they have revealed functions that are much more intriguing than the mere production of mirth, melancholy, and black bile. These splenic functions and the consequences of their absence are reviewed in this chapter.

RESERVOIR FUNCTION

A number of animals are able to sequester a large portion of their red cell mass within the spleen and, by contraction of smooth muscle, force intrasplenic blood into the circulation in response to various forms of stress (4,5). As much as one-third of the red cell mass, for example, may be sequestered in the spleen of anesthetized dogs (6). In contrast, the spleen of the average-sized adult human has no capsular muscle, contains only about 20-50 ml of blood, and does not act as a significant red cell reservoir (7-9). Patients with certain pathologic conditions that result in massive splenomegaly, however, may store large volumes of blood in the spleen (10). The sudden pooling of red cells within the spleen of patients with major sickle hemoglobinopathies may result in a marked increase in splenic size associated with severe and often life-threatening anemia (11).

Penny and co-workers (12) have shown that the spleen contains a pool of platelets. The size of this platelet pool is disproportionately greater than the amount of blood in the spleen. Intravenous infusion of epinephrine produces a transient increase in the number of circulating platelets, a response that is abolished by splenectomy (13,14). Although about one-third of the body's total platelet mass is normally pooled within the spleen, diseases that cause splenic enlargement may result in a marked increase in the splenic platelet pool, resulting in thrombocytopenia (14,15).

The spleen does not appear to act as a reservoir for easily mobilized granulocytes. The sudden increase in granulocytes and mononuclear leukocytes after epinephrine injection is no different in the normal and in the asplenic subject (16,17). Increased splenic pooling, however, may be responsible for the granulocytopenia of hypersplenism (18). There is evidence that the spleen stores factor VIII (anti-hemophilic factor) and will release it after exercise or challenge with any of a number of chemical agents (13,19).

BLOOD PRODUCTION

For years the spleen was believed to be an active site of hematopoiesis in the fetus. Hematopoiesis in the spleen was said to begin about the fifth month of gestation, with the production of erythroid, myeloid, and megakaryocytic cell lines (20), and then to decline and to be nearly absent by the time of birth. More recent studies have shown little evidence of hematopoiesis in the spleen of the human fetus. It has been proposed that the immature cells found in the spleen are trapped precursor cells that have been circulating in the fetal bloodstream (21).

Small clusters of hematopoietic cells also are present in the spleens of patients with disorders that place great stress on the bone marrow to increase blood cell production (22,23). Crosby believes that primary hematopoiesis does not occur in the spleen. He has proposed that immature cells escape from the marrow, are trapped in the filter of the spleen's red pulp and, because they have the potential for an additional few mitotic divisions, form a cluster that merely resembles a nest of erythropoiesis (24). Megakaryocytes and megakaryoblasts may also be removed from the blood in a similar manner (22). In some human neoplastic disease states, such as myeloid metaplasia associated with myelofibrosis, splenic hematopoiesis does occur (24,25). This does not appear to be a reactive or compensatory phenomenon in these disorders, for the spleen may be large and metaplastic even before there is fibrosis of the bone marrow (25).

DESTRUCTION OF BLOOD

As the red cell ages, the activity of a number of its enzymes diminishes (26). As a result, adenosine $5'$-triphosphate (ATP) production within the cell, an important determinant of erythrocyte deformability, decreases. The cell becomes thinner, brittle, and mechanically fragile (27,28). As the senescent red cell, with its compromised metabolism and reduced flexibility, tries to traverse the microcirculation of the spleen, which contains the narrowest vascular passages in the body, it becomes trapped and finally destroyed. Thus, the spleen has been called the "graveyard" for senescent red cells (29). However, red cell survival is not prolonged in the asplenic but otherwise normal individual. This function of red cell removal is also performed by reticuloendothelial cells in other organs of the body, such as the liver and bone marrow.

The clearance of erythrocytes that are severely damaged by any of several pathologic processes occurs not only in the spleen, but throughout the entire *reticuloendothelial system* (RES). Such red cell damage may be induced by heating (30), red cell antibodies (31), or may be due to a number of acquired or inherited disorders. The spleen, however, has a special ability to trap mildly damaged erythrocytes such as those treated with only brief heating (30) or exposed to tiny amounts of antibody (31). This function, referred to as "culling" (9), explains why some hemolytic disorders improve after splenectomy while others do not. Removal of the spleen, for example, is followed by remission of the hemolytic anemia present in patients with hereditary spherocytosis. The membrane defect of the erythrocyte is still present after splenectomy, but the one organ of the body capable of recognizing this defect and prematurely culling the abnormal red cells from the circulation is now gone. The remaining organs containing elements of the reticuloendothelial system apparently are not able to identify this subtle abnormality of the red cell membrane. No such response to splenectomy occurs in the patient with sickle-cell anemia. In other disorders, such as hereditary hemolytic elliptocytosis or autoimmune hemolytic anemia, the response to splenectomy is unpredictable.

Thrombocytosis and leukocytosis commonly occur after splenectomy. The platelet count, although often very high during the first few weeks after surgery, eventually falls, but remains above normal levels for years (32). This persisting thrombocytosis is due to the loss of the reservoir function the spleen normally provides. It has been suggested that the increased mortality from acute myocardial infarction reported in American servicemen after splenectomy for trauma during World War II may be due to this persistent elevation in the circulating number of platelets (33). Platelet survival, like red cell survival, remains unchanged after removal of the spleen in an otherwise normal person. Splenectomy often is successful in either curing or modifying the severity of chronic autoimmune thrombocytopenia. In this case, splenectomy eliminates not only a source of antibody production, but it eliminates a site of removal of the antibody-damaged platelets (34).

THE PITTING FUNCTION

"Pitting" refers to the ability of the spleen to remove particles from intact red cells without destroying the cells containing the particles. When blood with a large number of siderocytes (erythrocytes with iron-staining inclusions) is transfused into a normal recipient, the siderotic granules are removed within hours, yet the red cells remain in the circulation. These intracellular granules cannot be removed by the asplenic individual (35). Other intraerythrocytic inclusions, such as red cell nuclei, Howell-Jolly bodies (nuclear remnants), and Heinz bodies (denatured or precipitated hemoglobin granules) are also removed by splenic pitting, and normally are not found in the blood.

As the red cells with inclusion bodies travel through the narrow sinusoidal walls of the spleen, the highly deformable erythrocytes pass through, but rigid inclusions remain trapped. The red cell membrane apparently stretches, and a small portion with the inclusion is pinched off and remains in the spleen. The membrane then reseals itself, and the cell, now without the inclusion, returns into the circulation (36). The finding of erythrocytes containing Howell-Jolly bodies on examination of a blood smear suggests that the patient is either asplenic or has splenic dysfunction (37). Counting pocked erythrocytes (that is, red cells with indentations or craters on their surface) using phase-contrast interference microscopy is a simple method of determining the presence or absence of the pitting function of the spleen (38,39).

A number of studies indicate that the pitting function of the spleen is not fully developed in the premature and full-term infant. Padmanabhan and co-workers (40) reported finding occasional Howell-Jolly bodies in the blood smears of 1 out of 76 full-term neonates and in 4 out of 82 healthy prematures. Interference phase-contrast microscopy revealed many pocked red cells in neonates, especially in premature infants (38,41). Freedman et al. (39) found a significant linear correlation between the percent of pocked erythrocytes and gestational age, with the most premature infants having counts in the same range as asplenic individuals. The number of pocked red cells correlated better with gestational age than with birth weight, indicating that the ability of the spleen to cull pocked red cells improves with maturation.

THE SPLEEN AND INFECTION

Bacterial Infection and the Overwhelming Postsplenectomy Infection (OPSI) Syndrome

For years it has been known that the spleen plays an important role in the body's defense against infection. More than a century ago it was shown that intravenously injected bacteria disappeared from the bloodstream and then appeared in large numbers in the spleen (42). There is now little doubt that impaired function of the spleen or absence of the spleen increases susceptibility to bacterial sepsis. The great majority of these infections are caused by encapsulated strains of *Streptococcus pneumoniae, Hemophilus influenzae* type b, or *Neisseria meningitidis*, but other organisms also are occasionally responsible (43-46).

The classical picture of the clinical disorder called OPSI syndrome consists of abrupt onset, high incidence of disseminated intravascular coagulation, and death occurring within hours of onset. This has been reported not only in those who have undergone surgical splenectomy, but also in patients with congenital and functional asplenia. The mortality rate of patients with OPSI syndrome may be as high as 50-80% (47,48) even when the patient is treated with appropriate antibiotics. There is an enormous proliferation of bacteria in the bloodstream, and gram stain of the peripheral blood and urine may identify the responsible organisms (49,50). This syndrome was once thought to occur only in young children (usually under age 4 years) within two years of splenectomy, and in the patient who had undergone splenectomy for an underlying hematologic or malignant disorder. Although most persons who develop the syndrome fall in to one or more of these groups, a number of older children and adults with no underlying disease have developed this complication many years after splenectomy (33,51,52). Singer believed the incidence of this complication in individuals splenectomized after trauma to be at least 58 times that of the general population (43).

Most experimental work with laboratory animals has demonstrated the importance of the spleen in protecting the host against *Streptococcus pneumoniae* (53-55), the bacteria most commonly implicated in the OPSI syndrome. In these studies, bacteria inoculated by intravenous or intraperitoneal injections more frequently led to death in asplenic animals than in normal controls. Coil and co-workers (56) have shown that *Streptococcus pneumoniae* sepsis also can be induced in an animal model via the respiratory tract, a route of inoculation more closely resembling the route of infection that occurs in humans. This route of exposure also results in an increased mortality in splenectomized mice when compared to controls.

Moxon et al. (57), investigated the effect of splenectomy on the susceptibility of rats to intravenous and intranasal inoculation of *Hemophilus influenzae* type b. The 50% lethal dose (LD_{50}) for asplenic rats challenged either by intravenous injection or intranasal installation of bacteria was nearly identical, but was markedly lower than the LD_{50} for control animals. Thus, the presence or absence of the spleen was more important in determining the LD_{50} than was the route of administration of the bacteria. The mean survival time, however, was much longer for asplenic rats inoculated intranasally compared to asplenic rats inoculated intravenously (Figure 1).

Both groups of investigators believed that animals challenged with encapsulated bacteria via the respiratory tract were more biologically relevant experimental models for investigating the role of the spleen in defense against infection than were models using parenteral injection of organisms.

Other Infections

Several reports have noted an increased susceptibility of asplenic humans to viral infections. These have included cases of fulminant varicella (58-60), severe cytomegalovirus infection (61), and viral hepatitis (62). Stone and co-workers (62) reported an experimental study of viral hepatitis in weanling mice. They found that the mortality rate was increased 2.5 times by performing splenectomy befor inoculation of the virus. The spleen also acts as an important defense against intraerythrocytic parasitic infections with Bartonella, Plasmodia, and Babesia by pitting these organisms from the red cell (63). Nearly all cases of babesiasis reported in humans have occurred in asplenic individuals (64).

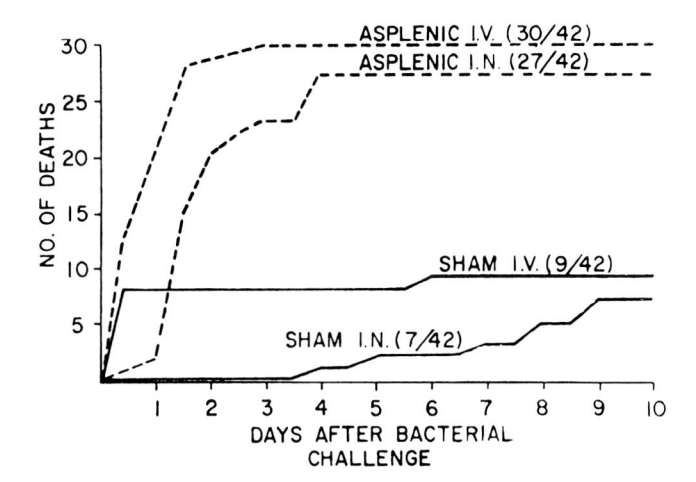

Figure 1 Number of deaths in asplenic and sham-operated rats after intravenous (I.V.) or intranasal (I.N.) challenge. No deaths occurred after day 9. (From Ref. 57, used with permission.)

Production of Antibody

Some insight into the mechanism of the spleen's protective effect was provided by Rowley in 1950 (65,66). He demonstrated that small doses of particulate antigen administered intravenously into laboratory rats or into humans was followed by an antibody response. Such a response could not be produced by an asplenic recipient. The asplenic animal, however, had a normal antibody response to particulate antigen when challenged intraperitoneally, intraportally, intramuscularly, subcutaneously, or intradermally. The route by which the particulate antigen was administered, therefore, appeared to be a critical factor in determining whether or not the splenectomized individual could produce antibody against the antigen.

This inability to respond with antibody production to intravenous challenge of small doses of particulate antigen also has been demonstrated in children with hereditary splenic hypoplasia (67) and in children who are functionally asplenic due to sickle cell anemia (68). Both of these groups are extremely susceptible to overwhelming sepsis in early childhood (69,70). This latter group of patients is unique. Young children with sickle-cell anemia and splenomegaly may have evidence of hypersplenic function with thrombocytopenia due to splenic pooling of platelets (15) and sequestration of red cells, resulting in life-threatening anemia (11), yet they are unable to pit Howell-Jolly bodies from erythrocytes, remove particulate matter such as $^{99}Tc_m$-sulfur colloid from the circulation (71), or produce antibodies in response to intravenous challenge with particulate antigen (68). This apparent paradox can best be explained by postulating that the splenic reservoir is independent of reticuloendothelial function.

The immunre response of the asplenic individual to a number of polysaccharide antigens administered intramuscularly also is not normal. Although early studies reported that pneumococcal vaccines stimulate a normal antibody response in asplenic children (72) and adults (73), Hosea et al. (74) found that their immune response was impaired. IgG and IgM responses were less than those found in controls in terms of absolute titer, relative rise in titer, and rates of rise. Others have reported that this response is also impaired in the asplenic child (75, 76). Hebert and co-workers (78), using a mouse model challenged with *Streptococcus pneumoniae* via the respiratory tract, demonstrated that immunization 7 days before splenectomy was much more effective in decreasing the mortality rate than was immunization after splenectomy.

Amlot and Hayes (78) used a synthetic polysaccharide antigen, dinitrophenyl (DNP)-ficoll, to which there is no natural exposure, to study antibody response in splenectomized individuals. They found that the speed of the antibody response to de novo exposure to this antigen is greatly impaired in asplenic patients. However, the effect of previous exposure was important in enabling asplenic patients to respond to the same antigen after splenectomy. The authors suggested that prior exposure leads to the generation of a population of B cells that leave the spleen and are later able to respond after restimulation.

Whatever the exact explanation for the suboptimal response might be, it is clear that polyvalent pneumococcal vaccine administered to the asplenic patient does not always lead to protective antibody levels to all of the pneumococcal types in the vaccine. Also, giving such a vaccine to the asplenic patient may be followed by a decline to subprotective levels of antibody 1-2 years after vaccination, even if the initial antibody response was good (75). Thus, a number of vaccinated asplenic patients have developed pneumococcal septicemia with serotypes contained in the vaccine (79-82). It is now recommended that immunization with bacterial polysaccharides should be given before splenectomy whenever possible.

Phagocytosis

Circulating encapsulated bacteria, such as pneumococci, become heavily coated with specific complement-fixing antibodies once they enter the blood stream of an animal that is already immunized against them. In such animals it has been shown that the liver, with its large mass of reticuloendothelial cells, is the most important organ for clearance of pneumococci (83). The fixed macrophages of the liver, however, depend heavily upon the presence of type-specific antibody to clear bacteria maximally (83,84). The spleen, gram for gram, has a much greater capacity than the liver for clearing bacteria from the bloodstream regardless of the immunologic status of the animal (83-85); thus the role of the spleen becomes extremely important in the nonimmune animal. Poorly opsonized organisms are trapped in the spleen as a consequence of its unique architecture (44). The very slow passage of blood through the splenic sinusoids contrasts with the rapid flow past the Kupfer cells of the liver. This decreased contact time of bacteria with hepatic phagocytes presumably can be compensated for by the presence of antibody, which increases the liver's efficiency for phagocytosis (84).

Thus, in the absence of the spleen, the nonimmune host is not only unable to respond to blood-borne bacteria with antibody production, but is also unable to optimally remove the organisms from the circulation. This is probably the major reason why the OPSI syndrome is more frequent in the younger child. Effective antibodies against *Hemophilus influenzae* type b cannot be demonstrated in 95% of children less than 2 years of age. In contrast, those over 2 years of age usually have high antibody titers (86,87). The antibacterial activity for pneumococci also is low before the age of 2 years (88). The report of severe infections in 50% of children who were splenectomized before 1 year of age therefore should not be surprising (89). A much smaller number of apparently normal adults do not have circulating antibodies against some of the common bacterial organisms, including the pneumococcus (88) or *H. influenzae* type b (90,91). Such an adult, after splenectomy, is very likely as susceptible to severe infection with these organisms as is the young asplenic child.

Ozoylu and co-workers (92) studied phagocytic function of the spleen in rats using $^{99}Tc_m$-sulfur colloid. They demonstrated markedly reduced phagocytic activity of the spleen at birth, but an increase to normal adult levels by 2-4 weeks of age. This decreased ability to clear particulate matter from the circulation may be one reason why bacterial infections in newborn babies are so severe.

Other Immune Defects

Deficiency of tuftsin, a phagocytosis-promoting tetrapeptide, has been reported in the majority of splenectomized patients studied (93). Individuals with congenital deficiency of tuftsin have repeated infections of the respiratory tract, of the lymph nodes, and of the skin, often caused by *Staphylococcus aureus* (94), but they do not appear prone to overwhelming infections with encapsulated bacteria. Asplenia does not predispose the patient to the usual types of infection found in the congenitally tuftsin-deficient patient. Therefore, the clinical importance of tuftsin deficiency in the asplenic patient remains unclear.

Properdin is a natural serum protein involved in association with magnesium and complement in the destruction of selected bacteria and viruses. This substance has been reported to be in lower concentration in splenectomized patients than in normal persons (95). Corry and co-workers (96) demonstrated deficiency of the alternate pathway of complement activation (the properdin system) in 6 out of 58 asplenic patients. However, Winkelstein and associates (97) could document no abnormalities in the properdin pathway in asplenic persons. As with tuftsin deficiency, the significance of these findings is not known.

A number of studies have reported low serum IgM levels in asplenic patients (98–100) but this has not been a consistent finding (73,101,102). Koren and associates (102) noted a significant decrease in IgM levels after splenectomy in children with thalassemia major and sickle-cell anemia. Levels remained low for as long as 2 years. In contrast to others (100), they were unable to demonstrate changes in the IgM levels in patients splenectomized for trauma except for a transient increase during the immediate postoperative period. It is possible that at least some of these conflicting observations may be due to the length of time between surgery and testing, or the possible implantation and growth of functional splenic tissue (splenosis) following trauma.

MANAGEMENT OF THE ASPLENIC STATE

The major concern regarding the asplenic person is the danger of developing severe infection. Although such individuals may be at risk for other problems, such as increased mortality from cardiovascular disease (33), these possible complications are still speculative and require further investigation. Clearly, one simple means of preventing problems is to avoid splenectomy; such a statement is easily made by the author, who is not a surgeon and who does not deal with trauma patients.

With the increasing acceptance of the fact that the asplenic state carries increased risk of severe infection, more conservative management of splenic trauma is now being advocated by surgeons in treating both children and adults. Nonoperative management, surgical repair of the spleen, and partial splenectomy have all been used successfully (103–106). Ratner and co-workers (107) reported that only 2 out of 17 children with blunt trauma to the spleen required splenectomy, while in the remainder the spleens were successfully repaired by surgery. No patient required reoperation, and follow-up isotopic scans were normal. A lacerated, almost transected spleen was repaired in a 3-day-old infant (108). Also, splenic repair was achieved in two hydropic neonates with splenic damage associated with massive splenomegaly due to erythroblastosis fetalis (109). Surgical methods for splenic preservation are now being advocated after blunt splenic trauma in adults (110).

Residual splenic tissue after less than total splenectomy has been shown to confer protection against pneumococcal challenge in animals (111–113). Reported cases of septicemia in children who had undergone staging laparotomy for Hodgkin's disease (114) have prompted some to advocate use of partial splenectomy when performing surgical staging in these children (115). One must weigh the danger of the asplenic state against the possibility of understaging by failing to detect splenic involvement, and the effect this failure may have on the outcome of therapy in these patients (116).

Prophylactic use of penicillin has been suggested after splenectomy, but the patient still remains prone to infection with penicillin-resistant organisms such as *Hemophilus influenzae*. Strains of pneumococci resistant to penicillin and other antibiotics have been reported within the last two decades (117-119). Most individuals who developed infections with these organisms had been treated with prophylactic penicillin and other antibiotics or had received multiple antibiotics in the past. This suggests that these persons either became colonized with resistant organisms because sensitive bacteria were eradicated while the resistant organisms were unaffected, or because the antibiotics themselves were responsible for the development of new resistant strains. Pneumococci grown in vitro in the presence of subinhibitory concentrations of penicillin will acquire resistance to this antibiotic (120). There is data, however, demonstrating that penicillin prophylaxis, in both the asplenic animal (121) and human (122,123) is effective in decreasing the incidence of fatal bacteria infection, although protection is not absolute (79,82,124). Prophylaxis is not effective when the patient does not take the medication as prescribed, which appears to be a common problem (125). In addition, penicillin prophylaxis may prevent the occurrence of minor pneumococcal infections that result in natural immunity, and the high risk of infection may resume once the antibiotic is discontinued (123,125).

It is recommended that polyvalent pneumococcal vaccine be given to asplenic individuals, but the vaccine does not protect against all pneumococcal subtypes. As discussed earlier, maximal production of protective antibody may not occur in the asplenic host. Although it has been suggested that the vaccine be administered before splenectomy, the most common reason for this surgical procedure is for trauma, not for treatment of a hematologic disorder or for staging of Hodgkin's disease. In addition, the antibody response to polysaccharide vaccines in children under 2 years of age is often suboptimal (72,126). This is the population at highest risk for serious infection. Reis and co-workers (127) reported that only 6 out of 138 patients they studied who had undergone splenectomy after 1975 had subsequently received pneumococcal immunization. Thus, even this simple procedure of immunization, despite its limitations, is often not used. Even more disconcerting was the fact that only 2 of these 138 asplenic patients had been given information by their physicians about the possibility that they might develop a severe infection.

One technique suggested as a means of preserving splenic function in the patient whose traumatized spleen cannot be salvaged is autoimplantation of splenic

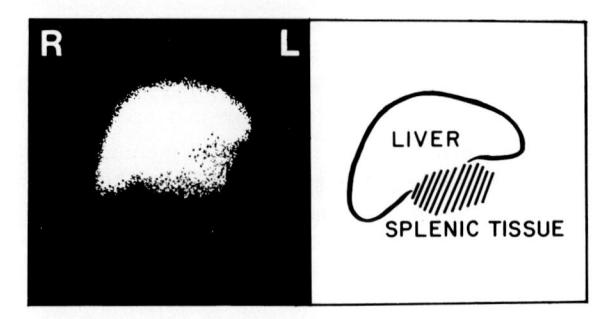

Figure 2 $^{99}Tc_m$-sulfur colloid scan 6 months postsplenectomy and implantation of splenic tissue into the omentum of a rat. Presence of active splenic tissue (cross-hatched area) is evident on the scan.

tissue into the peritoneal cavity. Regeneration of such tissue, referred to as splenosis, may commonly occur in persons splenectomized after trauma. It has been suggested by Pearson and co-workers (128) that the presence of this so-called "born-again spleen" may account for the lower incidence of OPSI syndrome in patients splenectomized because of trauma, as compared to those who have been splenectomized or have become asplenic for other reasons. Splenic autoimplants are capable of removing Howell-Jolly bodies (129,130) and surface indentations (128) from erythrocytes; they are also capable of clearing intravenously injected radiocolloid (128,130,131) (Figure 2) and of performing a number of immunologic functions (130-133).

The data regarding the protective effect of splenosis to parenteral challenge with *S. pneumoniae* (134-137) and with bartonella (138,139) have been conflicting. In an effort to use a model that more closely approximates the natural route of infection in humans, some investigators have challenged their experimental animals with bacteria via the respiratory tract. Two studies have shown that splenosis under these test conditions is remarkably successful in preventing death from infection with *S. pneumoniae* (140) or *H. influenzae* type b (141). Because peak bacteremia occurs significantly later after intranasal as opposed to intravenous inoculation (57), the host has time to mobilize a variety of immunologic responses that effect the ultimate outcome.

Many surgeons now advocate splenic replantation if the spleen cannot be salvaged after trauma (130,142). However, splenosis is not as effective in clearing the bloodstream of bacteria, producing antibodies, or increasing survival rates in the experimental animal as either the normal intact spleen or the impaired spleen after partial splenectomy. However, splenosis offers an advantage over the asplenic state (141,143). This defect in function may be because of lack of a critical mass of splenic tissue (144), interruption of the normal blood supply (145), or both. Whatever the reason, a number of deaths due to infection with encapsulated bacteria have been reported in patients found to have splenosis at postmortem examination (43,146,147).

There is presently no known infallible method for protecting the asplenic person from infection. Immunization, prophylactic antibiotics, and, in selected situations, splenosis, may lessen the dangers. Even those patients who are given the benefit of these preventive measures should be educated as to the small but very real risk of serious infection.

SUMMARY

Investigators have achieved some insight into the functioning of the spleen only within the last few decades. Under normal circumstances the human spleen is insignificant as a reservoir for erythrocytes and leukocytes, but does contain about one-third of the body's total platelet mass. It also stores factor VIII (antihemophilic factor). Despite earlier reports, there is little evidence to show that the spleen is responsible for significant hematopoiesis, either in the fetus or adult, except in some neoplastic states.

The spleen removes senescent and damaged erythrocytes from the circulation. Its unique ability to remove mildly damaged red cells, such as those found in patients with hereditary spherocytosis, is referred to as "culling." "Pitting" refers to the spleen's ability to remove particles from intact red cells without destroying the cells containing these particles. The absence of this function results in the presence of intracellular remnants, such as Howell-Jolly bodies, in the red cells, and an increased number of indentations on erythrocyte surfaces.

The spleen plays an important role in the body's defense against infection, especially against encapsulated bacteria. Its abilities to produce antibodies and to remove bacteria from the blood stream may be life-saving to the individual who has not been previously immunized against the infectious challenge. The asplenic host, however, does not appear to be as prone to severe infection by bacteria once he has been immunized against them.

A number of protective measures can be taken to protect the asplenic patient from severe infection, including the use of immunizations with pneumococcal vaccine, prophylactic antibiotics, and education of the patient to seek early medical help when evidence of infection occurs. Surgeons, now aware of the dangers of the asplenic state, are making a greater effort to salvage the spleen after trauma. A number of techniques, including the use of hemisplenectomy and the creation of splenosis offer protection, but nothing yet appears to protect against infection as well as does the normal spleen.

REFERENCES

1. Rosner F: The spleen in the Talmud and other early Jewish writings. *Bull Hist Med* 1972;46:82-85.
2. Gould GM, Pyle WL: *Anomalies and Curiosities of Medicine*. Philadelphia, W. B. Saunders Company, 1900, p. 461.
3. Holland P, Islip A (transl): *Naturall Historie*, London, 1601, p. 343.
4. Barcroft J, Stephens JG: Observations upon the size of the spleen. *J. Physiol* (Lond) 1927;64:1-22.
5. Toghill PJ, Prichard BNC: A study of the action of noradrenaline on the splenic red cell pool. *Clin Sci* 1964;26:203-212.
6. Motulsky AG, Casserd F, Giblett ER, et al: Anemia and the spleen. *N Engl J Med* 1958;259:1164-1169; 1215-1219.
7. Ebert RV, Stead EA Jr: Demonstration that in normal man no reserves of blood are mobilized by exercise, epinephrine, and hemorrhage. *Am J Med Sci* 1974;201:655-664.
8. Hedge UM, Williams ED, Lewis SM, et al: Measurement of splenic red cell volume and visualization of the spleen with technetium. *J Nucl Med* 1973;14:769-771.
9. Crosby WH: Normal functions of the spleen relative to red blood cells; a review. *Blood* 1959;14:399-408.
10. Jandl JH, Greenberg MS, Yonemoto RH, Castle WB: Clinical determination of the sites of red cell sequestration in hemolytic anemias. *J Clin Invest* 1956;35:842-867.
11. Emond AM, Collis R, Darvill D, et al: Acute splenic sequestration crisis in homozygous sickle cell disease: Natural history and management. *J Pediatr* 1985;107:201-206.
12. Penny R, Rozenberg MC, Firkin BG: The splenic platelet pool. *Blood* 1966;27:1-16.
13. Libre EP, Cowan DH, Watkins SP, Schulman NR: Relationships between the spleen, platelets and factor VIII levels. *Blood* 1968;31:348-368.
14. Aster RH: Pooling of platelets in the spleen; role in the pathogenesis of "hypersplenic" thrombocytopenia. *J Clin Invest* 1966;45:645-665.
15. Schwartz AD: The splenic platelet pool in sickle cell anemia. *Blood* 1972;40:678-683.
16. Raab SO, Athens JW, Haab OP, et al: Granulokinetics in normal dogs. *Am J Physiol* 1964;206:83-88.
17. Storti E, Lusvarghi E, Grignaffini GF, Sgandurra A: Biological and clinical significance of the adrenalin test in haematology. *Haematologia* 1967;1:27-34.
18. Brubaker LH, Johnson CA: Correlation of splenomegaly and abdominal neutrophil pooling (margination). *J Lab Clin Med* 1978;92:508-515.
19. Webster VP, Reddick RL, Roberts HR, Penick GB: Release of factor VIII (anti-haemophilic factor) from perfused organs and tissues. *Nature* (Lond) 1967;213:1146-1147.

20. Gilmour JR: Normal haemopoiesis in intra-uterine and neonatal life. *J Pathol Bactiol* 1941;52:25-55.
21. Wolf BC, Luevano E, Neiman R: Evidence to suggest that the human fetal spleen is not a hematopoietic organ. *Am J Clin Pathol* 1983;80:140-144.
22. Yam LI, McMillan R, Tavassoli M, Crosby WH: Splenic hemopoiesis in idiopathic thrombocytopenic purpura. *Am J Clin Pathol* 1974;62:830-837.
23. Rappaport H, Crosby WH: Autoimmune hemolytic anemia. II. Morphologic observations and clinicopathologic correlations. *Am J Pathol* 1957;33:429-449.
24. Crosby WH: Hematopoiesis in the spleen. *Arch Int Med* 1983;143:1321-1322.
25. Silverstein MN: *Agnogenic Myeloid Metaplasia*. Acton, MA, Publishing Sciences Group, 1975.
26. Allison AC, Burn GP: Enzyme activity as a function of age in the human erythrocyte. *Br J Haematol* 1955;1:291-303.
27. Singer K, Weisz L: The life cycle of the erythrocyte after splenectomy and the problems of splenic hemolysis and target cell formation. *Am J Med Sci* 1945;210:301-323.
28. Stewart WB, Stewart JM, Izzo MJ, Young LE: Age as affecting the osmotic and mechanical fragility of dog erythrocytes tagged with radioactive iron. *J Exp Med* 1950;91:147-159.
29. Rous P: Destruction of the red blood corpuscle in health and disease. *Physiol Rev* 1923;3:75-105.
30. Wagner HN Jr, Razzak MA, Gaertner RA, et al: Removal of erythrocytes from the circulation. *Arch Intern Med* 1962;10:90-97.
31. Jandl JH, Kaplan ME: The destruction of red cells by antibodies in man. III. Quantitative factors influencing the pattern of hemolysis in vivo. *J Clin Invest* 1960;39:1145-1149, 1156.
32. Davis WM, Ross AOM: Thrombocytosis and thrombocytopenia; the laboratory and clinical significance of an elevated platelet count. *Am J Clin Pathol* 1973;59:243-247.
33. Robinette CD, Fraumeni JR Jr: Splenectomy and subsequent mortality in veterans of the 1939-45 war. *Lancet* 1977;2:127-129.
34. McMillan R, Longmire RL, Yelenosky R, et al: Quantitation of platelet binding IgG produced in vitro by spleens of patients with idiopathic thrombocytopenic purpura. *N Engl J Med* 1974;291:812-817.
35. Crosby WH: Siderocytes and the spleen. *Blood* 1957;12:165-170.
36. Leblond PF: Etude au microscope electronizue a balayage, de la migration des cellules sanguines à travers les parois dessenusoides splenique et medullaires chez le rat. *Nouv Rev Fr Hematol* 1973;13:771-788.
37. Lipson RI, Bayrd ED, Watkins CH: The post splenectomy blood picture. *Am J Clin Pathol* 1959;32:526-532.
38. Holroyde CP, Oski FA, Gardner FH: The "pocked" erythrocyte; red-cell surface alterations in reticuloendothelial immaturity of the neonate. *N Engl J Med* 1969;281:516-520.

39. Freedman RM, Johnston D, Mahoney MJ, Pearson HL: Development of splenic reticuloendothelial function in neonates. *J Pediatr* 1980;96:466-468.
40. Padmanabhan J, Risemberg HM, Rowe RD: Howell-Jolly bodies in the peripheral blood of full-term and premature neonates. *Johns Hopkins Med J* 1973;132:146-150.
41. Preston EE, Shahani RT: Surface ultra microscopy of neonatal erythrocytes. *Lancet* 1970;1:1177-1178.
42. Wyssokowitsch W: Uber die Schicksale der in's Blut injizcirten Mikroorgismen im Korper der Warmbluter. *Z Hyg* 1886;1:3-45.
43. Singer DB: Postsplenectomy sepsis. *Perspect Pediatr Pathol* 1973;1:285-311.
44. Ellis EF, Smith RT: The role of the spleen in immunity; with special reference to the post-splenectomy problem in infants. *Pediatrics* 1966;37:111-119.
45. Eraklis AJ, Kevy SV, Diamond LK, Cross R: Hazard of overwhelming infection after splenectomy in childhood. *N Engl J Med* 1976;276:1225-1229.
46. Pearson HA, O'Brien RT, McIntosh LS, Aspnes GT: The spleen, asplenia and overwhelming penumococcal infection. In Robbins JB, Horton RE, Krause RM: Proceedings of symposium, *New Approaches fo Inducing Natural Immunity to Pyogenic Organisms*, publication No. 74-553. Washington, D.C., U.S. Dept. of Health, Education & Welfare, 1983, 9-16.
47. Lucas RV, Krivit W: Overwhelming infection in children following splenectomy. *J Pediatr* 1960;57:185-191.
48. Dickerman JD: Bacterial infection and the asplenic host; a review. *J Trauma* 1976;16:662-668.
49. Bisno AL, Freeman JC: The syndrome of asplenia, pneumococcal sepsis, and disseminated intravascular coagulation. *Ann Intern Med* 1970;72:389-393.
50. Torres J, Bisno AL: Hyposplenism and pneumococcemia; visualization of *Diplococcus pneumoniae* in the peripheral blood smear. *Am J Med* 1973; 55:851-855.
51. Balfanz JR, Nesbit ME, Jarvis C, Krivit W: Overwhelming sepsis following splenectomy for trauma. *J Pediatr* 1976;88:458-460.
52. Dickerman JD: Traumatic asplenia in adults—A definite hazard? *Arch Surg* 1981;116:361-363.
53. Leung LS, Szal GJ, Drachman RH: Increased susceptibility of splenectomized rats to infection with *Diplococcus pneumoniae. J Infect Dis* 1972; 126:507-513.
54. Rothberg H, Corallo LA: Influence of splenectomy on resistance to pneumococcal infection in rats. *Proc Soc Exp Biol Med* 1959;100:200-222.
55. Shinefeld HR, Steinberg CR, Kay D: Effect of splenectomy on the susceptibility of mice inoculated with *Diplococcus pneumoniae. J Exp Med* 1966; 123:777-794.
56. Coil JA, Dickerman JD, Boulton E: Increased susceptibility of splenectomized mice to infection after exposure to an aerosolized suspension of type III *Streptococcus pneumoniae. Infect Immun* 1978;21:412-416.

57. Moxon ER, Goldthorn JF, Schwartz AD: *Haemophilus influenzae* b in rats: Effect of splenectomy on bloodstream and meningeal invasion after intravenous and intranasal inoculations. *Infect Immun* 1980;27:872–875.
58. Forward AD, Ashmore PG: Infection following splenectomy in infants and children. *Canad J Surg* 1960;3:229–233.
59. Smith CH, Elundson MD, Stern G, Hilgartner MW: Post-splenectomy infection in Cooley's anemia; an appraisal of the problem in this and other blood disorders, with a consideration of prophylaxis. *N Engl J Med* 1962;266:737–743.
60. Diamond LK, Allen DM, Magill FB: Congenital erythroid hypoplastic anemia; a 25 year study. *Am J Dis Child* 1961;102:403–415.
61. Baumgartner JD, Glauser MP, Burgo-Black AL, et al: Severe cytomegalovirus infection in multiply transfused, splenectomized, trauma patients. *Lancet* 1982;2:63–66.
62. Stone HH, Stanley DG, DeJarnette RH: Postsplenectomy viral hepatitis. *J Am Med Assoc* 1967;199:851–853.
63. Schnitzer B, Sodeman TM, Mead ML, Contacos PG: An ultrastructural study of the red pulp of the spleen in malaria. *Blood* 1973;41:207–218.
64. Western KA, Benson GD, Gleason NN, et al: Babesiosis in a Massachusetts resident. *N Engl J Med* 1970;283:854–856.
65. Rowley DA: The effect of splenectomy on the formation of circulating antibody in the adult male albino rat. *J Immunol* 1950;64:289–295.
66. Rowley DA: The formation of circulating antibody in the splenectomized human being following intravenous injection of heterologous erythrocytes. *J Immunol* 1950;65:515–521.
67. Kevy SV, Tefft M, Vawter GF, Rosen FS: Hereditary splenic hypoplasia. *Pediatrics* 1968;42:752–757.
68. Schwartz AD, Pearson HA: Impaired antibody response to intravenous immunization in sickle cell anemia. *Pediatr Res* 1972;6:145–149.
69. Waldman JD, Rosenthal A, Smith AL, et al: Sepsis and congenital asplenia. *J Pediatr* 1977;90:555–559.
70. Powars DR: Natural history of sickle cell disease; the first 10 years. *Semin Hematol* 1975;12:267–285.
71. Pearson HA, Spencer RP, Cornelius EA: Functional asplenia in sickle-cell anemia. *N Engl J Med* 1969;281:923–926.
72. Ammann AJ, Addiego J, Wara DW, et al: Polyvalent pneumococcal polysaccharide immunization of patients with sickle cell anemia and patients with splenectomy. *N Engl J Med* 1977;297:897–900.
73. Sullivan JL, Ochs HD, Schiffman G, et al: Immune response after splenectomy. *Lancet* 1978;1:178–186.
74. Hosea SW, Burch CG, Brown EJ, et al: Impaired immune response of splenectomized patients to polyvalent pneumococcal vaccine. *Lancet* 1981;1:804–807.
75. Giebink GS, Le CT, Schiffman G: Decline of serum antibody in splenectomized capsular polysaccharides. *J Pediatr* 1984;105:576–582.

76. Pedersen FK, Hendricksen J, Schiffman G: Antibody response to vaccination with pneumococcal capsular polysaccharides in splenectomized children. *Acta Paediatr Scand* 1982;71:451-455.
77. Hebert JC, Gamelli RL, Dickerman JD, et al: Lack of protection by pneumococcal vaccine after splenectomy in mice challenged with aerosolized pneumococci. *J Trauma* 1983;23:1-6.
78. Amlot PL, Hayes AE: Impaired human antibody responses to the thymus independent antigen, DNP-ficoll, after splenectomy; implications for postsplenectomy infections. *Lancet* 1985;135:115-158.
79. Giebink GS, Schiffman G, Krivit W, Quie PG: Vaccine type pneumococcal pneumonia occurrence after vaccination in an asplenic patient. *JAMA* 1979; 141:2736-2737.
80. Iverturf GD, Field R, Edmonds R: Death from type 6 pneumococcal septicemia in a vaccinated child with sickle-cell disease. *N Engl J Med* 1979; 300:143.
81. Sumaya CV, Harbison RW, Britton HA: Pneumococcal vaccine failutes; two case reports and review. *Am J Dis Child* 1981;135:155-158.
82. Evans DIK: Fatal post-splenectomy sepsis despite prophylaxis with penicillin and pneumococcal vaccine. *Lancet* 1984;1:1124.
83. Schulkind ML, Ellis EF, Smith RT: Effect of antibody upon clearance of I^{131} labelled pneumococci by the spleen and liver. *Pediatr Res* 1967;1: 178-184.
84. Hosea SW, Brown EJ, Hamburger MI, Frank MM: Opsonic requirements for intravascular clearance after splenectomy. *N Engl J Med* 1981;304:245-250.
85. Benacerraf B, Sebestyen MM, Schlossman SL: A quantitative study of the kinetics of blood clearance of p^{32} labelled *Escherichia coli* and Staphylococci by the reticuloendothelial system. *J Exp Med* 1959;110:27-48.
86. Norden CW, Melish M, Overall JD Jr, Baum J: Immunologic responses to *Hemophilus influenzae* meningitis. *J Pediatr* 1972;80:209-214.
87. Greenfield S, Peter G, Howie VM et al: Acquisition of type specific antibodies to *Hemophilus influenza* type B. *J Pediatr* 1972;80:204-208.
88. Sutliff WD, Finland M: Antipneumococcic immunity reaction in individuals of different ages. *J Exp Med* 1932;55:837-852.
89. Horan M, Colebatch JH: Relation between splenectomy and subsequent infection; a clinical study. *Arch Dis Child* 1962;37:398-414.
90. Graber CD, Gershanik JJ, Levkoff AH, Westphal M: Changing pattern of neonatal susceptibility to *Hemophilus influenzae*. *J Pediatr* 1971;78:948-950.
91. Norden CW, Callerame ML, Baum L: Hemophilus influenzae meningitis in an adult; a study of bacteriocidal antibodies and immunoglobulins. *N Engl J Med* 1970;282:190-194.
92. Ozsoylu S, Hosain F, McIntyre PA: Functional development of phagocytic activity of the spleen. *J Pediatr* 1977;90:560-562.
93. Constantopoulos A, Najjar VA, Wish JB, et al: Defective phagocysosis due to tuftsin deficiency in splenectomized subjects. *Am J Dis Child* 1973;125: 663-665.

94. Najjar VA: Defective phagocytosis due to deficiencies involving the tetrapeptide tuftsin. *J Pediatr* 1975;87:1121-1124.
95. Carlisle HN, Saslaw S: Properdin levels in splenectomized persons. *Proc Soc Exp Biol Med* 1959;102:150-154.
96. Corry JM, Polhill RB Jr, Edmonds SR, Johnston RB Jr: Activity of the alternative complement pathway after splenectomy; comparison to activity in sickle cell disease and hypogammaglobulinemia. *J Pediatr* 1979;95: 964-969.
97. Winkelstein JA, Lambert GH, Swift A: Pneumococcal serum opsonizing activity in splenectomized children. *J Pediatr* 1975;87:430-433.
98. Claret I, Morales L, Montaner A: Immunologic studies in the postsplenectomy syndrome. *J Pediatr Surg* 1975;10:59-64.
99. Anderson V, Cohn J, Sorensen SF: Immunological studies in children before and after splenectomy. *Acta Paediatr Scand* 1976;65:409-415.
100. Schumaker MJ: Serum immunoglobulin and transferrin levels after childhood splenectomy. *Arch Dis Child* 1970;45:114-117.
101. Merikanto J, Ruuskanen O, Eskola J, et al: Immunological consequences of neonatal splenectomy. *Pediatr Res* 1979;13:83 (Abstr).
102. Koren A, Haasz R, Taitler A, Katzuni E: Serum immunoglobulin levels in children after splenectomy; a prospective study. *Am J Dis Child* 1984; 138:53-55.
103. Ein SH, Shandling B, Simpson JS, Stephens CA: Nonoperative management of traumatized spleen in children—How and Why? *J Pediatr Surg* 1978;13:117-119.
104. Howman-Giles R, Gilday DL, Venugopal S, et al: Splenic trauma-nonoperative management and long-term follow-up by scintiscan. *J Pediatr Surg* 1978;13:121-216.
105. Sherman NJ, Asch MJ: Conservative surgery for splenic injuries. *Pediatrics* 1978;61:267-271.
106. Burrington JD: Surgical repair of a ruptured spleen in children. *Arch Surg* 1977;112:417-419.
107. Ratner MH, Garrow E, Valda V, et al: Surgical repair of the injured spleen. *J Pediatr Surg* 1977;12:1019-1025.
108. Matsuyama S, Suzuki N, Nagamachi Y: Rupture of the spleen in the newborn; treatment without splenectomy. *J Pediatr Surg* 1976;11:115-116.
109. Simmons MA, Burrington JD, Wayne ER, Hathaway WE: Splenic rupture in neonates with erythroblastosis fetalis. *Am J Dis Child* 1973;126:679-681.
110. Mucha P Jr: Changing attitude toward the management of blunt splenic trauma in adults. *Mayo Clin Proc* 1986;61:472-477.
111. Goldthorn JR, Schwartz AD, Swift AJ, Winkelstein JA: Protective effect of residual splenic tissue after subtotal splenectomy. *J Pediatr Surg* 1978; 13:587-590.
112. Grosfeld JL, Ranochak JE: Are hemisplenectomy and/or primary splenic repair feasible? *J Pediatr Surg* 1976;11:419-424.

113. Coil JA Jr, Dickerman JD, Horner SR, Chalmer BJ: Pulmonary infection in splenectomized mice; protection by splenic remnant. *J Surg Res* 1980; 28:18-22.
114. Chilcote RR, Baehner RL, Hammond D: Septicemia and meningitis in children splenectomized for Hodgkin's disease. *N Engl J Med* 1976;295: 798-800.
115. Boles ET Jr, Haase GM, Hamoudi AB: Partial splenectomy in staging laparotomy for Hodgkin's disease: An alternative approach. *J Pediatr Surg* 1978;13:581-586.
116. Dearth JC, Gilchrist GS, Telander RL, et al: Partial splenectomy for staging Hodgkin's disease; risk of false-negative results. *N Engl J Med* 1978; 299:345-346.
117. Hansman D, Glasgow H, Sturt J, et al: Increased resistance to penicillin of pneumococci isolated from man. *N Engl J Med* 1971;284:175-177.
118. Hansman D, Devitt L, Miles H, Riley I: Pneumococci relatively insensitive to penicillin in Australia and New Guinea. *Med J Austral* 1974;2:353-356.
119. Jacobs JR, Koornhof HJ, Robins-Browne RM, et al: Emergence of multiply resistant pneumococci. *N Engl J Med* 1978;299:735-740.
120. Gunnison JW, Fraher MA, Pelcher EA, Jawetz E: Penicillin-resistant variants of pneumococci. *Appl Microbiol* 1968;16:311-314.
121. Dickerman JD, Bolton E, Coil JA, et al: Protective effect of prophylactic penicillin on splenectomized mice exposed to an aerosolized suspension of type III Streptococcus pneumoniae. *Blood* 1979;53:498-503.
122. Gaston MH, Verter JI, Woods G, et al: Prophylaxis with oral penicillin in children with sickle cell anemia; a randomized trial. *N Engl J Med* 1986; 314:1593-1599.
123. John AB, Ramlal A, Jackson H, et al: Prevention of pneumococcal infection in children with homozygous sickle cell disease. *Br Med J* 1984; 288:1567-1570.
124. Brivit F, Herer B, Fremaux A, et al: Fatal post-splenectomy pneumococcal sepsis despite pneumococcal vaccine and penicillin prophylaxis. *Lancet* 1984;2:356.
125. Buchanan GR, Smith SJ: Pneumococcal septicemia despite pneumococcal vaccine and prescription of penicillin prophylaxis in children with sickle cell anemia. *Am J Dis Child* 1986;140:428-432.
126. Cowan JJ, Amman AJ, Wara DW, et al: Pneumococcal polysaccharide immunization in infants and children. *Pediatrics* 1978;62:721-725.
127. Reis TC, Clark C, Burris O, et al: Case 19-1983: postsplenectomy sepsis. *N Engl J Med* 1983;309:926.
128. Pearson HA, Johnston D, Smith KA, Touloukian RJ: The born-again spleen: Return of splenic function after splenectomy for trauma. *N Engl J Med* 1978;298:1389-1392.
129. Widmann WD, Laubscher FA, Davidson SJ, Grenoble RA: Effects of splenectomy and splenosis on the blood and platelet count and red cell morphology. *Milit Med* 1971;136:15-19.

130. Velcek FT, Jongco B, Shaftan GW, et al: Posttraumatic splenic replantation in children. *J Pediatr Surg* 1982;17:879-882.
131. Schwartz AD, Dadash-Zadeh M, Goldstein R, et al: Antibody response to intravenous immunization following splenic tissue autotransplantation in Sprague-Dawley rats. *Blood* 1977;49:779-783.
132. Likhite VV: Opsonic and leucophilic γ-globulin in chronically splenectomized rats with and without heterotropic autotransplanted splenic tissue. *Nature* 1975;253:742-744.
133. Likhite VV: Evidence of immunological activity in heterotropic autotransplanted splenic tissue in DBA/Z mice. *Cell Immunol* 1974;12:382-386.
134. Likhite VV: Protection against fulminant sepsis in splenectomized mice by implantation of autochthonous splenic tissue. *Exp Hematol* 1978; 6:433-439.
135. Schwartz AD, Goldthorn JF, Winkelstein JA, Swift AJ: Lack of protective effect of autotransplanted splenic tissue to pneumococcal challenge. *Blood* 1978;51:475-478.
136. Cooney DR, Swanson SE, Dearth JC, et al: Heterotopic splenic autotransplantation in prevention of overwhelming postsplenectomy infection. *J Pediatr Surg* 1979;14:336-342.
137. Whiteside DC, Thomas CG Jr: Effect of splenectomy and autologous splenic implantation on a Streptococcus pneumoniae challenge. *Surg Forum* 1979;30:32-34.
138. Crosby WH, Benjamin NR: Frozen spleen reimplanted and challenged with Bartonella. *Am J Pathol* 1961;29:119-127.
139. Perla D, Marmorston-Gottesman J: Studies on *Bartonella muris* anemia of albino rats III; the protective effect of autoplastic splenic transplants on the *Bartonella muris* anemia of splenectomized rats. *J Exp Med* 1930; 52:131-143.
140. Dickerman JD, Horner SR, Coil JA, Gump DW: The protective effect of intraperitoneal splenic autotransplants in mice exposed to an aerosolized suspension of type III *Streptococcus pneumoniae*. *Blood* 1979;54:354-358.
141. Moxon ER, Schwartz AD: Heterotopic splenic autotransplantation in the prevention of *Haemophilus influenzae* meningitis and fatal sepsis in Sprague-Dawley rats. *Blood* 1980;56:842-845.
142. Benjamin JT, Komp DM, Shaw A, McMillan CW: Alternatives to total splenectomy; two case reports. *J Pediatr Surg* 1978;13:137-138.
143. Cooney DR, Dearth JC, Swanson SE, et al: Relative merits of partial splenectomy, splenic reimplantation, and immunization in preventing postsplenectomy infection. *Surgery* 1979;86:561-569.
144. Van Wyck DB, Witte MH, Witte CL, Thies AC Jr: Critical splenic mass for survival from experimental pneumococcemia. *J Surg Res* 1980;28:14-17.
145. Horton J, Ogden ME, Williams S, Coln D: The importance of splenic blood flow in clearing pneumococcal organisms. *Ann Surg* 1982;195:172-176.

146. Rice HM, James PD: Ectopic splenic tissue failed to prevent fatal pneumococcal septicaemia after splenectomy for trauma. *Lancet* 1980;1:565–566.
147. Case Records of the Massachusetts General Hospital (Case 36-1975). *N Engl J Med* 1975;293:547–553.

6
Hypersplenism

RICHARD H. SILLS
Children's Hospital of New Jersey, and University of Medicine and Dentistry-New Jersey Medical School, Newark, New Jersey

In contrast to hyposplenism, hypersplenism has been recognized for decades, but relatively little new information has become available in the last 10 years. The definition of hypersplenism and the clinical disorders associated with it will be reviewed in this chapter.

Hypersplenism is a clinical syndrome in which splenic function becomes excessive. It usually is the result of the function of a normal spleen becoming excessive (or harmful) simply as the spleen enlarges. By clinical examination alone, it is often difficult to determine when isolated splenomegaly results in hypersplenism. Crosby probably defined it most accurately, although not necessarily most practically, by stating: "When a person is hematologically better off without his spleen, he has hypersplenism" (1). The more specific, generally accepted definition of hypersplenism consists of four parts: (1) splenomegaly, (2) deficits in one or more cellular elements of blood, (3) hyperplasia or, at least, normocellular representation of precursors of the deficient cell line in the bone marrow, and (4) correction or improvement of the hematologic deficits following splenectomy. Individual elements of this definition may be missing, such as when the blood counts are normal because of bone marrow compensation or the concurrent presence of a hypocellular process in the marrow (1,2,3). Certainly, the diagnosis of hypersplenism is often made prior to splenectomy.

Many disorders are no longer considered to be hypersplenic. Prime examples of this are hematologic disorders in which destruction of abnormal blood cells occurs primarily in the spleen. Examples include hereditary sphereocytosis, autoimmune hemolytic anemia, and immune thrombocytopenic purpura. Although splenic destruction plays a critical role in the pathophysiology of these disorders, the destruction occurs because of an abnormality of the blood cell itself. The spleen is functioning normally and appropriately in removing these abnormal cells from the circulation. In true hypersplenism, excessive splenic function removes or sequesters normal cells from the circulation. It is also essential to remember that hypersplenism is a clinical syndrome resulting from an underlying disease process. It does not, in itself, represent an etiologic diagnosis.

PATHOPHYSIOLOGY OF HYPERSPLENISM

The pathophysiology of hypersplenism has been studied extensively. A limited discussion will be presented here, with references available if the reader wants further details (1,2,4,5). In response to infection or inflammation, the spleen increases its cellularity and vascularity by mechanisms that are poorly understood (5). When the spleen enlarges to the degree that its function becomes excessive, it is then capable of removing excessive numbers of normal blood cells.

Earlier theories suggested that hypersplenism resulted in bone marrow suppression as well as increased blood cell sequestration. Although there is a possibility that some bone marrow (hematopoietic) inhibition may occur, there is little supportive evidence for such a mechanism (5,6). The anemia of hypersplenism is predominantely due to a combination of sequestration and hemodilution. Under normal conditions, there is no significant sequestration of erythrocytes in the spleen. As the spleen enlarges, transit time of red cells through the spleen decreases and the percentage of red cell mass within the spleen becomes significant. From 10 to 45% of the body's total red cell mass can be found sequestered in the splenic pool in hypersplenism. Red cells in this splenic pool exist in slow equilibrium with the remainder of the circulation (1,7,8). Overall red cell survival is generally only slightly decreased and overt hemolysis is rarely seen (5,8). On occasion, however, up to 4% of the total red cell mass can be destroyed daily in the spleen (9).

As the spleen enlarges, blood volume expands because of the increased vascular compartment within the spleen and within the remainder of the splanchnic vasculature. This expansion of the splanchnic circulation is due to the increased portal venous pressure secondary to the augmented splanchnic blood flow. Plasma volume increases to compensate for the expansion of total blood volume. While the total red cell mass usually remains normal or even increases, hemoglobin concentration decreases as plasma volume expands. This component of the anemia represents a dilutional effect and is not a true decrease in red cell mass (5,8).

Thrombocytopenia is also the result of increased sequestration in the spleen. Normally up to one-third of platelets are sequestered in the spleen; these sequestered platelets are rapidly exchanging with the remaining two-thirds of platelets are rapidly exchanging with the remaining two-thirds of platelets in the general circulation. In hypersplenism, as many as 50 to 90% of the patient's platelets are found in the spleen. However, platelet survival remains normal or only slightly decreased and total body platelet mass remains normal (7,10).

The neutropenia of hypersplenism appears to be due to an increase in the marginal pool within the splenic circulation. The marginal pool increases from 50% of the total neutrophil pool to as much as 80% in hypersplenic patients. Infections on the basis of neutropenia in hypersplenic patients are rare because neutrophils in this marginal pool are readily available when needed (5,11,12).

LABORATORY EVALUATION OF THE HYPERSPLENIC STATE

A number of laboratory techniques have been used to evaluate the presence or degree of hypersplenism. Unfortunately, most are techniques better adapted for research studies and are less helpful as diagnostic tests for routine clinical use.

The epinephrine stimulation test has been advocated as a method to identify the presence of a hypersplenic states. In hypersplenism, greater increases in neutrophil counts were reported in response to epinephrine-induced release of the marginal pool (11). However, most investigators have not found this test to be clinically useful (13,14).

Comparison of total body hematocrit with venous hematocrit has also been used to evaluate hypersplenism. As the size of the spleen increases, the spleen predominantly sequesters more red cells than plasma. In response to increasing splenic sequestration, the blood volume is expanded, but outside of the spleen most of this volume expansion consists of plasma. Therefore, the venous hematocrit falls faster than total body hematocrit, providing a parameter that confirms the presence of hypersplenism. Unfortunately, the test requires radioisotopic labelling to determine total body hematocrit. The test also does not help in establishing a specific etiology of the hypersplenism (15), so its use is limited to confirming the presence of a hypersplenic state.

Radionuclide spleen scanning is the technique most commonly used to document the presence or severity of hypersplenism. Usually chromium-51-labelled, heat-damaged red cells are used for this imaging technique. The labelled, heat-damaged red cells are destroyed predominantly in the spleen. Both the survival of the red cells as well as surface scanning using scintigraphy can be measured using these labelled red cells. In hypersplenism, both a shortened heat-damaged red cell survival and excessive labelling of the spleen using scintigraphy are seen. Although this technique can provide useful information, its interpretation must consider several limitations. It is difficult to determine the relative uptake of red cells in the spleen compared to other sites, which is essential to confirm hypersplenism (5,16). Furthermore, it is likely that these scans simply reflect splenic blood flow as opposed to specific increases in macrophage activity within the spleen (5). This technique has not been able to reliably identify those patients with hypersplenism who will respond favorably to splenectomy (17).

None of these studies are helpful in establishing the specific cause of hypersplenism as opposed to simply documenting its presence. Although it may be important to confirm the presence of hypersplenism, it is usually more crucial to determine its underlying etiology.

ETIOLOGIES OF HYPERSPLENISM

Infectious Etiologies of Hypersplenism

Although splenomegaly is common in many infections, documented hypersplenism is rare. Chronic infections which are reported to cause hypersplenism include malaria, tuberculosis, leishmaniasis, schistosomiasis, trypanosomiasis and Q-fever (Table 1).

Malaria is the most common infectious cause of hypersplenism. Splenic enlargement and concomitant enhancement of splenic function may play an important role in host defense in these patients (18a). Unfortunately, the splenomegaly may be massive and can frequently cause hypersplenism in both children and adults. Anemia is present in most patients, with up to 40% of the red cell mass being sequestered in the spleen. Plasma volume usually expands, increasing the apparent severity of the anemia. Thrombocytopenia and leukopenia are also common (2,18).

Tuberculosis involvement of the spleen can be complicated by hypersplenism. This is most often seen in primary tuberculosis of the spleen, which is a rare presentation of this infection. The spleen in these patients may be massively enlarged. Leukopenia and anemia are the most common hematological changes, but thrombocytopenia can also occur. Primary splenic involvement by tuberculosis can be very difficult to diagnose. Calcifications of the spleen provide a helpful diagnostic clue. In several reports, splenectomy resulted in resolution of the hematological changes (2,19,20,21).

Leismaniasis, or kala-azar, can produce massive splenomegaly and hypersplenism in both children and adults. Hypersplenism occurs with both the Asiatic and the Mediterranean (or infantile) forms of leishmaniasis. Irregular fever and lymphadenopathy are often present. Pancytopenia becomes increasingly evident with increasing duration of disease and increasing size of the spleen. Leukopenia appears first, followed by anemia and finally thrombocytopenia. Anemia and leucopenia are most prominent. One-third of patients have hemoglobin levels less than 7 g/dl and almost 90% have white blood cell counts less than

Table 1 Etiologies of Hypersplenism

A. Infectious
   1. Malaria
   2. Tuberculosis
   3. Leishmaniasis
   4. Schistosomiasis
   5. Brucellosis *
   6. Candidiasis **
   7. Histoplasmosis **
   8. Syphilis **
   9. Q fever **
   10. Viral illness **
B. Inflammatory and collagen-vascular disorders
   1. Felty's syndrome *
   2. Sarcoidosis *
   3. Systemic lupus erythematosis *
C. Congestive Splenomegaly
D. Storage Diseases
   1. Gaucher's disease
   2. Niemann-Pick disease
   3. Amyloidosis *
   4. Glycogen storage disease **
   5. Tangier disease **
   6. Sea-blue histiocytosis
E. Hematologic disorders
   1. Sequestration crisis
   2. Myeloproliferative, lymphoproliferative and lymphomatous disorders
      a. Agnogenic myeloid metaplasia
      b. Polycythemia vera *
      c. Hematologic malignancies
         1-Hodgkin's disease
         2-Non-Hodgkin's lymphoma
         3-Chronic myelogenous leukemia *
         4-Chronic lymphocytic leukemia *
         5-Hairy cell leukemia *
   3. Primary hypersplenism
   4. Histiocytosis X
   5. Aplastic anemia **
   6. Red cell aplasia **
   7. Thrombotic thrombocytopenia purpura **
F. Non-hematologic neoplastic disorders
   1. Carcinomas *
   2. Isolated splenic cysts **

Table 1 (continued)

F. Non-hematologic neoplastic disorders (continued)
   3. Hamartomas **
   4. Malignant melanoma **
G. Miscellaneous conditions
   1. Tropical splenomegaly
   2. Hemodialysis *
   3. Thyrotoxicosis **
   4. Whipple's disease **
   5. Malignant mastocytosis **
   6. Progressive multifocal leucodystrophy **
   7. Syndrome of hypogammaglobuliemia, splenomegaly and hypersplenism**
   8. Splenic cyst
   9. Diabetes mellitus

---

*Reported in adults but not in children or adolescents.
**Based upon splace clinical data.

5,000/mm^3. All white cell types are reduced in numbers, but neutrophils are decreased most. The majority of patients have thrombocytopenia, with average counts of 103,000/mm^3 (1,22,23). The bone marrow is consistently hyperplastic. Effective therapy of the leishmania infection results in gradual resolution of the hypersplenism (22).

Infestation with schistosomiasis in both children and adults can be complicated by hypersplenism (22,24). Portal hypertension develops in these patients from embolism due to schistosomiasis ova that enter the hepatic portal system from the mesenteric circulation. The host responds to these ova retained in the liver with granuloma formation, which results in scarring. A perisinusoidal block to hepatic portal blood flow develops with resulting portal hypertension (25). Most of the patients with portal hypertension manifest hypersplenism.

Splenic involvement is common in brucellosis. The spleen is actually the most common site of chronic localized infection due to brucella organisms (26). Localized splenic infection is characterized by a chronic infection, extending over a period of years, with intermittent acute exacerbations. Calcifications of the spleen are often present. Hypersplenism causes anemia and thrombocytopenia in adults with brucellosis. Some reports noted that splenectomy was necessary to cure antibiotic resistant brucella infection localized to the spleen; anemia and thrombocytopenia disappeared following splenectomy (27).

A number of infections have occasionally been reported to cause hypersplenism. These include candidiasis (21,28), histoplasmosis (28), syphilis (especially the congenital form) (4,21,29,30), and endocarditis due to Q fever (Coxiella burnetti) (31,31a).

Acute infection is the most common cause of splenomegaly, but it is rarely mentioned as a cause of hypersplenism. It is likely that hypersplenism due to acute infection occurs but is not recognized. A combination of splenomegaly and deficits in one more cellular elements of blood are common in viral illnesses. Unfortunately, it is difficult to establish before the infection resolves whether the cytopenias are due to a suppressive effect of the infection on the marrow or due to hypersplenism. Increased sequestration of labelled erythrocytes in the spleen has been noted in individual patients with infectious mononucleosis, infectious hepatitis, subacute bacterial endocarditis, miliary tuberculosis, and psittacosis. A hypersplenic state was suggested by the presence of splenomegaly as well as by the finding of spherocytes in the peripheral blood of all of these patients. Thrombocytopenia and leukopenia were seen in some patients. All patients recovered once the primary infection and the associated splenomegaly resolved (4).

INFLAMMATORY AND COLLAGEN-VASCULAR DISORDERS AS ETIOLOGIES OF HYPERSPLENISM

These disorders include Felty's syndrome, sarcoidosis, and systemic lupus erythematosis.

Felty's syndrome is the classical collagen-vascular disease associated with hypersplenism. This variant of rheumatoid arthritis, which typically occurs in middle age, is associated with splenomegaly and leukopenia. The severity of the rheumatoid arthritis does not directly correlate with the severity of the hematologic changes. All patients are leukopenic and approximately 80% are granulocytopenic (32). Occasionally the leukopenia is cyclic (2). The pathophysiology of the leukopenia is complex, with evidence of increased margination, increased splenic sequestration, decreased survival and even marrow depletion of leukocytes. The precise mechanism or mechanisms responsible for the neutropenia remain to be elucidated (2,33-35). Leukocyte dysfunction is also present and is as important as the leukopenia in predisposing these patients to infections (32). As many as 90% of patients are anemic, and 40% are thrombocytopenic (32). The anemia is primarily due to splenic sequestration and decreased red cell survival (36,37). Hemolysis may be evident but is rarely severe. The bone marrow is hypercellular (2). Most patients demonstrate resolution of the anemia and leukopenia following splenectomy, although infectious complications may persist and the hematologic complications may recur (36-38). Treatment of the syndrome remains controversial.

Hypersplenism is a complication of sarcoidosis. Although 20% of patients with sarcoidosis manifest splenomegaly, most do not develop hypersplenism

(39). When hypersplenism occurs, leukopenia and thrombocytopenia are not uncommon, and deaths due to bleeding in thrombocytopenic patients have been reported. Anemia occurs less frequently and may respond to splenectomy. Severe thrombocytopenia or leukopenia may improve or resolve following splenectomy (21,40,41).

Systemic lupus erythematosis causes hypersplenism (5,42). However, most instances of splenomegaly associated with deficits in peripheral blood cells in lupus are caused by autoimmune-mediated hematologic disease and are not caused by true hypersplenism.

CONGESTIVE SPLENOMEGALY

Congestive splenomegaly is the most common cause of hypersplenism. There is an anatomic predisposition to portal hypertension because the hepatic portal vein has no valves. Any increase in pressure in the portal vein readily backs up and is reflected in the spleen. Portal hypertension and hypersplenism can then result (43).

Cirrhosis is the cause of 70% of portal hypertension in adults. Etiologies of cirrhosis include alcoholism, hepatitis, schistosomiasis, Wilson's disease, congenital disorders, neoplasms, and cystic fibrosis. The most common causes of portal hypertension in patients under the age of 18 years are extrahepatic in nature. The portal venous thrombosis syndromes are the most common of these extrahepatic etiologies. They include cavernous transformation due to systemic infections, gastroenteritis, dehydration, and trauma due to umbilical venous catheters. The next most common cause of portal hypertension in children is cirrhosis. This is most often due to intrinsic liver disease, biliary atresia, or metabolic disorders. Other extrahepatic etiologies of portal hypertension, seen in children, adults, or both, include congenital stenosis or atresia of the hepatic portal vein, thrombosis of the hepatic vein (Budd-Chiari syndrome), irradiation, splenic venous compression due to tumor or pancreatic fibrosis, and splenic artery aneurysm (2). In extrahepatic portal hypertension, there are likely to be few or no symptoms until gastrointestinal hemorrhage occurs. Normocytic, normochromic anemia, leukopenia, neutropenia and thrombocytopenia are common. In portal hypertension secondary to cirrhosis, target cells and teardrop poikilocytes are often noted as a result of the impairment of hepatic function.

Treatment of congestive splenomegaly is complex and controversial. Although splenectomy improves the pancytopenia, the risk of the surgery is high and splenectomy does little to alter the long-term prognosis. Improved survival depends upon preventing variceal hemorrhage. Once the first such hemorrhage occurs, there is little chance of surviving more than one or two years without therapy (2). If splenectomy is to be performed, it is often done as part of a shunt procedure to reduce the portal hypertension. Appropriate surgical textbooks provide the operative details of these shunting procedures together with the expected outcomes.

STORAGE DISEASES AS CAUSES OF HYPERSPLENISM

Storage diseases associated with hypersplenism include Gaucher's disease (44a), Niemann-Pick disease, amyloidosis, glycogen storage disease (1,2,44), Tangier disease (45), and sea blue histiocytosis (46). These are discussed in detail in Chapter 9 "Splenomegaly: Metabolic Disorders."

HEMATOLOGIC DISEASES AS CAUSES OF HYPERSPLENISM

Many hematologic disorders can cause hypersplenism. Those disorders in which the primary abnormality involves the circulating blood cell, and not primarily the spleen itself, are no longer considered to be examples of hypersplenism (2,4, 5,47). In these instances, the spleen is simply performing its normal function of removing abnormal cells. The primary problem is an excess of abnormal circulating blood cells and not an abnormality of the spleen. Examples of primary blood cell problems include congenital disorders, such as hereditary spherocytosis or elliptocytosis, and acquired disorders such as autoimmune hemolytic anemia or immune thrombocytopenic purpura.

Hematologic disorders included in this category are (1) acute splenic sequestration, (2) myeloproliferative, lymphoproliferative and lymphomatous disorders, (3) primary hypersplenism, (4) histiocytosis-X, and (5) other hematologic disorders.

Acute splenic sequestration is characterized by sudden and rapid enlargement of the spleen due to trapping of circulating erythrocytes. This type of sequestration can be considered an exception to the concept that defects of circulating hematologic cells do not cause hypersplenism according to the strict definition. In these instances, the abnormal erythrocytes produce an alteration in the spleen itself that then results in a form of hypersplenism. Sequestration crises most commonly complicate the sickle hemoglobinopathies, although sequestration is occasionally seen in patients with other hemolytic anemias such as hereditary sphereocytosis.

In sickle cell anemia, acute splenic sequestration is the second most common cause of death in young children. Little is known about the pathophysiology and virtually nothing is known of precipitating factors (48,49). Some acute alteration must occur in the red cells, in the spleen, or in both the red cells and spleen, that results in an abrupt increase in splenic congestion. As a consequence, large volumes of blood enter the spleen but fail to exit adequately. A large portion of the total circulating blood volume may be abruptly sequestered, with shock and even death occurring within hours. Sequestration crises in sickle cell anemia affect young children predominately, with most cases occurring in the first 6 years of life. Approximately one-quarter of episodes occur in the first 2 years of life, with some as early as 3 months (49). Acute splenic sequestration is the first major complication of sickle cell disease in approximately one-fifth of patients (50). The incidence has been reported to be as high as 11.3 episodes per 100 patient years, with 27% of children developing this complication (49). Paradoxically, acute sequestration crises often occur in patients who have already developed hyposplenism (51).

Children with sickle cell anemia and acute sequestration crises present abruptly without any recognizable prodrome or precipitating factors. They suddenly develop pallor, abdominal distention and polydipsia. Left-sided abdominal pain and vomiting are frequent. Loss of blood volume into the spleen soon results in shock, with marked dyspnea, profound weakness, tachypnea and tachycardia quickly developing. The spleen is markedly enlarged and tender. Laboratory findings include a significant decrease in hemoglobin level, an increase in reticulocytes, together with normoblastemia and often thrombocytopenia (52).

Mortality rates from acute splenic sequestration range from as high as 29.4 to as low as 3.1 per 100 events, with the latter (lower) rate thought to have resulted from intensive patient education (49). Death can occur within 4 hours of the first symptom and almost always occurs before transfusions can be started. Up to one-half of patients will have recurrences, usually within 4 months. Survivors show a greater than expected response to transfusion. Presumably, this enhanced response is due to liberation of sequestered red cells from the spleen once the circulatory impairment in the spleen has been improved by the transfusion of non-sickling red cells (49,52).

As many as 6% of Jamaican children with homozygous sickle cell anemia develop a chronic hypersplenic state. In one-half of these children chronic hypersplenism develops following an episode of acute splenic sequestration which unexpectedly fails to resolve. The spleen remains enlarged more than 4 cm below the left costal margin, the hemoglobin level remains below 6.5 g/dl and the platelet count is below 200,000/mm^3. An equal number of children have been reported to develop this chronic hypersplenic state without a pre-existing acute splenic sequestration. The natural history of this complication is poorly documented (51,53).

Acute splenic sequestration also occurs in patients with hemoglobin SC disease. Unlike the crises associated with homozygous (SS) sickle cell anemia, adults as well as children can develop this complication. This is probably related to the fact that patients with hemoglobin SC disease have persistence of splenomegaly into adolescence and adulthood, rather than undergoing complete splenic infarction at an early age, as occurs in most patients with homozygous sickle cell anemia (54).

Although aplastic crises are the most common cause of acute exacerbations of anemia in hereditary spherocytosis, splenic sequestration crises may also occur. Splenic sequestration is usually seen in association with viral illnesses which are often otherwise quite mild in presentation (4,55,56). The viral illness presumably stimulates the reticuloendothelial system, resulting in sequestration and increased hemolysis. An abrupt increase in splenic size is associated with a fairly sudden drop in the hemoglobin level. Jaundice is often noted. The sequestration crises of hereditary spherocytosis, however, do not tend to be as abrupt and life-threatening as those of sickle cell anemia.

Various myeloproliferative, lymphoproliferative, and lymphomatous disorders can be associated with splenomegaly and hypersplenism. Because the defect in these disorders involves hematopoietic cells, it is doubtful whether they should be considered as true examples of hypersplenism.

Agnogenic myeloid metaplasia (idiopathic myelofibrosis) is commonly associated with a hypersplenic state. The splenomegaly results from extramedullary hematopoiesis in the spleen and a marked increase in splenic blood flow through the celiac axis. Myeloid metaplasia is predominately a disorder of patients over the age of 50, rarely occurring in persons less than 30 years of age. However, children with idiopathic myelofibrosis as young as 13 months have been reported (57). All patients develop splenomegaly, with about one-third developing an enlarged spleen that fills the entire left side of the abdomen. Most patients have mild anemia and leukopenia (58-60). Splenectomy can improve the peripheral blood counts, decrease the portal hypertension, and relieve pain due to splenic enlargement. It is not clear whether splenectomy improves long-term survival (61). Furthermore, splenectomy is associated with significant complications in this group of patients. Early postoperative morbidity (56%) and mortality (28%) have been reported in the group (61a). Occasional patients also develop massive compensatory hepatic myeloid metaplasia following splenectomy (61b).

Polycythemia vera is another disorder occurring in adults associated with hypersplenism. The etiology of the hypersplenism in polycythemia vera remains undefined (62). Late in the clinical course of polycythemia vera, a "spent phase" occurs in at least 5% of cases. Hypersplenism is an important component of this phase. These patients tend to rapidly develop acute leukemia or splenic myeloid metaplasia. Whether splenectomy can prevent this progression of polycythemia to leukemia or myeloid metaplasia is unknown (63).

Overt hematologic malignancies may also cause hypersplenism. These include Hodgkin's disease (64), non-Hodgkin's lymphomas (65-68), chronic myeloid leukemia, chronic lymphocytic leukemia (1,2,67,69) and hairy cell leukemia (70,71). Although bone marrow failure is the usual cause of pancytopenia in these patients, hypersplenism can also occur and is usually difficult to diagnose.

In hairy cell leukemia, the pancytopenia is usually due to both hypersplenism and bone marrow failure. Splenectomy in these patients improves the pancytopenia by abolishing the hypersplenism (70).

The primary hypersplenism syndromes were first reported over 40 years ago. The adjective "primary" denoted the absence of an identifyable disorder causing the hypersplenism. Secondary hypersplenic disorders have well defined etiologies. Since the vast majority of published cases of primary hypersplenism were reported 30 to 40 years ago, it is likely that most of them were "secondary" to underlying disorders which could not be specifically diagnosed because of the limitations of diagnostic capabilities available at the time. Cases of primary hypersplenism, however, are occasionally still described. Many may represent pre-leukemic states. On this basis, the "primary" hypersplenic disorders have been classified as hematologic disorders.

The term primary splenic neutropenia was used to describe patients with isolated neutropenia, which usually was associated with splenomegaly, and which was cured by splenectomy (6,72). Clinical findings included recurrent fevers, pharyngitis, mucous membrane ulcerations, and bone marrow hyperplasia (43). Primary splenic pancytopenia was associated with a similar clinical picture, except for the presence of pancytopenia rather than isolated neutropenia. In both disorders, splenectomy was associated with improvement or cure (6,7,74).

In a recent article, the outcome of patients with massive splenomegaly and hypersplenism of unknown etiology was reviewed. Patients as young as 22 years were identified. Splenectomy corrected the pancytopenia, but 2 of the 5 patients developed non-Hodgkin's lymphoma within 6 years following surgery. In a review of published reports of primary hypersplenism, 9 out of 46 cases showed development of non-Hodgkin's lymphoma 8 to 80 months post-splenectomy. Although the pathophysiology is not clear, it is likely that cases of "primary splenomegaly" or "non-tropical idiopathic splenomegaly" represent a potentially pre-lymphomatous condition (75).

Histiocytosis X is associated with hypersplenism. Hypersplenism is usually a complication of the severe systemic form of the disease (Letterer-Siwe disease) that generally presents in the first year of life. The hypersplenism is usually a late complication of hepatic involvement. Healing of the liver often occurs with fibrosis. Cirrhosis, hypersplenism and portal hypertension can result and death may occur secondary to these complications (76). However, pancytopenia, due at least in part to hypersplenism, also appears to occur in association with splenomegaly during the acute phase of the disease. In this instance, the hypersplenism resolves following successful therapy of the histiocytosis (77,78).

Some patients with aplastic anemia have been thought to have a component of hypersplenism on the basis of a modest improvement in blood counts following splenectomy. It is not clear whether this actually represents a degree of hypersplenism (1,79). A patient with severe red cell aplasia and chronic active hepatitis also had hematologic improvement following splenectomy (80). However, this improvement may have been a response to an autoimmune process and not necessarily due to the presence of hypersplenism. There have also been reports of improvement following splenectomy in patients with thrombotic thrombocytopenic purpura. In these cases, however, it is likely that the improvement was due to a mechanism other than hypersplenism (1,81).

NEOPLASTIC CONDITIONS ASSOCIATED WITH HYPERSPLENISM

In addition to the hematologic malignancies discussed above, other neoplastic disorders have rarely been associated with hypersplenism. These include isolated splenic cysts (82), hamartomas (83), and carcinoma of the tail of the pancreas (84). All of these cases were in adults.

Malignant melanoma is associated with increased splenic uptake or technetium-99m sulfur-colloid, but true hypersplenism has not been reported. Furthermore, hemoglobin levels and leukocyte counts showed no relationship to the augmented sulfur-colloid splenic uptake on scan. The enhanced uptake of colloid is thought to be due to a potentiation of phagocytic activity, possibly due to stimulation by tumor antigens, immune complexes, or both (85). In the absence of any other evidence of hypersplenism, the significance of this increased splenic uptake of sulfur-colloid is unknown.

MISCELLANEOUS CONDITIONS ASSOCIATED WITH HYPERSPLENISM

Topical splenomegaly is an additional syndrome, which was labelled as a form of primary hypersplenism. Although some controversy still exists (86a) it now seems likely that the pathophysiology of this disorder involves infection with malaria. This syndrome probably represents an atypical immune response to the malarial organism (86). Tropical splenomegaly is characterized by massive splenomegaly which occurs only in areas where malaria is endemic. Children as well as adults are affected. Anemia is usually present and appears to be due to increased plasma volume and an expanded red cell pool. Leukopenia and thrombocytopenia are common (86,87). Anti-malarial chemotherapy as well as splenectomy have helped some patients (86).

Hemodialysis is also associated with hypersplenism. The multifactorial anemia of hemodialysis patients has a hemolytic component. Chromium-labelled red cell survival studies have documented excessive splenic uptake, and splenectomy has resulted in significant improvement in both the rate of hemolysis and anemia

(88,89). Further investigation has produced evidence suggesting that the hemolysis and resulting splenic sequestration of red cells may have been caused by chloramine contamination in the water source for dialysis fluid. No additional cases of anemia were observed once chloramine was removed from the water supply (88).

Hypersplenism has been reported to occur in association with a variety of other disorders. Most of these associations were based on single cases reports or very small studies which have not been confirmed. For this reasons, these entities will only be mentioned. Disorders reported to be associated with hypersplenism include thyrotoxicosis (90), Whipple's disease (intestinal lipodystrophy) (91), malignant mastocytosis (92), progressive multifocal leukoencephalopathy (93), the syndrome of hypogammaglobulinemia, splenomegaly and hypersplenism (94), and splenic cysts (94a). Diabetes mellitus was associated with an increased splenic uptake using technetium-99m sulfur-colloid, but no clinical evidence of hypersplenism was mentioned (95).

TREATMENT OF HYPERSPLENISM

Therapy is complex and varies considerably depending upon the specific etiology of the hypersplenism. Although splenectomy, by definition, should cure hypersplenism, the benefits and risks of the operation must be carefully considered. Some patients, such as those with Gaucher's disease and bleeding complications, may benefit greatly from splenectomy. Other patients, such as those with congestive splenomegaly, may derive less or little benefit from the operation. In congestive splenomegaly, the primary problems result from gastrointestinal bleeding due to portal hypertension, and not from pancytopenia. Any benefit to be gained from splenectomy must be carefully weighed against the immediate risk of the procedure, and the long-term risk of the post-splenectomy sepsis syndrome.

Considering the various disorders and therapeutic modalities now available, a detailed discussion of the therapy of hypersplenism is beyond the scope of this chapter. Information on the therapy of specific disorders causing hypersplenism is available in recent textbooks in internal medicine, pediatrics and surgery.

SUMMARY AND CONCLUSIONS

Hypersplenism is a clinical syndrome with a wide variety of causes. Unlike hyposplenism, in which the primary consequence is an increased risk of life-threatening infection, hypersplenism presents a more complex and varied clinical picture. Its direct hematologic effects, the deficits of one or more cellular blood elements, is a major concern. However, even more life-threatening are the portal hypertension and the risk of variceal hemorrhage which accompanies the congestive forms of hypersplenism

Hypersplenism is important for several reasons. It can be the presenting clinical picture of a wide variety of disorders which often present significant diagnostic dilemmas. Once the diagnosis is established, the difficult issue of therapy must be addressed.

REFERENCES

1. Crosby WH: Hypersplenism. *Ann Rev Med* 1962;13:127-146.
2. Wintrobe MM, Lee GR, Boggs DR, et al; (eds): *Clinical Hematology*, Lea and Febiger, Philadelphia, PA, 1981, pp. 1426-1446.
3. Crosby WH: Hypersplenism, In, Williams WJ, Beutler E, Erslev AJ, Lichtman MA, (eds): *Hematology*, McGraw-Hill, New York, 1983, pp 660-666.
4. Armorosi EL: Hypersplenism. *Semin Hematol* 1965;2:249-285.
5. Bowdler AJ: Splenomegaly and hypersplenism. *Clin Haematol* 1983;12: 467-488.
6. Crosby WH: Is hypersplenism a dead issue? *Blood* 1962;20:94-99.
7. Jandl JH, Aster RH: Increased splenic pooling and the pathogenesis of hypersplenism. *Am J Med Sci* 1967;253:383-398.
8. Christensen BE: Erythrocyte pooling and sequestration in enlarged spleens. *Scand J Haematol* 1973;10:106-119.
9. Christensen BE: Quantitative determination of splenic red blood cell destruction in patients with splenomegaly. *Scand J Haematol* 1975;14:295-302.
10. Aster RH: Pooling of platelets in the spleen; role in the pathogenesis of "hypersplenic" thrombocytopenia. *J Clin Invest* 1966;45:645-657.
11. Brubaker LH, Johnson CA: Correlation of splenomegaly and abnormal neutrophil pooling (margination). *J Lab Clin Med* 1978;92:508-515.
12. Bishop CR, Rothstein G, Ashenbrucker HE, et al: Leucokinetic studies, XIV, Blood neutrophil kinetics in steady state neutropenia. *J Clin Invest* 1971;50:1678-1689.
13. Joyce RA, Boggs DR, Hasiba U, et al: Marginal neutrophil pool size in normal subjects as measured by epinephrine infusion. *J Lab Clin Med* 1976; 88:614-620.
14. Chatteyea JB, Dameshek W, Stefanini M: The adrenalin (epinephrine) test as applied to hematologic disorders. *Blood* 1953;8:211-235.
15. Fudenberg H, Baldini M, Mahoney JP, et al: The body hematocrit/venous hematocrit ratio and the "splenic reservoir." *Blood* 1961;17:71-82.
16. Holzbach RT, Shipley RA, Clark RE, et al: Influence of splenic size and portal pressure on erythrocyte sequestration. *J Clin Invest* 1964;43:1124-1135.
17. Armos RR: Clinical studies with spleen-specific radiolabeled agents. *Semin Nucl Med* 1985;15:260-275.

18. Richmond J, Donaldsen GWK, Williams R, et al: Haematological effects of the idiopathic splenomegaly seen in Uganda. *Br J Haematol* 1967;13: 348-363.
18a. Looareesuwan S, Ho M, Wattanagoon Y, White NJ, Warrell DA, Bunnag D, Harinasuta T, Wyler DJ: Dynamic alteration in splenic function during acute falciparum malaria. *N Engl J Med* 1987;317:675-679.
19. Chapman AF, Reeder PS, Baker LA: Neutropenia secondary to tuberculous splenomegaly: Report of a case. *Ann Intern Med* 1954;41:1225-1231.
20. Chapman AF, Reeder PS, Baker LA: Neutropenia secondary to tuberculous splenomegaly; report of a case. *Ann Int Med* 1954;41:1225-1231.
21. Doan CA: Hypersplenism. *Bull NY Acad Med* 1949;26:625-650.
22. Cartwright GE, Chung HL, Chang A: Studies on the pancytopenia of Kala-azar. *Blood* 1948;3:249-275.
23. Burchenal JH, Bowers RF, Haedicke TA: Visceral leishmaniasis complicated by severe anemia; improvement following splenectomy. *Am J Trop Med* 1947;27:699-709.
24. Soto-Albors CE, Rayburn WF, Taylor L, Musselman M: Portal hypertension and hypersplenism in pregnancy secondary to chronic schistosomiasis. *J Reproduct Med* 1984;29:345-348.
25. Mahmoud AA: Trematodes (Schiostosomiasis, other flukes), In, GL Mandell, RG Douglas Jr, JE Bennett, (eds); *Principles and Practice of Infectious Disease*, John Wiley and Sons, New York, 1985, pp. 1573-1576.
26. MacDonald GF, Martin WJ, Wellman WE, Weed LA: Chronic localized brucellosis of the spleen. *Postgrad Med* 1966;40:703-707.
27. McGarity WC, Serafin D: Brucellosis; indications for splenectomy. *Am J Surg* 1968;115:355-363.
28. Bodey GP, De Johgh D, Isassi A, et al: Hypersplenism due to disseminated candidiasis in a patient with acute leukemia. *Cancer* 1969;24:417-420.
29. Ingall D, Musher D: Syphilis, In, Remington JS, Klein JO, (eds); *Infectious Diseases of the Fetus and Newborn Infant*, WB Saunders Co., Philadelphia, PA, 1983, pp 344-345.
30. Harmos O, Myers ME: Gummatous syphilitic splenomegaly. *Am J Clin Path* 1951;21:737-742.
31. Spring WJC, Hamspon J: Chronic Q fever endocarditis causing massive splenomegaly and hypersplenism. *Br Med J* 1982;285:1244.
32. Spivak JL: Felty's syndrome; an analytical review. *John Hopkins Med J* 1977;141:156-162.
33. Vincent PC, Levi JA, Macqueen A: The mechanism of neutropenia in Felty's syndrome. *Brit J Hematol* 1974;27:463-475.
34. Srodes CR, Hyde F, Chernvick PA, et al: Neutrophil kinetics of Felty's syndrome. *Blood* 1972;40:950A.
35. Abdou NI, N Pombejara C, Balentine L, Abdou NL: Suppressor cell-mediated neutropenia in Felty's syndrome. *J Clin Invest* 1978;61:738-743.
36. Hume R, Dogy JH, Fraser TN, et al: Anemia of Felty's syndrome. *Ann Rheum Dis* 1964;23:267-271.

37. Barnes CG, Turnbull AL, Vernon-Roberts B: Felty's Syndrome. *Ann Rheum Dis* 1971;30:359-374.
38. Ruderman M, Miller LM, Pinals RS: Clinical and serologic observations on 27 patients with Felty's syndrome. *Arthritis Rheum* 1968;11:377-384.
39. Longcape WT, Freiman DG: A study of sarcoidosis. *Medicine* 1952;31: 1-132.
40. Bertino J, Myersom RM: The role of splenectomy in sarcoidosis. *Arch Int Med* 1960;105:213-217.
41. Webb AK, Mitchell DN, Patricia CM, et al: Splenomegaly and splenectomy in sarcoidosis. *J Clin Path* 1979;32:1050-1053.
42. Dubois EL: *Lupus Erythematosis*, University of Southern California Press, Los Angeles, CA, 1974, pp 367-368.
43. Rogers HM, Hall BE: Primary splenic neutropenia. *Arch Int Med* 1945; 75:192-195.
44. Duckett JW: Splenectomy in treatment of secondary hypersplenism. *Ann Surg* 1963;157:737-746.
44a. Bar-Maor JA, Grovin-Yehudain J: Partial splenectomy in children with Gaucher's disease. *Pediatrics* 1985;76:398-401.
45. Linman JW: Hematology: *Physiologic, Pathophysiologic, and Clinical Principles*, Macmillan Publishing Co. Inc., New York, 1975, pp 823-848.
46. Silverstein MN, Ellefson RD: The syndrome of the sea-blue histiocyte. *Semin Hematol* 1972;9:299-307.
47. Dameshek W: Hypersplenism. *Bull New York Acad Med* 1955;31:113-136.
48. Serjeant GR: Treatment of sickle cell disease in early childhood in Jamaica. *Am J Pediatr Hematol Oncol* 1985;7:235-239.
49. Emond AM, Morais P, Venngopal S, et al: Role of splenectomy in homozygous sickle cell disease in childhood. *Lancet* 1984;1:88-90.
50. Bainbridge R, Higgs DR, Muade PH, Serjeant GR: Clinical presentation of homozygous sickle cell disease. *J Pediatr* 1985;106:881-885.
51. Serjeant GR: *Sickle Cell Disease*. Oxford University Press, Oxford, 1985, pp 115-123.
52. Seeler RA, Shwiaki MF: Acute splenic sequestration crisis (ASSC) in young children with sickle cell anemia. *Clin Pediatr* 1972;11:701-704.
53. Topley JM, Rogers DW, Stevens MCG, Serjeant GR: Acute splenic sequestration and hypersplenism in the first five years in homozygous sickle cell disease. *Arch Dis Child* 1981;56:765-769.
54. Sears DA, Udden MM: Splenic infarction, splenic sequestration and functional hyposplenism in hemoglobin S-C disease. *Am J Hematol* 1985;18: 261-268.
55. Krueger HC, Burgert EO: Hereditary spherocytosis in 100 children. *Mayo Cl Proc* 1966;41:821-828.
56. Lux SE, Glader BE: Disorders of the red cell membrane, In, Nathan DG, Oski FA, (eds); *Hematology of Infancy and Childhood*, WB Saunders, Philadelphia, PA, pp 498-499.

57. Rosenberg HS, Taylor FM: The myeloproliferative syndrome in children. *J Pediatr* 1958;52:407-423.
58. Ward HP, Block MH: The natural history of agnogenic myeloid metaplasia (AMM) and a critical evaluation of its relationship with the myeloproliferative syndrome. *Medicine* 1971;50:357-420.
59. Silverstein MN: Agnogenic myeloid metaplasia. In, Williams WJ, Beutler E, Erslev AJ, Lichtman MA, (eds): *Hematology* McGraw-Hill Book Co., New York, 1983, pp 214-218.
60. Silverstein MN: *Agnogenic myeloid metaplasia*, Publishing Science Corp., Boston, MA, 1975.
61. Benbasset J, Penchas S, Ligumski M: Splenectomy in patients with agnogenic myeloid metaplasia; an analysis of 321 published cases. *Br J Haematol* 1979;42:297-214.
61a. Malmaeus J, Akre T, Adami HO, Hagbery H: Early postoperative course following elective splenectomy in haematological disease: a high complication rate in patients with myeloproliferative disorders. *Br J Surg* 1986; 73:720-723.
61b. Towell BL, Levine SP: Massive hepatomegaly following splenectomy for myeloid metaplasia. *Am J Med* 1987;82:371-375.
62. Berg B, Stohl E, Soderstrom N: The cytology of spleen aspiration in uncomplicated polycythaemia vera. *Scand J Hematol* 1973;10:59-61.
63. Najean Y, Arrago JP, Rain JD, et al: The "spent" phase of polycythemia vera: Hypersplenism in the absence of myelofibrosis. *Br J Haematol* 1984; 56:163-170.
64. Rousselot LM, Rella AJ, Rottino A: Splenectomy for hypersplenism in Hodgkin's disease. *Am J Surg* 1962;103:769-774.
65. Hickling RA: Giant follicle lymphoma of the spleen; recovery after splenectomy. *Brit Med J* 1960;1:1464-1467.
66. Sheehan PL, Sokal JE: Thrombocytoepnia with marked reduction of megakaryocytes in a patient with lymphosarcoma-leukemia, treated by splenectomy. *New York State J Med* 1961;61:791-797.
67. McIntosh S, Rooks Y, Ritchey AK et al: Fever in young children with sickle cell disease. *J Pediatr* 1980;96:199-204.
68. Kraemer BB, Osborne BM, Butler JJ: Primary splenic presentation of malignant lymphoma and related disorders. *Cancer* 1984;54:1606-1619.
69. Fisher JH, Welch CS, Dameshek W: Splenectomy in leukemia and leukosarcoma. *N Engl J Med* 1952;246:479-484.
70. Catovsky D, Pettit JE, Galton DAG, et al: Leukaemic reticuloendotheliosis ("Hairy Cell Leukemia"): A distinct clinico-pathological entity. *Br J Haematol* 1974;26:9-27.
71. Golomb HM: Hairy Cell Leukemia, In, Williams WJ, Beutler E, Erslev AJ, Lichtman MA, (eds): *Hematology*, McGraw-Hill Book Co., New York, 1983, pp 999-1002.
72. Wiseman BK, Doan CA: Primary splenic neutropenia; a newly recognized syndrome, closely related to congenital hemolytic icterus and essential thrombocytopenic purpura. *Ann Int Med* 1942;16:1096-1117.

73. Reinhard EH, Loeb V Jr: Dyssplenism secondary to chronic leukemia or malignant lymphoma. *JAMA* 1955;158:629-634.
74. Doan CA, Wright CS: Primary congenital and secondary acquired splenic panhematopenia. *Blood* 1946;1:10-26.
75. Manoharan A, Bader LU, Pitney WR: Non tropical idiopathic splenomegaly (Dacie's Syndrome). *Scand J Haematol* 1982;28:175-179.
76. Grosfeld JL, Fitzgerald JF, Wagner VM, Newton WA, Baehner RL: Portal hypertension in infants and children with hystiocytosis X. *Am J Surg* 1976;131:108.
77. Lipton EL: Hemolytic and pancytopenic syndrome associated with Letterer-Siwe disease. *Pediatrics* 1954;14:533-541.
78. Porter FS: Histiocytosis (histiocytosis X, reticuloendotheliosis), In, William WJ, Beutler W, Erslev AJ, Lichtman MA, (eds): *Hematology*, McGraw-Hill Book Co., New York, 1983, p 877.
79. Scott JL, Cartwright GE, Wintrobe MM: Acquired aplastic anemia: An analysis of thirty-nine cases and review of the pertinent literature. *Medicine* 1959;38:119-172.
80. Faentz SD, Krantz SB, Sears DA: Studies on pure red cell aplasia VII. Presence of proerythroblasts and response to splenectomy; a case report. *Blood* 1975;46:261-270.
81. Cuttner J: Splenectomy, steroids, and dextran 70 in thrombotic thrombocytopenia purpura. *JAMA* 1974;227:397-402.
82. Steidl RM, Cardy JD: Solitary cyst of the spleen associated with hypersplenism: Report of a case. *Am J Surg* 1957;77:45-48.
83. Hardmeirer T: Hypersplenism bei einem Hamartom des Milz (Splenom). *Schweiz Med Wschr* 1962;92:1270-1271.
84. Carere RP, Clemes IL: An unusual cause of splenomegaly and pancytopenia (secondary hypersplenism). *Can Med Ass J* 1962;86:833-835.
85. Wagstaff J, Phadke K, Adam N, et al: The "Hot Spleen" phenomenon in metastatic malignant melanoma. Its incidence and relationship with the immune system. *Cancer* 1982;49:439-444.
86. Pitney WR: The tropical splenomegaly syndrome. *Trans R Soc Trop Med* 1968;62:717-728.
86a. Hesdorffer CS, Macfarlane BJ, Sandler MA, Grant SC, Ziady F. True idiopathic splenomegaly—A distinct clinical entity. *Scand J Haematol* 1986; 37:310-315.
87. Crane GG, Pryor DS, Wells JV: Tropical splenomegaly syndrome in New Guinea. II. Long term results of splenectomy. *Med J Aust* 1972;66:733-741.
88. Higgins MR, Grace M, Ulan RA, et al: Anemia in hemodialysis patients. *Arch Int Med* 1977;137:172-176.
89. Hartley LCJ, Innio MD, Morgan TO, et al: Splenectomy for anaemia in patients on regular haemodialysis. *Lancet* 1971;2:1343-1345.
90. Girsh LS, Myerson RM: Thyrotoxicosis associated with thrombocytopenia and hypersplenism. *Am J Clin Path* 1957;27:328-331.

91. Lundberg GD, Linder WR: Whipple's disease with associated splenomegaly and pancytopenia. *Arch Int Med* 1963;112:207-215.
92. Roth J, Brudler O, Henze E: Functional asplenia in malignant mastocytosis. *J Nucl Med* 1985;26:1149-1152.
93. Weinstein VF, Woolf AL, Meynell MJ. Progressive multifocal leucoencephalopathy and primary hypersplenism. *J Clin Path* 1963;26:405-418.
94. Prasad AS, Reiner E, Watson CJ: Syndrome of hypogammaglobulinema, splenomegaly and hypersplenism. *Blood* 1957;12:926-932.
94a. Marterre WF Jr, Sugerman HJ: True splenic cyst associated with hypersplenism. *Arch Surg* 1986;121:859.
95. Wilson GA, Keys JW Jr: The significance of the liver-spleen uptake ratio in liver scanning. *J Nucl Med* 1974;15:593-597.

7
Role of the Spleen in Autoimmune Disorders

WILLIAM G. MURPHY* and JOHN G. KELTON
McMaster University Medical Centre, Hamilton, Ontario, Canada

The spleen plays a pivotal role in autoimmune diseases in three ways. First, the spleen's unique architecture makes it the principal organ for clearance of antibody-sensitized platelets in idiopathic thrombocytopenic purpura, for clearance of sensitized red cells in autoimmune hemolytic anemia, and for clearance of sensitized neutrophils in cases of autoimmune neutropenia. Second, the autoantibody that causes the autoimmune disease may be synthesized exclusively or predominantly by the B lymphocytes of the spleen. Finally, there is evidence that the spleen plays an important role in antigen processing; thus, it is possible that defects in antigen recognition in the spleen could be important in causing autoimmune disease.

OVERVIEW OF THE PROCESS OF ANTIBODY AND COMPLEMENT-MEDIATED CELL CLEARANCE

Antibody-mediated cell clearance is a vital part of the host defense system. Foreign antigens are cleared from the body after the binding of antibody molecules to soluble or particulate antigens. These foreign antigens can include microorganisms (such as bacteria, protozoa, and viruses), as well as altered host antigens such as neoplastic transformed cells. Likewise, the body's own cells some-

---

*Current affiliation: Royal Infirmary, Edinburgh, Scotland

times behave as foreign antigens, as occurs in autoimmune disorders. Once an antibody has become bound to the cell or particle, a chain of events is initiated, with the endpoint being the clearance of that particle or cell. Therapeutic interventions that blunt this response will impair host resistance, and can result in infectious complications that may sometimes be life-threatening.

Role of IgG in Cell Clearance

IgG is the major immunoglobulin in human serum, and makes up about 20% of all plasma proteins. It is a bifunctional molecule with about one-quarter of the molecule (one-half of the Fab region) being extremely variable. The rest of the molecule is relatively constant. These properties give IgG a unique function. IgG acts as a bridge linking a large number of highly variable antigens to a limited number of immune effectors. Consequently, within the same molecule, there is one part that has a great deal of variability and another part with limited variability. The effector region of IgG is termed the Fc (or fragment crystallizable) portion. Each group of immunoglobulin molecules that has a common Fc structure is termed a class; the predominant immunoglobulin class is IgG (1-3).

IgG is made of four subclasses, which are found, in descending order from subclass 1 to 4, in the following proportions: IgG1, 66%; IgG2, 23%; IgG3, 7%; and IgG4, 4%. IgG1, IgG2, and IgG4 have the same molecular mass of 146 kD. IgG3 is slightly larger, at 170 kD. The IgG molecule is made of two identical heavy chains and two identical light chains. Small changes in the structure of the heavy chains are responsible for the class and subclass characteristics. IgG is mostly made of protein, but also contains 2-3% carbohydrate, with most of it found in one area, termed the Cγ2 domain (1,4). The IgG molecule contains several disulfide bonds, which act to hold the four chains together as well as to form loops within each of the chains (Figure 1). Each loop is made of about 110 amino acids and is termed a domain (1-4).

Different domains have different functions. The V$_H$ and V$_L$ domains of IgG are quite variable; this is the portion of the IgG molecule that binds to antigens (Figure 1). The Cγ1 region binds the fourth component of complement and also acts as a spacer between the antigen-binding terminus and the effector region on the molecule. The Cγ2 region is the binding site for complement C1q and also is the binding site for the Fc receptor (FcR) of phagocytic cells (1,5). Staphylococcal protein A binds to a small area between the Cγ2 and Cγ3 domains of IgG subclasses 1, 2, and 4. The precise role of the Cγ3 region is uncertain, but it probably helps hold the IgG molecule together. Most carbohydrate of IgG is located in the Cγ2 domain, and forms a pocket between the complimentary Cγ2 domains on the two heavy chains. This opening in the IgG molecule may permit access by the Fc receptors and C1q.

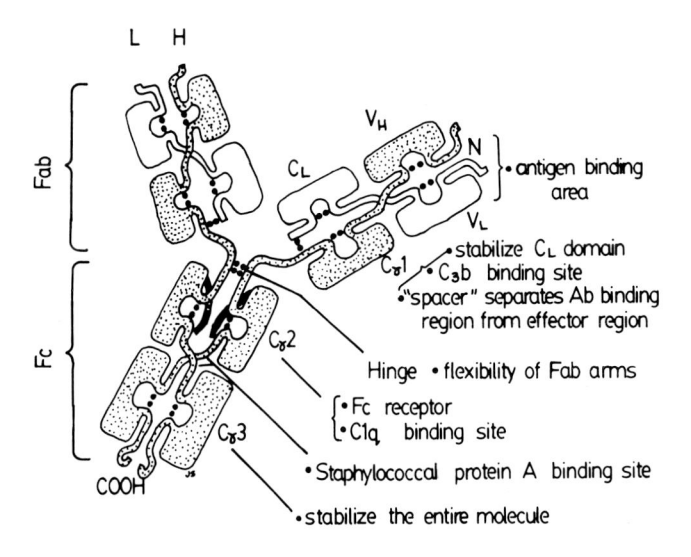

Figure 1 A schematic representation of the IgG molecule illustrating the different functional aspects of IgG. (From Kelton [18] with permission of the American Association of Blood Banks.)

The binding of IgG to the FcγR of the cells of the reticuloendothelial (RE) systems results in the clearance of the IgG-sensitized cells. This IgG-Fc interaction is not covalent. Therefore, the IgG-sensitized cells will bind to Fc-bearing cells that have the FcR with the highest affinity or number. The binding affinity of the FcR for IgG is lowest for platelets, higher for neutrophils, and highest for the monocytes and macrophages. The FcR-IgG binding affinity of monocytes and macrophages is about 1000 times higher than the binding affinity for platelets. From this, one would predict that all Fcγ binding sites on the monocytes and macrophages would have to be occupied before the platelet Fcγ binding sites could be occupied (1,6-9). Generally, this is correct. However, the binding of IgG complexes to Fc binding sites is exponentially proportional to the number of IgG molecules within the complex. Thus, those complexes that contain large numbers of IgG molecules can bind strongly to the low-affinity binding sites of the platelets, especially if there is a secondary binding site on the platelet that permits the complexes to be concentrated on the surface of the cell.

During the past several years, there have been important advances in our understanding of how IgG-sensitized cells interact with the Fc binding sites of the RE cells. Once it was thought that, after interaction of the IgG molecule with a cell or a particle, the IgG molecule underwent a conformational change in the Fc region. This change caused an increase in the binding affinity of IgG for the FcR on the phagocytic cell. This model, termed the allosteric or the associative model, was proposed to explain how IgG-sensitized cells are capable of binding to FcR in view of the very high concentrations of unbound IgG in the plasma. While this model presents an attractive explanation for the events observed in vivo, increasing evidence indicates that it is not correct. Indeed, there is virtually no experimental evidence to support the validity of this model (10-14).

It is now assumed that the interaction of an antigen with an antibody (in this case IgG) does not result in a conformational change in the Fc portion of the molecule. Thus, an antibody bound to an antigen is no more likely to interact with the FcR of the RE cell than is the uncomplexed (monomeric) IgG in the plasma (10-12,15). However, the multiple antigenic determinants present on most cells have the net effect of increasing the local concentration of IgG presented to the FcR of the RE system. As a result, the monomeric IgG is displaced from the FcR, and the complexed IgG binds. This model is termed the aggregative model. Our own studies support the aggregative model and, in addition, our studies suggest that in a healthy individual there is a delicate balance between IgG on the cell surface and IgG interacting with the RE cells. In other words, the serum concentration of IgG is directly related to the amount of IgG on circulating cells and indirectly related to the function of the RE system (16-18).

It is likely that the effectiveness of high-dose intravenous IgG (IV IgG) is related to a shift in this balance, because of the increased concentrations of IgG in the plasma (18). In contrast, patients with hypogammaglobulinemia have an increased rate of clearance of antigens by the RE system because these patients have lower concentrations of IgG in the plasma. Thus, patients with hypogammaglobulinemia have less monomeric IgG to compete with the cell bound IgG for the FcR. Later in this chapter, we will discuss how the unique architecture of the spleen skims the plasma away from the circulating cells. This results in a reduction in the concentration of monomeric IgG available to compete with cell-bound IgG for Fc binding sites.

The discussion so far has focused on IgG-mediated clearance in autoimmune diseases. Much less commonly, IgM causes rapid cell clearance. However, unlike IgG, there are no IgM receptors on the cells of the RE system, and IgM increases the rate of cell clearance by depositing complement on the surface of the cell, a process also termed complement activation. Both IgM and IgG can activate complement on the surface of a cell, although IgG is less efficient in activating complement than IgM. It is commonly believed that complement causes cell lysis. More frequently, however, complement causes the cells to adhere to specific complement binding sites on the RE cells. These binding sites have an especially high affinity for the third component of complement (C3b) and are found in high concentrations on the RE cells of the liver.

The complement system has three functions (1) cell lysis, (2) cell phagocytosis, and (3) nonspecific activation of the body's defense system. Complement activation is an enzymatic cascade, and each step activates many successive complement components; these in turn activate even more complement. Thus, the complement cascade, like the coagulation cascade, is an amplification system. In both systems, the dominant proteins (C3 for complement and fibrinogen for coagulation) are present in high concentrations and the other proteins are present in only trace amounts. And, just as a number of specific and nonspecific inhibitors control the rate and extent of coagulation, the complement cascade behaves similarly.

The C3b component of complement can bind to a particle (or cell) via an antibody (IgG or IgM), or it can bind directly after interaction with carbohydrates on the particle. This mechanism of complement activation is termed the alternate pathway. Many different proteases, including trypsin, plasmin, thrombin, and elastase, also can activate the C3 component of complement. After activation, C3 interacts with a stabilizing protein to form a complex termed factor C3b,B. Another protease (factor D) cleaves the C3b,B into C3b,Bb which is a potent activator of C3, and this results in a positive feedback with further generation of C3b.

C3 also can be deposited on the cell surface by IgG and IgM. Cell-bound IgG and IgM bind the first component of complement, termed C1q. C1q binds to several IgG molecules or to one IgM molecule. The binding kinetics are similar to that of IgG for FcR. Thus, the binding of C1q is exponentially related to the number of IgG molecules. Because IgM is made of five subunits, it is much more efficient than IgG at binding C1q. C1q is a unique molecule made of six linear filaments each attached to a globular head, so that the molecule resembles a bunch of tulips. In the presence of calcium, C1q binds to the $C\gamma 2$ domain of IgG and activates the two other components of the C1q complex, C1r and C1s. All of these reactions occur on the immunoglobulin molecule and away from the cell membrane. But once the C1 complex (C1qrs) is assembled, it has enzymatic activity that is capable of cleaving C4.

The larger portion of the C4 molecule (C4b) binds to both the cell membrane and C1qrs, and then activates C2 in the presence of magnesium that had been loosely associated with C4. The now strongly associated C4b2b complex is a potent activator of C3, cleaving it to C3b. Most of the cells sensitized by C3b are cleared by cells that have C3b receptors, especially those cells in the liver. The C3b binding sites of the RE cells in the spleen are either uncommon or have low affinity. Consequently, the spleen is relatively unimportant in complement-mediated cell clearance. Some of the C3b will escape clearance and, together with the C4b2b3b complex, C5b is activated. This is then followed by the sequential activation of the subsequent complement proteins (C6 to C9). This complex, termed the attack complex, polymerizes to form a tubule that penetrates and disrupts the cell membrane, resulting in lysis.

Recently, a role for the red cells in complement-mediated clearance has been proposed. Red cells have low-affinity C3b binding sites, but because of the enormous number of red cells, the overall impact of these C3b binding sites is considerable. C3b-sensitized particles and complexes bind to red cells. However, the interaction between C3b-sensitized particles and red cells has a low affinity. The C3b complexes can be stripped from the red cells as soon as the cells come in contact with the higher-affinity C3b receptors, most notably those C3b receptors in the liver.

IgM-mediated hemolysis, as in cold agglutinin hemolytic disease, illustrates the pathophysiology of complement-mediated cell clearance. Complement sensitization of the red cells causes them to attach to RE cells in the liver, and subsequently the red cells are phagocytosed in the liver. Only under unusual circumstances is the complement cascade "completed" with occurrence of intravascular hemolysis. Presumably, hemolysis only occurs when all of the RE cells carrying high-affinity C3b binding sites are saturated, and C3b-sensitized cells are allowed to circulate, which permits completion of the complement cascade. Because the spleen carries very few high-affinity C3b receptors, splenectomy is generally ineffective in a patient who has IgM-mediated hemolysis.

Recently, one group of investigators has reported a new type of IgM-mediated hemolysis in children (10). The IgM did not bind complement but resulted in a warm-type autoimmune hemolytic anemia, possibly due to agglutination of the sensitized red blood cells in the spleen.

ANATOMY OF THE SPLEEN AND ITS ROLE AS AN IMMUNE CLEARANCE ORGAN

The spleen weighs from 100 to 150 g in the adult. It contains a disproportionate amount of the total lymphatic tissue of the body (about 25%) and also receives a disproportionately large share of the cardiac output (6%). Arterial blood enters the spleen via the splenic artery, which branches into the trabecular arteries. The trabecular arteries in turn form the central arteries, which enter the white pulp.

ROLE OF THE SPLEEN IN AUTOIMMUNE DISORDERS

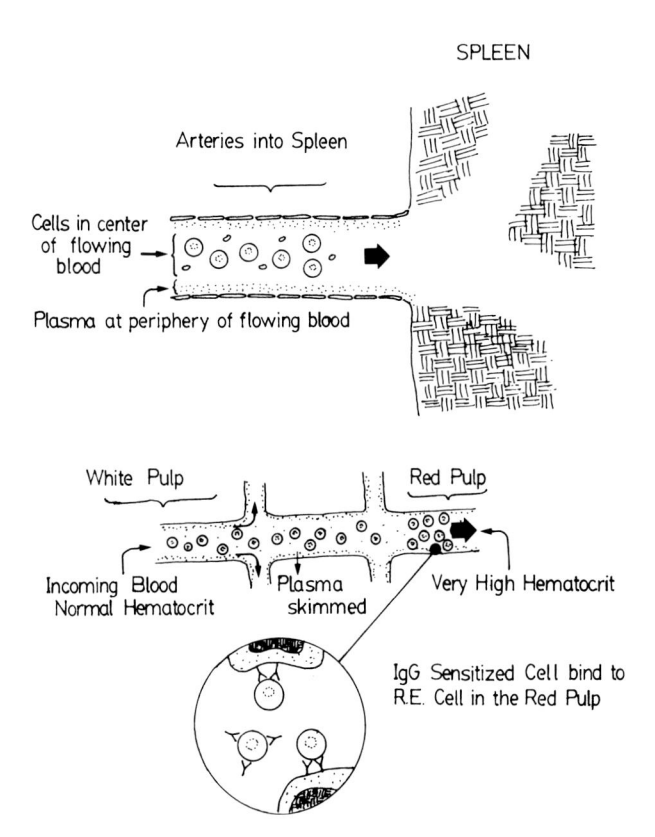

Figure 2 A schematic representation of the skimming effect of the spleen. In the top panel, the fast flowing arterial blood is moving into the spleen. Because of flow-density characteristics, the cells tend to lie in the center of the column of blood and the plasma is at the periphery. In the middle panel, the plasma is being skimmed off via the arteries, which exit perpendicularly to the main arteries in the white pulp. Within the red pulp the hematocrit is very high because most of the plasma has been removed. Because much of the plasma containing the inhibitory monomeric IgG has been removed, IgG-sensitized cells are more likely to interact with the Fc binding sites of the RE cells shown in the bottom panel.

The white pulp is so named because it consists mainly of lymphoid tissue, which gives it a pale appearance on the cut surface. The arteries in the white pulp of the spleen extend perpendicularly from the central arteries, and this anatomical configuration produces a unique effect. To understand how this happens, one must understand the flow characteristics of the arterial circulation. The rapid flow rate in the arteries causes the cellular elements to move to the middle of the column of blood, and the plasma moves centrifugally to the edges.

Because the splenic arteries extend perpendicularly, they draw off the plasma. This pattern of flow carries the soluble antigens into the lymphocyte-rich white pulp for processing by the dendritic cells and lymphocytes. The cellular elements remain and are carried into the red pulp, which is rich in macrophages and monocytes. The blood that is delivered to the red pulp has an exceptionally high hematocrit, being as high as 60-80%. More important, the plasma containing the inhibitory monomeric IgG has been removed (Figure 2). Consequently, any IgG-sensitive cellular components that flow through the red pulp are more likely to be cleared by the RE cells. The blood that enters the red pulp percolates slowly through vessels lined by RE cells (Figure 2). Again, this slow flow rate in the absence of inhibitory plasma IgG favors interaction of IgG-sensitized cells or particles with the RE cells. Finally, the cellular elements are filtered through endothelial sinus slits. This process serves as a final quality control for culling out cells with reduced deformability. Such cells include partially phagocytosed red cells that are sphere-shaped, which will be described later in this chapter. Cells that are engulfed by the monocytes and macrophages are destroyed.

THE SPLEEN IN IMMUNE THROMBOCYTOPENIC PURPURA

Morphological Considerations

Studies using the light microscope and the electron microscope have demonstrated characteristic changes in the spleens of patients with immune thrombocytopenic purpura (ITP). These changes are consistent with the spleen's dual role of antiplatelet antibody production and platelet destruction. There are two main changes. The first change is the presence of highly developed secondary lymphoid follicles with reactive germinal centers. In the marginal zones there is increased perivascular cuffing by plasma cells (20,21). Second, there is histological evidence of platelet destruction both within the splenic macrophages (20-28) and extracellularly within the splenic cords (20).

The reactive lymphoid changes that may reflect increased antibody synthesis (20) can vary, depending upon whether the patient received corticosteroid therapy (21,22). Thus, when the patient has had corticosteroid therapy before splenectomy, histological changes in the white pulp can be unremarkable. It is not known why these morphological changes are dependent on corticosteroid therapy. Corticosteroids in the therapeutic doses used in ITP have not been shown to interfere with IgG production in this disease (29). Likewise, in in vitro studies, corticosteroids have no effect on splenic synthesis of IgG (30). One study showed a decrease in anti-red cell antibody levels after corticosteroid therapy in autoimmune hemolytic anemia (31), but this observation could be due to increased catabolism of IgG (32).

Macrophage phagocytosis of platelets is detectable in all patients with ITP whether or not they are receiving corticosteroid therapy (21,22). The distinctive foamy histiocytes in the spleens of patients with ITP were first reported by Saltzstein and Landing (27,28). Subsequent study demonstrated that these cells were macrophages loaded with phospholipids from ingested platelet (25). Platelets in varying stages of destruction, from intact cells to phospholipid droplets can be identified within the splenic macrophages (20,25). Extracellular platelet degradation has also been observed in the splenic cords (20).

Platelet Kinetics in ITP

The rate of production and destruction of the platelets, as well as the sites of their destruction, can be best studied by the use of platelets labelled with ^{111}In (33-36). ^{51}Cr-labeled platelets have been used in studies of platelet kinetics in the past, but in comparative studies, ^{51}Cr-labeled platelets were shown to give an underestimate of the platelet mean life span (MLS), and an overestimate of platelet turnover (35,36). Release of ^{51}Cr from the platelets (possibly due to antiplatelet antibody) could account for the discrepancy between the two labels. Furthermore, the efficient gamma emissions of ^{111}In allow for wholebody counting, and enables one to avoid the inconsistencies of surface counting of low gamma emissions from ^{51}Cr (37,38). A third advantage of ^{111}In over ^{51}Cr as a platelet label is that the high labeling efficiency of ^{111}In allows the use of ^{111}In-labeled autologous platelets to determine platelet life span even in patients with severe thrombocytopenia (39,40).

Platelet production is regulated by the total platelet mass, that is, circulating platelets plus pooled platelets, rather than by the peripheral platelet count alone (40). When the rate of platelet destruction increases, the bone marrow responds with increased output up to an estimated maximum of eight times normal rate of platelet production (42). The thrombocytopenia of ITP occurs when the rate of destruction of platelets exceeds the maximum compensatory increase in platelet production that the bone marrow can achieve. Platelet destruction is always increased in ITP, and often the platelet lifespan is reduced to less than 24 hr (34,35,37,39). Some investigators have also reported underproduction of platelets in ITP (35,38,39,43). It is possible that this state of underproduction of platelets is due to antibody-mediated megakaryocyte destruction, as the autoantibody in ITP can recognize antigens on mature megakaryocytes (44,45).

The accelerated destruction of platelets in ITP takes place in two ways: in the spleen, and diffusely throughout the RE system. In most patients, platelet destruction occurs predominantly in the spleen. In a small proportion of patients, platelet destruction occurs diffusely throughout the RE system, including the liver, lungs, and bone marrow (36,39,46). The diffuse pattern of sequestration of ^{111}In-labeled platelets tends to occur in those patients with more severe disease; that is, those with lower platelet counts (35,39,47,48,49).

There is a slow transit time of about 10 min for platelets as they pass through the spleen (33). This slow passage permits long exposure of IgG-sensitized cells to the splenic RE cells (20). In contrast, the transit time of platelets through the liver is much shorter. Consequently, higher concentrations of IgG must be present on the platelet before the liver becomes a major site of cell destruction (50), even though the liver contains many more macrophages than the spleen. The degree of sensitization of the platelet by IgG correlates roughly with the severity of the immune thrombocytopenia.

ITP is not associated with splenomegaly. Thus, the presence of splenomegaly suggests another diagnosis (51). Therefore, the transit time of platelets through the spleen is not increased in ITP but remains at the normal time of 10 min (52). Similarly, there is no splenic pooling of platelets in ITP. Also, the spleen does not contribute to the platelet destruction by "conditioning" them in an unfavorable environment, as occurs with red cells in autoimmune hemolytic anemia.

Several authors have attempted to extrapolate the results of kinetic and sequestration studies to clinical outcome using ^{51}Cr and [111]In (34,46,49). In general, these tests have not reliably predicted response to splenectomy in an individual patient, although a pattern of predominant splenic destruction seems to indicate a better chance of favorable response to splenectomy. There are important reasons why kinetic and imaging studies cannot predict the outcome of splenectomy in any individual patient. First, in a patient with a diffuse pattern of destruction (possibly indicating more severe disease, or complement-mediated clearance), the spleen may be the prime site of antibody production (53,54,55), so that splenectomy could induce a remission. Conversely, if the antiplatelet antibody is primarily made by extrasplenic B lymphocytes, then the antibody will continue to be produced after splenectomy. Finally, it is possible that corticosteroid therapy during the isotope study period can influence the pattern of platelet sequestration (56-60).

Splenic Production of Antiplatelet Antibody in ITP

The increased rate of platelet destruction that occurs in ITP is caused by the sensitization of the platelets by antiplatelet autoantibody (51,54). The reason the autoantibody forms is not known. In children there is a close temporal relationship between a preceding viral illness and the development of ITP. This suggests that an antibody to a viral antigen also recognizes an antigen on the surface of the platelet, thus offering the possibility of crossreactivity. Alternatively, viral antigens could bind to the platelets, which in turn would result in the sensitization of platelets by IgG. However, in adults such a relationship is uncommon, and the appearance of the autoantibody in ITP usually arises as an apparently spontaneous event, presumably due to some perturbation of the recognition of self antigens. Sometimes antiplatelet autoantibodies develop in conjunction with a lymphoproliferate disorder (61-64), or as the initial manifestation of a more widespread autoimmune disorder (56).

Until recently, the antigenic specificity of the autoantibody of ITP was unknown for most ITP patients (65-68). Several studies have shown that the target antigen on the platelet membrane is not the same for all patients (65-69). Thus, in some patients the autoantibody recognizes an antigen on glycoprotein IIb/IIIa (65,66,69) or on the IIIa part of the IIb/IIIa complex (69). In another patient the antibody was directed against glycoprotein Ib (66). One study has suggested that the epitope recognized by the antiplatelet antibody may be present on more than one platelet membrane protein (65).

Karpatkin (55) and McMillan (53,54) demonstrated that lymphocytes from the spleens of patients with ITP produce large amounts of antiplatelet autoantibody. The titer of antiplatelet antibody almost always falls in ITP patients after splenectomy (70-74).

It is possible that the spleen is the only site, or it may be a major site, of antibody production in the early stages of ITP. With longstanding disease, B cells producing antiplatelet IgG may also be found in extrasplenic sites. Such a phenomenon could explain why some investigators have reported that splenectomy is more likely to induce complete remission of the disease if carried out early in its course (75), that is, while the spleen is still the sole producer of antiplatelet antibodies.

Unfortunately, it is not possible to determine the site of antibody production in ITP before splenectomy. However, even if such a capability were available it might not provide the complete answer on the likelihood of success of splenectomy in each individual patient.

Splenectomy in ITP

Although there are many macrophages in the liver, lung, and bone marrow, the spleen is the major site of destruction of circulating cells with antibody for two reasons. First, the slow transit time of platelets through the spleen (33), in conjunction with the skimming of the plasma from the cells, allows for prolonged contact between the antibody-sensitized cells and the FcR of the RE cells in the cords (Figure 2). With higher concentrations of IgG or C3b on the platelets, the phagocytic efficiency of the macrophages increases, and the liver increases in importance as a clearance organ (50). This probably explains the poorer response to splenectomy in patients with high concentrations of IgG on their platelets (76). The second reason the spleen is a major site for destroying platelets relates to antibody production in the spleen. The local production of antiplatelet antibody in the spleen ensures that the platelets are heavily sensitized by IgG as they pass through spleen tissue (52,53,54,55,77).

The natural history of ITP differs between adults and children. Most children with ITP have a spontaneous remission of their illness; only about 10% become chronic (78). In contrast, the majority of adults who develop ITP will not have a spontaneous remission of their disease (51). Apart from considerations of subsequent morbidity, splenectomy is more readily undertaken in adults at an early stage of the disease. About two-thirds of all adults who undergo splenectomy will have a remission of their disease.

About 10% of relapses after an initial favorable response to splenectomy are due to an accessory spleen (51,79,80). Many of these patients will respond to removal of the accessory spleen.

Use of Intravenous Immunoglobulin in ITP

Intravenous IgG, given at a dose of 1-2 g/kg, is effective in inducing remissions in ITP in both newly diagnosed patients and patients who are refractory to corticosteroids and splenectomy (81-88). The mechanism of action is not certain, but two possible explanations have been proposed: (1) occurrence of RE blockade by saturation of the FcR on the RE cells; and (2) antiidiotype antibody activity within the infused IgG that neutralizes the antiplatelet autoantibody.

It is likely that blockade of the RE system by saturation of RE FcR plays an important part in the efficacy of intravenous IgG in treatment of antibody-mediated disorders (20,85,88,89,90). Theoretically, intravenous IgG could be more effective than splenectomy in cases of ITP in two situations: (1) where large amounts of antiplatelet antibody are made in extrasplenic sites, and (2) where opsonization with antibody with or without complement is sufficient to induce significant extrasplenic macrophage-mediated platelet destruction. It has also been reported that intravenous IgG can result in a decrease in platelet associated IgG. Antiidiotypic antibody activity in the infused IgG could explain this phenomenon (18,91,92).

THE SPLEEN IN AUTOIMMUNE HEMOLYTIC ANEMIA

The pathophysiology of autoimmune hemolytic anemia (AIHA) closely parallels that of ITP, and the role of the spleen in AIHA is similar to its role in ITP. Thus, in AIHA the spleen serves as a site of antibody production and it is also an important site of removal of antibody-sensitized red cells. In addition, the spleen acts as a sieve and removes red cells with reduced deformability. Splenectomy is an effective treatment for autoimmune hemolytic anemia for probably the same reasons as it is effective in ITP. Prediction of the long-term response to splenectomy by isotope studies in AIHA is as unreliable as it is in ITP.

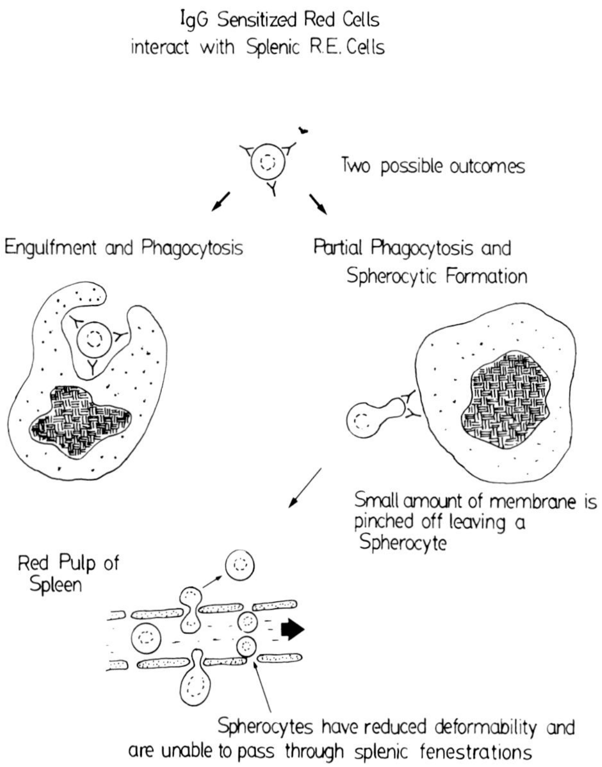

Figure 3 A schematic representation showing how immune hemolysis occurs in patients with autoimmune hemolytic anemia (AIHA). The top figure illustrates how many red cells sensitized by antibody will undergo only partial phagocytosis and will escape complete engulfment. However, they leave behind a portion of their membrane and consequently assume a spherical shape. The spherical shape and decreased deformability reduces the ability of the red cells to pass through the small openings within the red pulp of the spleen.

The spleen contributes to red cell destruction in another and a unique way. Red blood cells passing from the splenic cords into the sinuses must traverse the tiny fenestrations in the vessel walls. Only red cells with normal deformability are capable of undergoing these changes in shape (Figure 3). The normal red cell has excess membrane in relation to contents and assumes a biconcave disc shape. The loss of some of the red cell membrane results in a spherical shape because a sphere has the lowest ratio of surface to contents. A sphered red cell also has a markedly reduced deformability (93,94).

Sphering of the red cells characterizes AIHA and arises for two reasons. First, phagocytosis of opsonized red cells may fail to result in complete ingestion of the cell. Instead, a portion of the external membrane is ingested, and although the cell escapes from the phagocytic cell it assumes a spherical shape (95,96) (Figure 3). The sphered red cell is then mechanically trapped by the spleen. The loss of membrane deformability increases the transit time of the red cell through the spleen (97). Second, the spleen is usually enlarged in AIHA (98). As a result, the red cells have a slower transit time through the enlarged spleen (99, 100) and consequently they will be exposed for a longer time to the unfavorable environment of the spleen, with its low pH (101) and reduced glucose concentrations (102). The metabolic stress of the unfavorable environment of the spleen further damages the red cell (93,94,103).

Autoantibody in AIHA

The antibody responsible for AIHA is usually IgG, although it may be IgM, or very uncommonly IgA (19,104-107). As noted previously, IgM hemolysis presents a different clinical picture from IgG AIHA. Thus, the hemolysis induced by IgM (cold agglutinin disease) is due to complement deposition on the red cell membrane. This results either in intravascular hemolysis by the completed complement cascade, which is uncommon, or more frequently, in removal of the C3b-sensitized red cells from the circulation by the liver.

The spleen makes only a minimal contribution to the clearance of complement sensitized red cells in cold agglutinin disease, and therefore splenectomy is of little benefit (108,109). It is possible that reduction in autoantibody formation by the spleen in some patients with cold-type autoimmune hemolytic anemia can occasionally result in some improvement (110,111).

AIHA can be either acute or chronic. In children the acute type is most common. The hemolysis can be severe and life-threatening, and often follows an episode of infection or a vaccination. It is usually self-limited. In contrast, among adults and older children, a more chronic course is usual, with spontaneous remission of the disease being uncommon. The autoantibody is directed against an intrinsic red cell membrane antigen, most commonly a Rhesus (Rh) antigen (112), although in many cases the antigen cannot be identified. These antigens are almost always "public" antigens, being present on the cells of most normal individuals as well as on the patient's cells. Rarely, the autoantibody seems to be directed against antigens on red cell precursors, with resultant reticulocytopenia (112-115).

Studies implicating the spleen as a major site of autoantibody production in AIHA, as has been shown for ITP (53,55), are generally lacking. However, one early study showed that the splenic pulp from patients with AIHA synthesized a red cell agglutinin (116). Indirect evidence that the spleen is the major site of antibody production can be derived from studies that have shown disappearance of the autoantibody from the serum in patients after splenectomy (109, 117,118).

Splenic Destruction of Red Blood Cells

Red blood cells sensitized with IgG are sequestered in the spleen (119,120,121) by splenic RE cells binding the Fc terminus of IgG (122). The greater the amount of IgG sensitization of the red cell, the greater the efficiency of macrophage binding of the red cells (31,119). Complement activation by the IgG autoantibody enhances the phagocytic activity of the RE cells (119,123,124,125) and increases the contribution of extrasplenic macrophages to red cell destruction. As discussed in the section on ITP, high local concentrations of the antibody in the splenic cords (126) and diminished competition by plasma IgG for the FcR of the RE cells increase the efficiency of the splenic RE cells in opsonizing igG-coated cells. Because there is no free C3b in plasma, an inhibitory effect of plasma on C3b receptors does not occur.

Splenectomy in AIHA

Although about 80% of patients with chronic AIHA respond to treatment with corticosteroids (127), less than one-fourth of these will have a long-term treatment-free "cure" of the disease (109,118). About one-half of all patients require further therapy, such as splenectomy. Of those who undergo splenectomy, about 60% will benefit and have a complete or partial remission (127).

Can the effectiveness of splenectomy be predicted by laboratory studies? Studies of the pattern of clearance of radiolabelled red cells in AIHA have not been useful in predicting whether splenectomy will be beneficial (118,128,129, 130). Technical difficulties inherent in surface counting, plus the problem of red cell pooling in the spleen (131), create difficulties in data analysis. In addition, one cannot precisely determine the contribution of the spleen to autoantibody production. Consequently, the decision to perform splenectomy must be based on clinical findings, not on laboratory assessment alone.

THE SPLEEN IN AUTOIMMUNE NEUTROPENIA

It was long considered to be likely that idiopathic neutropenia was caused by an autoimmune disorder (132,133). However, the lack of an assay for antineutrophil antibodies delayed serological proof of the occurrence of autoimmune neutropenia until 1975 (134,135). Since then a number of assays have been described (136-140).

Autoimmune neutropenia affects patients of ages ranging from 3 months to over 70 years (141). In approximately 50% of cases, the specificity of the autoantibody, which may be IgG, IgM, or IgA (142), can be determined (141), with anti-NA_1 being the most common autoantibody (143).

Where treatment is required for severe neutropenia and recurrent infections, corticosteroids can be effective (136). As in AIHA and ITP, splenectomy can induce remission in primary autoimmune neutropenia (141). After splenectomy, there is disappearance of the antineutrophil IgG from the serum, suggesting that the antibody is produced in the spleen.

Destruction of Neutrophils in Primary Autoimmune Neutropenia

Over 90% of the neutrophils in the body are in the bone marrow; the remaining cells are distributed between the circulation and the extracellular space. The neutrophil spends only a few hours in the circulation. Neutrophil ingestion by splenic macrophages is sometimes observed in the spleen after splenectomy (135). Still, the neutropenia of primary autoimmune neutropenia could be related to impaired maturation of neutrophils due to intramedullary antibody-mediated destruction of myeloid precursors (131,144). Existence of such a mechanism would explain the occurrence of neutropenia in the absence of high antineutrophil antibody titers.

Autoimmune neutropenia also occurs in association with a number of other autoimmune diseases, including rheumatoid arthritis, AIHA, ITP, autoimmune thyroiditis, systemic lupus erythematosus, scleroderma, ulcerative colitis, and hairy-cell leukemia (142,143,145,146). Neutropenia in rheumatoid arthritis occurs in three different clinical settings, which can have a considerable degree of overlap. These are: (1) Felty's syndrome, that is, seropositive rheumatoid arthritis and neutropenia, with or without splenomegaly (140,147,148); (2) seropositive rheumatoid arthritis with neutropenia and splenomegaly and natural killer (NK) cell proliferation (149-151); and (3) chronic T cell lymphocytosis with seropositive rheumatoid arthritis, neutropenia and splenomegaly (152,153). The latter two categories may represent different stages of the same condition.

Felty's syndrome is often treated by splenectomy. The exact cause of the neutropenia remains unclear, although several investigators have observed increased granulocyte-bound IgG and antigranulocyte IgG in the serum in these patients (140,148,154,155). Response rates to splenectomy vary from 30 to 80% (156,157). Patients who respond favorably have a rise in neutrophil counts and a decrease in infections after splenectomy. Probably, the spleen in Felty's syndrome synthesizes autoantibody, as shown by the drop in antigranulocyte antibodies after splenectomy.

SUMMARY

The spleen contributes to the pathophysiology of idiopathic thrombocytopenic purpura (ITP), autoimmune hemolytic anemia (AIHA), and autoimmune neutropenia by acting as a site of autoantibody production and as a site of destruction of sensitized cells. The autoantibody in these diseases is usually IgG, although IgM and IgA autoantibodies can occur. IgG-sensitized cells are cleared via Fc receptors (FcR) by the cells of the reticuloendothelial (RE) system. FcR bind to IgG with equal affinity whether the IgG is bound to an antigen or free in the plasma. Therefore, the ability of the FcR to bind cell-bound IgG is inversely related to the concentration of plasma IgG.

Both IgG and IgM can also induce hemolysis through complement binding, with clearing of sensitized cells by the C3b receptors on RE cells or, less commonly, through completion of the complement cascade on the cell surface, which results in cell lysis. Some IgM autoantibodies can induce cell clearance by agglutination of the sensitized cells in the spleen.

The cellular components in the blood flowing through the central arteries of the spleen are separated from the plasma as a result of the anatomy of the spleen. The plasma is skimmed away from the cells via the arteries that leave the central splenic arteries. This results in plasma-poor cellular components being presented to the RE cells in the red pulp, while the plasma, carrying the soluble antigens, is diverted to the lymphocytes and dendritic cells of the white pulp. In the red pulp the phagocytic activity of the macrophages is enhanced by the sluggish blood flow, the close cell-to-cell contact, and by the depletion of the soluble IgG that would diminish the ability of the RE FcR to bind IgG-coated cells.

The spleen contributes to red blood cell destruction in another, unique, way. Red cells entering the red pulp must traverse the endothelium to leave the spleen via the venous sinuses. Red cells with impaired membrane deformability cannot easily pass through the endothelium, and are trapped in the unfavorable metabolic environment of the red pulp. Red cells that have lost part of their membrane due to partial phagocytosis by RE cells have reduced deformability, which causes them to be trapped and destroyed within the spleen.

The white pulp of the spleen is a major site of production of antibodies directed against intravascular antigens. In ITP, AIHA, and autoimmune neutropenia the spleen can be the primary or sole site of autoantibody production. Consequently, splenectomy results in remission of disease even if the spleen is not the major site of cell destruction. Although it is possible, by isotope labelling techniques, to estimate the relative amount of cell destruction within the spleen, it is not possible to determine whether most of the autoantibody is made by the spleen. For this reason, it is not possible to predict the response to splenectomy of a patient with autoimmune disease. Consequently, the decision to undertake splenectomy for a patient with ITP, AIHA, or autoimmune neutropenia is at present based on clinical considerations.

Splenectomy can be an effective therapy in those patients who develop chronic ITP, AIHA, or autoimmune neutropenia. Approximately two-thirds of patients who undergo splenectomy will have a prolonged remission of disease. Some pateints who relapse following an initial favorable response to splenectomy will be found to have an accessory spleen, and can have another remission after removal of the accessory spleen.

ACKNOWLEDGMENTS

Some of the studies described in this chapter were funded by the Medical Research Council of Canada and by a grant from the Research and Development fund of the Canadian Red Cross Blood Transfusion Service. The authors thank Mrs. Janice Butera and Mrs. Barb Lahie for typing the manuscript.

REFERENCES

1. Burton DR: Immunoglobulin G: Functional sites. *Mol Immunol* 1985; 22:161-206.
2. McClelland DBL, Yap PL: Clinical use of immunoglobulins. *Clin Haematol* 1984;13:39-74.
3. Heiner DC: Significance of immunoglobulin G subclasses. *Am J Med* 1984; 76:1-6.
4. Winkelhake JL: Immunoglobulin structure and effector functions. *Immunochemistry* 1978;15:695-714.
5. Schumaker VN, Calcott MA, Spiegelberg HL et al: Ultracentrifuge studies of the binding of IgG of different subclasses to the C1q subunit of the first component of complement, *Biochemistry* 1976;16:5175-5181.
6. Wright JK, Tschopp J, Jaton J-C, et al: Dimeric, trimeric and tetrameric complexes of immunoglobulin G fix complement. *Biochem J* 1980; 187: 775-780.
7. Kurlander RJ, Batker J: The binding of human immunoglobulin G1 monomer and small, covalently cross-linked polymers of immunoglobulin G1 to human peripheral blood monocytes and polymorphonuclear leukocytes. *J Clin Invest* 1982;69:1-8.
8. Fries LF, Hall RP, Lawley TJ, et al: Monocyte receptors for the Fc portion of IgG studied with monomeric human IgG1: normal in vitro expression of Fcγ-mediated in vivo clearance. *J Immunol* 1982;129:1041-1049.
9. Karas SP, Rosse WF, Kurlander RJ: Characterization of the IgG-Fc receptor on human platelets. *Blood* 1982;60:1277-1281.
10. Jaton J-C: Structural and biological effects of antigen binding to antibodies. A reevaluation of the data. In Nydegger UE (ed): *Immunohematotherapy. A Guide to Immunoglobulin Prophylaxis and Therapy*. London, Academic Press, 1981, 7-16.
11. Metzger H: The effect of antigen on antibodies: recent studies. In Reisfeld RA, Inman FP (eds): *Contemporary Topics in Molecular Immunology*. New York, Plenum Press, 1978, 119-152.

12. Metzger H: Effect of antigen binding on the properties of antibody. *Adv Immunol* 1974;18:169-207.
13. Dower SK, DeLisi C, Titus JA, et al: Mechanism of binding of multivalent immune complexes to Fc receptors. 1. Equilibrium binding. *Biochemistry* 1981;20:6326-6334.
14. Dower SK, Titus JA, DeLisi C, et al: Mechanism of binding of multivalent immune complexes to Fc receptors. 2. Kinetics of binding. *Biochemistry* 1981;20:6335-6340.
15. Segal DM, Dower SK, Titus JA: The role of non-immune IgG in controlling IgG-mediated effector functions. *Mol Immunol* 1983;20:1177-1189.
16. Kelton JG, Carter CJ, Rodger C, et al: The relationship among platelet-associated IgG, platelet life-span and reticuloendothelial cell function. *Blood* 1984;63:1434-1438.
17. Kelton JG, Singer J, Rodger C, et al: The concentration of IgG in the serum is a major determinant of Fc-dependent reticuloendothelial function. *Blood* 1985;66:490-495.
18. Kelton JG: The interaction of IgG with reticuloendothelial cells: Biological and therapeutic implications. In Garratty G (ed): *Current Concepts in Transfusion Therapy*. Arlington, American Association of Blood Banks, 1985, 51-107.
19. Salama A, Mueller-Eckhardt C: Autoimmune haemolytic anemia in childhood associated with non-complement binding IgM autoantibodies. *Br J Haematol* 1987;67-71.
20. Tavassoli M, McMillan R: Structure of the spleen in idiopathic thrombocytopenic purpura. *Am J Clin Pathol* 1975;64:180-191.
21. Hassan NMR, Neiman RS: The pathology of the spleen in steroid-treated immune thrombocytopenic purpura. *Am J Clin Pathol* 1985;84:433-438.
22. Luk SC, Musclow E, Simon GT: Platelet phagocytosis in the spleen of patients with idiopathic thrombocytopenic purpura (ITP). *Histopathology (Oxf)* 1980;4:127-136.
23. Kirstensen J, Myhre Jensen O: Splenic pulp, plasma cells and foamy histiocytes in immune thrombocytopenia: Combined morphometric, immunohistochemical and ultrastructural studies. *Scand J Haematol* 1985;34:340-344.
24. Ishihara T, Akizuki S, Yokota T, et al: Foamy cells associated with platelet phagocytosis. *Am J Pathol* 1984;114:104-111.
25. Firkin BG, Wright R, Miller S, et al: Splenic macrophages in thrombocytopenia. *Blood* 1969;33:240-245.
26. Cohn J, Tygstrup I: Foamy histiocytosis of the spleen in patients with chronic thrombocytopenia. *Scand J Haematol* 1976;16:33-37.
27. Saltzstein SL: Phospholipid accumulation in histiocytes of splenic pulp associated with thrombocytopenic purpura. *Blood* 1961;18:73-88.
28. Landing BH, Strauss L, Crocker AC, et al: Thrombocytopenic purpura with histiocytosis of the spleen. *N Engl J Med* 1961;265:572-577.
29. Karpatkin S: Autoimmune thrombocytopenic purpura. *Semin Hematol* 1985;22:260-288.

30. McMillan R, Longmire R, Yelenosky R: The effect of corticosteroids on human IgG synthesis. *J Immunol* 1976;116:1592-1595.
31. Rosse WR: Quantitative immunology of immune hemolytic anemia. II. The relationship of cell-bound antibody to hemolysis and the effect of treatment. *J Clin Invest* 1971;50:734-743.
32. Griggs RC, Condemi JJ, Vaughan JH: Effect of therapeutic dosages of prednisone on human immunoglobulin G metabolism. *J Lab Clin Med* 1972; 49:267-273.
33. Peters AM, Klonizakis I, Lavender JP, et al: Use of ^{111}Indium-labelled platelets to measure spleen function. *Br J Haematol* 1980;46:587-593.
34. Reiffers J, Vuillemin L, Broustet A, et al: Etude cinetique des plaquettes marquees a l'indium au cours des purpuras thrombopeniques idiopathiques. *Nouv Presse Med* 1982;11:2335-2338.
35. Heyns A du P, Badenhorst PN, Lotter MG, et al: Platelet turnover and kinetics in immune thrombocytopenic purpura: results with autologous ^{111}In-labelled platelets and homologous ^{51}Cr-labelled platelets differ. *Blood* 1986;67:86-92.
36. Schmidt KG, Ramussen JW: Kinetics and distribution in vivo of ^{111}In-labelled autologous platelets in idiopathic thrombocytopenic purpura. *Scand J Haematol* 1985;34:47-56.
37. Heyns A du P, Lotter MG, Badenhorst PN, et al: Kinetics, distribution and sites of destruction of ^{111}Indium-labelled human platelets. *Br J Haematol* 1980;44:269-280.
38. Ries CA, Price DC: [^{51}Cr] platelet kinetics in thrombocytopenia. Correlation between splenic sequestration of platelets and response to splenectomy. *Ann Intern Med* 1974;80:702-707.
39. Heyns A du P, Lotter MG, Badenhorst PN, et al: Kinetics and sites of destruction of ^{111}Indium-oxine-labelled platelets in idiopathic thrombocytopenic purpura: A quantitative study. *Am J Hematol* 1982;12:167-177.
40. Heyns A du P, Badenhorst PN, Wessels P, et al: Indium-^{111}-labelled human platelets: A method for use in severe thrombocytopenia. *Thromb Haemostas* 1984;52:226-229.
41. Harker LA, Finch CA: Thrombokinetics in man. *J Clin Invest* 1969;48:963-974.
42. Harker LA: Thrombokinetics in idiopathic thrombocytopenic purpura. *Br J Haematol* 1974;19:95-104.
43. Siegel RS, Coleman RE, Kurlander R, et al: Platelet turnover: An important factor in predicting response to splenectomy in autoimmune thrombocytopenic purpura. (Abstr) *Blood* 1984;64(Suppl):241a.
44. McMillan R, Luiken GA, Levy R et al: Antibody against megakaryocytes in idiopathic thrombocytopenic purpura. *JAMA* 1978;239:2460-2462.
45. Pizzi F, Carrara PM, Aldeghi A, et al: Immunofluorescence of megakaryocytes in the thrombocytopenic purpuras. *Blood* 1966;27:521-526.
46. Najean Y, Ardaillou N: The sequestration site of platelets in idiopathic thrombocytopenic purpura: its correlation with the results of splenectomy. *Br J Haematol* 1971;21:153-164.

47. Aster RH, Keene WR: Sites of platelet destruction in idiopathic thrombocytopenic purpura. *Br J Haematol* 1969;16:61-73.
48. Kernoff LM, Blake KCH, Shackleton D: Influence of the amount of platelet-bound IgG on platelet survival and site of sequestration in autoimmune thrombocytopenia. *Blood* 1980;55:730-733.
49. Gugliotta L, Isacchi G, Guarini A, et al: Chronic idiopathic thrombocytopenic purpura (ITP): Site of platelet sequestration and result of splenectomy. *Scand J Haematol* 1981;26:407-412.
50. Lockwood CM: Immunological functions of the spleen. *Clin Haematol* 1983;13:335-348.
51. McMillan R: Chronic idiopathic thrombocytopenic purpura. *N Engl J Med* 1981;304:1135-1147.
52. Peters AM, Saverymuttu SH, Wonke B, et al: The interpretation of platelet kinetic studies for the identification of sites of abnormal platelet destruction. *Br J Haematol* 1984;57:637-649.
53. McMillan R, Longmire RL, Yelenosky R, et al: Immunoglobulin synthesis in vitro by splenic tissue in idiopathic thrombocytopenic purpura. *N Engl J Med* 1972;286:681-684.
54. McMillan R, Longmire RL, Yelenosky R, et al: Quantitation of platelet-binding IgG produced in vitro by spleens from patients with idiopathic thrombocytopenic purpura. *N Engl J Med* 1974;291:812-817.
55. Karpatkin S, Strick N, Siskind GW: Detection of splenic anti-platelet antibody synthesis in idiopathic autoimmune thrombocytopenic purpura (ATP). *Br J Haematol* 1972;23:167-176.
56. Karpatkin S: The spleen and thrombocytopenia. *Clin Haematol* 1983;12:591-604.
57. McMillan R, Longmire RL, Tavassoli M, et al: In vitro platelet phagocytosis by splenic leucocytes in idiopathic thrombocytopenic purpura. *N Engl J Med* 1974;290:249-251.
58. Verp M, Karpatkin S: Effect of plasma, steroids or steroid products on the adhesion of human opsonized thrombocytes to human leucocytes. *J Lab Clin Med* 1975;85:478-485.
59. Rhinehart JJ, Balcerzak SP, Sagone AL, et al: Effects of corticosteroids on human monocyte function. *J Clin Invest* 1974;54:1337-1343.
60. Schreiber AD, Parsons J, McDermott P, et al: Effects of corticosteroids on the human monocyte IgG and complement receptors. *J Clin Invest* 1975;56:1189-1197.
61. Murphy WG, Allan NC, Perry DJ, et al: Hodgkin's disease presenting as idiopathic thrombocytopenic purpura. *Postgrad Med J* 1984;60:614-615.
62. Rudders RA: Autoimmune thrombocytopenic purpura in Hodgkin's disease. *N Engl J Med* 1974;291:49-50.
63. Fink K, Al-Mondhiry H: Idiopathic thrombocytopenic purpura in lymphoma. *Cancer (Phila)* 1976;37:1999-2004.
64. Weitzman S, Duilansky A, Yanai I: Thrombocytopenic purpura as the sole manifestation of recurrence in Hodgkin's disease. *Acta Haematol* 1977;58:129-133.

65. Mason D, McMillan R: Platelet antigens in chronic idiopathic thrombocytopenic purpura. *Br J Haematol* 1984;56:529-534.
66. van Leeuwen EF, van der Ven JThM, Engelfriet CP, von dem Borne AEGKr: Specificity of autoantibodies in autoimmune thrombocytopenia. *Blood* 1982;59:23-26.
67. Woods VL, Oh EH, Mason D, et al: Autoantibodies against the platelet glycoprotein 11b/111a complex in patients with chronic ITP. *Blood* 1984; 63:368-375.
68. Lynch DM, Howe SE: Antigenic determinants in idiopathic thrombocytopenic purpura. *Br J Haematol* 1986;63:301-308.
69. Beardsley DS, Spiegel JE, Jacobs MM, et al: Platelet membrane glycoprotein 111a contains target antigens that bind anti-platelet antibodies in immune thrombocytopenias. *J Clin Invest* 1984;74:1701-1707.
70. Karpatkin S, Strick N, Karpatkin MH, et al: Cumulative experience on the detection of anti-platelet antibody in 234 patients with idiopathic thrombocytopenic purpura, systemic lupus erythematosus and other clinical disorders. *Am J Med* 1972;52:776-785.
71. Dixon R, Rosse W, Ebbert L: Quantitative demonstration of antibody in idiopathic thrombocytopenic purpura: Correlation of serum and platelet antibody with clinical response. *N Engl J Med* 1975;292:230-236.
72. Hedge UM, Gordon-Smith EC, Worlledge S: Platelet antibodies in thrombocytopenic patients. *Br J Haematol* 1977;35:113-122.
73. Luiken GA, McMillan R, Lightsey AL et al: Platelet-associated IgG in immune thrombocytopenic purpura. *Blood* 1977;50:317-325.
74. Cines DB, Schreiber AD: Immune thrombocytopenia: Use of a Coomb's antiglobulin test to detect IgG and C3 on platelets. *N Engl J Med* 1979; 300:106-111.
75. Carpenter AF, Wintrobe MM, Fuller EA, et al: Treatment of idiopathic thrombocytopenic purpura. *JAMA* 1959;171:1911-1916.
76. Hedge UM, Ball S, Zviable A, et al: Platelet-associated immunoglobulins (PAIgG and PAIgM) in autoimmune thrombocytopenia. *Br J Haematol* 1985;59:221-226.
77. McMillan R, Martin M, Bakich MJ, et al: A new assay for the evaluation of antiplatelet antibody in idiopathic thrombocytopenic purpura. *Immunopharmacology* 1979;1:83-87.
78. Lusher JM, Iyer R: Idiopathic thrombocytopenic purpura in children. *Semin Thromb Hemostas* 1977;3:175-199.
79. Wallace D, Fromm D, Thomas D: Accessory splenectomy for idiopathic thrombocytopenic purpura. *Surgery (St Louis)* 1982;91:134-136.
80. Ambriz P, Munoz R, Quintanar E, et al: Accessory spleen compromising response to splenectomy for idiopathic thrombocytopenic purpura. *Radiology* 1985;155:793-796.
81. Seifried E, Pindur G, Stotter H, et al: Treatment of refractory chronic idiopathic thrombocytopenic purpura with high dose intravenous immunoglobulin. *Blut* 1984;84:369-376.

82. Uchino H, Yasunaga K, Akatsuka J-I: A cooperative clinical trial of high-dose immunoglobulin therapy in 177 cases of idiopathic thrombocytopenic purpura. *Thromb Haemostas* 1984;51:182-185.
83. Schmidt RE, Budde U, Broschen-Zyweitz C, et al: High dose gammaglobulin therapy in adults with idiopathic thrombocytopenic purpura (ITP) clinical effects. *Blut* 1984;48:19-25.
84. Abrams RA, Aster R, Anderson T: Intravenous gammaglobulin in refractory immune thrombocytopenic purpura: Efficacy with or without concomitant steroid therapy. *Am J Hematol* 1985;18:85-89.
85. Bussel JB, Schulman I, Hilgartner MW, et al: Intravenous use of gammaglobulin in the treatment of chronic immune thrombocytopenic purpura as a means to defer splenectomy. *J Pediatr* 1983;103:651-654.
86. Newland AC, Treleaven JG, Minchinton RM, et al: High-dose intravenous IgG in adults with autoimmune thrombocytopenia. *Lancet* 1983;1:84-87.
87. Lang JM, Faradji A, Giron C, et al: High-dose intravenous IgG for chronic idiopathic thrombocytopenic purpura in adults. *Blut* 1984;49:95-99.
88. Fehr J, Hofmann V, Kappeler V: Transient reversal of thrombocytopenia in idiopathic thrombocytopenic purpura by high-dose intravenous gammaglobulin. *N Engl J Med* 1982;306:1254-1258.
89. Morfini M, Vannucchi AM, Grossi A, et al: Direct evidence that high-dose intravenous gammaglobulin blocks splenic and hepatic sequestration of ^{51}Cr-labelled platelets in ITP. *Thromb Haemostas* 1985;54:554.
90. Kimberly RP, Salmon JE, Bussell JB, et al: Modulation of mononuclear phagocyte function by intravenous γ-globulin. *J Immunol* 1984;132:745-750.
91. Bussel JB, Kimberly RP, Inman RD, et al: Intravenous gammaglobulin treatment of chronic idiopathic thrombocytopenic purpura. *Blood* 1983;62:480-486.
92. Ljung R, Nilsson IM, Frohm B, et al: Platelet-associated IgG in childhood idiopathic thrombocytopenic purpura: Measurements on intact and solubilized platelets and after gammaglobulin treatment. *Scand J Haematol* 1986;36:402-407.
93. Chen LT, Weiss L: The role of the sinus wall in the passage of erythrocytes through the spleen. *Blood* 1973;41:529-537.
94. Leblond PF, LaCelle PL, Weed RI: Rheologie des erythroblastes et des erythrocytes dans la spherocytose congenitale. *Nouv Rev Fr d'Hematol* 1971;11:537-546.
95. Brown DL, Nelson DA: Surface microfragmentation of red cells as a mechanism for complement mediated immune spherocytosis. *Br J Haematol* 1973;24:301-305.
96. Ferrant A: The role of the spleen in haemolysis. *Clin Haematol* 1983;12:489-504.
97. Ferrant A, Leners N, Michaux JL et al: The spleen and haemolysis evaluation of the intrasplenic transit time. *Br J Haematol* 1987;65:31-34.

98. Myhre Jensen O, Kristensen J: Red pulp of the spleen in autoimmune haemolytic anemia and hereditary spherocytosis: Morphometric light and electron microscopic studies. *Scand J Haematol* 1986;36:263-266.
99. Motulsky AG, Casserd F, Giblett ER et al: Anemia and the spleen. *N Engl J Med* 1958;259:1164-1169.
100. Toghill PJ: Red cell pooling in enlarged spleens. *Br J Haematol* 1964;10:347-357.
101. Wennberg E, Weiss L: The structure of the spleen and hemolysis. *Annu Rev Med* 1969;20:29-40.
102. Jandl JH, Aster RH: Increased splenic pooling and the pathogenesis of hypersplenism. *Am J Med Sci* 1967;253:383-397.
103. Weed RI, LaCelle PL, Merrill EW: Metabolic dependence of red cell deformability. *J Clin Invest* 1969;48:795-809.
104. Clark DA, Dessypris EN, Jenkins DE, Krantz SB: Acquired immune hemolytic anemia associated with IgA erythrocyte coating: Investigation of hemolytic mechanisms. *Blood* 1984;64:1000-1005.
105. Stratton F, Rawlinson VI, Chapman SA, et al: Acquired hemolytic anemia associated wtih IgA anti-e. *Transfusion (Phila)* 1972;12:157-161.
106. Sturgeon P, Smith LE, Chun HMT, et al: Autoimmune hemolytic anemia associated exclusively with IgA of Rh specificity. *Transfusion (Phila)* 1979;19:324-331.
107. Suzuki S, Amano T, Mitsunaga M, et al: Autoimmune hemloytic anemia associated with IgA antibody. *Clin Immunol Immunopathol* 1981;21:247-256.
108. Lightsey AL, McMillan R: The role of the spleen in autoimmune blood disorders. *Am J Pediatr Hematol Oncol* 1979;1:331-341.
109. Dacie JV: Autoimmune hemolytic anemia. *Arch Intern Med* 1975;135:1293-1300.
110. Bell CA, Zwicker H, Sacks HJ: Autoimmune hemolytic anemia. *Am J Clin Pathol* 1973;60:903-911.
111. Evans RS, Turner E, Bingham M, et al: Chronic hemolytic anemia due to cold agglutinins. II. The role of C' in red cell destruction. *J Clin Invest* 1968;47:691-701.
112. Petz LD, Garratty G: Specificity of autoantibodies. In *Acquired Immune Hemolytic Anemias*. New York, Churchill Livingstone, 1980, 232-266.
113. Meyer RJ, Hoffman R, Zanjani ED: Autoimmune hemolytic anemia and periodic pure red cell aplasia in systemic lupus erythematosus. *Am J Med* 1978;65:342-345.
114. Pisciotta AJ, Hinz JE: Occurrence of agglutinins in normoblasts. *Proc Soc Exp Biol Med* 1956;91:356-358.
115. Hauke G, Fauser AA, Weber S, et al: Reticulocytopenia in severe autoimmune hemolytic anemia (AIHA) of the warm antibody type. *Blut* 1983;46:321-327.
116. Wagley PF, Shen SC, Gardner FJ et al: Studies on the destruction of red blood cells. VI. The spleen as a source of a substance causing agglutination of the red blood cells of certain patients with acquired hemolytic

jaundice by an antihuman serum rabbit serum (Coomb's serum). *J Lab Clin Med* 1948;33:1197-1203.
117. Habibi B, Homberg JC, Schaison G, et al: Autoimmune hemolytic anemia in children: A review of 80 cases. *Am J Med* 1974;56:61-69.
118. Allgood JW, Chaplin H: Idiopathic acquired autoimmune hemolytic anemia. *Am J Med* 1967;36:323-326.
119. Frank MM, Schreiber AD, Atkinson JP, et al: Pathophysiology of immune hemolytic anemia. *Ann Intern Med* 1977;87:210-222.
120. Jandl JH, Greenberg MS, Yonemoto RH, et al: Clinical determination of the sites of red cell sequestration in hemolytic anemias. *J Clin Invest* 1956; 35:842-867.
121. Goldberg A, Hutchinson HE, MacDonald E: Radiochromium in the selection of patients with haemolytic anemia for splenectomy. *Lancet* 1966;1: 109-113.
122. LoBuglio AF, Cotran RS, Jandl JH: Red cells coated with immunoglobulin G: Binding and sphering by mononuclear cells in man. *Science (Wash DC)* 1967;158:1582-1585.
123. Huber H, Polley MJ, Linscott WD, et al: Human monocytes: Distinct receptor sites for the third component of complement and for immunoglobulin G. *Science (Wash DC)* 1968;162:1281-1283.
124. Ehlenberger AG, Nussenzweig V: The role of membrane receptors for C3b and C3d in phagocytosis. *J Exp Med* 1977;145:357-371.
125. Mollison PL, Crome P, Hughes-Jones NC, Rochna E: Rate of removal from the circulation of red cells sensitized with different amounts of antibody. *Br J Haematol* 1965;11:461-470.
126. McMillan R: The pathogenesis of immune thrombocytopenic purpura. *CRC Crit Rev Clin Lab Sci* 1977;8:303-332.
127. Petz LD, Garratty G: Management of autoimmune hemolytic anemias. In *Acquired Immune Hemolytic Anemias*. New York, Churchill Livingstone, 1980, 392-440.
128. Crosby WH: Splenectomy in hematologic disorders. *N Engl J Med* 1971; 286:1252-1254.
129. Parker AC, MacPherson AIS, Richmond J: Value of radiochromium investigation in autoimmune haemolytic anaemia. *Br Med J* 1977;1:208-209.
130. Nightingale D, Prankers TAJ, Richards JDM, et al: Splenectomy in anemia. *Q J Med* 1972;41:261-267.
131. Bowdler AJ: The role of the spleen and splenectomy in autoimmune hemolytic disease. *Semin Hematol* 1976;13:335-348.
132. Wiseman BK, Doan CA: Primary splenic neutropenia; a newly recognized syndrome, closely related to congenital hemolytic icterus and essential thrombocytopenic purpura. *Ann Intern Med* 1942;16:1097-1117.
133. Hansen KB: Immunologic agranulocytosis; *Acta Med Scand* 1953;145: 169-174.
134. Lalezari P, Jiang A, Yegen L, et al: Chronic autoimmune neutropenia due to anti-NA2 antibody. *N Engl J Med* 1975;293:744-747.

135. Boxer LA, Greenberg MS, Boxer GJ, et al: Autoimmune neutropenia. *N Engl J Med* 1975;293:748-753.
136. Logue GL, Schimm DS: Autoimmune neutropenia. *Annu Rev Med* 1980; 31:191-200.
137. Harmon DC, Weitzman SA, Stossel TP: A staphlococcal slide test for detection of neutrophil antibodies. *Blood* 1980;56:64-69.
138. Van der Ween JPW, Hack CE, Engelfriet CP, et al: Chronic idiopathic and secondary neutropenia: Clinical and serological investigations. *Br J Haematol* 1986;63:161-171.
139. Hadley AG, Holburn AM, Bunch C, et al: Anti-granulocyte opsonic activity and autoimmune neutropenia. *Br J Haematol* 1986;63:581-589.
140. Blumfelder TM, Logue GL, Shimm DS: Felty's syndrome: Effects of splenectomy upon granulocyte count and granulocyte-associated IgG. *Ann Intern Med* 1981;94:623-628.
141. McCullough J: The clinical significance of granulocyte antibodies and in vivo studies of the fate of granulocytes. In Garratty G (ed): *Current Concepts in Transfusion Therapy*. Arlington, American Association of Blood Banks, 1985, 125-181.
142. Verheugt FWA, Borne AEGKr von dem, Noord Bokhorst JC, et al: Autoimmune granulocytopenia: The detection of granulocyte autoantibodies with the immunofluorescence test. *Br J Haematol* 1978;39:339-350.
143. Minchinton RM, Waters AH: The occurrence and significance of neutrophil antibodies. *Br J Haematol* 1984;56:521-528.
144. Fritchen JH, Cline MJ: Serum inhibitors of myelopoiesis. *Br J Haematol* 1980;44:7-16.
145. Pegels JG, Helmerhorst FM, Leeuwen EF van, et al: The Evan's syndrome: Characterization of the responsible autoantibodies. *Br J Haematol* 1982; 51:445-450.
146. Westbrook CA, Golde DW: Autoimmune disease in hairy-cell leukemia: Clinical syndromes and treatment. *Br J Haematol* 1985;61:349-356.
147. Felty AR: Chronic arthritis in the adult, associated with splenomegaly and leukopenia. *Bull Johns Hopkins Hosp* 1924;35:216-220.
148. Logue GL, Silberman HR: Felty's syndrome without splenomegaly. *Am J Med* 1979;66:703-706.
149. Wallis WJ, Loughran TP, Kadin ME, et al: Polyarthritis and neutropenia associated with circulating large granular lymphocytes. *Ann Intern Med* 1985;103:357-362.
150. Aisenberg AC, Wilkes BM, Harris NL, et al: Chronic T-cell lymphocytosis with neutropenia: Report of a case studied with monoclonal antibody. *Blood* 1981;58:818-822.
151. Chan WC, Check IU, Schick C, et al: A morphologic and immunologic study of the large granular lymphocyte in neutropenia with T lymphocytosis. *Blood* 1984;63:1133-1140.
152. Loughran TP, Kadin ME, Starkebaum G, et al: Leukemia of large granular lymphocytes: Association with clonal chromosomal abnormalities and

autoimmune neutropenia, thrombocytopenia, and hemolytic anemia. *Ann Intern Med* 1985;102:169-175.
153. Linch DC, Newland AC, Turnbull AL, et al: Unusual T cell proliferation and neutropenia in rheumatoid arthritis: Comparison with classical Felty's syndrome. *Scand J Haematol* 1984;33:342-350.
154. Logue G: Felty's syndrome: Granulocyte-bound immunoglobulin G and splenectomy. *Ann Intern Med* 1976;85:437-442.
155. Rosenthal FD, Beeley JM, Gelsthorpe K, et al: White cell antibodies and the aetiology of Felty's syndrome. *Q J Med* 1974;43:187-203.
156. Barnes CG, Turnbull AL, Vernon-Roberts B: Felty's syndrome. A clinical and pathological survey of 21 patients and their response to treatment. *Ann Rheum Dis* 1971;30:359-374.
157. Laslo J, Jones R, Silberman HR, et al: Splenectomy for Felty's syndrome. Clinico-pathologic study of 27 patients. *Arch Intern Med* 1971;75:381-385.

Part III

Splenomegaly

8
Splenomegaly
Diagnostic Overview

JAMES A. STOCKMAN III*

Northwestern University Medical School, Chicago, Illinois

Splenomegaly is a physical sign common to many disorders. Splenomegaly may also be viewed as a diagnostic clue to these disorders. Additionally, splenomegaly may pose problems related to the size or functioning of the spleen, such as by the occurrence of hypersplenism or hyposplenism. This chapter will provide a concise overall approach to the wide spectrum of possible causes of splenomegaly.

Despite the frequency with which splenomegaly is seen in clinical practice, it is often difficult to quickly isolate the cause of this finding. The spleen is truly an anomalous organ. It can be the cause of the principle difficulties associated with some disorders without being enlarged. An example of such a disorder is idiopathic immune thrombocytopenia. On the other hand, the spleen may be nonspecifically enlarged in serious disorders. In Hodgkin's disease, as an instance of this, the spleen may be enlarged but without histopathologic evidence of lymphoma (see Chapter 7).

Likewise, enlargement of the spleen may be a nonspecific finding, or it may be highly diagnostic of the etiology of the splenomegaly. Unfortunately, the hematologic features of many diseases or conditions characterized by splenic enlargement have not been well correlated with splenic morphology or histology. This lack of correlation leaves a large gap in our understanding as to the relationship between these conditions and the associated splenomegaly (1). Furthermore, the studies used to clinically define enlargement of the spleen are themselves, more often than not, nondiagnostic. Frequently, the diagnosis is

---

Current affiliation: Children's Memorial Hospital, Chicago, Illinois

established by studies of the blood, bone marrow, liver, or lymph nodes. Infrequently, splenic aspiration, biopsy, or splenectomy may be necessary for diagnostic purposes.

The greater challenge to the clinician is the initial need to decide whether the observation of a mildly enlarged spleen warrants immediate evaluation or merely careful observation. This is especially true in children. Although there are a few exceptions in older adults, clinically apparent splenomegaly should not be viewed as a trivial sign. In children and young adults, however, the spleen is a much more reactive organ and the diagnostic yield from careful assessment may be much lower. For example, at the time of admission to college, approximately 3% of students have a palpable spleen (2). Thus, the need for further testing for splenomegaly must be based on how the total appearance of the patient strikes the examiner, not just the notation of some degree of splenomegaly.

To properly frame the diagnostic overview of splenomegaly, the functions of the spleen will be briefly reviewed. It is usually some alteration of these functions that either produces splenomegaly or in some way provides an insight into the nature of the problem. In many instances, the spleen enlarges as it performs its normal functions. Among these important functions are synthesis of immunologic factors, destruction of senescent or abnormal circulating cellular elements, embryonic hematopoiesis, which may be reactivated in states associated with extramedullary hematopoiesis, and the clearance from the circulation of microorganisms or particulate matter.

FUNCTIONS OF THE SPLEEN

Antibody Formation

The spleen is capable of producing virtually all varieties of antibodies, especially after challenge with particulate antigens (3). In hyposplenic states, this function of the spleen is usually preserved, except in conditions associated with suppression of both cellular and humoral immunity. The ability to form specific antibody seems to be preserved longer in those conditions associated with functional hyposplenia than other functions of the spleen, such as removal of particulate material.

The unique microcirculation of the spleen also facilitates the immune response to intravenously administered particulate antigens. When blood enters the spleen, the soluble antigens are skimmed off, along with much of the plasma, to enter the right-angled arterioles supplying the germinal centers of the white pulp. But the particulare antigens, such as Samonella flagellar antigens, lodge first in the red pulp and within hours are transported, possibly by mobile macrophages, across the marginal zone into the germinal centers, where the IgM antibody response is initiated.

The spleen is also the major site of synthesis of tuftsin and properdin, two proteins that serve as opsonins. Serum levels of tuftsin, a basic tetrapeptide that coats blood polymorphonuclear leukocytes to promote phagocytosis, are subnormal after splenectomy (4,5). Serum levels of properdin, a vital component of the alternative pathway of complement activation, are also subnormal after splenectomy (6). Likewise, these abnormalities are present in functional hyposplenia. For example, children with sickle-cell anemia have subnormal levels of properdin and defective alternate pathway activity. This impairs their serum opsonization of pneumococci and, along with their functional asplenia, puts them back at risk for fatal pneumococcemia (7,8). It should be noted that after undergoing splenectomy for splenic trauma, normal children have normal pneumococcal serum opsonizing activity (9). Although partial deficiencies of tuftsin and properdin represent minor risk factors after splenectomy or with functional asplenia, it seems likely that the integrity of the microcirculation of the spleen is crucial to the survival of the immunologically compromised patient with pneumococcemia.

Except in the functional hyposplenic states in which certain of the above-mentioned proteins are deficient, defects in antibody formation are not associated with splenomegaly. Therefore, tests of antibody formation are not useful in determining the cause of splenomegaly.

Filtration Function of the Spleen

The spleen will remove normal but senescent cellular elements of the blood. It will also remove abnormal cells such as antibody-coated red blood cells, white blood cells, and platelets. This culling function appears to be done with a greater degree of precision by the spleen than can be accomplished by the liver in most instances (10,11).

This filtration process with regards to red blood cells involves several levels of activity. Entire cells may be culled from the circulation (12). Some pitting-out of inclusions may occur, with the polished cell reentering the circulation. Via this process, Howell-Jolly bodies, siderotic granules, Heinz bodies and the vacuoles of pocked cells are removed. For example, as the red cell moves through the stoma of a splenic sinus wall from the splenic cords to the sinus lumen, a Heinz body is trapped and then extruded from the "tail" of the cell. Parasites may be pitted from cells by this mechanism, allowing an intact red cell to migrate out of the spleen and resulting in the parasite being entrapped by phagocytes.

Splenic function and filtration depends critically upon the passage of cells through pulp cords rather than through open vascular pathways. Filtration is de-

Table 1 Diseases Associated with Hyposplenism

A. Atropic spleen
   Ulcerative colitis
   Celiac disease
   Dermatitis herpetiformis
   Thyrotoxicosis (Graves' disease)
   Hemorrhagic thrombocythemia
   Thorotrast

B. Normal-sized or enlarged spleen
   Sickle-cell anemia (early)
   Sarcoidosis
   Amyloidosis
   High-dose corticosteroids (?)

fective in functional asplenia (13). In a similar way, other types of cells may be removed. For example, acanthocytes will be removed if they pass through the splenic pulp. Spherocytes, such as in hereditary spherocytosis, are unable to pass through the spleen. Likewise, fixed sickled forms and hemoglobin C cells may be too rigid to pass through the splenic cores.

The presence of Howell-Jolly bodies in the peripheral blood of a patient with splenomegaly is a good indication of the cause of the splenomegaly, since relatively few disorders are associated with both splenomegaly and functional asplenia. Table 1 lists disorders associated with functional asplenia.

Phagocytosis

Phagocytosis in the spleen requires the interaction between the macrophage and the targeted cell to be removed. This mediation may be by surface immunoglobulin or complement, but erythrophagocytosis is also evident with red cells that are metabolically abnormal. Macrophages are easily shown to interact with red cells coated with 7 S IgG bound to specific receptors of monocytes. These cells then show vacuolization and fragmentation ultimately leading to spherocytosis (14). Thus far, most disorders associated with splenomegaly have not been demonstrated to exhibit secondary defects in splenic phagocytosis.

Hematopoiesis and Other Spleen Functions

The spleen normally is a hematopoietic organ in utero. In lower vertebrates, the spleen maintains this function. In human fetuses at 5 months gestation there is a switch to medullary hematopoiesis with discontinuation of blood cell generation in extramedullary sites. However, these sites of embryonic hematopoiesis can become active again at virtually any time of life by processes that are poorly understood. The spleen is particularly active in reactive hematopoiesis. In these instances, extramedullary splenic hematopoiesis may be compensatory or neoplastic. In most instances, however, it is characterized by ineffective hematopoiesis and abnormal red cell morphology (15).

In addition to the four major functions that have been ascribed to the spleen, the spleen has many other roles. The spleen is capable of helping to maintain the total blood pool volume. The normal red cell content of the spleen is 20-60 ml, or less than 5% of the total red cell mass. Thus, under most circumstances there is no significant red cell pool. When the spleen is enlarged, however, this pool will increase markedly and will contain a significant proportion of the overall red cell mass. The spleen is also capable of sequestering cellular elements without actually destroying these cells. In these instances, the cells are held temporarily in splenic sinuses before they are returned to the circulation. In contrast to sequestration, pooled cells in the spleen are in continuous exchange with the circulation. As blood flows through the sinuses and cords, effete and damaged cells and particulate foreign matter are phagocytosed by the endothelial macrophages and the reticulum cells. This is a delaying process that can result in some degree of pooling within the spleen.

The spleen also is capable of maintaining plasma volume control. The mechanism by which this occurs is not clear. Changes in plasma volume may lead to an apparent anemia, the so-called pseudoanemia or dilutional anemia of splenomegaly. Several mechanisms have been suggested to explain the expanded plasma volume in splenomegaly. These explanations include the possibility that the enlarged organ requires an expansion of blood volume to fill the additional intravascular space. In conditions where bone marrow erythropoietic activity is reduced, it may not be possible to maintain normal red cell plasma volume ratio. The additional volume is then provided by plasma alone.

Increased pressure in the portal vein has also been suggested as a triggering mechanism for plasma volume control. An increase in splanchnic blood volume resulting from obstructive or hyperkinetic portal hypertension may account for some of the plasma volume increases in splenomegaly. Protein alterations result in a change in colloid oncotic pressure. This has been suggested as a factor in tropical splenomegaly and in cirrhosis. There is even some evidence that plasma volume is controlled by osmoreceptors, but various sites where these are suspected to exist do not include the spleen.

Each of the above functions of the spleen, if aberrant, may result in some degree of splenomegaly. For these reasons, tests for splenic function sometimes are valuable clues as to the overall nature of the cause for splenomegaly.

Table 2 Biologic Substances Removed by the Spleen

A. In normal subjects
    Red blood cell membrane
    Red blood cell surface pits and craters
    Howell-Jolly bodies
    Heinz bodies
    Pappenheimer bodies
    Acanthocytes
    Senescent red blood cells

B. In those with diseases
    Spherocytes (hereditary spherocytosis)
    Sickled cells, hemoglobin C cells
    Antibody-coated red blood cells
    Antibody-coated platelets
    Antibody-coated white blood cells

Measurement of Splenic Function

A whole host of tests have been developed to measure splenic function. Radionuclide labeling provides a valuable procedure for studying various components of splenic function. These will be described in a subsequent section. Radiolabeling of cellular elements such as damaged erythrocytes may also give some information about the clearance function of the spleen. Simple examination of the peripheral blood smear for Howell-Jolly bodies or the use of interference-contrast microscopy to look for red cell pits is also helpful. If abnormalities with these tests are seen in the presence of enlargement of the spleen, specific diagnoses may be considered. In these cases, the number of possible diagnoses is small since relatively few causes of splenomegaly are associated with functional alterations of the spleen.

Table 2 lists the biological substances normally removed by the spleen.

DEFINITION OF SPLENOMEGALY

Physical Examination

A careful examination of splenomegaly should include palpation of the abdomen. The patient should be supine, in the right lateral decubitus position and with the knees up. This examination, of course, becomes somewhat easier as the child grows older, except in extremely muscular individuals. Only light fingertip pressure should be applied and the patient should inspire slowly. Some believe that splenic percussion can identify borderline enlargement in the presence of splenomegaly, whereas others have disputed this. If this technique is used, the percussion note in the lowest intercostal space in the left anterior auxillary line changes from resonant to dull with full inspiration.

Enlargement of the spleen is usually expressed by the number of centimeters the tip of the spleen is felt percussed below the left costal margin after deep inspiration. This measurement is most commonly made in a vertical plane roughly transecting the inferior tip of the spleen, if the spleen is lying in a normal position. It is clear that mild splenomegaly may not be detected with even the most careful physical examination. Also, there may be relatively poor correlation between the estimation of splenomegaly by physical examination and the estimation of splenic enlargement obtained with other diagnostic studies. Not infrequently, the spleen is misinterpreted as to whether it is large or normal depending on other associated factors. The spleen often is compressed against the abdominal wall or displaced inferiorly by the gastrointestinal tract or liver. Palpability, the first clue to splenomegaly, therefore can be an inaccurate monitor of splenic size.

Dell and Klinefelter (16) have shown that a palpable spleen certainly need not correspond to a radiologically enlarged spleen. Blackburn (17), in a study of subjects with experimentally induced malaria, has laid to rest the concept that the spleen, in order to be palpable, must be increased in size two to three times normal. He was able to detect by palpation an enlargement of the spleen of only 40% when spleen size was subsequently measured radiographically.

In the absence of an unusually displaced spleen, any palpability of a spleen may be a sign of splenomegaly. Depending on what other findings are present, it may then be necessary to verify enlargement of the spleen by some form of imaging technique. These techniques will now be discussed.

Diagnostic Imaging to Detect Splenomegaly

Because simple palpation of the spleen is often an inaccurate assessment of splenic size, we have come to rely on diagnostic imaging techniques to more accurately assess spleen size. In the pediatric age group, assessment by any of these imaging techniques is often difficult because of the uncertainty as to what constitutes a truly normal spleen size. The ability to localize or define a particular property of the spleen will vary considerably among different techniques. For example, the physical dimensions of the spleen may be measured with an accuracy of 1 or 2 cm by methods based on radionuclide studies, or with an accuracy of 1 or 2 mm by the x-ray techniques. The relative cost-benefit ratio and accuracy of each technique should be objectively judged when deciding what is the most appropriate test to determine spleen size and anatomy. In general, the question of whether the spleen is enlarged is one that has plagued clinicians and diagnostic imagers for many years.

Seldom are imaging studies performed simply to determine splenic size. Usually other information is sought as well. Currently, five techniques are available in most institutions to determine splenic size and architecture. These techniques vary in sensitivity and specificity. Which technique or techniques to use depends on what one is attempting to define. The methods include: (1) simple abdominal x-rays; (2) radionuclides, including conventional plain imaging, quantitative measurement, and *single-photon-emission computed tomography* (SPECT) computer reconstruction of the organ in three-dimensional planes; (3) ultrasound, including both static scanning and real-time sonography; (4) x-ray computed tomography; (5) nuclear magnetic resonance.

Roentgenographic examination of the abdomen can give a better evaluation of spleen size than simple physical examination, but this examination is of no help when the spleen is not well visualized. Unfortunately, a normal spleen length on roentgenographic examination does not exclude mild or even moderate splenomegaly. Occasionally a barium enema will help to outline an enlarged spleen.

Radionuclide imaging has perhaps been the most widely used technique for imaging of the spleen. The technique is relatively easy to perform and is atraumatic. The patient simply stands in front of the scanner for a relatively short period of time. However, injection of the radioactive material is required. With the widely available imaging equipment currently in use in the United States, records of the anatomy and some functions of the spleen related to pathology are demonstrable. For example, the spleen can be demonstrated to be the site of red blood cell destruction using denatured radiolabeled red blood cells. Extramedullary hematopoiesis in the spleen may be demonstrated using radioactive iron analogs. The size, integrity, shape, and relation of the spleen to other organs can be represented by visualizing the uptake of various colloid particles. Although the images are relatively crude compared to other modalities, this does not necessarily impair the usefulness of radionuclide imaging. A recent technique introduced to complement conventional planar radionuclide imaging is single-photon-emission computed tomography (SPECT) (18). This technique uses a succession of views taken at increments around the patient. A series of images of sections through the organ of interest are generated by means of a computer system. A three-dimensional representation of the spleen is thus achieved that may be superior to a set of conventional two-dimensional images. Volume of the spleen may be calculated directly without assumptions based on linear measurements. The site of space-occupying lesions in the spleen may be more accurately determined. The technique also offers the possibility of fairly accurate quantification of the amount of activity in terms of activity per unit volume of the spleen.

Technically, SPECT is carried out by obtaining camera views over 360° around the long axis of the body in examinations taking about 10 min. The corresponding profile extracted from each image is digitized, filtered back, and projected (19) by the computer to form a digital image of a section about 15 mm thick. This is repeated for all the sections through the organ. The additional equipment necessary for SPECT (other than the conventional camera and computer system) is a gantry capable of rotating the camera, a cantilevered couch, and a special computer program to carry out all the processing of the images.

The properties of both the radionuclide label used to perform a splenic scan and what the label is attached to must be considered when investigating the different functions of the spleen. The half-life of the radionuclide should be long enough to carry out the imaging procedure or to follow through a metabolic process, but not unnecessarily long so that a large radiation dose is given. $^{99}Tc_m$ is often considered an ideal radionuclide, with its half-life of 6 hr and its low associated radiation effects. Technetium is fairly economical since it is generated on site within nuclear medicine departments from a long-lived parent radionuclide, ^{99}Mb. ^{51}Cr was used in the past for blood labeling, but has a half-life of 28 days and produces few gamma rays in comparison to the relatively high radiation dose it delivers to the patient.

Technetium-labeled heat-damaged blood cells that are trapped in the splenic microcirculation offer a way of radionuclide imaging with little background interference (20). For spleen-related hematologic studies, the two radionuclides, ^{59}Fe and ^{52}Fe should be used for physiologic accuracy. In general, however, for splenic imaging with respect to size and simple function, most use technetium-labeled colloidal material. The radioisotopic spleen scan with $^{99}Tc_m$-sulfur colloid and the gamma scintillation camera technique gives a good index of splenic size, provided that careful measurements are made in both the lateral and posterior projections. With accurate measurements, mild splenomegaly can usually be distinguished from a normal size spleen, although normal values for children are quite scant. Usually, with splenic enlargement the lateral area increases more than the posterior area. This is not always so; thus, any two-dimensional measurement from scanning techniques may be subject to some degree of error.

Ultrasound imaging of the spleen with present-day instrumentation is relatively simple to perform. It is atraumatic and needs very little patient preparation. It is noninvasive and has no radiation hazards. Its major role is to provide information regarding spatial locations of the spleen and its anatomy. Less attention has been paid to this technique than to others. Unfortunately, ultrasonic imaging of the spleen has not received as wide a degree of acceptance as it might because the degree of quality and the amount of information derived from the images often depends on the skill of the operator. A number of artifacts are common to ultrasound images. These include artifactual echos caused by reverberation in which the echos rebound between structures and then return to the detector instead of returning directly. Acoustic shadows may also appear, cast by a structure such as bone or gas that strongly reflects or absorbs the ultrasound energy.

X-ray *computer-assisted tomography* (CAT scanning) gives very accurate representation of the anatomy of the spleen and its relationship to other adjacent organs such as the liver and kidneys (21). Lobulated or accessory spleens and subcapsular abscesses can be identified. The use of contrast material as a tracer of splenic function is limited, however, and few direct measurements of splenic function can be made with CAT scanning. Thus, CAT scans of the spleen have concentrated on size and shape determination, localization of benign lesions such as cysts, detection of certain malignant lesions such as lymphomas, and detection of trauma to the spleen (22). CAT scanning is noninvasive, atraumatic, and not particularly time consuming, though a significant radiation dose may be given.

Although CAT scanning has not been systematically applied to determine splenic size in children, it should be able to give a reasonable estimate of splenomegaly. The major advantage of CAT scanning is the architectural detail that may be provided. The CAT scan is probably more sensitive than radioisotopic scans in detecting small splenic lacerations, thus, it should be used when splenic trauma is being considered as a cause of splenomegaly. The major disadvantage of CAT scanning is that it gives no insight into reticuloendothelial function.

The attraction of nuclear magnetic resonance imaging (MRI) is that is offers a noninvasive investigation in comparatively fine detail, and in three dimensions, of a number of function-related parameters that are potentially sensitive to pathologic changes (23). In addition, MRI scanning is extremely simple to carry out from the patient-handling viewpoint, with no established consequent radiation sequelae or other known effects. Unfortunately, in view of the limited use of this technique in assessing spleens in children, the diagnostic usefulness of this technique is not yet established. Thus, the comparative abilities of MRI versus the techniques previously mentioned require further examination.

In general, the modality used to examine splenic size and function depends on availability of the equipment, the ease of its use, the cost of the tests, its influence on the patient management and its outcome in terms of morbidity and mortality. Nuclear medicine and ultrasound imaging are more widely available than CT. Strategies can be developed to make the most cost-effective use of available equipment. One such approach in adults has been proposed by Shirkhode et al. (24). These investigators recommend that a suspected splenic abnormality first be investigated by using a nuclear medicine technique with sulfur colloid. If a focal abnormality is found, an ultrasound test is proposed, otherwise splenic hematoma or trauma may be imaged using CAT scanning. If a focal lesion is confirmed by ultrasound, then further nuclear medicine tests with other radionuclides such as ^{67}Ga or CAT scanning should be carried out.

DIAGNOSTIC OVERVIEW

Background

Palpable spleens are not always abnormal, and hypersplenic spleens are not always palpable. As noted above, one study has shown that as many as 3% of 2200 healthy college freshmen had palpable spleens (2). In this report, all students were examined within several days of their arrival at Dartmouth College. The criterion for a palpable spleen was that the examiner's finger tips were struck and slightly raised ("flipped") by the descending spleen, and this finding was confirmed by a second examination within several days. Splenomegaly, according to the definition used, persisted over a 3-year period in approximately one-third of these students. The finding of a palpable spleen could not be explained on the basis of body habitus or the presence of infectious mononucleosis.

Of those with splenomegaly detected on routine examination, infectious mononucleosis was the only potential etiology detected upon subsequent evaluation. At best, however, infectious mononucleosis accounted for less than one-tenth of cases associated with "silent" splenomegaly. In the first 6 years of this study, there was no evidence for an increased prevalence of disease in the group of students with palpable spleens. 10 years later, a mail survey was conducted to detect possible differences in the health of those who earlier had splenomegaly in comparison to a matched control group (25). A significantly higher frequency of physician's office visits, infections other than "flu" or "cold," and infections including "cold or flu" were reported. It was concluded that asymptomatic splenomegaly in this age group was not associated with a higher risk of lymphoreticular malignancy, and that health in general, with the possible exception of an increased frequency of infection, was not impaired.

Thus, when one examines a patient and splenomegaly is detected, it is likely that the cause of the splenomegaly will be quite difficult to determine. Exceptions to this rule are patients in whom specific signs and symptoms are present, or other findings are illicited from the history and physical examination that indicate the cause of the splenomegaly.

Mild splenomegaly occurs with many diseases. It is probably more productive to list the mechanisms of splenomegaly and to provide examples of diseases associated with each mechanism than to discuss each disease. Table 3 indicates the six most common mechanisms of splenomegaly (26). These include work hypertrophy from excess immune response; work hypertrophy with rapid red cell destruction; plus congestive, myeloproliferative, infiltrative, and neoplastic disorders. Common examples of each of these are listed in the table.

Table 3 Classification and Etiology of Splenomegaly

Mechanism of splenomegaly	Common examples
Work hypertrophy: immune response	Subacute bacterial endocarditis; infectious mononucleosis; Felty's syndrome
Work hypertrophy: red cell destruction	Spherocytosis; thalassemia major; pyruvate kinase deficiency
Congestion	Hepatic cirrhosis; splenic vein thrombosis
Myeloproliferative disorders	Chronic myelocytic leukemia; myeloid metaplasia
Infiltrative diseases	Sarcoidosis; amyloidosis; Gaucher's disease
Neoplastic diseases	Lymphoma; chronic lymphocytic leukemia; metastatic cancer

Work hypertrophy resulting from a hyperimmune response is probably the most common cause of splenomegaly in children. It is often the most difficult to evaluate since so many nonspecific illnesses trigger a profound immune reaction in children. Work hypertrophy on the basis of a hyperimmune response is very typical in disorders such as subacute bacterial endocarditis, infectious mononucleosis, and Felty's syndrome. Work hypertrophy associated with red cell destruction is seen frequently in the hereditary hemolytic anemias, including hereditary spherocytosis and thalassemia. Congestive splenomegaly is usually the consequences of liver disease that has progressed to cirrhosis. It can result from malformations or thrombosis of the splenic vein. Other causes of conges-

Table 4 The Causes of Congestive Splenomegaly

A. Intrahepatic obstructive portal hypertension
   Portal cirrhosis; postnecrotic scarring; biliary cirrhosis
   Hepatolenticular degeneration
   Hemochromatosis
   Hepatic venous occlusion
   Sarcoidosis
B. Extrahepatic obstructive portal hypertension
   Venous malformation, thrombosis, stenosis, atresia, aneurysmal formation, and extrinsic occlusion of portal vein or splenic vein
C. Chronic passive congestion of cardiac origin

Table 5 Disorders Accompanied by Splenomegaly

A. Infections
  1. *Acute infections* Viral hepatitis infections, mononucleosis, septicemias (including tuberculosis), salmonellosis, relapsing fever, tularaemia, splenic abscess, cytomegalovirus infection, toxoplasmosis
  2. *Subacute and chronic infections* Subacute bacterial endocarditis, chronic septicemia, tuberculosis, brucellosis, syphilis, malaria[a], leishmaniasis[a], trypanosomiasis, histoplasmosis, and other systemic fungal diseases
B. Inflammatory and granulomatous conditions
  Felty's syndrome, systemic lupus erythematosus, rheumatic fever, serum sickness, sarcoidosis, and berylliosis
C. Congestive splenomegaly
  1. *Intrahepatic lesions* Portal cirrhosis, postnecrotic scarring, biliary cirrhosis, Wilson's disease, hemochromatosis, venoocclusive disease, congenital fibrosis, bilharziasis
  2. *Portal vein obstruction* Cavernous malformation; thrombosis, stenosis, or atresia; A. V. aneurysm, obstruction at porta hepatis
  3. *Splenic vein obstruction* Angiomatous malformation; thrombosis, stenosis or atresia; obstruction by pancreatic disease or splenic arterial aneurysm
  4. *Hepatic vein occlusion* Budd-Chiari syndrome
  5. *Cardiac* Especially chronic or recurrent congestive cardiac failure
D. Hematologic disorders
  1. *Red blood cell disorders* Hereditary disorders or red cell membrane, autoimmune haemolytic disease due to warm antibodies, thalassemia, sickle thalassemia, sickle-cell disease (early), haemoglobin-SC disease
  2. *Myeloproliferative disorders* Primary myeloid metaplasia[a], polycythemia vera (variable), essential thrombocythemia (variable)
  3. *Miscellaneous* Primary splenic hyperplasia, megaloblastic anemias, iron deficiency
E. Malignancy
  1. *Hematologic malignancy* Acute leukemias, chronic leukemias[a], leukemic reticuloendotheliosis[a], malignant lymphoma[a], malignant histiocytosis, myelomatosis
  2. *Intrinsic malignancy*
  Primary
  Lymphosarcoma, plasmacytoma, fibrosarcoma, angiosarcoma
  Secondary
  Cardinoma or melanoma
  Benign
  Hamartoma, fibroma, haemangioma, lymphangioma

Table 5 (continued)

F. Storage disease
   Gaucher's disease[a], Niemann-Pick disease, histiocytosis-X, Tangier disease, Hurler's syndrome
G. Miscellaneous
   Cysts
   Parasitic cyst, pseudocysts, amyloidosis, Albers-Schonberg disease, splenic mastocytosis, hereditary hemorrhagic telengiectasia, hyperthyroidism

[a]Major causes of marked splenomegaly.

tive splenomegaly is much less common in children comapred to adults but does occur. This can result from myelocytic leukemia or myeloid metaplasia. A number of infiltrative disorders such as sarcoidosis, amyloidosis, and storage diseases, particularly Gaucher's disease, can produce splenomegaly in children.

Table 5 provides a broad overview of the many different causes of splenomegaly in both children and young adults. Two findings, if present, are especially helpful in rapidly making a diagnosis of the cause of splenomegaly. One is the presence of giant splenomegaly. The other is the presence of hematologic signs of hypersplenism in the presence of splenomegaly. Each of these has a relatively restricted number of specific etiologies.

Giant Splenomegaly

Relatively few diseases in the United States cause giant splenomegaly as a presenting or consistent feature of the disorder. The largest of spleens in children may be caused by the myeloproliferative disorders, the most common of which would be chronic myelocytic leukemia. Leukemic reticuloendotheliosis (hairy-cell leukemia), a relatively newly recognized cause of giant splenomegaly does occur in children, but infrequently (27). Massive splenomegaly may occasionally be the presenting feature of Gaucher's disease. Isolated splenic lymphoma can also cause giant splenomegaly.

In the tropics, giant splenomegaly may be seen as a result of a hyperimmune response to malaria. In these cases, often called tropical splenomegaly, serum IgM levels are notable elevated (28). An interesting counterpart, idiopathic nontropical splenomegaly, exists in which no obvious cause for massive splenomegaly is found. This was thought to be a benign problem until several patients were observed years later to develop lymphoma (29). Thalassemia major is capable of producing massive splenomegaly in children, as can sarcoidosis on rare occasions (30).

Table 6 Disorders Associated with Hypersplenism

A. Primary hypersplenism
Primary splenic hyperplasia; simple splenic hyperplasia; nontropical idiopathic splenomegaly; primary splenic neutropenia; primary splenic panhematopenia; splenic anemia, thrombocytopenic type
B. Secondary hypersplenism
1. Acute infections with splenomegaly
2. Chronic infections; tuberculosis, brucellosis, malaria, kala-azar
3. Inflammatory conditions and granulomas; Felty's syndrome, sarcoidosis, systemic lupus erythematosus
4. Congestive splenomegaly
5. Storage disorders
6. Malignant disorders; leukemias, lymphomas, secondary carcinoma
7. Chronic hemolytic disorders
8. Myeloproliferative disorders
9. Splenic malformations, hyperthyroiditis, hypersplenism-hypogammaglobulinemia syndrome

Hypersplenism

It is clinically useful to recognize the presence of hypersplenism in association with splenomegaly. Most causes of splenomegaly do not result in hypersplenism. Because the list of causes of hypersplenism is relatively restricted, the presence of splenomegaly and any combination of anemia, leukopenia, and/or thrombocytopenia should lead one to examine the potential causes of splenomegaly related to hypersplenism.

Hypersplenism is an imprecise term. However, typically it refers to (1) splenomegaly; (2) any combination of anemia, leukoepnia, and/or thrombocytopenia; (3) compensatory bone marrow hyperplasia; and (4) improvement after splenectomy. The most common causes of hypersplenism may be seen in Table 6. The most interesting of these diseases associated with hypersplenism is Felty's syndrome, the triad of chronic rheumatoid arthritis, splenomegaly, and granulocytopenia. This is a truly unique variant of hypersplenism in which the spleen appears to be acting as if it were a giant lymph node. This disorder, of course, is relatively uncommon in children. There are several theories for the granulocytopenia of Felty's syndrome. These theories apply to both children and adults. The mechanism of granulocytopenia include (1) decreased marrow granulopoiesis, (2) increased margination of granulocytes from the peripheral pool, (3) increased splenic sequestration of granulocytes, and (4) the presence of antigranulocyte antibodies. There is an increased marginated pool of granulocytes

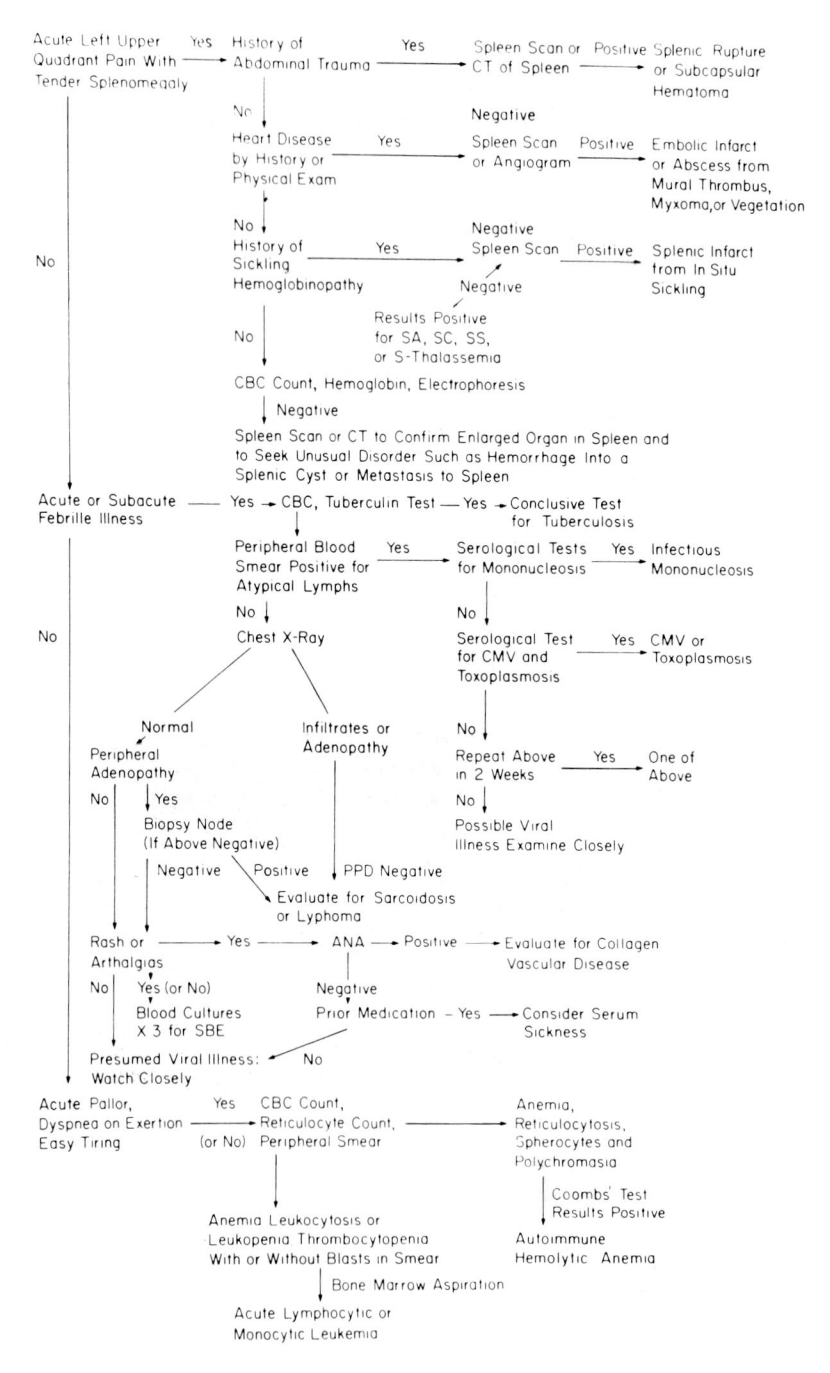

Figure 1 Algorithm for determining the cause of acute splenomegaly. (Modified from Ref. 33.)

SPLENOMEGALY: DIAGNOSTIC OVERVIEW

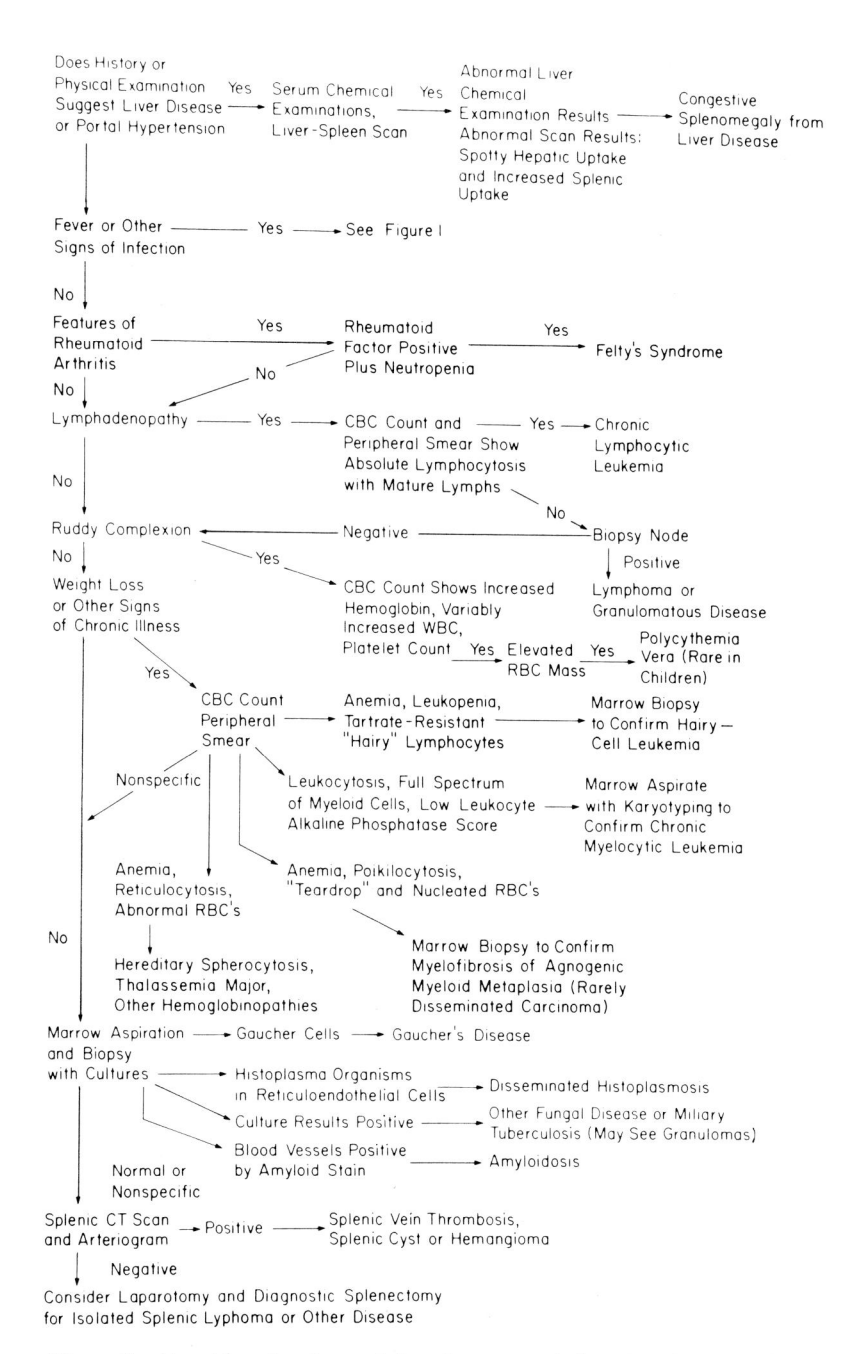

Figure 2 Algorithm for determining the cause of chronic splenomegaly. (Modified from Ref. 33.)

in this disorder (31). T cell suppression of bone marrow granulopoiesis has also been documented (32). Granulocytes in Felty's syndrome may be coated with immunoglobulin as part of a pan-autoimmune process. Immunoglobulin titers may decrease after splenectomy.

Diagnostic Approach to Splenomegaly

As has been suggested, clues to the cause of splenomegaly are more often found in sites distant to the spleen than in the spleen itself. The clues that determine the approach to be followed must be provided from the history and physical examination.

Figures 1 and 2 represent an algorithm approach to the diagnosis of acute or subacute splenomegaly. The strategies suggested are based on whether splenomegaly is associated with an acute or subacute illness, as opposed to a chronic illness or asymptomatic splenomegaly. The approaches illustrated in Figures 1 and 2 have been modified from Eichner et al. (33). Modifications emphasize the disorders more commonly seen in infants and children. As with the use of any algorithm, common sense and clues provided from the history and physical examination are more important than any standardized approach.

One of the most important questions in evaluating the child with acute splenomegaly is whether the enlargement of the spleen is associated with significant tenderness over the spleen. This finding can be a sign of subcapsular hematoma or frank rupture of the spleen. The same symptoms, however, can be seen with infectious mononucleosis and in a variety of other infectious states. A rapidly progressive leukemia can likewise cause rapid enlargement of the spleen and pain. Any patient with acute or newly recognized splenomegaly who has palpable tenderness over the spleen and for whom simple tests such as a complete blood count, heterophile agglutination, etc., fail to yield a diagnosis, should have the anatomy of the spleen examined.

The splenic scan remains the mainstay for detecting subcapsular hematoma or rupture of the spleen, but occasionally it is associated with false negative findings. As noted, the CAT scan may be as or more useful in detecting subcapsular hematoma or splenic rupture. Other causes of acutely tender, enlarged spleens include embolic infarction, multiple abscesses (such as in acute bacterial endocarditis), and in situ infarction as in sickle-cell disease. Splenic abscesses, usually in association with bacterial endocarditis, or after seeding of the spleen from peritonitis or postoperatively, are usually detected with routine splenic scanning. If a splenic abscess or abscesses are suspected, a ^{67}Ga scan may be particularly useful.

The most common occurrence is that of a child who is found to have painless splenomegaly on routine examination or during an examination for illness. In this instance, if a thorough and careful history and physical examination fails to provide any clue to the etiology of the splenomegaly, a logical approach to achieve a diagnosis should be used if the size and feel of the spleen warrants further evaluation. It is not necessary to further examine every child with splenomegaly at the time it is first noted. If the enlargement is barely detectable and there are no associated problems such as hepatomegaly, lymphadenopathy, and rash, for instance, it may be appropriate simply to reexamine the child after 1-2 weeks. If the diagnostic studies appear warranted, the initial test of greatest yield is a complete blood count, including a reticulocyte count, a platelet count, and a careful review of the peripheral blood smear. It is most simple to include a diagnostic test for infectious mononucleosis and to place a tuberculin test at this time as well.

If there is no answer provided by these studies in a child with an acute or subacute febrile illness it may be necessary to determine antibody titers against other infectious agents, particularly cytomegalovirus, toxoplasmosis, and if indicated, human immunodeficiency virus (HIV). Further studies are warranted depending on the level of concern. A chest x-ray is particularly useful to detect areas of lymphadenopathy not observable on physical examination and to exclude pulmonary parenchymal disease. If splenomegaly is persistent, a bone marrow examination, including both aspiration and biopsy, may be indicated to diagnose malignancy or storage diseases. If enlargement of a peripheral lymph node is present, biopsy may provide a ready histopathologic diagnosis.

In patients with chronic splenomegaly but without specific symptoms, a different variety of disorders is usually found. In particular, liver disease with portal hypertension, Gaucher's disease, anatomical defects of the spleen, sarcoidosis, collagen-vascular disease, and the hemolytic anemias should be considered as possibilities. Testing will include studies such as a complete blood count, reticulocyte count, platelet count, tuberculin testing, rheumatoid factor antinuclear assay (ANA), fungal testing, bone marrow examination, chest x-ray, and liver function studies. If no diagnosis is achieved, a study to define the anatomy of the spleen may be indicated. This would usually include a radionuclide scan, a CT scan, or both, to locate "filling" defects within the spleen, such as cysts, hemangiomas, infiltrative processes, etc. A splenic arteriogram may be necessary to complement these studies, particularly to exclude vascular malformations or splenic vein thrombosis.

When all else fails and the diagnosis of the cause of splenomegaly remains unknown, one may need to consider splenectomy or partial splenectomy as a diagnostic technique. Surgery should not be recommended lightly, for obvious reasons. In the vast majority of instances, it should be possible to make a diagnosis without resorting to such a dramatic procedure. In a patient who otherwise appears well and in whom none of the studies outlined above or in Figures 1 and 2 have provided any answers, expectant or observant management may be in order, assuming the patient does not have giant splenomegaly. In a study some 20 years ago, Herman et al. (34), reported that in only 9% of a series of 582 cases in which splenectomy was performed was the cause of splenomegaly unknown before operation. It is likely that the figures from a similar series today would show that in even fewer cases the cause of splenomegaly is not known before splenectomy. However, the value of a histologic examination of the spleen is that it not only provides a clear-cut diagnosis, but also may add further information of therapeutic and prognostic value.

Unlike with other lymphohemopoietic organs, splenic aspirations or biopsy are not performed frequently in the United States, largely because of the fear of hemorrhage. There are data to suggest that splenic aspiration and biopsy may be safe techniques when the spleen is the only organ capable of yielding a diagnosis (35-38). These studies showed only 4 or 5 minor complications resulting from splenic aspiration or biopsy in over 1600 procedures in adults. Lampert carefully reviewed the splenic pathology seen in many varieties of disorders associated with splenomegaly (39). Unfortunately the role of diagnostic splenic biopsy or puncture in children has never been well-examined in terms of yield or safety.

While splenectomy is still indicated as treatment for many cases, it has only a small role as a diagnostic procedure in children. Careful attention to all of the diagnostic techniques available to the clinician should enable one to establish a cause for splenomegaly in most cases. Radiologic imaging techniques will provide considerable information as to the nature of the pathologic processes in the spleen, whereas previously splenectomy may have been required for this purpose.

SUMMARY

The overall approach to the child with enlargement of the spleen is hampered by many factors. The spleen, especially in the younger child, is a very reactive organ. Relatively simple infections can cause enlargement of the spleen detectable on physical examination. Fortunately, resolution of splenomegaly under these circumstances can be just as rapid. We are additionally hampered by having relatively little information regarding truly normal splenic size for age, and the correlation of this size with findings on physical examination. In children, unlike adults, the presence of an isolated splenic malignancy such as Hodgkin's disease or non-Hodgkin's lymphoma is extremely rare. This factor alone permits a noninvasive approach to have a potentially higher diagnostic yield. It is useful to determine whether hypersplenism is present and whether giant splenomegaly exists, since each of these suggest a relatively restricted number of diagnostic possibilities.

When all else fails, a tincture of time will often provide a diagnosis if not a cure.

REFERENCES

1. Robb-Smith AHT: Pathologic lesions in surgically removed spleens. *Br J Hosp Med* 1970;3:19-22.
2. McIntyre OR, Ebaugh FG: Palpable spleens in college freshmen. *Ann Intern Med* 1976;66:301-306.
3. Battisto JR, Cantor LC, Borek F, et al: Immunoglobulin synthesis in hereditary spleenless mice. *Nature (Lond)* 1969;222:1196-1198.
4. Constantopoulos A, Naggar VA, Wish JB, et al: Defective phagocytosis due to tuftsin deficiency in splenectomized subjects. *Am J Dis Child* 1973; 125:663.
5. Spier Z, Zakuth V, Diamant S, et al: Decreased tuftsin concentrations in patients who have undergone splenectomy. *Br Med J* 1977;2:1574.
6. Carlisle HN, Saslaw S: Properdin levels in splenectomized persons. *Proc Soc Exp Biol Med* 1959;102:150.
7. Kabins SA, Lerner C: Fulminant pneumococcemia and sickle cell anemia. *JAMA* 1970;211:467.
8. Wilson WA, Hughes GR, Lachman PG: Deficiency of factor b of the complement system in sickle cell anemia. *Br Med J* 1976;1:367.
9. Winkelstein JA, Lambert GH: Pneumococcal serum opsonizing activity in splenectomized children. *J Pediatr* 1975;87:430.
10. Rosse WF: Quantitative immunology of immune hemolytic anemia. II. The relationship of cell-bound antibody to hemolysis and the effect of treatment. *J Clin Invest* 1971;50:734.
11. Wagner HN, Razzak MA, Gaertner RA, et al: Removal of erythrocytes from the circulation. *Arch Intern Med* 1962;110:90.
12. Crosby WH: Normal functions of the spleen relative to red blood cells; a review. *Blood* 1959;14:399-408.
13. Chen LT, Weiss L: Electron microscopy of the red pulp of human spleen. *Am J Anat* 1972;134:425.
14. LoBuglio AF, Cotrine RS, Jandl JH: Red cells coated with immunoglobulin G; sphering by mononuclear cells in man. *Science (Wash DC)* 1967;158: 1582-1585.
15. Ward HP, Block MH: The natural history of agnogenic myeloid metaplasia and a critical evaluation of its relationship wht the myeloproliferative syndrome. *Medicine (Baltimore)* 1971;50:357.
16. Dell JM, Klinefelter HF: Imaging studies of the spleen. *Am J Med* 1946; 211:437.
17. Blackburn CRD: On the clinical definition of enlargement of the spleen. *Aust Ann* 1953;2:78.

18. Budinger TF: Physical attributes of single photon tomography. *J Nucl Med* 1980;21:579-592.
19. Brooks RA: A quantitative theory of the Hounsfield unit and its applications to dual energy scanning. *J Comput Assist Tomogr* 1977;1:487.
20. Bowring CS: *Radionuclide Tracer Techniques in Hematology*. London, Butterworths, 1981.
21. Heymsfield SB, Fulenwider T, Nordlinger B, et al: Accurate measurement of liver, spleen and kidney size by CAT. *Ann Intern Med* 1979;90:185.
22. Kuhn JP, Berger PE: Computed tomography and the evaluation of abdominal trauma in children. *Radiol Clin N Am* 1981;19:503-513.
23. Crooks LE, Miller CM, Davis PL, et al: Visualization of cerebral and vascular anomalies by NMR imaging. *Radiology* 1982;144:843-852.
24. Shirkhode A, McCartney WH, Staab EV, Mittelstaedt CA: Imaging of the spleen; a proposed algorithm. *Am J Radiol* 1980;135:195.
25. Ebaugh FG, McIntyre DR: Palpable spleens; a 10 year followup. *Ann Intern Med* 1979;90:130.
26. Eichner E: Splenic functions; normal, too much, and too little. *Am J Med* 1979;66:311.
27. Cassiere SG, Gregg R, Eichner EF: Hairy cell leukemia. *Postgrad Med* 1977; 61:231.
28. Ziegler JL, Steuviver PC: Tropical splenomegaly syndrome. *Br Med J* 1972; 3:79.
29. Dacie JV, Galton DAG, Gordon-Smith ED, et al: Tropical idiopathic splenomegaly; a follow-up of 10 patients described in 1969. *Br J Haematol* 1978; 36:27.
30. Burt RW, Kuhl DE: Giant splenomegaly in sarcoidosis demonstrated by radionuclide scantiphotography. *JAMA* 1981;215:2110.
31. Vincent PC, Levi JA, Macqueen A: The mechanism of neutropenia in Felty's syndrome. *Br J Haematol* 1974;17:482.
32. Abdou NI, Napombejara C, Balentine L, et al: Suppression of granulopoiesis in Felty's syndrome. *J Clin Invest* 1978;61:738.
33. Eichner ER, Witfield CL: Splenomegaly; an algorithmic approach to diagnosis. *J Am Med Assoc* 1981;246:2858.
34. Herman RE, DeHaven K, Hawk WA: Splenectomy for the diagnosis of splenomegaly. *Ann Surg* 1968;168:896-900.
35. Lampert IA: Splenectomy as a diagnostic tool. *Clin Haematol* 1982;12:535-563.
36. Moeschlein S: *Splenic Puncture*. London, W. Heineman, 1957.
37. Sodestrom N: Cytologie der mitz in punktatin. In Lennert K, Harms D (eds): *Der Milz*. Berlin, Springer-Verlag, 1970.
38. Dameshek W, Gunz I: *Leukemia*, 2nd ed. New York, Grune and Stratton, 1964.
39. Lampert IA: Splenectomy as a diagnostic technique. *Clin Haematol* 1983; 12:535.

9
Splenomegaly
Infectious Etiologies

KAREN L. KOTLOFF and MARGARET B. RENNELS
University of Maryland School of Medicine, Baltimore, Maryland

Considered worldwide, infection is the most common cause of splenomegaly. The particular infections encountered vary from one region to another. Although slight enlargement of the spleen occurs commonly as an immunologic response to many types of antigenemia, in some infections, such as kala-azar and malaria, the splenomegaly may be quite massive. In this chapter we will discuss the mechanisms responsible for enlargement of the spleen during infection, and we will indicate those infections that are commonly accompanied by splenomegaly. Finally, we will suggest an approach to the diagnosis of a patient who has splenomegaly thought to be of infectious etiology.

NORMAL ANATOMY AND PHYSIOLOGY

Normal host defense functions of the spleen include clearance of microorganisms and particulate antigens from the bloodstream and participation in the immune response. The bulk of the spleen is composed of red pulp, which contains numerous vascular sinusoids separated by the splenic cords. These sponge-like splenic cords consist of a maze of macrophages connected by their dendritic processes. Foreign matter, including bacteria, is removed by phagocytosis as blood passes through this "macrophage filter."

The white pulp of the spleen consists of small white nodules, distributed throughout the spleen, that are composed of lymphoid tissue with numerous germinal centers intimately associated with the arterial circulation. The white pulp of the spleen is a major repository of lymphocytes, enabling the spleen to function immunologically as the lymphoid tissue of the blood. The reticular network of the white pulp traps antigen, allowing it to come in contact with lymphocytes. Both T and B cells are present in the periarterial sheaths of lymphoid tissue. Thus, the spleen may contribute to both humoral immunity and cell-mediated immunity.

PATHOPHYSIOLOGY

Splenic enlargement during infection may be due either to hyperplasia of normal structures or due to infiltration by microorganisms, which causes an associated inflammatory reaction. Histopathologic examination of spleens enlarged in response to infection shows reactive hyperplasia. This condition is also called acute inflammatory splenomegaly, septic splenitis, and acute splenic tumor. In the red pulp, there is an increase of both plasma cells and macrophages. The macrophages contain ingested debris from dead leukocytes and sometimes contain microorganisms. The lymphoid follicles in the white pulp are hyperplastic and show formation of germinal centers. Splenic hyperplasia may be a reaction to the presence of pathogenic organisms or it may simply be a reaction to the products of inflammation. These general features are modified slightly in various infections, but the changes are usually not sufficient to allow an etiologic diagnosis based solely on morphology.

Infiltrative processes in the spleen may be either diffuse or focal. Focal lesions secondary to infection consist of granulomas, areas of necrosis, and abscesses.

INFECTIONS THAT CAUSE SPLENOMEGALY

The list of infections commonly associated with splenomegaly is quite extensive (Table 1). However, presence of an enlarged spleen may be a useful clue to the etiology of the patient's illness. Following is a brief description of infectious diseases in which splenomegaly may be encountered.

Congenital (TORCH) Infections

The congenital, or TORCH infections (toxoplasmosis, rubella, *cytomegalovirus* (CMV), Herpes simplex, and syphilis) may all present with hepatosplenomegaly, thrombocytopenic purpura, *central nervous system* (CNS) disease, anemia, and jaundice (Table 2). It is frequently difficult or impossible to differentiate between the various etiologies solely on clinical grounds. Potentially helpful differential points are that Herpes simplex commonly presents with skin lesions,

Table 1 Infections That Cause Splenomegaly

1. Congenital (TORCH) infections
    a. Toxoplasmosis
    b. Rubella
    c. Cytomegalovirus
    d. Herpes simplex virus
    e. Syphilis
2. Infectious mononucleosis syndromes
3. Acute viral hepatitis
4. Human immunodeficiency virus (HIV) infection
5. The systemic mycoses
6. Spirochettsial infections
    a. Syphilis
    b. Borelia
7. Rickettsial infections
    a. Scrub typhus
    b. Q fever
    c. Rocky Mountain Spotted Fever
8. Ornithosis
9. Tuberculosis
10. Infective endocarditis
11. Splenic abscesses
12. The zoonoses
    a. Tularemia
    b. Brucellosis
13. Cat-scratch disease
14. Tapeworm infestations
    a. Cysticercosis
    b. Echinococcus
15. Infections in travelers and immigrants
    a. Typhoid fever
    b. Malaria
    c. Schistosomiasis
    d. Leishmaniasis

Table 2 Infectious Causes of Splenomegaly

Microbial etiology	Historic clues	Major clinical findings	Laboratory diagnosis
Congenital infections			
Toxoplasmosis	Contact with cats, eating meat	Chorioretinitis, HSM[a], intracranial calcifications	Serology, histology
Rubella	Susceptible mother	Intrauterine growth retardation, cataracts, congenital heart defects, deafness, mental retardation, HSM	Serology, culture
Cytomegalovirus (CMV)	Usually absent	HSM, thrombocytopenia purpura, chorioretinitis, periventricular calcifications	Serology, histology, culture
Herpes simplex virus (HSV)	Genital HSV infection in mother	Skin vesicles, hepatitis, encephalitis, pneumonia	Culture, immunofluorescence
Syphilis	Untreated maternal syphilis	Osteochondritis, periostitis, snuffles, HSM, rash, mucous patches, nephrosis	Serology

SPLENOMEGALY: INFECTIOUS ETIOLOGIES

Infectious mononucleosis			
Epstein-Barr virus (EBV)	First two decades	Fever, pharyngitis, adenitis, HSM	Serology
Cytomegalovirus (CMV)	First two decades	Fever, pharyngitis, adenitis, HSM	Serology, culture
Toxoplasmosis	Contact with cats, eating raw meat	Fever, pharyngitis, adenitis, HSM	Serology
Acute viral hepatitis			
Hepatitis A	Contaminated food and water, day care, institutional	Constitutional symptoms, abdominal discomfort, jaundice	Serology
Hepatitis B	Transfusion, sexual contact, health care worker, intravenous durg abuser	Same as for hepatitis A, but more insidious onset	Serology
Human Immunodeficiency	Member of an AIDS risk group	Lymphadenopathy, fever, wasting, diarrhea, opportunistic infections, Kaposi's sarcoma	Serology

whereas petechia and purpura are rare in toxoplasmosis, and bone lesions do not occur in herpetic infection.

Congenital toxoplasmosis may develop in infants of women who acquire infection with *Toxoplasma gondii* during pregnancy by eating undercooked meat or handling cat feces. Infected neonates may be totally asymptomatic or may suffer from severe generalized infection with CNS damage. The most constant physical finding in symptomatic infants with toxoplasmosis is chorioretinitis, which develops within a few weeks of birth. Unfortunately, the chorioretinitis usually involves the macula in addition to the periphery of the retina, and is typically bilateral. Other common features include hepatomegaly, splenomegaly, anemia, jaundice, convulsions, and diffuse intracranial calcifications. The majority of infants with CNS manifestations have abnormal cerebrospinal fluid findings, including xanthochromia, pleocytosis, and elevated protein; occasionally the microorganisms can be seen on a Wright's stain cytologic preparation of the spinal fluid. The diagnosis of toxoplasmosis can be made histologically by demonstration of the microorganisms in infected tissue, or by serological studies.

Congenital rubella syndrome is a risk for infants whose mothers have become infected with rubella in the first trimester of pregnancy. Classical characteristics of the congenital rubella syndrome include: intrauterine growth retardation, cataracts, congenital heart disease, deafness, microcephaly, and mental retardation. The infection may affect any organ, however. A variety of transient clinical manifestations may be present in the first weeks of life, including hepatitis, splenomegaly, bone lesions, hemolytic anemia, thrombocytopenic purpura, and pleocytosis of the cerebrospinal fluid. The diagnosis of rubella can be established either serologically or by isolation of the virus.

Symptomatic congenital invection occurs in infants of women who experience a primary reactivated CMV infection during pregnancy. Most infections are asymptomatic or mild, but fulminant, even fatal, infections occasionally occur. Hepatosplenomegaly is the most common manifestation of full-blown congenital CMV infection; other characteristic findings are jaundice and thrombocytopenic purpura. Additional findings include chorioretinitis, anemia, elevation in the white blood cell count and protein level of the cerebrospinal fluid, and periventricular calcifications. In infants who survive CMV infection, the thrombocytopenia and jaundice typically subside within a few weeks. The hepatosplenomegaly may actually increase over the first few months of life and persist for many months (1). Postmortem examination has revealed that the splenomegaly is due to extramedulary hematopoiesis. As in the other congenital infections, the diagnosis of CMV infection is usually confirmed by serology. Tissues removed by biopsy or autopsy may show characteristic inclusion bodies. This best way to make the diagnosis is by recovery of virus from the blood, urine, or other body fluids during the first week of life.

Neonatal infection with herpes simplex virus usually occurs at the time of delivery, although congenital and postnatal infection may occur. The clinical manifestations are similar regardless of when the infection was acquired. Neonatal infection is most commonly with type 2 herpesvirus, which is the usual case of genital herpes. Infection may be confined to a single organ (skin, mucous membranes, or CNS), or the infection may disseminate throughout the body. A child with disseminated disease typically appears well for the first few days or weeks of life and then develops fever or hypothermia, lethargy, progressively increasing icterus, and hepatosplenomegaly. Respiratory distress, bleeding, and circulatory collapse may ensue. Serologic studies have no role in the diagnosis of neonatal herpes infection. The diagnosis is made by immunoflorescent stain of scrapings of skin lesions, by culture, or both.

Transplacental *Treponema pallidum* infection can occur throughout pregnancy and during any stage of syphilis in the mother to cause congenital syphilis in the infant. The clinical findings in congenital syphilis are variable, and include bone changes (osteochondritis and periostitis), hepatosplenomegaly, generalized adenitis, rhinitis, rash (maculopapular or bullous), mucous patches, nephritis or nephrosis, and abnormal findings in the cerebrospinal fluid. Pathologic examination of the spleen in fatal cases of congenital syphilis shows splenic enlargement, with the presence of numerous spirochetes. Hyperplastic changes in the red pulp of the spleen are seen. These consist of an increased number of granulocytes, plasma cells, and phagocytic histiocytes.

Infectious Mononucleosis Syndromes

Beyond the neonatal period, several agents responsible for TORCH infections can produce a clinical picture resembling infectious mononucleosis, an acute viral infection most commonly caused by the Epstein-Barr virus (EBV).

In infectious mononucleosis, fever, pharyngitis, lymphadenopathy, splenic enlargement, and the presence of abnormal lymphocytes in the peripheral blood are the characteristic clinical features. The spleen is enlarged in about 50% of cases (2,3). Abnormalities of liver function tests are common, but clinical jaundice is rare. Complications are unusual, but may include airway obstruction secondary to hyperplasia of the lymphoid tissue in Waldeyer's ring, splenic rupture, myocarditis, pericarditis, meningoencephalitis, and mild degrees of neutropenia and thrombocytopenia. Asymptomatic infection frequently occurs. The clinical manifestations of infectious mononucleosis are usually less severe in young children than in older children or young adults. Absolute lymphocytosis (greater than 50%) with at least 10% atypical lymphocytes, is a hallmark of this disease. EBV accounts for over 90% of cases of the mononucleosis syndrome (4).

A syndrome resembling infectious mononucleosis may be produced by cytomegalovirus, toxoplasmosis, and certain other viral infections such as rubella and adenovirus. Differentiation depends on results of serologic studies; only EBV elicits the heterophile antibody. Young children may not show an elevated titer of heterophile antibody and further serologic confirmation may be necessary. CMV, which is responsible for most cases of mononucleosis seen among seronegative adults (4), can be isolated from body fluids (urine, saliva, cervical secretions, semen, or breast milk) or from tissue.

Acute Viral Hepatitis

Acute viral hepatitis is accompanied by mild (fingertip) splenomegaly in 5-25% of patients. Initial signs and symptoms are malaise, weakness, anorexia, vomiting, and vague, dull, right-upper-quadrant pain. Unless icterus ensues, this infection is commonly mistaken for flu; however, in hepatitis, increased levels of transaminase enzymes are invariably seen. Definitive diagnosis of hepatitis A, hepatitis B, and delta hepatitis can be made by serologic studies.

Human Immunodeficiency Virus (HIV) Infection

HIV is a retrovirus that infects the thymus-derived (T) lymphocytes. HIV preferentially infects the subset of T lymphocytes known as helper T lymphocytes, which augment the immune response. The infection is spread by contact with infected body fluids. Groups at high risk for acquiring infection with human immunodeficiency virus are homosexual of bisexual men, intravenous drug abusers, hemophiliacs, heterosexual partners or persons with the *acquired immunodeficiency syndrome* (AIDS) or at risk for AIDS, recipients of transfusions of blood or blood components, and infants born to parents at risk for developing AIDS (5). The clinical syndrome that emerges results from the underlying defect in cellular immunity. An acute, transient mononucleosis-like illness with or without aseptic meningits may occur in association with seroconversion for HIV antibody (6,7).

Symptomatic patients are classified by the Centers for Disease Control according to the following symptom complexes: First, persistent generalized lymphadenopathy, and second, other disease caused by HIV infection, which includes (1) constitutional disease, (2) neurologic disease, (3) secondary infectious disease, (4) secondary cancers, and (5) other conditions related to HIV infection or cellular immunodeficiency (8). The incidence of hepatosplenomegaly in adults with infections due to human immunodeficiency virus is unknown; however, enlargement of the liver and spleen is present in the vast majority of children presenting with AIDS or AIDS-related conditions (9-11). The etiology of enlargement of the liver, spleen, or both is generally related to the presence of various opportunistic infections to which these patients are susceptible (12). There is presently no diagnostic test specific for AIDS. Techniques for serologic diagnosis and viral culture are commercially available; however, diagnosis depends on the case definition of the Centers for Disease Control for national reporting (13-15).

The Systemic Mycoses

Systemic candidiasis has been reported with increasing frequency in recent years, occurring mostly in the immunocompromised host. Factors predisposing to candidiasis include immunosuppressive therapy, broad-spectrum antibiotics, intravascular catheters, prosthetic implantations, and intravenous hyperalimentation. When candida disseminates, many organs are usually involved, with the kidney, brain, myocardium, and eye being the most commonly affected. Infection of the liver and spleen can occur, particularly in cancer patients receiving extensive immunosuppressive therapy (16,17) (Table 3). On histopathologic examination, diffuse microabscesses with a combined supurative and granulomatous reaction and small microabscesses are seen.

The diagnosis of disseminated candidiasis may be difficult to make premortem; blood cultures are frequently negative and a reliable serologic test is not available. Computerized tomography and ultrasonography may allow visualization of the abscesses. Tissue should be obtained fro culture and histopathologic examination whenever possible.

Histoplasma capsulatum is endemic to the United States and to a lesser extent is endemic throughout the temperature and tropical regions of the world. In areas where the soil is heavily contaminated with excrement of birds and bats, virtually the entire population can become infected. Once inhaled, the spores germinate. The yeast-forms infect macrophages, which migrate to the lymphatics and reticuloendothelial systems, where caseating granulomas are formed. Most infections are asymptomatic. When symptoms occur, fever and headache are the most common complaints, followed by chills, cough, and chest pain. Although the liver and spleen are occasionally palpable in adults with heavy infection, hepatosplenomegaly is more common and more marked in infected infants and young children. Enlargement of the liver and spleen is most striking in disseminated histoplasmosis; this is a rare condition usually seen in individuals with immune deficits, including small infants (18).

The diagnosis of acute pulmonary histoplasmosis is made when the characteristic radiographic appearance of the chest is seen, consisting of small scattered pulmonary infiltrates associated with hilar adenopathy, these findings are present in a patient from an endemic area, who has a high or rising complement-fixation titer. Demonstration of either histologically compatible intracellular organisms or a positive culture of blood or tissue confirms the diagnosis of disseminated disease. However, these findings are rarely present in acute pulmonary histoplasmosis.

Table 3 Infectious Causes of Splenomegaly. Part II.

Microbial etiology	Historical clues	Major clinical findings	Laboratory diagnosis
Systemic mycosis			
Candidiasis	Immunosuppressed, iatrogenic risk factors	Endophthalmitis, abscesses in viscera	Histology
Histoplasma capsulatum	Endemic area	Fever, headache, pneumonia, HSM	Serology
Histoplasma duboisii	Endemic area	Lesions of skin, subcutaneous tissue, bone	Histology
Blastomyces dermatitidis	Endemic area	Pneumonia, skin lesions	Histology, culture
Coccidiodomycosis immitis	Endemic area	Pneumonia, lesions of skin, bones, testes, thyroid, meninges, subcutaneous tissue	Histology, culture
Sprichetes			
Syphilis			
Secondary	Sexually active	Rash, arthralgias, adenopathy, HSM, meningitis	Serology

Late	Not applicable	Visceral gummas	
Borrelia	Tick or louse exposure	Conjunctivitis, rash, HSM, tender abdomen, relapsing fever	Blood smear
Rickettsia			
Scrub typhus	Endemic area, chigger bite	Skin ulcer, regional adenopathy, systemic illness 1–3 weeks later	Serology
Q fever	Veterinarians, meat packers, dairy workers, farmers	Acute febrile illness, pneumonia	Serology
Rocky Mountain spotted fever	Endemic area, tick bite	Fever, headache, myalgia, petechial rash	Serology, immunoflorescence
Ornithosis	Exposure to birds	Systemic illness, atypical pneumonia	Serology
Tuberculosis	Exposure to infected person	Fever, cough, constitutional symptoms	Skin test, culture

Histoplasma duboisii infections are seen almost exclusively in central Africa. Occasional cases are imported into the United States. The clinical illness may consist of only a single lesion, most commonly of the skin, bone, or subcutaneous tissues. On the other hand there may be many lesions of the bone and skin accompanied by fever, anorexia, weight loss, lymphadenopathy, hepatosplenomegaly, and often death (19). Histologically, both suppurative and granulomatous lesions are seen. Diagnosis of histoplasma infection is made by culture; the organism must be differentiated from *Histoplasma capsulatum* by identifying the characteristic yeast-forms in tissue.

Blastomyces dermatitidis is endemic to North America, with cases being reported from Africa and South America as well. Infection is initiated by inhalation of spores, which germinate in the lungs. In the majority of cases, an asymptomatic or unrecognized pulmonary infection ensues. However, both acute and, more commonly, subacute infections can occur that, without therapy, follow a progressive course with or without extrapulmonary manifestations. The skin is the most common extrapulmonary focus of infection with blastomyces; lesions can be varrucous or ulcerative. Bone, reticuloendoethelial system, genitourinary system, CNS, and subcutaneous tissues are also frequently involved in this suppurative and granulomatous (noncaseating) process. When splenic involvement is found, it is usually a postmortem finding in a patient with widely disseminated disease (20). Definitive diagnosis requires the growth of the organism from clinical specimens. A presumptive diagnosis can be made by visualization of the characteristic yeast organisms in pus, sputum, secretions, or histopathologic sections.

Coccidioidomycosis immitis is a systemic mycosis that begins as a respiratory infection. Seen commonly in the southwestern United States, most infections go unrecognized. Clinically apparent primary infections resemble influenza by the presence of fever, chills, cough, and pleural pain. Disseminated coccidioidomycosis is a progressive, frequently fatal, but uncommon granulomatous disease seen most commonly in nonwhites. The disease is characterized by pulmonary lesions and the presence of abscesses and granulomata throughout the body, especially in the skin, subcutaneous tissues, bone, meninges, testes, and thyroid. Other sites of involvement by coccidioidomycosis, seen less frequently, are spleen, liver, kidney, and conjunctiva (21). Diagnosis is made by demonstrating the fungus microscopically or by culture of body fluids or tissues. Conversion of skin test or serologic response are supportive evidence of recent infection.

Spirochettsial Infections

Splenomegaly may be seen in either secondary or late syphilis. In secondary syphilis, systemic symptoms include fever, malaise, and anorexia. The most common manifestations are skin lesions. Macular, maculopapular, papular, pustular, and papular-pustular lesions may be present and may become widely distributed. The papules may coalesce in the intertriginous areas to produce plaques called condyloma lata. Mucous patches, which are silvery-gray erosions of the mucous membranes, may also be seen. Other manifestations of secondary syphilis include arthralgias, generalized adenopathy, splenomegaly, hepatitis, glomerulonephritis, nephrotic syndrome, and meningitis. Histologically the enlarged spleen shows follicular hyperplasia and the presence of many plasma cells in the red pulp. During late syphilis, gummatous lesions may develop in any organ, including the spleen. A gumma is a granulomatous lesion that varies in size from microscopic to large tumor-like masses that cause local destruction of adjacent tissues.

Borrelia or relapsing fever, which occurs throughout the world, is caused by arthropod-borne spirochetes of the genus *Borrelia*. There are two forms: (1) tick-borne disease, which is caused by several species and is relatively mild, and (2) the louse-borne form, caused by *Borrelia recurrentis* which can be quite severe. Borrelia is clinically characterized by recurrent episodes of fever and spirochetemia. Illness begins with an acute onset of high fever with rigors, severe headaches, myalgias, arthralgias, lethargy, photophobia, and cough. The most consistent physical findings in the initial febrile phase are conjunctival suffusion, petechiae, and diffuse abdominal tenderness with hepatomegaly and splenomegaly. A truncal rash, which may be petechial, macular, or papular, commonly appears at the end of the primary febrile episode. Pneumonia, bronchitis, and otitis media may occur, and death may result from myocarditis, shock, or hepatic failure in the louse-borne form.

In fatal cases the spleen is found to be moderately enlarged; focal necrosis and scattered collection of inflammatory cells and organisms are seen on histopathologic examination. In milder cases the primary febrile episode usually ends abruptly in 3-6 days. Louse-borne relapsing fever is usually associated with only one relapse, whereas multiple relapses of illness occur in the tick-borne disease. The severity of symptoms decrease with each relapse. The diagnosis of relapsing fever is established by the demonstration of borreliae in a peripheral blood smear of a febrile patient.

Rickettsial Infections

Splenomegaly may be detected in infections caused by *Rickettsia tsutsugamushi* (scrub typhus), *Coxiella burnetii* (Q fever), and *Rickettsia ricketsii*. Scrub typhus is a rickettsial infection seen in eastern Asia and in the western Pacific region. The organism is transmitted to man by the bite of chiggers. At the site of the bite a papule forms, ulcerates, and develops an eschar. Regional lymphadenopathy occurs. Six to 18 days after the bite, systemic symptoms develop, including high fever, severe headache, myalgia, apathy, and cough. Approximately 5 days later a rash begins on the trunk and spreads to the extremities. The exanthum is initially macular but may become papular as it evolves. At the height of the illness, lymphadenopathy occurs and splenomegaly can be detected in 25–40% of patients (22). Confirmation of the diagnosis can be made serologically.

Hepatosplenomegaly is present in approximately 50% of patients with Q fever (23). Unlike most other rickettsial infections, Q fever is virtually worldwide in distribution and is not accompanied by a rash. Illness begins with a sudden onset of severe headache, spiking fevers, chills, and myalgias. Pneumonia develops in 5–20% of patients, and endocarditis may ensue. Diagnosis is primarily by serology.

Rocky Mountain spotted fever is the most common rickettsial infection in the United States. The disease is most prevalent in the southeastern states but cases occur virtually throughout the country. Illness begins in a similar manner as with the other rickettsial infections; there is a sudden onset of fever, chills, headache, and myalgias. Rash appears on the third to fifth day. The lesions begin as macules on the distal extremities and spread towards the trunk in a centripedal manner. If the infection is not treated the rash will become petechial, then purpuric, and diffuse edema will develop from capillary leakage. Some degree of splenomegaly is commonly encountered. The diagnosis of Rocky Mountain spotted fever can be established serologically or by fluorescent stain of a biopsy of a skin lesion.

Ornithosis

Ornithosis, also called psittacosis, is a disease of birds that can be transmitted to man. It is caused by *Chlamydia psittaci*, which has a worldwide distribution. The microorganism causes a systemic infection; however, the lung is the organ most prominently involved. Illness begins with fever, malaise, and a severe diffuse headache. The pneumonitis is manifested by persistent cough and tachypnea. Splenomegaly is inconsistently seen. In fatal cases examination of the spleen reveals only diffuse reticuloendothelial hyperactivity. The combination of atypical pneumonia and splenomegaly should prompt one to consider a diagnosis of ornithosis, particularly if there is history of exposure to birds. Diagnosis can be confirmed serologically.

Tuberculosis

A silent bacillemia probably routinely occurs during primary tuberculosis. During this spread in the bloodstream, the spleen may become seeded with tubercle bacilli. Primary tuberculosis of the spleen is a rare entity that presents as a fever of unknown origin associated with anemia and splenomegaly. Splenomegaly is commonly in miliary tuberculosis, however, occurring in up to 50% of cases (24). The splenic enlargement is due to both infiltration by tubercular granulomas and inflammatory hyperplasia. The degree of splenomegaly varies, but the enlargement may be quite massive, with the spleen weighing as much as 4000 g (24). In pulmonary tuberculosis the spleen may be enlarged simply as part of the generalized reaction to severe acute infection. Diagnosis is by a combination of clinical and laboratory findings, including chest radiography, skin testing, and culture of sputum and urine.

Infective Endocarditis

Infective endocarditis, an infection of the endocardium, most commonly affects the heart valves, although the mural endocardium and the site of most congenital cardiac defects may be involved as well. Predisposing factors include congenital cardiac defects, acquired valvular heart disease (in particular rheumatic heart disease), degenerative cardiac lesions, prosthetic intracardiac implantations, intravenous drug abuse, and the presence of indwelling intravascular catheters. This disease may manifest as an acute, subacute, or chronic presentation. Because multiple organs may be involved in the disease process, including the lungs, eyes, CNS, kidney, and joints, diagnosis may be elusive. The classic syndrome consists of fever, a heart murmur, splenomegaly, and petechia in a patient who has several blood cultures positive for the same organism (Table 4).

The clinical presentation depends to a large extent on the infecting organism. The most common etiologic agent of acute endocarditis involving previously normal heart valves is *Staphylococcus aureus*. In most cases of acute endocarditis, the duration of the disease is too brief for detectable splenomegaly to develop (25). *Streptococcus viridinas* and group D streptococcus are found more commonly in cases of subacute endocarditis. Endocarditis due to these streptococci usually involves previously abnormal valves, has an indolent presentation, and is more commonly associated with splenomegaly. Although *Staphylococcus aureus* is the principal agent causing endocarditis in the drug addict, *Pseudomonas aeruginosa, Serratia marcescens,* and Candida species are seen with increased frequency in certain geographic locations. *Staphylococcus epidermis* and gram-negative bacilli are the principal etiologic agents in endocarditis associated with prosthetic valves.

The spleen is commonly involved in endocarditis; splenic enlargement is present in 20–57% of cases (26,27), primarily as a result of chronic antigenic stimulation. Histopathologic examination reveals hyperplasia of lymphoid and reticuloendothelial tissues, and scattered focal necrosis (28). Splenic infarctions have been reported in 44% of the autopsy cases, but evidence of such infarctions is rarely detected clinically (29). Abscess formation and rupture of the spleen are uncommon.

Splenic Abscesses

Splenic abscesses are uncommon lesions. They are seen most frequently as a complication of bacteremia or, less commonly, as a direct extension from a con-

Table 4 Infectious Causes of Splenomegaly. Part III.

Microbial etiology	Historical clues	Major clinical findings	Laboratory diagnosis
Infectious endocarditis	Dental procedure, cardiac lesion, IV drug abuse	Fever, heart murmur, splenomegaly, petechia	Blood culture, cardiac sonogram
Splenic abscess	Endocarditis, IV drug abuse, splenic injury	Fever, tender spleen	Blood culture, sonogram or computed tomography
Zoonoses			
Tularmeia	Tick bite, hunter	Systemic illness, local lesion in eye, skin, pharynx, or lung, with regional adenopathy	Serology
Brucellosis	Veterinarians, farmers, abattoir workers	Acute febrile illness, orchitis, vertebral osteomyelitis	Serology
Cat-scratch disease	Cat scratch	Primary skin papule with regional lymphadenopathy	Histology

Tapeworms			
Cysticercosis	Ingestion of raw or undercooked pork	Depending on site of infection, calcified mass may be seen radiographically	Microscopy
Echinococcosis	Sheep and cattle raisers	Osseous cysts in the viscera	Radiography, histology
Travelers and immigrants			
Typhoid fever	Contaminated food and water	Fever, constitutional symptoms, rose spots, adenopathy, splenomegaly	Culture
Malaria	Endemic area	Fever, constitutional symptoms, splenomegaly	Blood smear
Schistosomiasis	Swimming in contaminated water	Diarrhea, abdominal pain, HMS (S. mansoni); Dysuria, urinary frequency, hematuria (S. japonicum)	Microscopy
Leishmaniasis	Endemic area	Constitutional symptoms, debility, HSM	Microscopy

aHSM = hepatosplenomegaly.

tiguous focus of infection. Factors predisposing to splenic abscesses include bacterial endocarditis, intravenous drug abuse, splenic injury (both traumatic and surgical), and splenic infarction such as that seen in sickle-cell anemia. Clinical manifestations characteristic of splenic infection include fever and left-upper-quadrant pain. Sometimes the left-upper-quadrant pain is associated with left shoulder discomfort resulting from diaphragmatic irritation. A tender, enlarged spleen can be palpated in most instances. Auscultation of the abdomen may reveal a splenic rub. Localizing clinical signs may be totally absent in the patients with multiple small splenic abscesses (30). Solitary abscesses occur in one-third of patients, but in most cases multiple small abscesses are seen, usually as a complication of uncontrolled sepsis (30). In the early 1900s, typhoid fever was the most common cause of splenic abscess, followed in frequency by malaria. More recently, anaerobes, gram-negative fecal flora, and *Staphylococcus aureus* were reported as the principal etiologic agents. Blood cultures are positive in 70% of patients with multiple splenic abscesses, but cultures are positive in only 14% of those with solitary abscesses (30). Ultrasonography and computed tomography are the preferred diagnostic techniques.

The Zoonoses

Tularemia is an acute febrile illness caused by the organism *Francisclla tularensis*. The organism is ubiquitous in the Northern hemisphere during the summer months. The usual sources of infection are contact with infected animals or their carcasses (most commonly rabbits), bites by ticks or deer flies, and less often by inhalation of aerosolized organisms.

The disease has been classified according to the portal of entry into four types: (1) the ulceroglandular type (53% of cases) consists of a primary peripheral ulcer, often of the hand, with regional adenopathy, (2) the typhoidal type (30% of cases) is an acute illness usually following inhalation of the agent, consisting of a fulminant systemic infection frequently accompanied by pneumonia, (3) the glandular type (13% of cases) is a vague illness associated with lymphadenopathy, and (4) the oculoglandular type (4% of cases) is an acute ocular infection associated with conjunctival irritation, photophobia, dimness of vision, increased lacrimation, and local adenopathy (31).

Regardless of the portal of entry, the mode of onset and general features are the same: there is abrupt onset of fever, chills, headache, myalgias, vomiting, and photophobia. Lymphadenopathy and hepatosplenomegaly are common. A variety of skin rashes may appear during the second or third week of illness. Diagnosis can be made by serology. Culture of infected material should be performed only in specialized laboratories because of the risk of infection to personnel.

Brucellosis is a systemic bacterial disease with acute or insidious onset characterized by fever, malaise, chills, profuse sweating, fatigue, weight loss, and arthralgias. The disease occurs worldwide, predominantly in those working with infected animals or their tissues, especially in farmers, veterinarians, and abattoir workers (those engaged in the slaughter of animals and the handling of meat products. The microorganism, which gains access to the body through abraded skin or conjunctiva, or by ingestion or airborne spread, resides intracellularly within cells of the reticuloendothelial system. Lymphadenopathy is common. Splenomegaly is present in 10-15% of cases (32). Localized infection can occur in almost any organ, being found most commonly in bone, brain, heart, lungs, spleen, testes, liver, gallbladder, and prostate. The spleen is a frequent site of chronic localized brucellosis, most often due to *Brucella suis*, which can be detected radiographically by the presence of multiple calcifications. Hypersplenism, which can be severe, has resulted in pancytopenia (33). Diagnosis is made serologically or by culture of normally sterile body fluids or tissue.

Cat-Scratch Disease

Splenomegaly was found in 18% of a large series of patients with cat-scratch disease (34). This is usually a benign infection characterized by regional lymphadenopathy after the scratch of a cat, usually a kitten. Three to 10 days after the scratch, a primary skin papule forms followed by the development of adenopathy. About a quarter of the patients will experience mild systemic symptoms, including malaise, fatigue, headache, and low-grade fever. A clinical diagnosis is usually adequate. When more severe symptoms are present and a definitive diagnosis is sought, the diagnosis can be confirmed by demonstration of the organism in a node biopsy using Warthin-Starry silver impregnation stain (35). The cat-scratch antigen skin test is positive in 90% of patients; however, the test material, which is prepared from the purulent material aspirated from an involved lymph node, is not standardized or generally available.

Tapeworm Infestations

Cysticercosis is an infection with the pork tapeworm, *Taenia solium*, which is acquired by ingestion of contaminated human feces. The infestation occurs most commonly in Mexico and in certain parts of Africa and South America. The cysticercosis can develop in virtually any tissue of the body, including the spleen; the most common location of the infection is in the brain. The clinical manifestations of cysticercosis are a reflection of the organ involved. Diagnosis is sometimes suggested by the presence of a calcified mass on radiographs. Serologic tests for cysticercus antibodies are of value in confirming the diagnosis; however, there is frequently no detectable antibody response in cases of neurocysticercosis.

Man may become infected with the dog tapeworm, *Echinococcus granulosus*, by contact with contaminated dog feces. Sheep and cattle become the intermediate hosts when they ingest the infested feces. Therefore, echinococcosis is seen in most sheep- and cattle-raising areas of the world. When man ingests the eggs, oncospheres penetrate the mesenteric vessels and are carried to various organs, where they develop into hydatid cysts. The liver and lungs are most commonly infected, but hydatids may also be found in the spleen, kidney, brain, or bone. Radiographs may reveal a tumor mass outlined by a rim of calcification. Eosinophilia is common and diagnosis may be strengthened by the demonstration of antibodies to *Echinococcus granulosus*.

Infections in Travelers and Immigrants

Endemic malaria no longer occurs in many temperate-zone countries, but it is still a major cause of morbidity in many parts of the tropics and subtropics. Falciparun and vivax malaria are found in many endemic areas; ovale malaria is seen mainly in west Africa, where *Plasmodium vivax* is almost absent. Falciparum malaria, the most serious form, has a variable clinical presentation that may include fever, chills, sweats, and headache, and may progress to irreversible shock and coma. An increase in the size of the spleen accompanies most malaria infections secondary to immune-mediated lymphoid and reticuloendothelial hyperplasia (36). The spleen usually remains enlarged during chronic and repeated infections, but if the infection is eradicated the spleen size rapidly returns to normal. Laboratory confirmation is made by demonstration of malaria parasites in blood smears.

Typhoid fever is a systemic disease caused by the bacteria *Salmonella typhi*. Public health measures and modern sanitation have virtually eliminated the disease from the United States. The disease is endemic worldwide; however, most cases diagnosed in this country now represent importations or laboratory accidents. Transmission is by ingestion of food or water contaminated by the feces or urine of an infected person. Ingested microorganisms pass through the intestinal mucosa to the lamina propria where they are phagositized by mononuclear cells and transported to the lymphoid system. Once the microorganisms gain entry to the bloodstream they are removed by reticuloendothelial cells in the liver, spleen, and bone marrow, where hyperplasia occurs.

The ensuing illness is characterized by the insidious onset of sustained fever, headache, malaise, and anorexia. Constipation is present more often than diarrhea. Rose spots, lymphadenopathy, and splenomegaly can be found on physical examination. Localization of salmonella in bone, meninges, heart, lungs, kidneys, spleen, and other organs or tissues can lead to focal abscesses, which are characterized by a polymorphonuclear response. The presence of preexisting disease resulting in necrotic, scarred, or hyperplastic tissue favors localization of blood-borne organisms in these sites. *Salmonella typhi* can be isolated from the blood early in the disease, and it can be cultured from urine and feces after the first week. Although it is of limited sensitivity and specificity, serology may aid in diagnosis.

Any parasite that infects the mononuclear cells of the reticuloendothelial system can result in splenomegaly. *Leishmania donovani*, a tissue flagellate, is an intracellular parasite transmitted primarily by the bite of the sandfly. There are three main epidemiologic patterns of visceral leishmaniasis (kala-azar): the classical, the infantile, and the Sudanese types. Classic kala-azar of India affects chiefly adults. Mediterranean or infantile kala-azar is sporadic in children throughout the Mediterranean countries, China, Middle Asia, and Central and South America. Sudanese kala-azar only affects adults.

After inoculation, the parasite is phagocytized by mononuclear cells and transported to the reticuloendothelial cells of the spleen, liver, lymph nodes, bone marrow, intestinal mucosa, and other organs, where marked hyperplasia occurs. The clinical illness that ensues is characterized by fever, chills, sweating, diarrhea, and progressive debility. The infected liver and spleen gradually enlarge and can reach massive proportions. A marked leukopenia develops, associated with a relative monocytosis and lymphocytosis, anemia, and thrombocytopenia. Visualization of the parasite in blood or tissues by smear, culture, or inoculation of animals establishes the diagnosis.

Schistosomiasis is a blood fluke (trematode) infection found widely in Africa, South America, the Middle East, Asia, and in the Caribbean area. *Schistosoma mansoni, S. haematobium*, and *S. japonicum* are the major species causing human disease. Although man is the principal reservoir of infection, persistence of the parasite depends on the presence of an appropriate freshwater snail as the intermediate host. Infection is acquired from water containing free-swimming larval forms that have developed in snails. The parasites penetrate the skin, enter the bloodstream, and are carried to blood vessels of the lungs. They then migrate to the liver, where they develop to maturity, and then migrate to veins of the abdominal cavity. Symptoms result from adult male and female worms living in mesenteric or vesical veins of the host for many years. The female worms produce eggs that incite minute granulomata and scar formation in organs where they lodge. Diarrhea, abdominal pain, and hepatosplenomegaly are seen most commonly in infestations with *Schistosoma mansoni* and *S. japonicum*, while dysuria, urinary frequency, and hematuria most often accompany infections with *S. haematobium*. Definitive diagnosis depends on the demonstration of eggs in the stool, in urine, or in the biopsy specimens. Serology can be a helpful adjunct in diagnosis.

DIAGNOSTIC APPROACH TO THE PATIENT WITH SPLENOMEGALY

In most instances, a determination of the infectious etiology of splenomegaly can be obtained by history and physical alone. Several facts in the patient's medical history can offer clues to the diagnosis. Appreciation of the importance of the age of the patient is critical. TORCH infections (toxoplasmosis, rubella, CMV, herpes simplex, and syphilis) are the primary diagnostic considerations when splenomegaly is detected in the neonate. Most cases of infectious mononucleosis occur in the first two decades of life, whereas infections due to HIV predominate in the third decade. The systemic mycoses are more likely to disseminate at the extremes of age, in the very young and the very old. Knowledge of associated conditions is important. An immunodeficiency syndrome could predispose the patient to a disseminated viral or fungal infection, a damaged or prosthetic heart valve could lead to endocarditis, and recent abdominal surgery could be the nidus of infection for a splenic abscess. In otherwise healthy individuals, splenomegaly is usually a benign condition (37).

Facts in the patient's history regarding social behaviors, for example, homosexual or bisexual practices or intravenous drug abuse, suggest the possibility of HIV infection, infectious endocarditis, or splenic abscess. Occupational and recreational hazards are also important risk factors. Abattoir work increases the likelihood of brucellosis, bird exposure suggests the possibility of ornithoses, rabbit hunting causes exposure to tularemia, and contact with cats raises the risk of cat-scratch disease and toxoplasmosis. A history of a tick bite is often obtained from patients with Rocky Mountain spotted fever, scrub typhus, and tularemia. A history of travel to areas endemic for the agents responsible for tropical splenomegaly (such as malaria, schistosomiasis, and leishmaniasis), rickettsial infections, and tapework infectations can be the key to the diagnosis. Even patterns of travel within the United States can be helpful in diagnosing conditions such as the systemic mycoses and tularemia.

Repeated physical examination is important when the etiology of splenomegaly is elusive. Schistosomiasis, malaria, and in certain circumstances histoplasmosis produces the most massively enlarged spleens. Tenderness of the spleen is frequently seen when a splenic abscess is present. Careful examination of the patient for associated clinical signs should be performed. Cutaneous lesions can be seen in endocarditis, TORCH infections, secondary syphilis, blastomycosis, and tularemia, as well as in rickettsial infections and infections due to *Histoplasm duboisii* and borrelia. The conjunctiva can be involved in tularemia, cat-scratch disease, syphilis, the systemic mycoses (especially histoplasmosis) and tuberculosis. Petechial hemorrhages associated with bacterial endocarditis are often found on the conjunctiva as well. Careful examination of the eyes may reveal uveitis in cases of toxoplasmosis and syphilis; there may be cataracts in congenital rubella, and retinal changes in cases of endocarditis and in infections due to CMV and HIV. Associated lymphadenopathy can be seen in the systemic mycoses, syphilis, tularemia, infections mononucleosis, and tuberculosis.

The clinical laboratory can aid in the diagnosis of specific infections. Absolute lymphocytosis with at least 10% atypical lymphocytes is the hallmark of infectious mononucleosis. Lymphopenia may be seen in adults with HIV infection. The agents responsible for malaria and relapsing fever can be identified on blood smears. The etiologic agent of bacterial endocarditis, splenic abscesses, and disseminated mycoses can frequently be recovered from blood cultures. Presence of increased levels of hepatocellular enzymes alerts the clinician to the presence of acute viral hepatitis, infectious mononucleosis (usually a mild elevation), a TORCH infection, or secondary syphilis. Serologic assays are useful in the diagnosis of many of the infectious causes of splenomegaly, including the TORCH infections (at any age), EBV infection, hepatitis A and B, tularemia, brucellosis, and HIV infection. Recovery of the etiologic agent by a noninvasive technique for microbiologic examination can lead to the diagnosis of tuberculosis and typhoid fever.

Noninvasive techniques can be useful in determining the site and nature of infection. The presence of atypical pneumonia on radiographs of the chest can suggest the diagnosis of tuberculosis, fungal infection, tularemia, Q fever, or ornithosis. Cranial calcifications are seen radiographically in congenital CMV infection and toxoplasmosis, splenic calcifications can be seen in brucellosis, and calcific masses of various viscera may occur in echinococcosis and cysticercoses. Computerized tomography is one of the more important noninvasive techniques for the detection of splenic abscesses. Sonography of the heart may reveal an endocardial vegetation in a patient with endocarditis.

Skin testing is of limited diagnostic value in most circumstances. Conversion of skin tests to positive in patients whose skin tests were previously nonreactive can be supportive evidence of acute infection in patients with tuberculosis and the systemic mycoses.

Some of the infectious causes of splenomegaly require tissue diagnosis, and hence an invasive procedure is needed. Histopathologic examination is frequently necessary to determine the etiology of visceral lesions in disseminated fungal and viral infections, especially in the immunocompromised host. Definitive diagnosis of cat-scratch disease requires direct examination of the involved lymph node.

SUMMARY

The most frequent cause of splenomegaly worldwide is infection. In this chapter we outlined the mechanisms of splenic enlargement during infection, discussed the infections that are commonly accompanied by splenic enlargement, and commented upon the approach to the diagnosis of a patient with splenomegaly of infectious cause.

REFERENCES

1. McCracken GH, Shinefield, HR, Cobb K, et al: Congenital cytomegalic inclusion disease; a longitudinal study of 20 patients. *Am J Dis Child* 1969; 117:522–539.
2. Henke CE, Kurland LT, Elveback LR: Infectious mononucleosis in Rochester, Minnesota, 1950 through 1969. *Am J Epidemiol* 1973;98:483–490.
3. Baehner RL and Shuler SE. Infectious mononucleosis in childhood. Clinical expressions, serologic findings, complications, prognosis. *Clin Pediatr* 1967; 6:393–399.
4. Horwitz CA, Henle W, Henle G, et al: Heterophile-negative infectious mononucleosis-like illnesses; laboratory confirmation of 43 cases. *Am J Med* 1975;58:330–338.
5. Centers for Disease Control. Update: Acquired immunodeficiency syndrome in the United Stated. *Morbid Mortal Weekly Rep* 1986;35:757–766.
6. Cooper DA, Gold J, Maclean P, et al: Acute AIDS retrovirus infection. Definition of a clinical illness associated with seroconversion. *Lancet* 1985. 1985;I:537–540.
7. Ho DD, Sarngadharan MG, Resnick L, et al: Primary human T-lymphotropic virus type III infection. *Ann Intern Med* 1985;103:880–883.
8. Centers for Disease Control. Classification system for Human-T-lymphotropic-virus Type III/lymphadenopathy-associated virus infections. *Morbid Mortal Weekly Rep* 1986;35:334–339.
9. Shannon KM, Ammann AJ: Acquired immune deficiency syndrome in childhood. *J Pediat* 1985;106:332–342.
10. Pahwa S, Kaplan M, Fikrig S, et al: Spectrum of human T-cell lymphotropic virus type III infection in children. Recognition of symptomatic, asymptomatic, and seronegative patients. *J Am Med Assoc* 1986;255:2299–2305.
11. Scott GR, Buck BE, Leterman JG, et al: Acquired immunodeficiency in infants. *N Engl J Med* 1984;310:76–81.
12. Lebovics E: The liver in the acquired immunodeficiency syndrome; a clinical and histologic study. *Hepatology* 1985;5:293–298.
13. Centers for Disease Control. Update: acquired immunodeficiency syndrome (AIDS) in the United States. *Morbid Mortal Weekly Rep* 1983;32:688–691.
14. Selik RM, Haverkos HW, Curran JW: Acquired immunodeficiency syndrome (AIDS) trends in the United States, 1978-1983. *Am J Med* 1984;76:493–500.
15. Centers for Disease Control. Revision of the case definition of acquired immunodeficiency syndrome for national reporting—United States. *Morbid Mortal Weekly Rep* 1985;34:373–375.
16. Miller JH, Greenfield LD, Wald BR: Candidiasis of the liver and spleen in childhood. *Radiology* 1982;142:375–380.
17. Wald BR, Ortega JA, Ross W: Candidal splenic abscesses complicating acute leukemia of childhood treated by splenectomy. *Pediatrics* 1981;67:296–299.

18. Goodwin RA Jr, Shapiro SL, Thurman GH, et al: Disseminated histoplasmosis; clinical and pathologic correlations. *Medicine (Baltimore)* 1980; 59:1-33.
19. Cockshott WP, Lucas AO: Histoplasmosis duboisii. *Q J Med* 1964;33:223-238.
20. Busey JF, Baker Rd, Birch L, et al: Blastomycosis. I. A review of 198 collected cases in Veterans Administration Hospitals. *Am Rev Respir Dis* 1964;89:659-672.
21. Kafka JA, Catanzaro AC: Disseminated coccidioidomycosis in children. *J Pediatr* 1981;98:355-361.
22. Sheehy TW, Hazlett D, Turk RE: Scrub typhus; a comparison of chloramphenicol and tetracycline in its treatment. *Arch Intern Med* 1973; 132:77-80.
23. Spelman DW: Q fever; a study of 111 consecutive cases. *Med J Aust* 1982; 1:547-553.
24. Sharma SK, Shamim SQ, Bannerjee CK, et al: Disseminated tuberculosis presenting as massive hepatosplenomegaly and hepatic failure has been reported. *Am J Gastroenterol* 1981;76:153-156.
25. Watanakurakorn C: Prosthetic valve infective endocarditis. *Progr Cardiovasc Dis* 1973;16:239-274.
26. Weinstein L, Rubin RH: Infective endocarditis—1973. *Progr Cardiovasc Dis* 1973;16:239-274.
27. Pelletier LL, Petersorf RG: Infective endocarditis; a review of 125 cases from the University of Washington Hospitals, 1963-72. *Medicine (Baltimore)* 1977;56:287-313.
28. Krause JR, Levison SP' Pathology of infective endocarditis. In Kay D (ed): *Infective Endocarditis*. Baltimore, University Park Press, 1976, p. 55.
29. Weinstein L, Schlesinger JJ: Pathoanatomic, pathophysiologic, and clinical correlations in endocarditis (second of two parts). *N Engl J Med* 1974; 291:112-1126.
30. Gadacz T, Way LW, Dunphy JE: Changing clinical spectrum of splenic abscess. *Am J Surg* 1974;128:182-187.
31. Dienst FT Jr: Tularemia; a perusal of 3339 cases. *J Louisiana State M Soc* 1963;115:114-127.
32. Buchanan TM, Faber LC, Feldman TM: Brucellosis in the United States, 1960-1972; an abattoir-associated disease. Part I. *Medicine (Baltimore)* 1974;53:403-413.
33. Lynch EC, McKechnie JC, Alfrey CP: Brucellosis with pancytopenia. *Ann Intern Med* 1968;69:319-322.
34. Margileth AM: Cat scratch disease; a bacterial infection. In Mandell GL, Douglas RG Jr, Bennett JE (eds): *Principles and Practices of Infectious Diseases*, 2nd ed. New York, John Wiley and Sons, 1985, 1381-1383.
35. Wear DJ, Margileth AM, Hadfield TL, et al: Cat scratch disease; a bacterial infection. *Science (Wash DC)* 1983;221:1403-1405.
36. Voller A: Immunopathology of malaria. *Bull WHO* 1974;50:177-186.

37. McIntyre OR, Ebaugh G Jr: Palpable spleens in college freshman. *Ann Intern Med* 1967;66:301–306.

10
Splenomegaly
Neoplastic and Histiocytic Causes

RENÉE V. GARDNER*
University of Florida College of Medicine, Gainesville, Florida

In contemplating the causes of splenomegaly, geography is an important factor. When considered on a global scale, parasitic infestations and hemoglobinopathies must be given a very prominent place in the differential diagnosis. However, in the United States and Europe malignant neoplasms, and especially those of a myeloproliferative and lymphoproliferative nature, are pre-eminent considerations, despite their rarity.

Hirst and Bullock, in 1952, estimated the incidence of histologically confirmed cases of metastasis to the spleen to be 0.33% of the total number of autopsies performed, while 2.3% of carcinomas were found to metastasize to the spleen (1). Other early estimates of microscopic spread of malignant tumors to the spleen have ranged from 10% to almost 40% (1,2).

Slightly over 200 cases of primary non-lymphoreticular neoplasms of the spleen have been reported in the world literature (3). However, among these reported cases, various benign lesions are also included. A compilation of medical case records over a 50 year period at the Mayo Clinic revealed only 9 cases of primary non-lymphoreticular malignancies in the spleen in which the diagnosis could be confirmed (3).

For practical purposes, the list of potential diagnoses in cases of primary tumors of the spleen is quite similar for children and adults. However, malignant

---
*Current affiliation: National Institutes of Health, Bethesda, Maryland

Table 1 Neoplastic Causes of Splenomegaly

A. Benign tumors
   1. Hemangioma
   2. Lymphangioma
   3. Hamartoma
   4. Localized reactive lymphoid hyperplasia
   5. Inflammatory pseudotumor
B. Malignant tumors
   1. Malignant vascular tumors
      a. Hemangiosarcoma (angiosarcoma)
      b. Lymphangiosarcoma
      c. Hemangioendothelial sarcoma
   2. Lymphoid malignancies
      a. Lymphoma, both Hodgkin's and non-Hodgkin's varieties
      b. Plasmacytoma
   3. Leukemia
      a. Myeloid and lymphoid variants
   4. Non-lymphoid malignancies
      a. Fibrosarcoma
      b. Malignant histiocytoses
      c. Malignant fibrous histiocytoma
      d. Leiomyosarcoma
      e. Malignant teratoma
      f. Kaposi's sarcoma
      g. Metastatic tumors

involvement of the spleen in children is even more rare, with lymphoproliferative diseases seen most commonly (Table 1).

ROLE OF THE SPLEEN IN ANTI-TUMOR IMMUNITY

The mechanisms involved in restricting splenic involvement by malignant neoplasms are neither well understood nor widely studied. Only speculation as to the causes of the spleen's relative immunity to malignant dissemination of malignant tumors can be offered at this time. It is possible that certain mechanical factors are primarily responsible for this phenomenon. These include capsular resistance to direct tumoral spread, and the tortuosity, length and angle of the splenic artery from celiac axis which make metastatogenesis (seeding of metastases) a difficult process.

Animal studies, in which serial semi-thin spleen sections were obtained from hamsters inoculated with SV40-transformed cells, have shown that, from the earliest stages of neoplasia, neoplastic cells are present microscopically throughout the splenic reticulum (4). Despite an increase in malignant cell numbers which is proportional to the weight of the primary tumor, these cells remain relatively isolated. This finding leads one to assume the presence of undefined cytostatic factors within the spleen itself.

Could certain humoral or cell-mediated events take place after tumorigenesis has occurred? These events might restrict spread of tumor, if only transiently. What happens in the spleen after the organism undergoes "neoplastic transformation?" Both animal and human models have been used to study splenic changes in the presence of tumors. Oisgold-Daga, in examining mice with large tumor burdens, observed that spleen cells from such mice maintained responsiveness to exogenous migration inhibitory factor (MIF), but lymphocytes from these animals were unable to produce MIF in vitro (5). Whether this phenomenon was due to suppression of MIF production, or failure of response to MIF by the target cell population, is uncertain.

Spleens from patients with gastric carcinoma contain suppressor cells capable of inhibiting nonspecific immune responses (6). The presence of these suppressor cells in the spleen is dependent upon the extent of cancerous invasion of lymph node chains and the primary location of the malignancy. Blocking antibody and antigen-antibody complexes have also been detected in the blood of patients with gastric carcinoma (7), and are present in greatest amounts in those individuals having the most advanced disease. Since these substances are found in higher concentrations in blood obtained from the splenic vasculature as opposed to the peripheral blood, the spleen is believed to be the source of these inhibitory factors.

Data from patients with Hodgkin's disease support such observations gathered from murine and human experiments (8). When the spleen of patients with Hodgkin's disease is not involved by the malignancy, natural killer cell activity is increased. Natural killer cell activity is capable of lysing tumor cells in experimental systems and thus providing a possible first line of antitumor defense (9). This activity is reduced when histologically recognized tumor is present in the spleen, or when B symptoms (indicating widespread dissemination of Hodgkin's disease) develop. Local spontaneous activation of T cells within the spleen can be detected initially, but this activation soon disappears with increasing tumor dissemination. Again, this seems to indicate the late appearance of cells which are able to modulate cytotoxic natural killer cell activity.

Yet, reactivity to phytohemagglutinin (PHA) and the percentage of T cells among spleen cells of patients with advanced gastric carcinoma are actually comparable to that of patients with benign disorders who were studied concomitantly (7). This fact suggests that changes in lymphocytic subsets in the spleen that lead to immunosuppression are late events.

The findings of Dent and others lend corroboration to these findings (10). After animals are experimentally inoculated with tumor, T cell dependent antitumor activity is noted. This antitumor activity offers early anti-tumor protection which is of statistical significance, as indicated by decreased tumor weight at autopsy and a reduced tumor incidence. This antitumor activity is lost from the spleen of animals bearing large tumors, but can be restored after whole body irradiation is administered.

More studies will be needed to further delineate the role of the spleen in tumor immunity and in preventing tumor spread from the confines of its own parenchyma. Certainly, the models and data discussed above could be consistent with the patterns of spread seen clinically. In human cancers, metastasis to the spleen usually occurs late in the course of the disease, after malignant tumor dissemination is widespread and the tumor burden correspondingly large. However, such an explanation may not always be applicable since concomitant tumor immunity cannot be induced by all tumors.

CLINICAL PRESENTATION

Almost all pathologic conditions involving the spleen induce splenic enlargement. However, a lack of a palpable spleen does not rule out the possible presence of a malignant process or presence of tumors in that organ. In adults, the spleen must have increased one and one-half to two times its normal size to become palpable. It must also be remembered that approximately 10% of children normally may have a palpable spleen (11). The diversity of the pathologic spectrum of splenic tumors precludes the presence of any constant clinical feature. Likewise, symptoms caused by splenomegaly itself may be obscured by those symptoms due to the primary underlying pathologic condition. On the other hand, patients with splenomegaly may remain totally asymptomatic.

When present, symptoms of splenomegaly are often related to size of the spleen and are perceived as a feeling of left-sided fullness, dragging, or heaviness. Occasional pain occurring with inspiration or during exercise may be present, indicating perisplenitis or pleural effusion. Complaints may be of a more nonspecific or constitutional nature, consisting of weight loss, generalized fatigue, cachexia, weakness and fever. Massive enlargement of the spleen, causing displacement or compression of adjacent viscera can produce symptoms of dyspnea, early satiety, constipation, referred pain to the shoulder, or pedal edema. Rarely, there may also be problems resulting from accompanying leukopenia, thrombocytopenia, or anemia, such as weakness, bleeding tendency, or infection.

The anemia associated with hypersplenism may be moderate or marked, and associated with a low grade reticulocytosis (5 to 10%). Such an anemia may be accompanied by erythroid hyperplasia of the bone marrow and may be caused by any of several factors. Increase in total plasma volume may occur, with concurrent splenic plasma volume changes being only a minor component of such increase (12). Increased pooling of red blood cells within the spleen, with ensuing sequestration by the spleen of these cells, is frequently observed. Such red cell sequestration is demonstrated by increased radioactivity of the spleen during spleen imaging after ^{51}Cr-labelled autologous red cells have been injected into individuals with splenomegaly (3,13-15).

Despite the absence of overt signs of red blood cell destruction, hemolysis may also be present. Such destruction of red cells may be the result of (1) hypersplenism, (2) changes in red cell lifespan attributable to the underlying pathologic process, (3) the presence of abnormal vascular channels within the spleen, such as with angiosarcoma and its variants, or (4) autoimmune hemolytic processes that are sometimes seen with lymphomatous disorders (17). Excessive blood loss due to thrombocytopenia may contribute to this anemia. In such cases, thrombocytopenia may result from excessive pooling and subsequent sequestration of platelets, without concurrent lessening of the size of the total platelet pool. Also, spontaneous, nontraumatic splenic rupture may indicate the presence of splenic pathology (18).

Involvement of the bone marrow by a metastatic neoplasm may cause anemia, leukopenia and thrombocytopenia. Lastly, megaloblastic or macrocytic anemias can sometimes be a part of the presenting complex of signs associated with certain neoplasms. The reason for megaloblastosis remains obscure, since cytotoxic antitumor treatment cannot always be implicated as a cause. Some investigators have postulated increased utilization of folic acid or vitamin B_{12}, while others have suggested the presence of tumor-elaborated substances which may interfere with intestinal absorption of these cofactors. Extramedullary hematopoiesis, while contributing little in the way of effective hematopoiesis, may also play a role in the enlargement of the spleen.

Conversely, circulatory disturbances may be caused by the primary disorder of the spleen, and dysfunction of the reticuloendothelial system may result from direct infiltration by a malignant tumor (15,16). Defective uptake of radiocolloid by the spleen may be the result. This functional asplenia, commonly associated with a variety of autoimmune disorders (17), may be selective, as in the case of Sézary syndrome, where splenic uptake of ^{99m}technetium sulfur colloid is impaired (14). Examination of peripheral blood smears may reveal no clues signalling splenic hypofunction; thus, Howell-Jolly bodies may be absent. However, Wilkinson and others reported 3 patients in whom hyposplenism manifested itself as a lymphocytosis so marked as to suggest chronic lymphocytic leukemia (19).

DIAGNOSIS

There is no substitute for biopsy in obtaining a specific diagnosis of neoplasia-related splenomegaly. Metastasis to the spleen usually appears quite late in the course of a malignant neoplasm. However, a high index of suspicion and judicious use of diagnostic tools may allow early diagnosis of splenic pathology. This would avoid postmortem diagnosis, which occurs all too frequently. The constellation of symptoms with which the patient presents may sometimes offer a hint of a specific clinical entity, giving direction to the work-up. For instance, presence of night sweats, fever, and weight loss may prompt the clinician to perform a battery of radiographic examinations, as well as to do a bone marrow aspiration and biopsy. These bone marrow specimens are examined for detection of abnormal cellular infiltration bearing specific morphologic or histochemical features, as may be seen in non-Hodgkin's lymphoma. When the results of these studies are known, splenectomy and pathologic examination of the spleen may be unnecessary. Yet, as mentioned above, patients with splenomegaly usually have no specific complaints.

Among the various radiologic techniques now available (2,20-29), plain x-ray of the abdomen offers little useful information. The median border of the spleen is rarely seen on plain radiographs, and splenic contour is better visualized on conventional tomograms done in combination with the excretory urogram. Percutaneous splenoportogram is definitely contraindicated. Even with a normal clotting profile, 50 ml of blood or more may be found in the abdomen after this procedure. Percutaneous splenoportogram in many patients having malignancy and significant thrombocytopenia carries prohibitive dangers of intraabdominal hemorrhage. Selective splenic angiography, via the transfemoral or transaxillary approach, is now mainly performed for the study of the portal circulation only in cases where surgery is planned (29).

These procedures have been suppressed by new and more precise imaging techniques. Ultrasonography, although it is noninvasive and carries a low-risk of adverse effects, does not permit exact delineation of splenic topographic anatomy. However, ultrasound examination does allow visualization of the normal spleen as consisting of homogeneous tissue, shown by the appearance of low level echo throughout the parenchyma. These echoes tend to be of lower intensity than those seen in normal hepatic tissue. Normally, splenic trabeculae can be seen. These structures are delineated as resolvable scattering centers by use of mean scatter spacing measurements (28). Larger than normal separations among these "tissue scatterers" may indicate the presence of metastatic nodules or collagen deposition within the parenchyma of the spleen. This finding is not specific to any one disease process.

The internal vascular structure of the spleen is not readily identified by ultrasonographic visualization. Nonetheless, splenic hilar vessels can sometimes be demonstrated when splenomegaly is present. Measurements of the size of the spleen, longitudinal and transverse diameters, and thickness of the spleen can be obtained by real-time ultrasonographic imaging. Also, ultrasonography can be useful in the detection of cystic lesions. However, in most cases ultrasound does not distinguish between the various types of focal defects. Furthermore, very obese patients, or those having bony fractures or skin wounds in the left upper quadrant of the abdomen, may not be able to benefit from the use of this diagnostic modality.

General topography of the spleen and the location of a lesion within the spleen can be determined by liver-spleen scanning, but this is an imprecise technique. In one study, radionuclide imaging was found to be an inaccurate means of estimating spleen size or of detecting variations in spleen position. Correlation between radiographically-derived estimation of spleen mass and actual mass was not possible through use of the liver-spleen scan (26). As occurs with hamartomas of the spleen, the pattern of uptake of colloid by the spleen may vary, preventing identification of the lesion or a narrowing down of diagnostic possibilities (20).

Gallium scanning has been used in the diagnostic work-up of splenic tumors, as well as for diagnosis of infection (23). However, this technique only offers an overall true positive detection rate for splenic involvement of 2%, with a false positive rate of 12% (11). This unacceptably high failure rate for gallium scan is probably due to (1) the technique's failure to detect all filling defects, and (2) the normal accumulation of gallium in the liver, colon, bone, and spleen.

At the present time, computerized tomography (CT) displays the greatest accuracy among radiographic imaging techniques at our disposal for diagnosis of splenic tumors. In the future, it may be that magnetic resonance imaging (MRI) may yield even greater diagnostic detail, and have the advantage of avoiding radiation exposure and the use of intravenous contrast material. Presently, the scope of usefulness of MRI is unclear. CT best demonstrates the changes in shape associated with splenomegaly, such as loss of visceral surface concavity, while allowing cross-sectional examination of the spleen and other abdominal structures. Focal defects of the spleen are also detected with a fairly high degree of accuracy. This accuracy may be enhanced by the use of contrast agents, such as ethiodol oil emulsion (EOE-13) (11). CT also enables one to determine the size and nature of lesions, their relationship to adjacent viscera, involvement of lymph nodes and the liver by the disease process, and associated abnormalities of the pleura and of the abdominal cavity. Pathology demonstrated by CT has, at times, been the first and only manifestation of splenic involvement.

In summary, CT scanning has the advantages of reliability, reproducibility, greater ease of interpretation for the nonradiologist than other modalities such as ultrasound, high spatial resolution, and less operator dependency.

Biopsy of the spleen and concurrent accurate study of peripheral blood, bone marrow and liver remain absolute requisites for diagnosis. In one study, aspiration biopsy of liver and spleen suspected of malignant involvement was performed, after heterogeneity in the liver scan, elevation of transaminase, or both were noted (30). Ultrasonography in each instance was interpreted as normal. In 32 patients diagnosed as having carcinoma of varying histologic type, spread of malignancy to the spleen was not detected by aspiration biopsy. In 97 patients diagnosed as having Hodgkin's disease and non-Hodgkin's lymphoma, in whom aspiration biopsy of the spleen was performed, 11 biopsy specimens (approximately 11%) were found to be positive for neoplastic infiltration. An additional 9 samples were considered to be suspicious for malignancy although a definitive diagnosis could not be made. Thus, clinical staging alone is inadequate.

When splenic metastasis is only one part of a widely disseminated metastatic process, the information obtained from splenic biopsy may have little impact on therapeutic decisions. In non-Hodgkin's lymphomas, clinical and pathologic staging rarely differ significantly and biopsy of the spleen or diagnostic splenectomy are seldom necessary for staging. Splenectomy is reserved as treatment for symptomatic splenomegaly or hypersplenism (31).

Recently, it has been debated as to whether partial splenectomy can prevent the occurrence of overwhelming postsplenectomy infection, a complication seen in a significant proportion of asplenic individuals, especially children (32). Some investigators have suggested that partial splenectomy may accurately establish a diagnosis of splenic involvement by a number of neoplasms and still preserve splenic function (34). However, preliminary results suggest that partial splenectomy in Hodgkin's disease may be an inappropriate approach since splenic involvement can be limited to a few nodules in a localized distribution with no visible subcapsular lesions to attract the eye of the surgeon at the time of laparotomy (35). This results in a significant rate of failure of detection. Hodgkin's disease is highly curable and almost a third of individuals with Hodgkin's disease have upgrading of staging, i.e., are found at the time of splenectomy to have dissemination to the spleen despite absence of clinically evident disease (36). These facts dictate at this time that total splenectomy should be done for diagnostic purposes. Use of pneumococcal and hemophilus vaccines, together with penicillin prophylaxis and close supervision, are advised in post-splenectomy patients.

LEUKEMIAS

In both myelogenous and lymphoid leukemias, the spleen may act as a significant repository or reservoir of leukemic cells. Even minimal enlargement of the spleen may be a sign of splenic involvement. Rupture of the spleen, which occurs in 1% of leukemic patients, is seen more commonly in acute leukemias, both myeloid and lymphoid, and in hairy cell leukemia (37). Infarction of the spleen, on the other hand, is more frequently associated with chronic leukemia.

Chronic lymphocytic leukemia (CLL) is the most common leukemia among Caucasian adults. Splenomegaly is seen in 50% of patients with CLL upon presentation (38), usually accompanied by adenopathy, although enlargement of lymph nodes may be absent. With progression of the disease, splenomegaly becomes universal. Massive splenomegaly in the absence of peripheral adenopathy sometimes can mean the existence of a transitional type of chronic lymphocytic leukemia, which generally is resistant to cytostatic therapy.

A subset of CLL patients with isolated splenic involvement has also been identified (39). Patients diagnosed with this pure splenic form of CLL have been shown to have a slow, uneventful course even in the absence of therapy, with an overall median duration of survival of almost 10 years. However, another group of patients who are generally elderly males have only splenic involvement. These patients have the highest number of complications, in particular complications relating to hypersplenism, which, in turn, are associated with a low probability of survival (40).

Chronic lymphocytic leukemia can also have T cell origin; this variant is rare in Western countries and is associated with cutaneous involvement and significant splenomegaly. Other hematologic malignancies, in which splenomegaly is a conspicuous finding, such as hairy cell leukemia or prolymphocytic leukemia, rarely may be confused with the pure splenic form of CLL.

Prolymphocytic leukemia is characterized by marked splenomegaly, anemia, thrombocytopenia, and an aggressive, rapidly fatal course. The lymphocytic cells of the diseases are distinguished by their large vesicular nucleoli, relatively well-condensed nuclear chromatin, and large cell size. The cells in prolymphocytic leukemia are associated with a variable population of mature small lymphocytes having numerous antigenic sites on the cell surface, as well as blastic cells.

Hairy cell leukemia (HCL), representing about 2% of adult leukemias, is a disorder predominantly occurring in males. The abnormal cell population consists of circulating mononuclear cells whose prominent hair-like cytoplasmic projections give them a distinctive appearance. These hairy cells can be identified occasionally as having receptors for cytophilic antibodies characteristic of monocytes (41), and sometimes the cells exhibit phagocytic capabilities. Phenotypically, cells of hairy cell leukemia are believed to be B lymphocytes. They are further characterized by the presence of tartaric acid-resistant acid phosphatase.

Little or no adenopathy may be detected in hairy cell leukemia. Splenomegaly is seen commonly and early. Obliteration of the red pulp architecture occurs after sinusoidal infiltration by hairy cells, and cordal widening takes place. The total amount of white pulp is diminished and normal follicles are few in number. The total amount of periarteriolar lymphocyte sheath (PALS) is also decreased, but remains relatively well-preserved. Dilated pseudo-sinuses and blood lakes may be observed. In a recent immunohistochemical study of the spleens of patients with hairy cell leukemia, it was determined that these structures were lined by hairy cells, the underlying cells which ordinarily line the sinuses having been destroyed (42). The study also revealed that the $T_4:T_8$ (helper:suppressor) ratio, while inverted among peripheral blood lymphocytes, remains normal in primary follicles and in the periarteriolar lymphocyte sheath.

Splenomegaly is a common finding in children diagnosed with acute leukemias. Over 50% of children presenting with acute myelogenous leukemia are found to have significant hepatosplenomegaly (43). In the child diagnosed with acute lymphocytic leukemia (ALL), the spleen, along with the liver, lymph nodes and bone, are the extramedullary sites infiltrated by leukemic blasts. However, massive splenomegaly is not characteristic of the null cell variant of ALL. Presence of massive splenomegaly should indicate a more aggressive and prognostically unfavorable form of leukemia, such as the T cell or B cell type. Marked enlargement of the liver and spleen have been predictive of poor outcome (43), but multivariate analysis does not demonstrate independent significance for this variable. Also described is a leukemia-lymphoma syndrome in which patients are likely to be discovered after lymphomatous dissemination. These patients have a combination of three or more features, including mediastinal mass, hepatomegaly, splenomegaly, massive adenopathy, or hemoglobin level above 10 g/dl (43).

In chronic myeloid leukemia (CML) appearing in adults (44,45), disease for the most part is confined to the spleen, bone marrow and liver in the chronic phase. During the chronic phase of CML, myeloid cells proceed through normal maturational stages, exhibiting minimal invasiveness. There are only subtle functional abnormalities of platelets and granulocytes. Usually the spleen is palpable only when the white blood cell count is 50,000 to 150,000/mm^3, and the spleen increases in size as the white cell count rises. Red cell pooling, plasma volume changes, and impaired erythropoiesis in the bone marrow result in falling hemoglobin levels. Granulopoiesis increases in the spleen (44).

The acute or blastic phase of chronic myeloid leukemia, indicating transformation to an acute leukemic form, may be heralded by the evolution of extramedullary disease. Most patients with CML, especially after the first year, are at a constant risk of developing blast crisis. A number of factors, including a rising white cell count with an increasing population of immature cells, splenomegaly and hepatomegaly, or eosinophilia and basophilia, are associated with early transformation of CML to blastic crisis. The total dosage of busulfan required for control during the first year after diagnosis also has prognostic significance, as does the cellular karyotype. A normal karyotype indicates a poor prognosis. Since there is some evidence that bone marrow transplantation increases the chance of cure when the patient is still in the chronic phase (46), it is advantageous to have a scheme for prognosis whereby patients likely to undergo transformation will be identified early.

Chronic myeloid leukemia assumes two distinct forms in childhood, the classic adult type and the juvenile form. The adult type is characterized by presence of the Ph[1] (t(9;22) (q34.1;q11.21) chromosome and the concomitant translocation of proto-oncogenes, c-*abl* and c-*cis*, in up to 95% of patients (45). The age of onset of children with the adult type of CGL is usually above 2 years, with adenopathy occasionally seen. Marked splenomegaly is accompanied by upper abdominal fullness or a dragging sensation in the left upper quadrant. Hypersplenism may be present. The white blood cell count is usually greater than 100,000/mm^3. Monocytosis of peripheral blood and bone marrow is not observed and thrombocytopenia is not prominent initially. The median survival of children diagnosed with this form of CGL is two and a half to three years.

The juvenile form of chronic myeloid leukemia is characterised by very young age at onset, patients usually being less than 2 years of age (47). Lymphadenopathy is frequent, and splenomegaly is an inconsistent feature. The white cell count usually is under 100,000/mm^3 and the patients are usually Ph[1] chromosome negative. Response to chemotherapy is poor and the median survival is less than 9 months.

Some have proposed that the spleen is the site of origin for blastic crisis in chronic myeloid leukemia. However, no benefit has accrued from splenectomy with regard to duration of the chronic phase, length of survival, or success of chemotherapy (44). Instead, splenectomy has served as a valuable adjunctive therapy in not only CML but also in hairy cell leukemia, chronic lymphocytic leukemia, and in other types of leukemia in which splenomegaly, as a major disease component, is responsible for hypersplenic effects, severe pain or mass effect.

Patients with hairy cell leukemia have derived great benefit from splenectomy; those having undergone the operation demonstrate a definite survival advantage over those that have not (48). Approximately 80% of the patients have a good clinical response following removal of the spleen. This includes hematocrit of 35% or greater, white blood cell count of less than 100,000/mm^3, and a platelet count of over 100,000/mm^3. These patients also show prolonged survival (49,50). In CGL, splenectomy has ameliorated the complications seen in the terminal stages of the disease, but it has neither improved response to chemotherapy administration in the blastic phase nor influenced the duration of survival (51).

Only a minority of individuals with chronic lymphocytic leukemia experience complications necessitating splenectomy. Complications of the chronic lymphocytic leukemia requiring splenectomy include severe thrombocytopenia, autoimmune hemolytic anemia which has proven to be refractory to low dose corticosteroids, or massive splenomegaly causing fear of splenic rupture or other difficulties.

However, splenectomy is a procedure which should not be undertaken lightly in patients with leukemia. It should be performed only after careful consideration has been given to the part hypersplenism and marrow replacement each play in producing hematologic disturbances. Failure of hematologic responses may be seen after splenectomy, if bone marrow infiltration has been largely responsible for the patient's pancytopenic complications. Morbidity and mortality form splenectomy can be significant, stemming briefly from bleeding complications, post-splenectomy infection, pulmonary embolism, and exaggerated degrees of postsplenectomy thrombocytosis. Obviously, such complications can be avoided if the operation is performed early in the course of leukemia in chronic myeloid leukemia in chronic lymphocytic leukemia and in hairy cell leukemia.

Steinherz and co-workers reported performance of uncomplicated splenectomy in children with juvenile subacute myelomonocytic leukemia following angiographic splenic artery embolization (27). However, others have used splenic irradiation (52) for control of the underlying disease and hypersplenic complications in patients with chronic lymphocytic leukemia who were refractory to chemotherapy. Irradiation of the spleen was used in patients who were deemed unfit for surgical intervention. Low-dose irradiation to the splenic region can relieve the pain and discomfort of splenic enlargement, occasionally providing rapid control of these and other symptoms in disorders such as chronic granulocytic leukemia. However, splenic irradiation has no established superiority over use of cytostatic drugs, such as busulfan, in treatment of CGL.

In summary, splenectomy is usually indicated for cases of massive splenomegaly or hypersplenism where symptomatic relief can be accomplished without undue risk or morbidity. It should be realized, however, that for most leukemias splenectomy does not prolong life and is thus only an adjunctive measure.

Treatment of Leukemias

Chemotherapy remains the mainstay of treatment for most hematologic malignancies. Most notable have been the successes encountered in the treatment of childhood acute leukemias, in particular acute lymphoblastic leukemia (ALL). In ALL, use of relatively low toxicity chemotherapeutic regimens for remission-induction, consolidation and maintenance has resulted in a complete remission (CR) rate of at least 90%; cure is achieved in more than 50% of children with the illness (53). Attempts have been made to "fine-tune" chemotherapeutic protocols to lessen the immunosuppressive effects of the drugs employed, but these trials disappointingly have resulted in reduced efficacy (54).

Efforts to improve the disease-free survival (DFS) of children considered to be at high risk for early relapse or to salvage those who have relapsed have produced exciting results (55-57). The Children's Cancer Study Group recently reported that 96% of children receiving an intensive multiagent regimen with irradiation of bulky disease-bearing regions entered complete remission status (55). Seventy-four percent of their patients remained in continuous complete remission (CCR) for a median of 44 months and by life-table analysis were projected to have an event-free survival rate of 69% 48 months from diagnosis (55). Employing four-agent induction therapy and intensive L-asparaginase, other investigators have obtained an event-free survival rate at 4 years of almost 80% for children having high-risk ALL (57). In a Pediatric Oncology Group Study, Rivera and others reported that intensive chemotherapy utilizing rapid rotation of non-cross-resistant agents induced complete remission in 31 out of 39 patients (56). The probability of these responders remaining in remission was assessed as 0.29 for two years, and 5 patients were in second CCR for periods of 17 to 20 months after cessation of treatment.

Until now, survivors among adults have been, for the most part, individuals less than 50 years. But drawing on lessons derived from the therapeutic trials of childhood acute lymphoblastic leukemia, attempts have recently been made to emulate the pediatric treatment successes. Of 81 patients receiving multi-agent chemotherapy, 76 patients entered CR, with 40 remaining in continuous complete remission for periods extending up to 52 months (58). The median follow-up period was 16 months.

Of course, as implied earlier, chemotherapy does not have an accepted role in the treatment of all leukemias. In chronic lymphocytic leukemia, where the median survival period overall and for those over 70 years of age is 6 years and 30 months, respectively, it has not yet been shown that chemotherapy brings about improved or prolonged survival (59). Also, chemotherapeutic intervention has, at times, proven deleterious, especially in the elderly who may not tolerate the myelosuppressive effects of anti-neoplastic drugs (59). For example, whereas 50% of patients splenectomized for hairy cell leukemia may require no further therapy (60), those patients displaying signs of progressive disease after removal of the spleen present a special management problem. The administration of low-dose chlorambucil to these individuals has led to occasional clinical improvement, but in failing to bring about resolution of granulocytopenia, its use has been associated with a 25% mortality rate because of complicating infections (60).

Dismal results with chemotherapy and prohibitive deleterious side-effects have therefore led to intensified efforts to find alternative treatment measures. Trials incorporating immunotherapy with more conventional chemotherapeutic usage (61-63) have had mixed, and generally unimpressive, results. Recently, favorable results have been achieved in hairy cell leukemia with use of alpha-interferon, whether in partially purified human leukocyte or recombinant forms. Investigators have reported that 70 to 100% of patients receiving alpha-interferon show return of normal blood counts (64-76). Also observed have been an increase in helper/suppressor cell ratios (73), activation in vitro of natural killer cell activity (77), down-regulation of alpha-interferon receptors on tumor cells (77a), improvement of platelet-acquired defects (78), and clonal elimination (79). However, very few patients have actually had complete eradication of hairy cells from the peripheral blood or bone marrow, despite prolonged administration. The volume of bone marrow occupied by hairy cells is merely reduced, as assessed by stereologic analysis of semi-thin bone marrow biopsy sections or imputed by the hairy cell index (80).

Nor is there evidence of hairy cell maturation. Furthermore, control of the disease may necessitate continuous therapy for periods of up to 12 months. Deterioration of the hematologic parameters with slow increase in hairy cell numbers follows discontinuation of treatment. A majority of patients are amenable to reinduction with alpha-interferon once clinical deterioration is evident. Its toxicities include fever, flu-like symptoms and neurotoxicity which are mild in comparison to those seen with use of conventional chemotherapy. Nevertheless, interferon, while highly effective, remains an agent for palliation rather than cure in hairy cell leukemia. Its use may eventually be supplanted by that of pentostatin or 2'-deoxy-coformycin, an agent which in inhibiting adenosine deaminase activity is lymphocytotoxic. This drug, currently undergoing trials has resulted in normalization of peripheral blood counts, bone marrow profile, and spleen size (81); 7 of 9 patients receiving it in low dose were in unmaintained remission for a median duration of 6.2 months. At this time, it is difficult to judge which agent, interferon or pentostatin, should become the first choice of clinicians for patients with hairy cell leukemia requiring systemic therapy. However, pentostatin offers the distinct advantage of producing durable complete bone marrow remission.

The success of interferon seen in hairy cell leukemia has prompted its use in other forms of leukemia. Minimal clinical and hematologic improvement was noted in the patient with chronic lymphocytic leukemia after 2 weeks of interferon administration (74). In a phase II trial of interferon, clinical response, two of which were complete, were observed in 55 patients with advanced chronic myelogenous leukemia (82). Hematologic remission was attained by 24 of 27 patients receiving partially purified human leukocyte interferon (83). Remission state was indicated by decreased peripheral blood white count and lactate dehydrogenase levels, reduction of splenic size and reduction in both bone marrow cellularity and relative Ph-chromosome positivity (83). Ochs et al., treated 20 children with refractory lymphoproliferative diseases, primarily ALL, with recombinant alpha-interferon (70). One of 17 children with ALL was successfully reinduced into remission and remained in CR for 11 months, while 3 more patients reached a stabilization of their disease. These results, however, do not duplicate successes seen in hairy cell leukemia, and overall the verdict seems that interferon will have only a "fair" track record in the treatment of other hematologic malignancies.

Increasingly, bone marrow transplantation (BMT) has been applied to the treatment of relapsed refractory, or high-risk leukemias (84-97). Patients with ALL undergoing bone marrow transplantation in second remission have disease-free survival rates of 20 to 30% for over 3 years, while the survival rate for those transplanted in third or greater remission, or with advanced or resistant disease is 10 to 20% at 5 years (85). With AML, disease-free survival rates of 45 to 55% have been accomplished when patients have been transplanted in first complete remission (94). Patients transplanted in first chronic phase of CML have a 60% disease free survival rate, while the survival rate for those engrafted in accelerated or blastic crises declines correspondingly to 40% and 16%, respectively (94). Although bone marrow transplantation has been termed the treatment of choice, for pediatric patients at least, for second or subsequent remission of ALL, first or subsequent remission of AML, and CML in stable or accelerated phase (84), its usage does evoke some controversy. Not all transplantation studies have demonstrated a clearly significant survival advantage of BMT over use of conventional chemotherapy. Chessels and others were unable to detect any significant benefit of marrow transplantation in the treatment of second remission of ALL. They concluded that bone marrow transplantation's role in prolonging remission, and concomitant survival, in these children is limited (86). Critics of this analysis have referred to the small number of patients used in the study and the method of analysis (98). In AML, data accrued from intensive chemotherapy trials indicate that the results of chemotherapy and transplantation are equivalent (99).

Also, the application of allogeneic bone marrow transplantation in treatment of leukemia is definitely limited by donor non-availability. Also, its complications can be prohibitive. Attempts to increase donor selection possibilities include the use of unrelated histocompatible donors, the development of T-cell depletion techniques (in the hope of lessening the incidence of graft-vs-host disease in transplant recipients), and the performance of autologous bone marrow transplants.

Patients receiving allogeneic grafts from unrelated volunteers and those receiving HLA-mismatched marrow from family donors had comparable survival rates of 29% and 36%, respectively (87). This approach is unfortunately restricted by the median time needed to locate or select unrelated volunteer donors (about 4 months) and the multi-ethnicity of the donor pool.

Transplantation after T lymphocyte depletion, while occasionally lessening the risk of GVHD (100,101), has been associated with an increased rate of graft failure, with 10 to 35% of HLA-identical T-cell depleted grafts and up to 50% HLA-nonidentical grafts failing to take (101). There may also be a concurrent rise in the actuarial relapse rate (101). Sondel and coworkers have reported recovery of autologous bone marrow hematopoietic function, without observed chimerism in the intervening period, after T-cell depletion of donor marrow in leukemic patients (102). Obviously, the problems associated with this approach are far from solved.

Autologous bone marrow transplantation, with in vitro treatment of marrow with monoclonal antibodies and/or drugs has been developed as an alternative treatment. Thus far, the majority of patients receiving autografts have achieved complete remission status but have relapsed fairly rapidly (103-108). Few patients have become long-term survivors. Gorin and colleagues reported an overall disease-free survival rate of 52% at 560 days for all patients having acute leukemia and receiving autografts (103). Although there was a slight trend pointing towards a beneficial effect of marrow purging with either drugs or monoclonal antibodies, the difference between purged or non-purged marrow autografting in terms of survival for AML or ALL was not statistically significant. Autologous marrow transplantation was performed in 25 patients with AML in second or third complete remission after ex vivo marrow treatment with 4-hydroxy-peroxycyclophosphamide (105). Eleven patients remained in remission for a median of greater than 400 days; an actuarial relapse rate of 46% was computed, leading the investigators to conclude that autologous bone marrow transplantation could yield disease-free survival statistics comparable to those of syngeneic or allogeneic transplantation.

Most results, however, have not been so sanguine. Whereas 30 to 50% of patients with acute lymphoblastic leukemia treated with autologous marrow transplants are survivors at 2 years, results have been disappointing in AML and CML, with survival rates of 20 to 30%, and 10 to 20%, respectively. Eleven of 24 poor-risk patients with ALL treated with autograft relapsed within a median of 3 months (107). Three were in complete remission for 14 to 24 months after transplantation. Noting that all of his patients undergoing autologous transplantation, receiving cryopreserved marrow harvested during remission had relapsed, Gorin referred to the remission induced by autologous transplantation as a "chronologic chimera" (108). Autologous bone marrow transplantation in chronic myeloid leukemia has resulted in only a modest prolongation in long-term survival and has been characterized by rapid recurrence of blasts (85,106).

Thus, the search for improved salvage methods and increased survival continue, with some breakthroughs and many painful disappointments.

LYMPHOMAS: HODGKIN'S DISEASE AND NON-HODGKIN'S LYMPHOMA

Splenomegaly is not a usual presenting feature of lymphomas. It is estimated that only 1% of all lymphomas present with splenomegaly, in the absence of significant peripheral lymphadenopathy (109,110). Splenomegaly is more prominent in non-Hodgkin's lymphoma (NHL) than in Hodgkin's disease.

Splenomegaly in itself is an unreliable indicator of involvement in Hodgkin's disease. Instead, splenomegaly may result from reactive hyperplasia of splenic tissue. Granulomas are sometimes seen in the spleen and may have favorable prognostic significance (38). During laparotomy, downstaging is possible after a negative histologic evaluation, even though the spleen may have appeared by clinical examination to have lymphomatous involvement. As many as 42% of patients with Hodgkin's disease were proven by laparotomy findings to have abdominal disease which otherwise was not suspected on clinical grounds (111).

In Hodgkin's disease, involvement of para-aortic lymph nodes, celiac nodes, liver and bone marrow is associated with a high probability of involvement of the spleen. Also, left-sided cervical adenopathy is more frequently associated with involvement of the spleen in Hodgkin's disease. Nodular metastases to the spleen are initially present as focal lesions in the follicular marginal zones. The probability of dissemination to the spleen is influenced greatly by histologic subtype. The incidence rates of splenic involvement for the various histologic subtypes of Hodgkin's disease are as follows: lymphocyte predominant 16%, nodular sclerosis 35%, mixed cellularity 59%, and lymphocyte-depleted 83% (38).

In non-Hodgkin's lymphoma, about a third of adult patients will be diagnosed as having disease within the spleen, which may rarely be the only intraabdominal site of lymphoma. Prominent splenomegaly is believed by many to be an invariable indicator of widespread dissemination in NHL (112). Over 50% of individuals with splenic involvement will have concomitant hepatic involvement (113). Spleens weighing more than 400 grams are associated with a high probability of positive liver biopsy. A palpable spleen coupled with a positive lymphangiogram indicates a 100% incidence of hepatic dissemination in patients with non-Hodgkin's lymphoma (111). Bone marrow involvement and splenomegaly also have a significant correlation with subsequent leukemic transformation (112).

Histologically, any subtype of non-Hodgkin's lymphoma can present with spread to the spleen. In one survey of cases of malignant lymphoma with primary splenic presentation, the small lymphocytic type comprised 55%, large cell type 15%, and mixed cell type 15% of cases. The intermediate cell and the small non-cleaved cell types of lymphoma each represented 5% of patients in the series (113). No significant correlation exists between histologic type of NHL and clinical symptomatology, splenic size, involvement of lymph nodes, or peripheral blood abnormalities. But survival of patients does vary according to histopathologic subtype.

With involvement by any lymphoma, the spleen's capsule may be smooth, focally thickened or impressed from beneath by tumor mass. Breitfeld and Lee identified four distinct types of gross splenic involvement in lymphomas: (1) microscopic, without grossly visible defects, (2) a diffuse miliary pattern, (3) well-circumscribed nodules, with small nodules compacting to form the larger, and, least commonly, (4) single small or large tumor masses (114). Hodgkin's disease, whose earliest involvement is often at the outer edge of the marginal zone, rarely presents with the type 1 pattern (that is, with microscopic findings only). Large cell lymphomas, previously termed histiocytic lymphomas, tend to form large tumors which displace splenic parenchyma (109). Involvement of the spleen by the large cell type of lymphoma is less common than in lymphocytic or follicular types. A diffuse or miliary distribution is more likely to be observed with other forms of non-Hodgkin's lymphoma.

The mass of neoplastic cells of lymphoma initially expands in a nodular fashion within the spleen, compressing the surrounding red pulp without necessarily destroying it. Later, the spleen's architecture may be completely obliterated by the infiltrating cells. It has been said that the anatomic pattern of involvement within the spleen in lymphomas is determined primarily by the splenic microenvironment, rather than by any inherent growth determinant or pattern of the primary disease process.

Primary splenic lymphoma (113,115,116) is extremely uncommon, and is seen in only 1 to 2% of all patients with non-Hodgkin's lymphoma. Its exact incidence is difficult to determine since, until recently, the diagnosis of primary lymphoma of the spleen was sometimes made when generalized disease was actually present. The diagnosis of splenic lymphoma is definitively established when disease is confined to the spleen and existence of neoplasm in liver, mesenteric lymph nodes, paraaortic nodes, bone marrow, etc., is excluded by means of appropriate biopsies. Also, there should be no clinical, biochemical, hematologic, or radiographic evidence of spread of the lymphoma. Absence of detectable disease in extrasplenic sites 6 months following diagnosis is used as a prerequisite for confirming a diagnosis of primary splenic lymphoma (115).

All histologic subtypes of non-Hodgkin's lymphoma have been observed in primary splenic lymphomas, although small lymphocytic lymphomas are most common (113). Survival varies according to histologic type, as in other forms of NHL. The symptoms of primary and secondary lymphomatous involvement of the spleen do not differ greatly. Nonspecific symptoms of chills, fever, night sweats, fatigability, malaise, and weight loss may develop 2 to 12 months prior to diagnosis. Hypersplenism may cause major hematologic compromise, indicating the need for splenectomy, and a mild normocytic-normochromic anemia may be present. The erythrocyte sedimentation rate is usually elevated. Patients may present with left upper quadrant pain and mass. Pleural effusion is not uncommon. Rupture of the spleen or necrosis with superimposed infection may also occur.

Usually the histopathologic diagnosis of primary splenic lymphoma should present no great difficulties. However, included in the differential diagnosis are such benign lesions as reactive lymphoid hyperplasia, giant follicular pseudolymphoma (Castleman's tumor), inflammatory pseudotumor, hematoma, splenic cyst, and splenic abscess.

Of special interest is the entity of non-tropical idiopathic splenomegaly or primary hypersplenism (31,117). Diagnosed in adults, this term refers to splenomegaly associated with hypersplenism with no evidence on examination of the peripheral blood of leukoerythroblastosis or other obvious morphologic or clinical features of myeloproliferative disease. Slight to moderate hepatomegaly is observed, without accompanying cirrhosis or portal hypertension, and the lymph nodes are not enlarged. Upon removal of the spleen, histologic examination demonstrates only moderate to marked hyperplasia of splenic tissue. A significant proportion of these patients are later found to have non-Hodgkin's lymphoma.

With the majority of patients presenting with Hodgkin's disease and non-Hodgkin's lymphoma now becoming long-term survivors (118,126), attention is being centered on refining treatment regimens, developing adequate means of treating those patients who relapse or become refractory to therapy, and minimizing toxicities. The latter concern is a pressing one. By analyzing the results of treatment of 320 patients with Hodgkin's disease over a 25 year period, Rubin noted a marked incearse in the observed-to-expected ratio of second malignancies in patients who received both combination chemotherapy and irradiation (127). These results are in accordance with those previously recorded (128,129).

Individuals with Hodgkin's disease who relapse may be salvaged by use of alternative chemotherapeutic regimens. But the refractory patient with Hodgkin's disease or non-Hodgkin's lymphoma may require use of various therapeutic innovations. Interferons have been shown to be active in the treatment of non-Hodgkin's lymphoma (130,131). Further study will be required to determine their usefulness in Hodgkin's disease.

Both allogeneic and autologous bone marrow transplants have been used in the treatment of malignant lymphomas (132,136). Performing allogeneic transplants in 17 patients with non-Hodgkin's lymphoma, 85% of whom were in relapse at the time of transplantation, Phillips noted 4 prolonged survivors who were disease-free for 11 months, 17 months, 21 months, and 41 months (132). Autografting after administration of high-dose chemotherapy, Anderson and his coworkers reported that two of four patients with non-Hodgkin's lymphoma were alive at 874 days and 448 days, and one patient was alive and well at 446 days (133). Comparable results have been noted by others (134,135), but morbidity, which has included failure of reconstitution and the ensuing complications, late pulmonary toxicity, cardiotoxicity, etc., has been high, and remission unsustained. It has been suggested that poor-risk patients might benefit from transplantation during earlier stages of disease, but the appropriate time to undertake the procedure has not been agreed upon.

MYELOFIBROSIS

Myelofibrosis refers to a spectrum of myeloproliferative diseases arising from disordered proliferation of one or more hematopoietic cell lines as a result of a multipotential stem cell defect. It is distinguished by its monoclonality (136) and presence of reactive bone marrow fibrosis. Uncertainty exists as to whether this entity should be classed as a neoplasm or a secondary phenomenon. Myelofibrosis can be a reactive component of bone marrow injury due to chemicals, physical trauma, infectious agents, malignant tumors, or infarction. The myelofibrosis of myeloproliferative disease is characterized by the monoclonal nature of blood cell production and the accompanying reactivation of hematopoietic sites active during fetal life, such as in the liver and spleen.

Occurring usually in middle-aged or elderly individuals, the clinical presentation of myelofibrosis is heterogeneous and dependent upon the amount of remaining normal functioning hematopoietic tissue present. The disease rarely occurs in young adults and children (137). Three patients reported by Shalev and others (137) had a stable or slowly progressive course without significant morphologic abnormalities of the peripheral blood or bone marrow, or presence of severe organomegaly. Although clinical variants cannot always be clearly categorized, Gilbert recently divided myelofibrosis into three basic groupings: (1) reactive myelofibrosis with marrow hyperplasia, (2) reactive myelofibrosis with marrow dysplasia, and (3) reactive myelofibrosis with aplastic or hypoproliferative bone marrow (138).

Patients falling within the first category (reactive myelofibrosis with marrow hyperplasia) have variable marrow fibrosis and excessive megakaryocyte production. They show normal blood cell differentiation and maturation with hyperplasia of one or more hematopoietic cell lines. Centrifugal expansion of bone marrow occurs, along with progressive myeloid metaplasia. It is important to note that the proliferative features of this variant are prominent, since the disorder arises de novo or as an expression of preexisting disease, such as polycythemia vera.

Splenomegaly resulting from fibrosclerotic obliteration of the bone marrow space can be severe and progressive. Hepatomegaly is usually less impressive. The spleen is found to have areas of reticulum cell hyperplasia and active hematopoiesis. The course of this disease is often indolent, with a median survival of 8 years, but there is the risk of progression and subsequent development of overt malignancy, such as acute leukemia. Therapy is frequently aimed at amelioration of complications, mainly those resulting from splenic enlargement and increased cellular turnover or cytopenias (such as anemia, leukopenia, and thrombocytopenia). Specific therapeutic modalities include allopurinol to combat hyperuricemia, myelosuppressive drugs for shrinkage of the enlarged spleen, diuretics to reduce volume overload, and repeated transfusions for treatment of anemia.

In reactive myelofibrosis with dysplastic marrow function, marrow fibrosis is accompanied by normal or increased proliferation of one or more hematopoietic cell precursors (such as presence of marked megakaryocytopoiesis), together with abnormal differentiation and maturation of hematopoietic cells. Pancytopenia may result, due to hypersplenism coupled with ineffective hematopoiesis and intramedullary hemolysis. Bone marrow expands centrifugally resulting in axial bone marrow fibrosis. About one-third of the patients have osteosclerosis, seen on radiographs as new bone deposition. The total hematopoietic cell mass in the bone marrow is diminished. Within the bone marrow, erythroid hyperplasia with sideroblastic proliferation may be evident. Increased proportions of fetal hemoglobin give evidence of a reversion to fetal patterns of erythropoiesis. Splenomegaly is progressive.

Tear drop cells, reticulocytes, and ovalocytes are prominent; ineffective erythropoiesis is seen as an elevation in indirect bilirubin and lactate dehydrogenase, with decreased serum haptoglobin levels. A left-shift is evident in the maturational status of leukocytes, with circulating myeloblasts and promyelocytes being noted in the peripheral blood smear. The emergence of abnormal clones of cells can give rise to either paroxysmal nocturnal hemoglobinuria, or various forms of leukemia. The median duration of disease in myelofibrosis is approximately 3 years. A variable response has been seen when patients are treated with androgens or testosterone. However, treatment may ultimately be aimed at the effects of complications of myelofibrosis rather than at its underlying defect or cause.

The third variant of myelofibrosis is characterized by generalized marrow fibrosis, retention of clusters of atypical megakaryocytes, and hyperplasia and immaturity of all three hematopoietic cell lines. Myeloid metaplasia and resulting splenomegaly are usually minimal. Splenomegaly may even be absent. Circulating myeloid precursors may be present. The clinical course of this variant of myelofibrosis is acute and progressive, the patients ordinarily surviving less than one year. Bone and joint pains, and generalized wasting are present. The primary therapeutic approach is supportive. Transfusions of red cells, white cells, and platelets ultimately are ineffective as macrophages destroy both autologous and transfused cells. Treatment with androgens and cytotoxic drugs has also proved to be unsuccessful. There has been recent success with allogeneic bone marrow transplantation (139), but the application of this therapeutic modality to myelofibrosis is presently limited. Death results from hemorrhagic or infectious complications.

Recent studies have led to a better understanding of the pathogenetic mechanisms of myelofibrosis. Although the fibroblasts are not abnormal, the excessive amount of collagen produced by them during the course of the disease impedes normal bone marrow proliferation. In myelofibrosis, serum levels of aminoterminal procollagen type III peptide, specific to the reticulin network of bone marrow sinuses and periosteum, are elevated. These levels are higher in the more advanced stages than in early stages of disease (140). Type I collagen may be increased during the later stages as well (141). In some patients with myelofibrosis, increased levels of platelet-derived growth factor have been detected. This factor, when it is inappropriately released, leads to fibroblastic cell division and secretion of collagen. Then inhibition of collagenase occurs due to the simultaneous release of platelet factor V which prevents the degradation of the newly-formed collagen.

In cases where myelofibrosis is a reactive component of the disease process, vitamin D_3 metabolites cause a regression of myelofibrosis (142). The active hormonal metabolite, 1,23-dihydroxy vitamin D_3, inhibits human megakaryocytopoiesis in vitro, inducing differentiation of myeloid cells along the monocyte/macrophage lineage. The macrophages and monocytes thus induced are responsible for collagen degradation. However, clinical use of vitamin D_3 metabolites is not yet practical, nor of proven benefit.

Perhaps a more practical result of our increased knowledge of the pathophysiology of myelofibrosis is the proposed use of pharmacologic agents which inhibit collagen metabolism or secretion of collagen (143). These agents include (1) vinblastine, colchicine, and cytochalasin B, which are inhibitors of collagen secretion via microtubules and filaments, (2) proline analogs to prevent collagen metabolism, and (3) D-penicillamine and β-aminopropionitrile (BAPN), both of which interfere with collagen cross-linkage formation. Experience in humans has been limited, but results of studies using animal models and in vitro testing are promising.

It is not clear what role the spleen may play in the development of myelofibrosis. Even when it exceeds 3 kilograms in weight, the enlarged spleen retains its basic anatomy without distortion. Hemosiderosis resulting from intensive transfusion therapy can sometimes be seen together with infarction, hemorrhage, and inflammation of the fibrous capsule, causing the discomfort of perisplenitis. Although it is the site of extramedullary hematopoiesis, the spleen's contribution to blood proliferation in most cases is negligible.

The rate of plasma iron turnover is increased and the spleen has an increased uptake of iron. Both of these findings point to ineffective erythropoiesis. Shortened red cell survival time, increased plasma volume, and sequestration of red cells in the spleen combine to give rise to a diagnosis of hypersplenism. In some variants of myeloproliferative disease the spleen may have an inhibitory effect on the bone marrow's proliferative capacity (46).

The spleen may also play a minor role, through hyposplenia or asplenia, in the development of immune compromise in patients with myelofibrosis, compounding the immunodepressive effects of pancytopenia and abnormalities of the alternate complement pathway. Such abnormalities in immunity are responsible for bacterial infections which occur in a significant proportion of patients with myelofibrosis and are a major cause of death.

Most interesting are those studies which point to the spleen as the source of colony-forming cells in myelofibrosis (143). Progenitor cells of patients with myelofibrosis are generally found in increased numbers relative to the control or normal population (144). However, myeloid colony-forming units (CFU-C) have been detected in greater numbers in blood obtained from the splenic vein at the time of splenectomy than in blood in the systemic circulation. Cells bearing cytogenetic abnormalities have occasionally been discovered first in the spleen and circulation, appearing only later in the bone marrow (143). This finding gives credence to the idea that the spleen in myelofibrosis is the site of origin of both normal and neoplastic stem cells.

Splenectomy usually causes a decrease in the number of circulating progenitor cells, in rare instances being associated with loss of the abnormal clone (143). Low-dose X-irradiation of the spleen has also produced significant pancytopenia; the mechanism for this reduction in circulating blood cells is unclear. Thus, there is increasing evidence for a prominent role of the spleen in the etiology of at least some myeloproliferative disorders. However, more data is needed to further elucidate the spleen's pathophysiologic role.

At present, splenic irradiation offers only temporary control of symptoms for most patients with myelofibrosis. Splenectomy is indicated for patients with repeated splenic infarction, mechanical embarrassment due to massive splenomegaly, and for complications of hypersplenism or hydremia. Splenectomy is contraindicated in the event of enhanced megakaryocytopoiesis, since resultant post-splenectomy thrombocythemia can pose serious thrombotic problems.

HISTIOCYTOSIS

Histiocytic tumors occur with a frequency of 0.3% (145). These tumors include the entities malignant histiocytosis, histiocytosis-X, and malignant fibrous histiocytoma. They are not to be confused with the variant of lymphoma, previously classified as histiocytic lymphoma, but now established as a tumor of B cell origin.

Malignant Histiocytosis

Malignant histiocytosis is defined as a progressive systemic proliferation of immature or malignant histiocytes. The diagnosis is frequently made with great difficulty, as a second-guess (or not at all) during life. However, it has been noted that the number of cases of malignant histiocytosis has been rapidly increasing recently (145), probably due to the availability of more sophisticated immunochemical or enzymologic technology for diagnosis.

Clinical presentation of this neoplasm is insidious and the course is highly aggressive. Without treatment, death within 6 months is a virtual certainty. The usual duration of symptoms prior to diagnosis is less than 2 months (146). Although all age groups are affected, series of cases of malignant histiocytosis limited to children have been compiled (147,148).

Most frequently, patients with malignant histiocytosis present with wasting, anorexia, bone pain or muscular pain, malaise, and weight loss. The presence of fever is a sine qua non; its absence decreases the likelihood of a diagnosis of malignant histiocytosis. Hepatosplenomegaly is a common finding, with spleens having a median weight of 1080 grams and sometimes weighing over 2000 grams (149). Jaundice, either a result of liver damage by histiocytic infiltration or hemolysis may also be prominent. Increased numbers of mitotic figures in hepatocytes may be seen in patients with malignant histiocytosis (150). This finding suggests the existence of a factor produced by the infiltrating cells which is toxic to hepatocytes and causes dysfunction of the liver.

Usually, pulmonary lesions and lytic bone lesions are absent, but both have been reported (147). Similarly, oral (146), nasal and sinus (151), small bowel (152), pancreatic (147), adrenal and kidney involvement (147) are rare. Central nervous system (CNS) involvement can be seen with or without cerebral hemorrhage. Incidence of CNS disease has obvious therapeutic implications and is an important cause of death in patients with malignant histiocytosis.

Convulsions and clinical evidence of meningeal involvement were a notable feature in at least one series, occurring in 4 out of 10 patients during the course of illness (153). In analyzing prognostic indicators, the investigators found that the development of seizures was the only indicator of poor outcome, since all children with CNS involvement died, despite the administration of aggressive treatment which in two cases included intrathecal drug dosing and cranial irradiation. Two out of four patients were examined at autopsy and discovered to have had meningeal infiltration by atypical histiocytes. Cutaneous nodules, pleural effusion and widespread lymphadenopathy may also be features of this disease.

Significant bleeding may occur from the gastrointestinal tract, or there may be intracerebral or intraabdominal bleeding. The bleeding diathesis is caused by (1) hepatic failure with its resultant impaired synthesis of coagulation factors, (2) thrombocytopenia, the result of hypersplenism or bone marrow replacement by malignant histiocytes, or (3) disseminated intravascular coagulation (154).

Lymphopenia and neutropenia may lead to recurrent infection. Anemia is frequent and usually is the result of bone marrow involvement. Erythrophagocytosis or other cytophagocytosis is of no clinical significance. In itself this finding causes no hematologic disturbance. Various serologic abnormalities have also been identified, including a polyclonal hypergammaglobulinemia (146), positive rheumatoid factor determination (146), positive heterophil antibody titer (150), and the presence of cold agglutinins (155). It is not known whether the presence of positive cold agglutinin or heterophil titers indicates coincident infection of the immunocompromised host or is actually a hallmark of malignant histiocytosis.

However, it must be mentioned that, although cases of malignant histiocytosis in children and adults share certain features, there are distinctive features that characterize presentation of this disease in children. Whereas lymphadenopathy is frequently absent or develops as a late feature of the disease in adults, adenopathy is a presenting sign in two-thirds of children with malignant histiocytosis. Lymphadenopathy is extensive, most often seen in the supraclavicular and axillary regions. In contrast to other malignancies in which lymph node spread is characterized by matted, non-tender, enlarged nodes, malignant histiocytosis is typified by extensive inflammation, induration and tenderness of the lymph nodes. Mediastinal and para-aortic nodes are enlarged with similar frequency. Mediastinal adenopathy was observed in 12 of the 22 pediatric cases described by Zucker and coworkers (147); mediastinal adenopathy was bilateral, causing respiratory obstruction in one-third of affected patients. Subsequent to nodal compression, ureteral obstruction and hydronephrotic changes were also present in 3 of the children included in this series.

Adults are stricken in a male:female ratio of 2.5:1 (145). No sexual predilection was evident in children. Cutaneous and subcutaneous lesions are characteristic of malignant histiocytosis of childhood. These skin lesions are inflamed and indurated. They are commonly seen in the cervicothoracic region, infiltrating deeply into the dermis, muscle and underlying nodes. The lesions may have a yellowish or red-purple hue, a maculopapular or micronodular appearance, and sometimes are accompanied by itching.

Hepatosplenomegaly was infrequent among the pediatric patients of Zucker but was present in Jurco's patients (148). Half of Jurco's patients, a very small series accumulated over a 10 year period by Texas Children's Hospital, presented with small peribronchial histiocytic infiltrates of the lung. One patient had a substernal mass consisting of a mixed infiltrate of atypical histiocytes, as well as benign histiocytes, plasma cells, and lymphocytes.

Traditionally, erythrophagocytosis has been considered an essential criterion for diagnosis. However, the presence of erythrophagocytosis can no longer be considered evidence for specific identification of malignant histiocytosis. Erythrophagocytosis has also been observed in lymphomas, of both B cell and T cell origin (156), and in some non-lymphoid tumors (157), as well. Reactive macrophages capable of cytophagocytosis have also, at times, been noted in various infectious disorders (158). Extensive sinusoidal infiltration, a feature of malignant histiocytosis, and phagocytosis of erythrocytes can also occur among T cell populations, causing considerable diagnostic confusion (156). Finally, it is even possible that erythrophagocytosis is not a property of those cells which comprise the bulk of the malignant cellular population. Instead, it is more likely a property to be shared by well-differentiated, non-neoplastic cells (145).

Although biopsy of all involved organs may be useful in making the diagnosis, histologic examination of the liver has often been most helpful in establishing a diagnosis in children (145). In adults, however, diagnosis of malignant histiocytosis is made by bone marrow examination. This technique is especially useful when serious illness of the patient or the presence of coagulation disturbances prevent the performance of a closed liver biopsy or splenectomy for histopathologic evaluation. Diagnosis of malignant histiocytosis was confirmed by bone marrow aspiration in about 50% of adult patients studied (144). In one pediatric series, no bone marrow involvement could be discovered (145); in another, less than one-fourth of the patients studied had evidence of bone marrow infiltration (148).

Examination of lymph nodes involved by malignant histiocytosis shows diffuse disaggregated infiltration by malignant histiocytes which are characterized by cellular atypia, frequent mitoses, and erythrophagocytosis. The capsule of the lymph node is spared, but there is displacement or compression of the follicles caused by infiltration of the medullary region. The portal tracts and sinusoids of the liver are invaded by tumor cells and marked steatosis of hepatocytes is present. Abnormal and normal mitoses are visible in both hepatocytes and malignant histiocytes. The normal architecture of the spleen may be completely destroyed by diffuse infiltration by tumor, as the neoplastic cells proliferate in the red pulp and, to a lesser extent, in the white pulp.

The difficulty of making the diagnosis must be stressed. Malignant histiocytes can often be distinguished from their reactive or normal counterparts by having a higher nuclear:cytoplasmic ratio, presence of irregularly clumped chromatin, large, (often multiple and irregular) nucleoli, and frequent mitoses. However, similar appearing histiocytes are occasionally seen in preterminal stages of leukemia (158-164). Reactive histiocytes capable of cytophagocytosis also can be present in numerous other disorders (166), including mycobacterial and fungal infections, typhoid fever, sarcoidosis, and in certain viral infections, such as in viral-associated hemophagocytic syndrome (161,165-167).

Immunocytologic methods have been devised to eliminate some of the diagnostic confusion. Malignant and normal histiocytes bear cytochemical similarities. They both contain diffusely distributed cytoplasmic acid phosphatase, as well as acid nonspecific esterase which is sensitive to sodium fluoride treatment. Neoplastic cells may sporadically be found to have more focal or granular distribution of these enzymes. The presence of lysozyme within the cytoplasm of the tumor cell is a diagnostic tool, a positive test facilitating the diagnosis of malignant histiocytosis. α-1-Antitrypsin synthesis by histiocytes is a property which can help in the separation of tumors of histiocytic and lymphoid origin, but is not necessarily specific to histiocytic neoplasms, since it can also be seen with T cell lymphomas.

The presence or absence of immunoglobulin can also render diagnostic assistance. Thus a follicular center cell lymphoma or large cell lymphoma should be considered if surface immunoglobulin is detected on the cells studied. Monocyte-specific antibodies are present on the cells of malignant histiocytosis, but cross-reactivity with B cell or T cell antigens (Ia, OKT11, Leu3, and B1) is sometimes demonstrable (168-170).

Recently, cytopathologic studies have revealed two groups of histiocytes that may be responsible for neoplasia: T-zone histiocytes and mononuclear phagocytes (158). Malignant histiocytes were considered to represent lysozyme negative T-zone histiocytes. These histiocytes also react to antibodies to a protein termed S100. However, the existence of these two distinctive populations of phagocytic cells is not universally accepted. Some T cells react with anti-S100 antibodies; they stain for α-1-antitrypsin, non-specific esterase, etc. Other T cells sharing histiocytic mononuclear antigenic determinants can sometimes also be identified.

The differential diagnosis of malignant histiocytosis can be kept reasonably limited. Large cell ("histiocytic") lymphomas generally have cells with a single nucleolus, absence of esterase, a uniform appearance, and positive stain for immunoglobulin. The rare discovery of Reed-Steinberg-like cells in malignant histiocytosis sometimes causes difficulty in distinguishing between this disease and lymphocyte-depleted Hodgkin's disease. However, the sinusoidal distribution of malignant histiocytosis should facilitate the diagnosis. Metastatic tumors, such as malignant melanoma, can be differentiated by the cellular aggregation of metastatic melanoma cells in nests separated by reticulin fibers. The aggressive and disseminated nature of the Letterer-Siwe variant of histiocytosis X also may cause confusion. But usually individuals afflicted with this disorder are much younger, the histiocytes are benign in appearance, the skin involvement is more prominent, and the lesions are not perivascular or periappendicular in nature.

Hemophagocytosis can be a part of the histologic spectrum, and histiocytes are sometimes visualized on the peripheral blood smear.

Familial erythrophagocytic lymphohistiocytosis appears clinically to be identical with malignant histiocytosis, but it is distinguished by its familial association and a lack of nuclear atypia in its infiltrating cells. There is limited experience with the use of chemotherapy in this disorder. In 4 patients treated there was survival for up to 27 months after initiation of treatment with combination chemotherapy which included epidophyllotoxin and CNS prophylaxis (179).

Familial erythrophagocytic lymphohistiocytosis (FEL) is an autosomal recessive disorder usually diagnosed during the first 6 months of life. This disease is rare and almost always fatal. Patients with FEL usually have a rapidly progressive lymphohistiocytic infiltration of viscera and CNS, which produces symptoms of fever, irritability, pallor, and edema. Pancytopenia, liver dysfunction and coagulopathy are seen, and death due to hemorrhage, sepsis or histiocytic infiltration of the CNS usually ensues within 3 months of the initial presentation.

In malignant histiocytosis, therapeutic trials have been frustrating. The number of patients treated have been small, preventing the use of controlled or multi-institutional protocol studies. In rare instances splenectomy alone has produced lengthening of survival (149), but has offered only temporary or moderate benefit at best. Because of the aggressive, systemic character of the disease, recent attention has focused on the use of antitumor drugs.

Retrospective analysis of cases of malignant histiocytosis showed that 50% of patients who received chemotherapy died within one year of diagnosis. However, chemotherapy encompassing a wide range of agents (171), given singly or in combination, induced "good" initial clinical response in a significant number of patients (171). Patients who responded to treatment had a median survival of 23 months from onset of symptoms, which was a significant improvement over that of non-responders (172), most promising results were seen in those patients given the CHOP regimen (cyclophosphamide, Adriamycin, vincristine and prednisone).

These studies have recently been updated (173). CHOP remained the standard chemotherapy regimen, with modification to include bleomycin, high-dose methotrexate, or both. A complete remission rate of 68% was seen, and partial remission was seen in an additional 23% of those treated. The median duration of complete remission was over 30 months. All patients who attained only partial remission died. The median survival for the group of 24 patients reviewed retrospectively was 2 years, with a 5 year actuarial survival rate of 40%.

Lampert also used the CHOP regimen in 7 patients with malignant histiocytosis (150). Six patients had clinical and hematologic responses, including 4 with complete remission. Three patients remained relapse-free for over 14, 18 and 19 months after discontinuation of therapy. Good objective responses were seen in an additional 7 patients in a trial of chemotherapy with adriamycin, vincristine and prednisone (HOP), although only one patient actually achieved complete remission (101).

Simon and coworkers at Roswell Park Memorial Institute most recently reported two patients with this disorder who achieved long-term DFS after undergoing aggressive treatment with a CHOP regimen which included intrathecal prophylaxis (174). Pizzuto reported continuous complete remission of 3 years in a patient whose treatment consisted of splenectomy in combination with Adriamycin given as a single agent (174a). Good objective responses were seen in an additional 7 patients in a trial of chemotherapy with Adriamycin, vincristine and prednisone (HOP), although only one patient actually achieved complete remission (175). In children, the median survival of patients receiving chemotherapy in a regimen consisting of vincristine, cyclophosphamide, Adriamycin and prednisone was over 2 years (147).

Including Adriamycin in intensive chemotherapy regimens has greatly improved the chances of therapeutic success with malignant histiocytosis. However, alternative drugs are sought when anthracycline resistance is shown. Amsacrine (mAMSA) (176), and cytosine arabinoside (177) have been variably successful in achieving remission and disease control.

Epipodophyllotoxins also have had demonstrable efficacy in the treatment of this malignancy (161). Ten patients were aggressively treated for periods ranging from 6 to 24 months with combination chemotherapy which included both CHOP and VP16-213. Five patients achieved CR and remained in remission off therapy for periods of 23 to 48 months from the onset of disease.

The results of these treatment efforts are obviously encouraging. Yet, the evolution of this disease in the post-chemotherapy era may prove to be analogous to that of acute leukemia, where improved survival was attended by an increased incidence of CNS involvement. In malignant histiocytosis, cerebral involvement, at times accompanied by hemorrhage, is a common cause of death (145), and several investigators have recommended the use of CNS prophylaxis. In fact, Tseng noted that the addition of mid-cycle high-dose methotrexate with leucovorin rescue to the CHOP regimen apparently has produced improved survival (173). But, because only a small number of patients was studied, a definite survival benefit cannot yet be established.

Attempts are also being made to identify those diagnostic and treatment variables which are useful in determining prognosis. Several factors have been proposed as having independent prognostic significance. They include an initial platelet count of less than 150,000/mm^3 and the drug doses actually delivered

(173); hepatic and/or pulmonary involvement and dysfunction (based upon a modification of the Lahey scoring system) (7); chromosomal abnormalities (such as aneuploidy or balanced (8;16) translocation (178); extensive bone marrow involvement by malignant histiocytosis or predominance of immature hematopoietic cells (150); and vascular invasion of small perionodal vessels (147). However, it cannot yet be judged which clinical or laboratory features will be verified as being significant prognostic indicators.

Histiocytosis-X

Landing proposed two categories of disseminated or visceral infiltrative processes involving histiocytes (180). Included in the first category were patients with disseminated histiocytosis-X (HX), also known by its eponym Letterer-Siwe disease. Malignant histiocytosis, familial erythrophagocytosis and X-linked lymphoproliferative syndromes comprised the second group and were collectively referred to as lymphohistiocytoses. Both categories of disease involve the same spectrum of organ involvement and may be morphogenetically related, as suggested by the presence of Langerhans granules in some cases of malignant histiocytes. However, patterns of organ involvement in the two diseases (HX and MH) are different (Table 2).

There has long been controversy as to the exact nature of histiocytosis-X. This disease encompasses different degrees of clinical severity and ranges from the limited form of unifocal or multifocal bone involvement (as in eosinophilic granuloma) to the disseminated and aggressive Letterer-Siwe disease. Thus, various authors have argued that histiocytosis-X represents an inflammatory process rather than a neoplastic process (181,182). They point to several factors which they feel support this contention. Their arguments include (1) lack of consistent evidence of uncontrolled proliferation of a uniform cellular population in situ, (2) the lack of reliable correlation between the degree of differentiation and the clinical outcome, (3) the relatively high rate of spontaneous remission, and (4) the benign appearance of infiltrating histiocytes.

An immunological basis of this disease has been suggested by some. In the majority of patients with histiocytosis-X, a deficiency of T-suppressor cells with an increased $T_4:T_8$ (helper:suppressor) ratio in the peripheral blood has been detected (182). This immunologic abnormality disappears with spontaneous resolution of the disease. This finding prompted some to speculate that failure of normal cellular homeostatic mechanisms occurs, resulting in abnormal macrophage behavior and a breakdown in normal intercellular "conservation" (182, 183). A verdict regarding the true nature of histiocytosis-X has not yet returned. In this chapter we follow tradition by considering at least the disseminated form of the disorder a malignant neoplasm.

Table 2 Comparison of Organ Involvement Seen in Malignant Histiocytosis and Histiocytosis-X

Organ	Histiocytosis-X	Malignant histiocytosis
Kidney	+/−	+++
Lungs	+++ (septal/perilobular)	+++ (peribronchial/perivascular/centrilobular)
Spleen	+++	+++
Gastrointestinal tract	++ (↑ parenchymal destruction)	++
Liver	+++	+++ (portal triad infiltration)
Gonads	+/−	++
Urinary bladder	+/−	++
Thymus	++	++
Central nervous system	++ (pituitary:epidural/dural)	++ (cerebellar/hypothalamic; arachnoidal/perivascular)
Bone marrow	+++	+++

Disseminated histiocytosis-X is characterized by a granulomatous infiltration of many organs including the tonsils, thymus, pancreas, lungs, liver, spleen, myocardium, bone, etc. Diagnosis can be made by biopsy of any accessible organ. Biopsy of bone, bone marrow, liver or subcutaneous nodules will usually result in an accurate diagnosis. Radiographic examination of the skeleton reveals osteolytic lesions, usually with a sclerotic border and occasionally with periosteal new bone formation. Plain X-rays can be obtained rather than radionuclide scans for the purpose of evaluating the skeleton in patients with histiocytosis-X (184). This recommendation is based on the fact that only 35% of individual bone lesions can be detected by radionuclide scan, and the poorest correlation between plain x-rays and bone scans is seen in those individuals having the greatest number of lesions.

The histiocytes responsible for widespread proliferation or infiltration appear cytologically benign, containing an abundant pale-staining cytoplasm, subtly present nucleoli, and an ovoid or leaf-shaped nucleus with fine chromatin. These cells are often admixed with eosinophils, lymphocytes and mononuclear cells of uncertain origin. Cytophagocytosis is occasionally seen, as are multinucleated histiocytes. Necrosis of the lesions is not infrequent, and intersinusoidal infiltration by histiocytes has been observed.

The histiocytes in this disorder, like their more neoplastic counterparts in malignant histiocytosis, have certain features in common with normal histiocytes. That is, they have F_c, C_3, Ia antigenic, and T6 antigenic markers (185, 186). Also described in cells of histiocytosis-X are Birbeck or Langerhans granules, which are possibly analogous to granules contained within the Langerhans cells of the skin. However, cells of histiocytosis-X lack lysozyme and nonspecific crossreacting antigen with carcino-embryonic antigen (CEA), which are considered macrophagic markers. They have therefore been designated by some as T-zone histiocytes (186) see above).

Disseminated histiocytosis-X has been reported in adults (181), although doubt has been cast on the validity of the diagnosis of systemic giant cell histiocytosis, otherwise known as the adult form of Letterer-Siwe disease (187). Most of the cases of disseminated histiocytosis-X occur in children under the age of 2 years, and one-third of these children present in the first 6 months of life (188). Twenty cases have been reported as congenital.

Both mortality and morbidity, to a large extent, are dependent upon the interrelated factors of age, organ involvement and dysfunction. For instance, those children surviving Letterer-Siwe disease are more likely to have had more complaints of skeletal involvement, such as pain of the affected bone or bones and swelling or mass. As many as 38% of survivors had multiple bony lesions; 35% of survivors had accompanying diabetes insipidus (189). However, diabetes insipidus and bony lesions frequently occur late in the course of disease, with the diabetes insipidus not identified as a presenting symptom in patients under 4 years of age (181), and bony lesions being more common in the older child (190).

Sixty percent of children presenting when less than 3 years of age had more than 3 organ systems which were involved by disease (190). Skin involvement, common in the Letterer-Siwe variant of histiocytosis-X, is more apt to be seen in children under 3 years of age.

Thus, the observation that the disseminated form of this disorder was most characteristically seen in the young child, in whom it took on its most aggressive and widespread behavior, forms the basis for numerous staging systems. The most widely used staging system is the Lahey system (191,192).

Lahey observed the highest mortality among the very young (202). Children diagnosed before their third birthday had a mortality rate of 50%, and 70% of those presenting before the age of 6 months died. A scoring system has been devised based upon the number of organ systems identified with disease-related dysfunction. Dysfunction of one or two organ systems, giving a score of 1 or 2 is coupled with a mortality rate of 5%, and a 20% chance of developing sequelae (186). Dysfunction of 5 or more organ systems is associated with a mortality rate of 80 to 100%. Occasionally, patients may present with a low score; however, at a later date they develop a greater degree of organ involvement (186). Thus, the Lahey system is not infallible in its prognostication.

Greenberger has presented a staging system, similarly based upon organ involvement (194), whereby patients with advanced stages of disease were found to have a correspondingly poor prognosis. In this system, patients 2 years or older who have liver and/or spleen involvement, massive adenopathy, infiltration of the lung ("honeycomb lung"), or bone marrow involvement were classified as having stage III disease. Those with the spleen enlarged to 6 cm below the costal margin or with fever lasting longer than one month, with or without adenopathy, lung, bone marrow or liver involvement, were said to be stage IV patients. A separate category, stage V, was used for individuals who have clinical findings consistent with stage III or stage IV, while having more than 20% monocytes on their peripheral blood smear. Stage IV disease was associated with 100% mortality.

Patients with disseminated histiocytosis-X often present with nonspecific complaints, such as fever, diarrhea, and otitis media. Fifty percent of cases have cutaneous manifestations at the onset (188). Skin findings include a seborrheic eruption on the scalp, appearing in successive crops; a petechial or hemorrhagic rash on the palms and soles; rose-yellow, translucent papules on the trunk or scalp; and xanthomatous or eczematoid lesions. Subcutaneous nodules may occur as histiocytes invade subcutaneous fatty tissues or as a result of direct extension of granulomatous tumors from bony lesions. There may also be ulceration of the mucous membranes.

Involvement of the bones, most frequently the flat bones, vertebrae, and cranium, is more frequently seen in cases having a favorable course, appearing in later stages of the disorder. Bony involvement can occasionally mean premature loss of teeth. In the older child and adult, a possible correlation exists between sites of bone disease and outcome (182); involvement of the distal bones of the extremity appeared to indicate poorer prognosis in some of the patients studied. Generally, distal bones of the extremity were not affected in adulthood.

As previously mentioned, splenomegaly, occurring in a third of those children with histiocytosis-X (195), is an ominous sign, with less than a third of those children so affected surviving the disease (188). Adenopathy is not usually prominent but has been noted in 25 to 75% of fatal cases. Marked hepatomegaly is frequent. Progressive hepatic fibrosis and cirrhosis has been reported in association with obstructive jaundice (196). This complication is the result of extensive histiocytic infiltration of the portal regions and sinusoids, sometimes with primary bile duct involvement and signals a very poor prognosis.

Hypoproteinemia, without a reversed albumin/globulin ratio, is most likely the result of hepatic dysfunction. However, hypoproteinemia also could be secondary to histiocytic intestinal infiltration with resultant protein-losing enteropathy, or hypercatabolism of serum proteins by abnormal histiocytes. When hyperbilirubinemia is observed, the serum bilirubin is usually less than 3 mg%. The serum cholesterol may be low; no abnormal lipid fraction is noted. Serum haptoglobin levels are diminished, but not absent. Patients may also have severe deficiencies of fibrinogen and other clotting factors; these deficiencies may cause severe hemorrhagic complications (197).

Histiocytic infiltration of the lungs generally signals poor outcome. However, some believe that pulmonary disease alone probably has little prognostic significance in the child with histiocytosis-X; the lung infiltrates at times are asymptomatic and without detectable clinical evidence of sequelae (181). Yet pulmonary infiltration alone could be a major factor causing mortality in adults, in whom symptoms and disability are common.

In the bone marrow of patients with histiocytosis-X, proerythroblasts predominate and reticulocytosis and erythroblastosis can be significant. Pancytopenia is frequent. It is due to histiocytic infiltration of the bone marrow and indicates a grave prognosis. Pancytopenia may also be treatment-induced. Reduced red cell survival has been detected along with concomitant increases of urinary urobilinogen. In addition, some have postulated a role for neutrophils and platelets, as well as red blood cells (cytophagocytosis) in producing pancytopenia (186). But it seems improbable that cytophagocytosis is a prominent mechanism in causing pancytopenia.

Spontaneous remission of histiocytosis-X, either permanent or punctuated by periods of exacerbation, has been notable (198,199). However, patients spontaneously remitting with this disease may have multiple sites of involvement, but lack hepatosplenomegaly or evidence of organ failure, which is a significant distinction. Numerous cytotoxic agents have been used as chemotherapy for the disseminated disease and have been proven to be effective when given as single drug therapy (200). Thus, vincristine, vinblastine, and cyclophosphamide have produced response rates of 50, 63, and 55%, respectively. In most cases, use of combinations of effective agents have not proven to be superior to these agents given singly (201,202).

Low-dose irradiation of symptomatic, isolated or multiple bony lesions is an accepted practice. However, local injections of methylprednisolone has supplanted irradiation in some centers for those patients having involvement of only a single-system, such as the skeleton or lymph nodes (182). Giving a total dose of 900 rad in two courses with a 4 week hiatus between courses, Griffen treated an infant with disseminated histiocytosis-X with sequential hemibody irradiation. He found no evidence of disease within the treated fields upon subsequent autopsy examination (203). The cause of death in this infant was severe neuropathy secondary to vinca alkaloid therapy.

It has been urged by some that the use of irradiation be reserved for those patients whose lesions are not readily accessible to treatment approaches such as local steroid injection, or in whom there is compromise of function, such as that due to spinal cord compression or optic nerve compression (182). It is argued that the beneficial effects of current chemotherapy regimens are outweighed by the untoward, harmful side-effects. It is asserted that high-dose prednisolone (2 mg/kg) given over a period of several months is as effective as combination chemotherapy for this disease.

A trial of thymic extract was conducted on 17 patients with biopsy-proven multiple site histiocytosis-X (183). Ten responded favorably. A significant correlation between response and prior detection of immunologic abnormality, such as evidence of defective functional suppressor cell activity, was observed. Favorable response, however, was not seen in patients under two years of age, or in patients with dysfunction and involvement of more than 4 organs. Response was also less likely in the patient group that had had prior chemotherapy. A smaller trial of thymic hormone treatment in children with multisystem disease did not yield such favorable results (204), since 3 out of 4 children showed progression of disease while undergoing therapy. Instead, beneficial effects were seen after conventional therapy was instituted (213a).

One patient with progressive histiocytosis-X resistant to chemotherapy received a graft from an HLA-matched sibling after conditioning with cyclophosphamide, melphalan, fractionated total-body irradiation and intrathecal methotrexate (205). No complications were subsequently observed and the patient has been well, with no evidence of disease recurrence for 2 1/2 years. Considering the patient's previous refractory and progressive clinical course, these results may be viewed as encouraging, but overoptimism is cautioned against, since very late disease recurrence is a feature of this disorder.

Malignant Fibrous Histiocytoma

Malignant fibrous histiocytoma (MFH) (206) is rare, but it is being diagnosed with increasing frequency. This disease denotes a pleomorphic sarcoma, preiously classified as pleomorphic rhabdomyosarcoma or pleomorphic liposarcoma, and it is usually found in the soft tissues. A true histiocytic malignancy, malignant fibrous histiocytoma has more in common with the clinical and morphologic features of sarcomas.

Histologically, the distinctive feature of MFH is the infiltration of affected organs by fibroblastic-appearing and histiocytic-appearing cells in clusters or sheets (storiform pattern), in conjunction with foam cells, inflammatory cells, and multinucleated giant cells. Clinically, patients may present with systemic symptoms of fever, sweats and malaise. The disease may occur in children, as well as adults, although usually individuals with malignant fibrous histiocytoma are over 40 years of age. Although splenectomy has resulted in effective control of the disease, the clinical course appears to be one of inexorable progression, with recurrence, metastasis to numerous sites, including lungs, lymph nodes, liver, peritoneum and cerebrum, and finally death. Chemotherapy has been used with a reported response rate of 33% (207).

ANGIOSARCOMA

This tumor is also called hemangiosarcoma, hemangio-endotheliosarcoma, hemangioblastoma, or malignant endothelioma. Among non-lymphoreticular malignant neoplasms affecting the spleen, angiosarcoma ranks first as a neoplasm primarily affecting the spleen (34). In the Mayo Clinic series, 67% of those patients confirmed as having primary splenic malignancies had angiosarcoma (3). However, it remains a rare entity, with angiosarcoma of any site comprising less than 3% of all soft tissue sarcomas (208), and to date only 57 patients with primary splenic angiosarcoma have been reported in the world literature (16). Most angiosarcomatous involvement of the spleen will represent metastasis, with the liver being the usual primary site (34).

The tumor is unique in having a proven environmentally-related or occupational cause. Hepatic angiosarcoma has been associated with previous exposure to thorium dioxide (thorotrast) (209), arsenic (210), or vinyl chloride (34). However, histologic examination of spleens taken from workers exposed to vinyl chloride, with or without development of angiosarcoma, revealed follicular enlargement and proliferation of red pulp cells (211). These changes could not be attributed to portal hypertension. Instead the changes appeared to be due to a primary stimulus, probably related to toxic exposure of splenic lymphoid and reticuloendothelial cells.

The histological appearance of angiosarcoma consists of disorganized vascular channels or anastamoses with areas of solid spindle-cell proliferation. Endothelial cells appear malignant and sometimes budding. Degenerative changes, including hemorrhage and necrosis may be present. Extra-medullary hematopoiesis is occasionally seen in the primary tumor and in its associated liver metastases. It is paradoxical that anaplasia may sometimes be more histopathologically exaggerated in the metastatic hepatic lesions than in the primary splenic tumor (3).

This tumor spares no age group, but appears with greatest frequency during the fifth and sixth decades, a characteristic which might be expected if environmental exposures cause a neoplasm of the spleen or liver. No sexual predilection is evident. Presenting complaints include nonspecific abdominal pain and distension, cachexia, weakness, and weight loss. Dyspnea may occur as a result of pleural effusion of metastases to the lungs. On physical examination, splenic tenderness, ascites, or left upper quadrant mass may be evident.

A presenting problem of catastrophic proportions is spontaneous splenic rupture. This occurs in almost a third of patients with angiosarcoma of the spleen (18). This complication bears no relationship to age or sex of the patient, or size of the spleen. A high index of clinical suspicion is essential since over 50% of patients with splenic rupture were diagnosed at post-mortem (16). The mean duration of survival was only 4.4 months in patients with angiosarcoma of the spleen whose diagnosis was unsuspected and in whom splenectomy was performed after spontaneous rupture (16). This compares with a mean duration of 14.4 months if the spleen is removed prior to splenic rupture (16).

In greater than 70% of patients with splenic angiosarcoma, anemia, typically of a normocytic, normochromic nature, is present. Coagulation abnormalities vary. Microangiopathic hemolysis results from the highly irregular vascular endothelial network and fibrous stranding within the spleen.

Diagnosis can be assisted by the imaging techniques discussed above, in conjunction with findings of physical examination and history. Findings in plain x-rays may be nonspecific, but an elevated left hemidiaphragm may suggest a left upper quadrant mass. The liver-spleen scan may be characterized by nonvisualization of the spleen or by filling defects within spleen or liver parenchyma. Computerized tomography results may at times be misleading, but diffuse infiltration or solitary lesions may be visible. The angiographic appearance of angiosarcoma bears a similarity to that of cavernous hemangioma; thus, the intense peripheral tumor stain appears late in the arterial phase, lasting 30 to 40 seconds. Ultrasonography at times can also be useful in rendering a diagnosis of angiosarcoma.

Clinically, the tumor's behavior is unpredictable and often extremely aggressive. The prognosis is universally poor, with only 20% of patients with this neoplasm surviving as long as 6 months.

Angiosarcoma is a radiosensitive tumor and response to radiotherapy has been noted in some cases of angiosarcoma of the breast and extremities (134, 135). However such responses are generally short-lived, with the tumor recurring and metastasizing to lungs, liver, and nodes. Chemotherapy and immunotherapy have also been proposed as a treatment, but the rarity of the tumor precludes their use in clinical trials. This is especially true of splenic angiosarcoma in which isolated trials of anticancer agents have been unsuccessful.

Angiosarcomas of the spleen must be distinguished from benign hemangioendotheliomas which may be congenital lesions, usually with multiple sites. Benign hemangioendotheliomas are frequently symptomatic and may be complicated by hemodynamic or coagulation disorders. Splenic hemangiomas must also be differentiated from angiosarcoma. The absence of atypical or malignant appearance of the anastomotic vascular channels should enable such diagnosis to be made with relative ease. Hamartomas and organizing hematomas rarely cause diagnostic confusion. The macroscopic appearance of organizing hematomas occasionally resembles that of an angiosarcoma, and the proliferating endothelial cells may have some histologic atypia. The mitotic activity of the tumor, and the presence of endothelial cell piling and neovascular anastamoses should dispel any doubts about the diagnosis of angiosarcoma. Similarly, angiosarcoma-like changes in thrombosed vessels, lymphangioma, and angiolymphoid hyperplasia with eosinophilia, which features ill-defined lesions composed of numerous proliferative vascular channels, should all be distinguished from angiosarcoma by the distinctive histopathologic characteristics of this tumor.

Hairy cell leukemia with its vascular pseudosinuses, hemangiopericytoma, Kaposi's sarcoma, and spindle-cell tumors having vascular components can also cause diagnostic problems. However, spindle-cell tumors usually have some focal epithelial features, and demonstrate continuity with the basal layer of the epidermis. Kaposi's sarcoma is not seen as a primary splenic tumor but usually as part of a widespread process. It is increasingly seen among homosexuals with AIDS (acquired immunodeficiency syndrome), in whom it is becoming a major health concern.

MISCELLANEOUS

Occasionally, benign neoplastic lesions must be distinguished from metastatic and primary splenic malignancy. In children, splenic cysts are the most common primary lesions of the spleen. In the United States, such cysts are commonly congenital, representing embryonic dysaggregation of mesodermal islets that form the anatomic spleen in the dorsal mesogastrium. Splenic cysts are mostly epidermoid in individuals less than 20 years of age, and usually present as a mass. Symptomatology is minimal, although left upper quadrant fullness or pain, with radiation to the back, shoulder or chest, can be a presenting complaint. Usually solitary, the cysts leave the remaining splenic architecture intact. Infrequently, true dermoid cysts may occur within the spleen. Pseudocysts developing after intrasplenic hemorrhage can also be observed.

Parasitic cysts, uncommon in the United States, are most frequently hydatiform, due to Echinococcus. However, rapidly changing demographic profiles in this country indicate that questions regarding exposure in areas endemic for this and other parasites should be included in the history. If a positive history is elicited, then an eosinophil count, erythrocyte sedimentation rate, Casoni's test and the complement fixation test, the latter being positive in 80% of individuals with echinococcal cyst, will confirm the clinical diagnosis of ecchinococcosis. Direct splenic infection is unusual in this country, especially in children. Most cases of infection or abscess formation involve the immunocompromised host or the individual with an underlying infection, such as pneumonia, empyema or osteomyelitis, or the intravenous drug abuser.

Cystic lymphangioma, a benign lymphatic malformation not ordinarily associated with systemic complaints, can rarely present in the spleen. On ultrasound, cystic lymphangioma is visualized as multiloculated cystic lesions. Radioisotopic uptake is diminished. Hamartoma, the most common benign splenic neoplasm, is a well-circumscribed lesion which is often unencapsulated and appears darker than the surrounding spleen. Since it is the only splenic tumor which contains functioning splenic tissue, its capacity to sequester erythrocyes or to take up ^{99m}technetium sulfur colloid allows its distinction from other splenic neoplasma [20]. Usually an incidental surgical finding, hamartomas of the spleen are rarely of clinical importance.

Lesions metastatic to the spleen have been found in up to 9% of autopsy cases where patients have been diagnosed with cancer [3,213]. The splenic metastases are microscopic in 33% of those cases identified and they are grossly visible at autopsy in 67% [21]. It has been stated that in considering the relative weights of liver and spleen, metastases must be considered as common to the spleen as to the liver [214]. However, the spleen is still a relatively uncommon site of metastasis despite its large lymphoid tissue mass and its role as a filtration site for systemic blood flow.

Particularly frequent in showing metastatic spread to the spleen are carcinomas of the breast, lung, and cervix [1], and malignant melanoma. Direct extension to the spleen from pancreatic carcinoma, or from gastric, colonic or retroperitoneal tumors may also take place.

Mastocytosis, a disorder consisting of abnormal proliferation of tissue mast cells, may involve the spleen. This tumor has onset during any decade, but is most often diagnosed in early childhood [215]. There is no evidence of a neoplastic mast cell clone giving rise to this disorder, the process usually being self-limited, but rarely adults may develop a malignant mast cell proliferation. Generally, mastocytosis is characterized by persistent cutaneous lesions. However, in systemic mastocytosis, affecting about 10% of patients, the presence of extracutaneous disease is indicated by the occurrence of fever, cognitive disorganization, malaise, weight loss, bone pain, or epigastric pain. About half of patients with systemic mastocytosis have splenic infiltration by mast cells. Changes of splenic architecture may be negligible or extensive, and hypersplenism is rarely a complication. Functional asplenia has been observed in patients diagnosed with the malignant variant of this disorder, malignant mastocytosis (216).

Primary plasmacytoma of the spleen is rarely diagnosed. More commonly, splenic infiltration is part of a generalized myelomatosis and no one dominant site can be identified.

Hepatosplenomegaly and subsequent dysfunction can sometimes originate from nonmetastatic tumor (217) or splenic vein thrombosis. However, enlargement of the liver and spleen usually are the result of cancer spread to these organs, and all malignant neoplasms have, at one time or another, been implicated.

SUMMARY

The spleen is an uncommon site of metastatic disease, and is even more infrequently the origin of primary malignant neoplasm. The rarity of neoplastic involvement of the spleen may be due to (1) the presence of mechanical factors, such as capsular resistance to tumoral spread, or certain architectural features of the splenic artery which make direct seeding of tumor difficult, and (2) humoral and cell-mediated immunologic responses by the lymphocytes within the spleen which might prevent initial proliferation and spread of tumor cells.

The clinical features of splenic tumors are not constant but dependent, to a large extent, upon the tumor's histopathology. However, symptoms when present may relate to the size of the spleen and may indicate perisplenitis, mass effect, or pleural effusion. Nonspecific or constitutional complaints may also be made. Red cell, leukocyte, and platelet sequestration by the spleen, and/or spontaneous splenic rupture can be observed. Concomitant hemolysis, megaloblastosis or bone marrow replacement may act to compound already existent anemia or thrombocytopenia, with the attendant clinical problems of bleeding, weakness or infection.

Occasionally, benign neoplastic lesions are confused with metastatic and primary splenic malignancy. Such lesions include hamartoma, the most common benign neoplasm; pseudotumor, true dermoid cyst, or splenic cyst, the most common primary lesion of the spleen in children. Splenic cysts, in the United

States and Europe, are most often congenital, although parasitic infestation is a primary cause of splenic cysts in underdeveloped regions of the world. Direct splenic infection is unusual in the industrialized nations, and usually indicates an immunocompromised or underlying infectious state.

Malignant neoplasms, when present in the spleen, are most often myeloproliferative or lymphoproliferative disorders. This is especially true in the pediatric patient. In adults, splenomegaly is a particularly prominent feature in chronic lymphocytic leukemia, hairy cell leukemia, prolymphocytic leukemia and chronic granulocytic leukemias. In the latter disorder, the development of extramedullary disease, such as dissemination to the spleen with associated enlargement, marks the transformation of the chronic phase to an acute or blastic form of the disease. In childhood, significant hepatosplenomegaly is more likely to accompany acute myelogenous leukemia or indicate the more prognostically unfavorable B cell or T cell leukemias.

Only 1% of all lymphoid malignancies present with splenomegaly as an initial finding, in the absence of significant peripheral lymphadenopathy. Splenomegaly itself is an inconsistent indicator of neoplastic involvement. In Hodgkin's disease, splenic enlargement may denote reactive hyperplasia of splenic tissue. However, a large spleen almost invariably signifies widespread dissemination of malignancy in non-Hodgkin's lymphoma.

While all neoplasms have the capability of metastasizing to the spleen, carcinomas of the breast, lung, and cervix, as well as malignant melanoma metastasize most often. Primary malignancy of the spleen is rare, with just over 200 cases of primary nonlymphoreticular neoplasms of the spleen reported in the world literature. Among nonlymphoreticular splenic neoplasms, angiosarcoma, a tumor with aggressive clinical course and universally poor prognosis, is the most frequently occurring primary neoplasm.

Myelofibrosis, a spectrum of myeloproliferative diseases stemming from a defect in the multipotential hematopoietic stem cell, is characterized by monoclonality and reactive bone marrow fibrosis. Rarely diagnosed in children and young adults, it features severe and progressive splenometaly, with the spleen containing areas of active hematopoiesis.

Among the histiocytoses marked by disseminated or visceral infiltration, histiocytosis-X and malignant histiocytosis figure most prominently, while malignant fibrous histiocytoma is being increasingly diagnosed. Malignant histiocytosis X and disseminated histiocytosis-X have a similar spectrum of organ involvement and may be morphogenetically related. However, the patterns of organ involvement for the two disorders differs. Until recently, the prognosis in these disorders has been very poor, but advances in chemotherapy have brought about improved survival in a significant proportion of patients.

In most malignant neoplastic involvement of the spleen, chemotherapy, immunotherapy or radiotherapy, singly or in combination, form the mainstay of treatment. However, splenectomy, although not always necessary for diagnosis or staging, may provide a therapeutic benefit to the patient. Specifically, patients in whom massive splenomegaly causes significant mass effect of hypersplenism results in severe hematologic compromise, may derive symptomatic relief from splenectomy. Occasionally, as in hairy cell leukemia, a definite survival advantage can be demonstrated after the performance of splenectomy. However, careful consideration should be given to the part hypersplenism and marrow replacement each play in causing hematologic disturbance. Performance of splenectomy early in the course of leukemias such as hairy cell leukemia or chronic granulocytic leukemia may prevent complications and achieve the greatest clinical benefit.

REFERENCES

1. Hirst AE Jr, Bullock WK: Metastatic carcinoma of the spleen. *Am J Med Sci* 1952;223:414–417.
2. Krumbhaar EB: The incidence and nature of splenic neoplasms. *Ann Clin Med* 1927;5:833–860.
3. Wick MR, Smith SL, Scheithauer BW, Beart RW Jr: Primary nonlymphoreticular malignant neoplasms of the spleen. *Am J Surg Pathol* 1982;6:229–242.
4. Zuinghedau J, Duthu A, DeVaux S, Cry C: Presence and significance of tumor cells in the spleen of tumor-bearing hamsters. *Br J Cancer* 1979; 39:594–597.
5. Oisgold-Daga S, Janis MS, Klein S, deBonaparte YP: Immune reactivity of spleen cells in advanced stages of tumor growth. *Biomed Pharmacother* 1982;36:319–323.
6. Kurosu Y, Fukamachi S, Moritak: The significance of relationship of the presence of nonspecific suppressor cells in spleens with gastric cancer-related pathology. *Jap J Surg* 1984;14:293–298.
7. Kanayama H, Hamazae R, Osaki Y, et al: Immunosuppressive factor from the spleen in gastric cancer patients. *Cancer* 1985;56:1963–1166.
8. Al Sam S, Jones DB, Payne SV, Wright DH: Natural killer (NK) activity in the spleen of patients with Hodgkin's Disease and controls. *Br J Cancer* 1982;46:806–810.
9. Ames IH, Garcia AM, John PA, et al: Decreased natural cytotoxicity in mice with high incidence of mammary adenocarcinoma. *Clin Immunol Immunopath* 1986;38:265–273.
10. Dent LA, Jones F: In vivo detection and partial characterization of effector and suppressor cell populations in spleens of mice with large metastatic fibrosarcomas. *Br J Cancer* 1985;51:533–541.
11. Sty J, Conway JJ: The spleen; development and functional evaluation. *Semin Nucl Med* 1985;15:276–298.

12. Donaldson GWK, McArthur M, Macpherson AIS, Richmond J: Blood volume changes in splenomegaly. *Br J Haematol* 1970;18:45-55.
13. Christensen BE: Erythrocyte pooling and sequestration in enlarged spleens. *Scand J Haematol* 1973;10:106-119.
14. Bowring CS, Ferrant AE, Glass HI, et al: Quantitative measurement of splenic and hepatic red-cell destruction. *Br J Haematol* 1975;31:467-477.
15. Eichner ER: Splenic function; normal, too much and too little. *Am J Med* 1979;66:311-320.
16. Smith VC, Eisenberg BL, McDonald EC: Primary splenic angiosarcoma. *Cancer* 1985;55:1625-1627.
17. Lockwood CM, Worlledge S, Nicholas A, et al: Reversal of impaired splenic function in patients with nephritis or vasculitis (or both) by plasma exchange. *N Engl J Med* 1979;300:524-530.
18. Popper H, Selikoff IJ: Spontaneous rupture of hepatic and splenic angiosarcoma demonstrated by CT. *AJR* 1982;138:965-966.
19. Wilkinson LS, Tang A, Gjedsted A: Marked lymphocytosis suggesting chronic lymphocytic leukemia in three patients with hyposplenism. *Am J Med* 1983;75:1053-1056.
20. Kuykendall JD, Shanser JD, Sumner TE, Goodman LR: Multimodal approach to diagnosis of hamartoma of the spleen. *Pediatr Radiol* 1977;5:239-421.
21. Federle M, Moss AA: Computerized tomography of the spleen. *CRC Crit Rev Diag Imaging* 1983;19:1-16.
22. Groshar D, Israel O, Front D: Spleen imaging—enlargement of the spleen. *Semin Nucl Med* 1983;13:295-297.
23. Meyers MJ: Spleen imaging. *Clin Haematol* 1983;12:395-420.
24. Biemer JJ: Hepatic manifestations of lymphomas. *Ann Clin Lab Sci* 1984;14:252-260.
25. Hermann GS, Fogh J, Graem N, et al: Primary hemangiosarcoma of the spleen with angioscintigraphic demonstration of metastases. *Cancer* 1984;1682-1685.
26. Hagenberg HJA, Muller CJ: Accuracy or inaccuracy of spleen mass measurements from radionuclide images. *Diag Imag Clin Med* 1984;53:288-291.
27. Lindfors KK, Meyer JE, Palmer EL III, Harris NL: Scintigraphic findings in large-cell lymphoma of the spleen; concise communication. *J Nuc Med* 1984;25:969-971.
28. Sommer FG, Hoppe RT, Fellingham L, et al: Spleen structure in Hodgkin's Disease; ultrasonic characterization. *Radiology* 1984;53:219-222.
29. Steinherz PG, Exelby PR, Young J, Watson RC: Splenectomy after angiographic embolization of the splenic artery in patients with massive splenomegaly and severe thrombocytopenia, in juvenile subacute myelomonocytic leukemia. *Med Pediatr Oncol* 1984;12:28-32.
30. Jansson SE, Bondestam S, Heinonen E, et al: Value of liver and spleen aspiration biopsy in malignant diseases when these organs show no signs of involvement in sonography. *Acta Med Scand* 1983;213:279-281.

31. Mitchell A, Morris PJ: Splenectomy for malignant lymphoma. *World J Surg* 1984;9:444-448.
32. Kitchens CS: The syndrome of post-splenectomy fulminant sepsis; case report and review of the literature. *Am J Med Sci* 1977;274:303-310.
33. Chilcote RR, Baehner RL, Hammond D: The Investigators and Special Studies Committee of the Children's Cancer Study Group; septicemia and meningitis in children splenectomized for Hodgkin's disease. *N Engl J Med* 1976;295:798-800.
34. Morganstern L, Rosenberg J, Geller SA: Tumors of the spleen. *World J Surg* 1885;9:468-478.
35. Dearth JC, Gilchrist GS, Telander RL, et al: Partial splenectomy for staging Hodgkin's disease; risk of false-negative results. *N Engl J Med* 1978;299: 345-346.
36. Goffinet DR, Warnke R, Kunnick NR, et al: Clinical and surgical (laparotomy) evaluation of patients with non-Hodgkin's lymphomas. *Cancer Treat Rep* 1977;61:981-992.
37. Maurer R: The role of the spleen in leukemias and lymphomas including Hodgkin's disease. *Experientia* 1985;41:215-224.
38. Christensen BE, Jonsson V, Videbaek A: The spleen in lymphoproliferative disorders. *Clin Haematol* 1983;12:517-533.
39. Dighiers G, Charron D, Debre P, et al: Identification of a pure splenic form of chronic lymphocytic leukemia. *Br J Haematol* 1979;41:169-176.
40. Paolino W, Infelise V, Levis A, et al: Adenosplenomegaly and prognosis in uncomplicated and complicated chronic lymphocytic leukemia. *Cancer* 1984;54:339-346.
41. Golde DW: Disorders of mononuclear phagocyte proliferation, maturation and function. *Clin Haematol* 1975;4:705-721.
42. Meijer CJLM, Albeda FF, Van Der Valk P, et al: Immunohistochemical studies of the spleen in hairy-cell leukemia. *Am J Pathol* 1984;115:266-274.
43. Quinn JJ: The lymphoproliferative disorders. In, Altman AJ, Schwartz AD, eds; *Malignant Diseases of Infancy, Childhood, and Adolescence*, Philadelphia, W.B. Saunders, 1983;239-206.
44. Goldman JM, Nolasco I: The spleen in myeloproliferative disorders. *Clin Haematol* 1983;12:505-516.
45. Champlin RE, Golde DW: Chronic myelogenous leukemia; recent advances. *Blood* 1985;65:1039-1047.
46. Castro-Malaspina H, Schaison G, Passe S, et al: Subacute and chronic myelomonocytic leukemia in children (juvenile CML). Clinical and hematologic observations, and identification of prognostic factors. *Cancer* 1984;675: 686.
47. Fefer A, Cheever MA, Greenberg PD, et al: Treatment of chronic granulocytic leukemia with chemoradiotherapy and transplantation of marrow from identical twins. *N Engl J Med* 1982;306:63-68.

48. Golomb HM, Vardiman JW: Response to splenectomy in 65 patients with hairy cell leukemia; an evaluation of spleen weight and bone marrow involvement. *Blood* 1983;61:349-352.
49. Garrison RN, McCoy M, Winkler C, et al: Splenectomy in hematologic malignancy. *Am Surg* 1984;50:428-432.
50. Coon WW: The limited role of splenectomy in patients with leukemia. *Surg Gynecol Obstet* 1985;160:291-294.
51. Ihde DC, Canellos GP, Schwartz TW, DeVita VT: Splenectomy in the chronic phase of chronic granulocytic leukemia. *Ann Intern Med* 1976;84:17-21.
52. Aabo K, Walton-Jorgensen S: Spleen irradiation in chronic lymphocytic leukemia (CLL): palliation in patients unfit for splenectomy. *Am J Hematol* 1985;19:177-180.
53. Miller DR, Leikin S, Albo V, et al: Prognostic factors and therapy in acute lymphoblastic leukemia of childhood: CCG-141. *Cancer* 1983;51:1041-1641.
54. Chessells JM, Durrant J, Hardy RM, Richards S: Medical Research Council Leukaemia Trial—UKALL V: An attempt to reduce the immunosuppressive effects of therapy in childhood acute lymphoblastic leukemia. *J Clin Oncol* 1986;4:1758-1764.
55. Steinherz PG, Gaynon P, Miller DR, et al: Improved disease-free survival of children with acute lymphoblastic leukemia at high risk for early relapse with the New York regimen—A new intensive therapy protcol: A report from the Childrens Cancer Study Group. *J Clin Oncol* 1986;4:744-752.
56. Rivera GK, Buchanan G, Boyett JM, et al: Intensive retreatment of childhood acute lymphoblastic leukemia in first bone marrow relapse. A Pediatric Oncology Group Study. *N Engl J Med* 1986;315:273-278.
57. Clavell LA, Gelber RD, Cohen HJ, et al: Four-agent induction and intensive asparaginase therapy for treatment of childhood acute lymphoblastic leukemia. *N Engl J Med* 1986;315:657-663.
58. Linker CA, Levitt LJ, O'Donnell M, et al: Improved results of treatment of adult acute lymphoblastic leukemia. *Blood* 1987;69:1242-1248.
59. Kennedy BJ: Leukemia and lymphoma in the elderly. *Front Radiat Ther Oncol* 1986;20:150-156.
60. Golomb HM, Ratain MJ: Recent advances in the treatment of hairy-cell leukemia. *N Engl J Med* 1987;316:870-872.
61. Jim RTS: Failure of immunotherapy to prolong survival in chronic myeloid leukemia. *Hawaii Med J* 1985;44:471-472.
62. Advani SH, Gulwani B, Ghogale SG, et al: Effects of administration of BCG, levamisole and irradiated leukemic cells on immune status and remission status in chronic myelogenous leukemia. *Oncology* 1985;42:275-281.
63. Ota K, Kurita S, Yamada K, et al: Immunotherapy with bestatin for acute nonlymphocytic leukemia in adults. *Cancer Immunol Immunother* 1986;23:5-10.
64. Bennett CL, Westbrook CA, Gruber B, Golomg HM: Hairy cell leukemia

and mucormycosis. Treatment with alpha-2 interferon. *Am J Med* 1986; 81:1065-1067.
65. Ehmann WC, Silber R: Recombinant alpha-2 interferon for treatment of hairy cell leukemia without prior splenectomy. *Am J Med* 1986;80:1111-1114.
66. Quesada JR, Gutterman JU, Hersh EM: Treatment of hairy cell leukemia with alpha interferons. *Cancer* 1986;57:1678-1680.
67. Castaigne S, Sigaux F, Cantell K, et al: Interferon-alpha in the treatment of hairy cell leukemia. *Cancer* 1986;57:1681-1684.
68. Flandrin G, Sigaux F, Castaigne S, et al: Treatment of hairy cell leukemia with recombinant alpha interferon. I. Quantitative study of bone marrow changes during the first months of treatment. *Blood* 1986;67:817-820.
69. Golombe HM: Interferons: present and future use in cancer therapy. *J Clin Oncol* 1986;4:123-125.
70. Ochs J, Abromowitch M, Rudnick S, Murphy SB: Phase I-II study of recombinant alpha-2 interferon against advanced leukemia and lymphoma in children. *J Clin Oncol* 1986;4:883-887.
71. Merz B: Interferon's track record; good in hairy-cell leukemia, fair in other hematologic cancers, poor in solid tumors. *JAMA* 1986;256:1242-1244.
72. Gastl G, Aulitzky W, Margreiter R et al: Recombinant alpha-2 interferon for induction and maintenance of remission in hairy cell leukaemia. *Br J Haematol* 1985;61:581-582.
73. Worman CP, Catovsky D, Bevan PC, et al: Interferon is effective in hairy-cell leukaemia. *Br J Haematol* 1985;60:759-763.
74. Janssen JTP, Ludwig H, Scheithauer W, et al: Phase I study of recombinant human interferon alpha-2C in patients with chemotherapy-refractory malignancies. *Oncology* 1985;42(suppl 1):3-6.
75. Huber C, Glener R, Gastl G: Interferon-alpha-2C in the treatment of advanced hairy cell leukaemia. Results of a phase II trial. *Oncology* 1985; 42(suppl 1):7-9.
76. Rohatiner AZS, Richards MA, Barnett MJ, et al: Chlorambucil and interferon for lowgrade non-Hodgkin's lymphoma. *Br J Cancer* 1987;55:225-226.
77. Semenzato G, Pizzolo G, Agostino C, et al: Alpha-interferon activates the natural killer system in patients with hairy cell leukemia. *Blood* 1986;68: 293-296.
77a. Billard C, Sigaux F, Castaigne S, et al: Treatment of hairy cell leukemia with recombinant alpha interferon: II. In vivo down-regulation of alpha interferon receptors on tumor cells. *Blood* 1986;67:821-826.
78. Dupuy E, Sigaux F, Bryokaert MC, et al: Platelet acquired defect in PDGF and beta thromboglobulin content in hairy cell leukaemia: improvement after interferon therapy. *Br J Haematol* 1987;65:107-110.
79. Raghavachar A, Dartram CR, Porzsolt F: Eradication of one clone in biclonal hairy cell leukaemia. *Lancet* 1986;ii:516.
80. Bardawil RG, Groves C, Ratain MJ, et al: Changes in peripheral blood and bone marrow specimens following therapy with recombinant alpha interferon for hairy cell leukemia. *Am J Clin Pathol* 1986;85:194-201.

81. Foon KA, Nakano GM, Koller CA, et al: Response to 2'-deoxycoformycin after failure of interferon-alpha in nonsplenectomized patients with hairy cell leukemia. *Blood* 1986;68:297-300.
82. Talpaz M, McCredie KB, Mavliget GM, Gutterman JU: Leukocyte interferon-induced mycloid cytoreduction in chronic myelogenous leukemia. *Blood* 1983;62:689-692.
83. Talpaz M, McCredie K, Kantarjian H, et al: Chronic myelogenous leukaemia; haematological remissions with alpha-interferon. *Br J Haematol* 1986; 64:87-95.
84. Parkman R: Current status of bone marrow transplantation in pediatric oncology. *Cancer* 1986;58:569-572.
85. Gale RP: Clinical trials of bone marrow transplantation. *Isr J Med Sci* 1986;22:260-263.
86. Chessels JM, Rogers DW, Leiper AD, et al: Bone-marrow transplantation has a limited role in prolonging second marrow remission in childhood lymphoblastic leukaemia. *Lancet* 1986;i:1239-1241.
87. Hows JM, Yin JL, Marsh J, et al: Histocompatible unrelated volunteer donors compared with HLA nonidentical family donors in marrow transplantation for aplastic anemia and leukemia. *Blood* 1986;68:1322-1328.
88. Lehn P, Devergie A, Benbunan M, et al: Bone marrow transplantation for chronic granulocytic leukemia. *J Natl Cancer Inst* 1986;76:1301-1305.
89. Fefer A, Clift RA, Thomas ED: Allogeneic marrow transplantation for chronic granulocytic leukemia. *J Natl Cancer Inst* 1986;76:1295-1299.
90. Blume KG, Forman SJ, Synder DS, et al: Allogeneic bone marrow transplantation for acute lymphoblastic leukemia during first complete remission. *Transplantation* 1987;43:389-392.
91. Ringden O, Zwaan F, Hermans J, Gratwohl A for the Leukemia Working Party of the European Group for Bone Marrow Transplantation: European experience of bone marrow transplantation for leukemia. *Transplant Proc* 1987;19:2600-2604.
92. Herzig RH, Bortin MM, Barrett AJ, et al: Bone-marrow transplantation in high-risk acute lymphoblastic leukaemia in first and second remission. *Lancet* 1987;1:786-789.
93. Forman SJ, Krance RA, O'Donnell MR, et al: Bone Marrow transplantation for acute nonlymphoblastic leukemia during first complete remission. *Transplantation* 1987;43:650-654.
94. O'Reilly RJ: Current developments in marrow transplantation. *Transplant Proc* 1987;19:92-102.
95. Blume KG, Forman SJ, O'Donnell MR, et al: Allogeneic bone marrow transplantation for acute lymphoblastic leukemia during first complete remission.
96. Verdirame JD, Bruckman JE, Feagler JR, Commers JR: Bone marrow transplantation for good-risk patients with leukemia in a university affiliated hospital. *Am J Hematol* 1986;22:365-373.
97. Fefer A, Cheever MA, Greenberg PD: Identical-twin (syngeneic) marrow transplantation for hematologic cancers. *J Natl Cancer Inst* 1986;76:1269-1273.

98. Trigg ME: Role of bone-marrow transplantation as retrieval therapy for acute lymphoblastic leukaemia in childhood. *Lancet* 1986;ii:102.
99. Sanders JE, Thomas ED, Buckner CD, et al: Marrow transplantation for children in first remission of acute nonlymphoblastic leukemia: an update. *Blood* 1985;66:460–462.
100. Herve P and the Cooperative Study Group on T Cell Depletion: Depletion of T-lymphocytes in donor marrow with pa-T monoclonal antibodies and complement for prevention of acute graft-versus-host disease: A pilot study on 29 patients. *J Natl Cancer Inst* 1986;76:1311–1316.
101. Champlin RE, Ho WG, Mitsuyasu R, et al: Graft failure and leukemia relapse following T lymphocyte-depleted bone marrow transplants: effect of intensification of immunosuppressive conditioning. *Transplant Proc* 1987;19:2616–2619.
102. Sondel PM, Hank JA, Trigg ME, et al: Transplantation of HLA-haploidentical T-cell-depleted marrow for leukemia: autologous marrow recovery with specific immune sensitization to donor antigens. *Exp Hemat* 1986;14:278–286.
103. Gorin NC, Herve P, Aegerter P, et al: Autologous bone marrow transplantation for acute leukaemia in remission. *Br J Haematol* 1986;64:385–395.
104. Ito T, Ishikawa Y, Noda M, Fujii R: Preliminary clinical trial of autologous bone marrow transplantation after in vitro monoclonal antibody and complement treatments in null cell-type acute lymphocytic leukemia. *Jpn J Cancer Res* (Gann) 1985;76:1222–1229.
105. Yeager AM, Kaizer H, Santos GW, et al: Autologous bone marrow transplantation in patients with acute nonlymphocytic leukemia, using ex vivo marrow treatment with 4-hydroxyperoxycyclophosphamide. *N Engl J Med* 1986;315:141–147.
106. Reiffers J, Gorin NC, Michallet M, et al: Autografting for chronic granulocytic leukemia in transformation. *J Natl Cancer Inst* 1986;76:1307–1310.
107. Pico JL, Hartmann O, Maraninchi D, et al: Modified chemotherapy with carmustine, cytarabine, cyclophosphamide and 6-thioguanine (BACT) and autologous bone marrow transplantation in 24 poor-risk patients with acute lymphoblastic leukemia. *J Natl Cancer Inst* 1986;76:1289–1293.
108. Gorin NC: Autologous bone marrow transplantation in acute leukemia. *J Natl Cancer Inst* 1986;76:1281–1287.
109. Harris NL, Aisenberg AC, Meyer JE, et al: Diffuse large cell (histiocytic) lymphoma of the spleen. *Cancer* 1984;54:2460–2467.
110. Narang S, Wolf BC, Neiman RS: Malignant lymphoma presenting with prominent splenomegaly. *Cancer* 1985;55:1948–1957.
111. Biemer JJ: Hepatic manifestation of lymphomas. *Ann Clin Lab Sci* 1984;14:252–260.
112. Ture S, Mazza P, Lauria F, et al: Non-Hodgkin's lymphomas in leukemic phase: incidence, prognosis and therapeutic implications. *Scand J Haematol* 1985;35:123–131.

113. Spier CM, Kjeldsberg CR, Eyre HJ, Behn FG: Malignant lymphoma with primary presentation in the spleen. *Arch Pathol Lab Med* 1985;109:1076-1080.
114. Breitfeld V, Lee RE: Pathology of the spleen in hematologic disease. *Surg Clin NA* 1975;55:233-251.
115. Das Gupta T, Coombes B, Brasfield RD: Primary malignant neoplasms of the spleen. *Surg Gynecol Obstet* 1965;120:947-960.
116. Skarin AT, Davey FR, Moloney WC: Lymphosarcoma of the spleen. *Arch Intern Med* 1971;127:259-265.
117. Dacie JV, Brain MC, Harrison CV, et al: "Non-Tropical idiopathic splenomegaly" ("primary hypersplenism"): a review of ten cases and their relationship to malignant lymphomas. *Br J Haematol* 1969;17:317-333.
118. Koziner B. Myers J, Cirrincione C, et al: Treatment of stages I and II Hodgkin's disease with three different therapeutic modalities. *Am J Med* 1986;80:1067-1078.
119. Rubin P, Constine L, Bennett J: Hodgkin's disease IIB or not to be—using irradiation alone or in combination with chemotherapy? That is the question! *J Clin Oncol* 1986;4:455-457.
120. Crnkovich MJ, Hoppe RT, Rosenberg SA: Stage IIB Hodgkin's disease; the Stanford experience. *J Clin Oncol* 1986;4:472-479.
121. Lampkin BC, Wong KY, Kalinyak K, et al: Solid malignancies in children and adolescents. *Surg Clin N Am* 1985;64:1351-1386.
122. Vinciguerra V, Proper KJ, Coleman M, et al: Alternating cycles of combination chemotherapy for patients with recurrent Hodgkin's disease following radiotherapy; a prospectively randomized study by the Cancer and Leukemia Group B. *J Clin Oncol* 1986;4:838-844.
123. Behrendt H, van Bunningen BNFM, van Leeuwen EF: Treatment of Hodgkin's disease in children with or without radiotherapy. *Cancer* 1987;59:1870-1873.
124. Sullivan MP, Boyett J, Pullen J, et al: Pediatric Oncology Group experience with modified LSA_1-L_2 therapy in 107 children with non-Hodgkin's lymphoma (Burkitt's lymphoma excluded). *Cancer* 1985;55:323-336.
125. Skarin AT: Diffuse aggressive lymphomas: a curable subset of non-Hodgkin's lymphomas. *Semin Oncol* 1986;4(suppl 5):10-25.
126. Rusthoden JJ: Current approaches to the treatment of advanced-stage non-Hodgkin's lymphoma. *Can Med Assoc J* 1987;136:29-36.
127. Rubin P, Zagars G, Cheang C, Thomas EM: Hodgkin's disease; is there a price for successful treatment? A 25 year experience. *Int J Radiation Oncology Biol Phys* 1986;12:153-166.
128. Boivin JF, Hutchinson GB: Leukemia and other cancers after radiotherapy and chemotherapy for Hodgkin's disease. *J Natl Cancer Inst* 1981;67:751-758.
129. Nelson DF, Cooper S, Weston MG, Rubin P: Second malignant neoplasms in patients treated for Hodgkin's disease with radiotherapy or radiotherapy and chemotherapy. *Cancer* 1981;48:2386-2393.

130. Smyth JF, Balkwill FR, Cavalli F, et al: Interferons in oncology: current status and future directions. *Eur J Clin Oncol* 1987;23:887-889.
131. Horning SJ, Merigan TC, Krown SE, et al: Human interferon alpha in malignant lymphoma and Hodgkin's disease. *Cancer* 1985;56:1305-1310.
132. Phillips GL, Herzig RH, Lazarus HM, et al: High-dose chemotherapy, fractionated total-body irradiation, and allogeneic marrow transplantation for malignant lymphoma. *J Clin Oncol* 1986;4:480-488.
133. Anderson CC, Goldstone AH, Souhami RL, et al: Very high dose chemotherapy with autologous bone marrow rescue in adult patients with resistant relapsed lymphoma. *Cancer Chemother Pharmacol* 1986;16:170-175.
134. Jagannath S, Dicke KA, Armitage JO, et al: High-dose cyclophosphamide, carmustine, and etoposide, and autologous bone marrow transplantation for relapsed Hodgkin's disease. *Ann Int Med* 1986;104:163-168.
135. Dumont J, Teillet F: Autologous bone marrow transplantation in Hodgkin's disease. *Blood Transfusion Immunohaemat* 1985;28:531-538.
136. Kahn A, Bernard JF, Cottreau D, Marie J, Bowin P: A deficient G-6PD variant with hemizygous expression in blood cells of a woman with primary myelofibrosis. *Hemangenetik* 1975;30:41-46.
137. Shalev O, Goldfarb A, Ariel I, Rachmilewitz E: Myelofibrosis in young adults. *Acta Haematol* 1983;70:396-399.
138. Gilbert HS: Myelofibrosis revisited: characterization and classification of myelofibrosis in the setting of myeloproliferative disease. *Progr Clin Biol Res* 1984;154:3-17.
139. Wolf JL, Spruce WE, Bearman RM, et al: Reversal of acute ("malignant") myelosclerosis by allogeneic bone marrow transplantation. *Blood* 1982; 59:191-193.
140. Hahn EG, Hochweiss S, Berk PD: Diagnostic parameters of altered collagen turnover. *Progr Clin Biol Res* 1984;154:335-343.
141. McCarthy DM: Fibrosis of the bone marrow: content and causes. *Br J Haematol* 1985;59:1-7.
142. Fruchtman SM: Therapeutic implications of collagen metabolism in myelofibrosis. *Prog Clin Biol Res* 1984;154:467-474.
143. Adamson JW, Powell JS: The spleen as a source of colony-forming cells in myelofibrosis. *Progr Clin Biol Res* 1984;154:323-334.
144. Hibbin JA, Njoku OS, Matutes E, et al: Myeloid progenitor cells in the circulation of patients with myelofibrosis and other myeloproliferative disorders. *Br J Haematol* 1984;57:495-503.
145. Van Heerde P, Feltkamp CA, Hart AAM, et al: Malignant histiocytosis and related tumors. A clinicopathologic study of 42 cases using cytological, histochemical and ultrastructural parameters. *Hematol Oncol* 1984; 2:13-32.
146. Esseltine DW, DeLeeuw NKM, Berry GR: Malignant histiocytosis. *Cancer* 1983;52:1904-1910.
147. Zucker JM, Caillaux JM, Vanel D, Gerard-Marchant R: Malignant histiocytosis in childhood. *Cancer* 1980;45:2821-2829.

148. Jurco S, Starling K, Hawkins EP: Malignant histiocytosis in childhood: morphologic considerations. *Hum Pathol* 1983;14:1059–1065.
149. Goldman JM, Jacobson BM, James GW III: Splenectomy for histiocytic medullary reticulosis. *Postgrad Med J* 1971;47:671–686.
150. Lambert IA, Catovsky D, Bergier N: Malignant Histiocytosis: a clinicopathological study of 12 cases. *Br J Haematol* 1977;40:65–77.
151. Mogi G, Maeda S, Yoshida T: Histiocytic medullary reticulosis with involvement of the nose. *Laryngoscope* 1976;86:1752–1756.
152. Chawla SK, Lopresti PA, Burdman D, et al: Diffuse small bowel involvement in malignant histiocytosis. *Am J Gastroenterol* 1975;63:129–134.
153. Esumi N, Hashida T, Matsumura T, et al: Malignant histiocytosis in childhood. Clinical features and therapeutic results by combination chemotherapy. *Am J Ped Hem/Onc* 1986;8:300–307.
154. Salz-Steiner D, Eldor A, Vangrover D, et al: Disseminated intravascular coagulation in two patients with histiocytic medullary reticulosis. *Am J Clin Pathol* 1984;82:119–123.
155. Williams DM, Clement JR: Malignant histiocytosis appearing as cold-agglutinin disease. *South Med J* 1985;78:1373–1376.
156. Isaacson PG: Histiocytic malignancy. *Histopathology* 1985;9:1007–1011.
157. Falini B, Bucciarelli E, Grignani F, Martelli MF: Erythrophagocytosis by undifferentiated lung carcinoma cells. *Cancer* 1980;46:1140–1145.
158. Theodorakis ME, Zamkoff KW, Davey FR, et al: Acute nonlymphocytic leukemia complicated by severe cytophagocytosis of formed blood elements by nonmalignant histiocytes: cause of significant clinical morbidity. *Med Pediatr Oncol* 1983;11:20–26.
159. Jaffe ES, Costa J, Fauci AS, et al: Malignant lymphoma and erythrophagocytosis simulating malignant histiocytosis. *Am J Med* 1983;75:741–749.
160. Kim TH, Chan WC, Alvarado C, et al: Malignant histiocytosis after lymphoblastic lymphoma. *Am J Dis Child* 1983;137:474–476.
161. Heiman DF, Haas M, Griffiths JK, Bia FJ: Fever, jaundice and histiocytic erythrophagocytosis: fulminant infection or malignancy? *Yale J Biol Med* 1984;57:787–795.
162. Rubin M, Rothenberg SP, Panchacaharam P: A histiocytic medullary reticulosis-like syndrome as the terminal event in lymphocytic lymphoma. *Am J Med Sci* 1984;287:60–62.
163. O'Brien CJ, Child JA, Stark A, et al: Concurrent T-cell lymphocytic lymphoma and malignant histiocytosis. *Histopathology* 1985;9:977–986.
164. Yin JAL, Kumaran TO, Marsh GW, et al: Complete recovery of histiocytic medullary reticulosis-like syndrome in a child with acute lymphoblastic leukemia. *Cancer* 1983;51:200–202.
165. Danish EH, Dahms BB, Kumar ML: Cytomegalovirus-associated hemophagocytic syndrome. *Pediatrics* 1985;75:280–283.
166. Davson J: Virus-associated hemophagocytic syndrome or malignant histiocytosis? *J Pediatr* 1985;107:989.

167. Sullivan JL, Woda BA, Herrod HG, et al: Epstein-Barr virus-associated hemophagocytic syndrome: virological and immunopathological studies. *Blood* 1985;65:1097-1104.
168. Tubbs RR, Sheibani K, Sebek BA, Savage RA: Malignant histiocytosis. Ultrastructural and immunocytochemical characterization. *Arch Pathol Lab Med* 1980;104:26-29.
169. Vilpo JA, Klemi P, Lassila O, et al: Cytological and functional characterization of three cases of malignant histiocytosis. *Cancer* 1980;46:1795-1801.
170. Plous R: Malignant histiocytosis. *Mt Sinai J Med (NY)* 1985;52:496-498.
171. Warnke RA, Kim H, Dorfman RF: Malignant histiocytosis (histiocytic medullary reticulosis). I. Clinico-pathologic study of 29 cases. *Cancer* 1975;35:215-230.
172. Alexander M, Daniels JR: Chemotherapy of malignant histiocytosis in adults. *Cancer* 1977;39:1011-1017.
173. Tseng A Jr, Coleman CN, Cox RS, et al: The treatment of malignant histiocytes. *Blood* 1984;64:48-53.
174. Simon JH, Tebbi CK, Freeman AI, et al: Malignant histiocytosis. Complete remission in two pediatric patients. *Cancer* 1987;59:1566-1570.
174a. Pizzuto J, Aviles A, Conte G, et al: Adriamycin and splenectomy in the treatment of histiocytic medullary reticulosis. *Med Pediatr Oncol* 1980; 8:41-46.
175. Tirelli U, Veronesi A, Galligioni E, et al: Adriamycin, vincristine, and prednisone (HOP) in the treatment of malignant histiocytosis. *Am J Clin Oncol* 1983;6:605-606.
176. Abrams RA, Hanson G, Hansen R, et al: Malignant histiocytosis resistant to anthracycline. Response to intensive treatment with etoposide and amsacrine. *Arch Intern Med* 1985;145:742-743.
177. Vera R Jr, Bertino JR, Cadman E, Waldron JA: Malignant histiocytosis. Response to VP-16-213 and cytosine arabinoside. *Cancer* 1984;54:991-993.
178. Schouten TJ, Hustinix TWJ, Scheres JMJC, et al: Malignant histiocytosis. Clinical and cytogenetic studies in a newborn and a child. *Cancer* 1983; 52:1229-1236.
179. Fischer A, Virelizier JL, Arenzama-Seisdedos F, et al: Treatment of four patients with erythrophagocytic lymphohistiocytosis by a combination of epipodophyllotoxin, steroids, intrathecal methotrexate, and cranial irradiation. *Pediatrics* 1985;76:263-268.
180. Landing B: Distribution of involvement in Letterer-Siwe Disease and lymphohistiocytosis. *Pediatr Pathol* 1984;2:395-399.
181. Enriquez P, Dahlin DC, Hayles AB, Henderson ED: Histiocytosis X: A clinical study. *Mayo Clin Proc* 1967;42:88-99.
182. Broadbent V, Pritchard J: Histiocytosis X—current controversies. *Arch Dis Child* 1985;60:605-607.
183. Osband ME, Lipton JM, Lavin P, et al: Histiocytosis X. Demonstration of

abnormal immunity, T-cell histamine H_2-receptor deficiency, and successful treatment with thymic extract. *N Engl J Med* 1981;304:146-153.
184. Parker BR, Pinckney L, Etcubanas E: Relative efficacy of radiographic and radionuclide bone surveys in the detection of the skeletal lesions of histiocytosis X. *Radiology* 1980;134:377-380.
185. Nezelof C, Diebold N, Rousseau-Merck MF: Ig surface receptors of erythrophagocytic activity of histiocytosis X cells in vitro. *J Pathol* 1977; 122:105-113.
186. Tsunematsu Y, Koide R, Watanabe S, et al: A clinicopathological study of histiocytosis X. *Japan J Clin Oncol* 1984;14:633-646.
187. Wolfson WL, Gossett T, Pagani J: Systemic giant cell histiocytosis—report of a case and a review of the adult form of Letterer-Siwe Disease. *Cancer* 1976;38:2529-2537.
188. Gianotti F, Caputo R: Histiocytic syndromes: A review. *J Am Acad Dermatol* 1985;13:383-404.
189. Sims DG: Histiocytosis X. *Arch Dis Child* 1977;52:433-440.
190. Talbot ML: Histiocytosis X. *Amer Surg* 1974;40:89-96.
191. Lahey ME: Histiocytosis X—comparison of three treatment regimens. *J Pediatr* 1975;87:179-183.
192. Lahey E: Histiocytosis X—an analysis of prognostic factors. *J Pediatr* 1975;184-189.
193. Lahey E: Prognostic factors in histiocytosis. *Pediatr Pathol* 1984;2:383-387.
194. Greenberger J: Clinical evolution of the histiocytoses. *Pediatr Pathol* 1984; 2:383-387.
195. Murphy SB: The lymphomas, lymphadenopathy, and histiocytoses. In, Nathan DG, Oski FA, (eds.): Hematology of Infancy and Childhood. Philadelphia. W. B. Saunders Company, 1981, pp. 1051-1065.
196. LeBlanc A, Hadchouel M, Jehan P, et al: Obstructive jaundice in children with histiocytosis X. *Gastroenterology* 1981;80:134-139.
197. Donati MB, Casteels-VanDaele M, et al: Hypofibrinogenemia in Histiocytosis X, type Letterer-Siwe Disease. *Helv Paediat Acta* 1973;28:603-609.
198. Lichtenstein L: Histiocytosis X. Integration of eosinophilic granuloma of bone, "Letterer-Siwe disease," and "Schüller-Christian Disease" as related manifestations of a single nosologic entity. *Arch Pathol* 1953;56:84-102.
199. Broadbent V, Davies EG, Heaf D, et al: Spontaneous remission of multisystem histiocytosis X. *Lancet* 1984;1:253.
200. Starling KA, Donaldson MH, Haggard ME, et al: Therapy of histiocytosis X with vincristine, vinblastine, and cyclophosphamide. *Am J Dis Child* 1972;123:105-110.
201. Komp DM, Silva-Sosa M, Miale T, et al: Evaluation of a MOPP-type regiment in histiocytosis X—A Southwest Oncology Group study. *Cancer Treat Rep* 1977;61:855-859.
202. Komp DM, Trueworthy R, Hvizdala E, Sexauer C: Prednisolone, methotrexate, and 6-mercaptopurine in the treatment of histiocytosis X. *Cancer Treat Res* 1979;63:2125-2126.

203. Griffin TW: The treatment of advanced histiocytosis-X with sequential hemibody irradiation. *Cancer* 1977;39:2435-2436.
204. Davies EG, Levinsky RJ, Butler M, et al: Thymic hormone therapy for histiocytosis X? *N Engl J Med* 1983;309:493-494.
205. Ringden O, Ahstrom L, Lonnqvist B, et al: Allogeneic bone marrow transplantation in a patient with chemotherapy-resistant progressive histiocytosis X. *N Engl J Med* 1987;316:733-735.
206. Kearney MM, Soule EH, Ivins JC: Malignant fibrous histiocytoma. A retrospective study of 167 cases. *Cancer* 1980;45:167-178.
207. Govoni E, Bazzocchi F, Piler S, Martinelli G. Primary malignant fibrous histiocytoma of the spleen. *Histopathology* 1982;6:351-361.
208. Fletcher CDM, McKee PH: Sarcomas—a clinicopathological guide with particular reference to cutaneous manifestation. III. Angiosarcoma, malignant hemangiopericytoma, fibrosarcoma and synovial sarcoma. *Clin Exp Dermatol* 1985;10:332:349.
209. Silverman PM, Ram PC, Korobkin M: CT appearance of abdominal thorotrast deposition and thorotrast-induced angiosarcoma of the liver. *J Comput Assist Tomogr* 1983;7:655-658.
210. Fawcett FJ, Easterbrook P, Smerdon GR: Angiosarcoma of liver and spleen in a scrap metal merchant. *Br J Ind Med* 1983;40:113-114.
211. Morales PH, Lindsberg RD, Barkley HT Jr: Soft tissue angiosarcoma. *Int J Radiat Oncol Biol Phys* 1981;7:1655-1659.
212. Graham WJ, Bogardus CR Jr: Angiosarcoma treated with radiation therapy alone. *Cancer* 1981;48:912-914.
213. Scully RE, Mark EJ, McNeely BU: Case records of Massachusetts General Hospital. 15-1982. *N Engl J Med* 1982;306:918-925.
214. Butler JJ: Pathology of the spleen in benign and malignant conditions. *Histopathology* 1983;7:453-474.
215. Tharp MD: Southwestern internal medicine conference: The spectrum of mastocytosis. *Am J Med Sci* 1985;289:119-132.
216. Roth J, Brudler O, Henze E: Functional asplenia in malignant mastocytosis. *J Nucl Med* 1985;26:1149-1152.
217. Conroy B: Primary adrenal carcinoma as a cause of non-metastatic hepatosplenomegaly and liver dysfunction syndrome. *J Roy Nav Med Serv* 1984;70:163-165.

11

Splenomegaly
Storage Disorders

IRENE N. SILLS
Diabetes Program Children's Hospital of Buffalo, Buffalo, New York

Storage disorders usually are due to specific inherited enzyme deficiencies in the degradation of products of cellular metabolism. As a consequence of these deficiencies, there is accumulation of that substrate which occurs prior to the missing enzyme in the metabolic pathway. Many of the storage disorders represent lysosomal enzyme deficiencies, since the lysosomes are key in the catabolism of cellular waste. Continuous uptake in the lysosomes of non-metabolizable substrate leads to lysosomal overload and eventual cell dysfunction.

This macromolecular accumulation does not occur uniformly in all tissues. Instead, the accumulations occur only in locations where there is abundant substrate and where degradation of the substrate occurs at the usual rate. Therefore, because of the variable rate of accumulation of substrate, cell dysfunction and organ damage that results differs among the various storage diseases.

The spleen plays an important role in phagocytosing many products of cellular metabolism, especially glycolipids in the membranes of circulating blood cells. It will enlarge secondary to intrinsic lysosomal enzyme deficiencies. The spleen, however, has powerful capabilities for phagocytosis of particulate matter. Thus, it will enlarge secondary to enzymatic deficiencies outside the spleen, as in the lipoprotein lipase deficiency in type 1 hyperlipoproteinemia. Finally, congestion secondary to storage and damage in the liver may cause splenomegaly due to portal hypertension.

The storage disorders discussed in this chapter are rare diseases (Table 1). However, familiarity with them is necessary in the evaluation of a patient at any age with splenomegaly. The dysmorphic phenotypes in the mucopolysac-

---

Current Affiliation: Department of Pediatric Endocrinology, Children's Hospital of New Jersey, Newark, New Jersey

Table 1 Storage Disorders Causing Splenomegaly

Disorders of carbohydrate metabolism
   Glycogen storage disease
   Diabetes mellitus

Disorders of lipoprotein metabolism
   Type I hyperlipoproteinemia
   Analphalipoproteinemia (Tangier disease)

Disorders of sphingolipid metabolism
   Gaucher disease
   Niemann-Pick disease
   Sea-blue histiocyte disease

Mucopolysaccharidoses
   Hurler syndrome
   Hunter syndrome
   Sanfilippo disease
   Maroteaux-Lamy disease
   Sly syndrome

Sulfatide lipidosis

Generalized gangliosidosis

Mucolipidosis II (I-cell disease)

Disorders of glycoprotein degradation
   Mannosidosis
   Fucosidosis
   Sialidosis

Neutral lipid storage diseases
   Wolman's disease
   Cholesteryl ester storage disease

Amyloidosis

Cystinosis

Hemochromatosis

---

charidoses, the recognizable storage changes in the histology of the peripheral blood smears and bone marrow preparations, and the pertinent findings in family histories all aid in diagnosing these disorders. However, modern biochemical capabilities for specifically assaying the deficient enzyme have made more exact diagnosis possible. Furthermore, it is likely that our understanding of the initial clinical manifestations and subsequent courses of these diseases will change. Continued biochemical research and new technology may reveal new categories of these clinical syndromes.

DISORDERS OF CARBOHYDRATE METABOLISM

Glycogen Storage Disorders

The glycogen storage disorders are a heterogeneous group of diseases which are considered together because the enzyme defect is associated with the accumulation of normal or abnormal glycogen. The glycogen storage disease most often accompanied by splenomegaly is the rare type IV glycogenosis (Figure 1), which is also referred to as amylopectinosis and Andersen disease (1). More than 15 infants with this form of glycogenosis have been reported (2). The spleen is only rarely enlarged in glucose-6-phosphatase deficiency (type I glycogenosis); it is occasionally enlarged in amylo-1,6-glucosidase deficiency (type III glycogenosis).

The biochemical defect in type IV glycogen storage disease is an absence of the brancher enzyme amylo-1,4-1,6-transglucosylase which is required for formation of branches in glycogen synthesis (3). Thus, abnormal forms of glycogen are synethesized and stored. The storage of abnormal glycogen is mainly in the liver, but abnormal glycogen can also be found in the spleen, heart and muscle (4). The brancher enzyme has been shown to be absent in patients with the disease, and activity of the enzyme is reduced by about half in skin fibroblasts of the parents of such a patient (3).

Patients with type IV glycogenosis acquire the disease through autosomal recessive inheritance. They are normal at birth but soon fail to thrive, exhibiting progressive hepatosplenomegaly, cirrhosis and cardiac failure. Neurologic dysfunction becomes evident by the lack of normal development, hypotonia, muscular atrophy, and decreased or absent deep tendon reflexes (5). Death occurs before the third year of life due to hemorrhage from esophageal varices or due to cardiac failure.

The definitive diagnosis of type IV glycogenosis is made by measurement of the brancher enzyme activity in leukocytes (6). Biopsy of the liver shows cirrhosis and serum transaminase levels are increased.

Type I glycogenosis (glucose-6-phosphatase deficiency) is only rarely accompanied by splenomegaly. It is characterized by hepatomegaly, hypoglycemia, acidosis, and failure-to-thrive presenting at about 6 months of age. The glucagon stimulation test reveals no rise in blood glucose but there is a rise in blood lactate.

Type III glycogenosis (amylo-1,6-glucosidase deficiency) is clinically similar to type I glycogenosis, but the spleen is more likely to be enlarged. Fasting hypoglycemia is present in 80% of patients. The blood glucose response after glucagon is abnormal in the fasting state, but it may be normal shortly after eating. Blood lactate is normal (2).

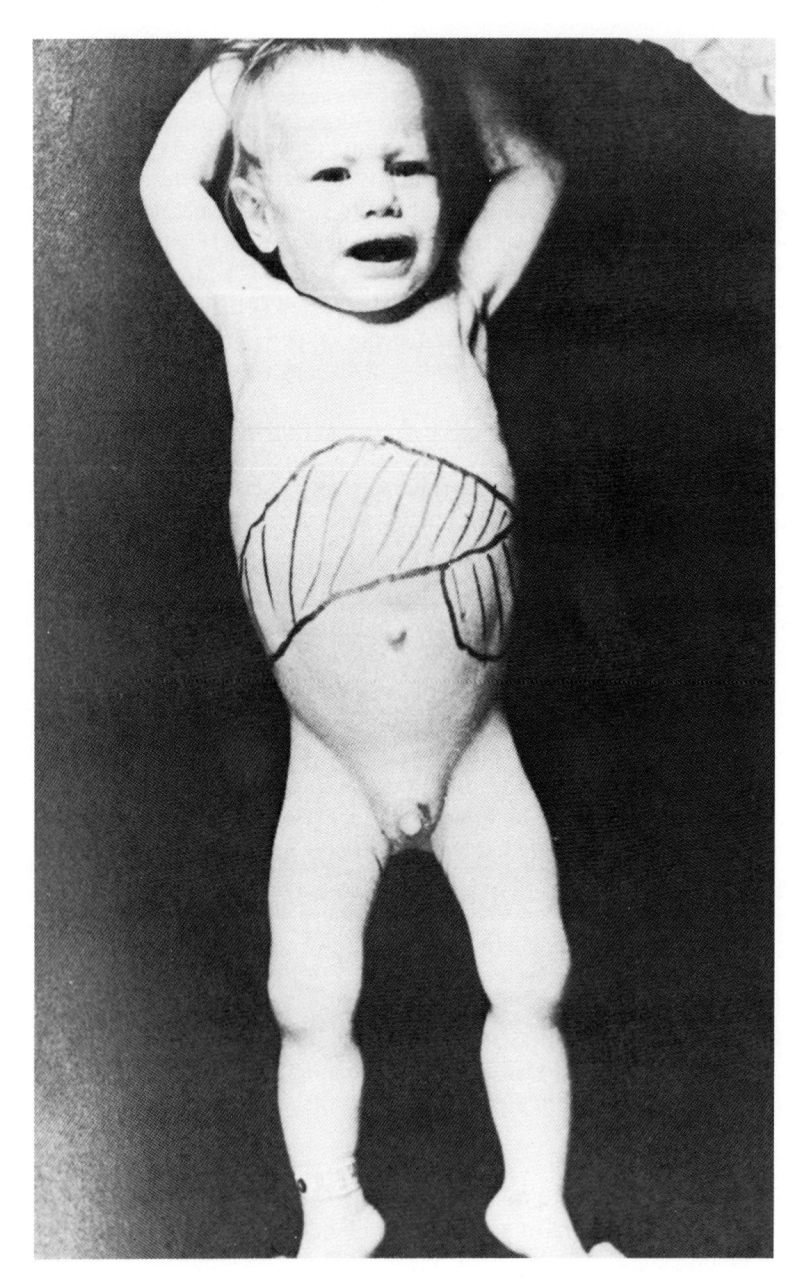

Figure 1 Fifteenth-month old boy with type IV glycogenosis. Markings identify hepatic and splenic enlargement. (Reproduced with permission from Stanbury et al., *Metabolic Basis of Inherited Disease*, 3rd ed., McGraw-Hill, New York, 1972, p. 165.)

Diabetes Mellitus

Diabetes mellitus may be associated with splenomegaly secondary to fatty infiltration of the spleen. Lipid-containing cells have been observed by light microscopy in the spleen of patients with uncontrolled diabetes mellitus and hyperlipidemia of undetermined type (7). Hyperlipidemia can develop in the diabetic patient who has either type I (insulin dependent-ketosis prone) or type II (non-insulin dependent) diabetes (8).

DISORDERS OF LIPOPROTEIN METABOLISM

The plasma lipoproteins are macromolecular complexes that represent the functional unit for the transport of water-insoluble lipids in blood. The lipoproteins vary on the basis of their lipid and protein composition. Normal subjects have four classes of lipoproteins: (1) chylomicrons, (2) very low density lipoproteins (VLDL), (3) low density lipoproteins (LDL), and (4) high density lipoproteins (HDL). These classes of lipoproteins are separated on the basis of their density. Lipoproteins may also be designated according to their electrophoretic mobility.

The protein portion of the lipoprotein molecule that regulates lipoprotein metabolism is called the apoprotein. The apoproteins are positioned on the outside surface of the lipoprotein molecule. Apoproteins bind the lipoprotein to specific cellular receptors, they activate or inhibit plasma enzymes involved in lipid breakdown, formation, or transfer. The better characterized apoproteins are designated A through E.

Type I Hyperlipoproteinemia (Hyperchylomicronemia)

This rare type of hyperlipidemia is commonly accompanied by splenomegaly. The disease is associated with a reduction in chylomicron removal. The major function of chylomicrons is transport of dietary or exogenous triglycerides. Chylomicrons carry dietary triglyceride in the lymph to the thoracic duct where it enters the blood stream. Normally, chylomicrons can not be detected in plasma 10 to 12 hours after intake of food because they are cleared from the circulation by hydrolysis of triglyceride. This reaction is carried out on the capillary endothelial cell membrane by the enzyme lipoprotein lipase. The enzyme activity of lipoprotein lipase is deficient in type I hyperlipoproteinemia and, therefore, removal of chylomicrons is impaired. In type I hyperlipoproteinemia large numbers of chylomicrons persist for more than 14 hours (9).

The excess chylomicron fat accumulates in the lysosomes of histiocytes, macrophages, and Kupfer cells in the liver, spleen and bone marrow. Ferrans et al. (9), reported the histochemical, biochemical, microfluorometric, and electron microscopic changes in the spleen of a patient with type I hyperlipoproteinemia.

Pathologic study of the spleen revealed lipid droplets in the walls of blood vessels, congestion of the red pulp, and infiltration of the red pulp by polymorphonuclear leukocytes and foam cells. The foam cells contained non-birefringent granules with autofluorescent ceroid. Results of the study suggested that the splenic foam cells contained the end products of the chylomicrons that could not be physiologically metabolized in this disorder (9). Similar appearing foam cells were seen in the bone marrow (10). The splenomegaly was felt to be secondary to congestion of the spleen rather than due to foam cell infiltration since there were insufficient foam cells present to account for the increase in spleen size (9).

Type I hyperlipoproteinemia is usually manifested in childhood with recurrent abdominal pain that varies in intensity, duration, and localization. Severity of the abdominal pain is related to the plasma triglyceride concentration and may at times be severe enough to prompt surgical exploration. The pain may also be secondary to pancreatitis (11). Hepatosplenomegaly is a common physical finding, and acute hepatic enlargement may occur during periods of rapid decline in triglyceride concentration.

Eruptive xanthomas occur frequently in patients with sustained triglyceride concentrations in excess of 2000 mg/dl. These lesions are small, elevated, white to yellow papules with an erythematous base and are not infrequently mistaken for furuncles. The lesions usually occur over the extensor surfaces but may appear on any cutaneous surface. The lesions may come and go spontaneously over a period of weeks or months. The arteries and veins in the retina may appear yellowish-pink instead of bright red. This retinopathy is called lipemia retinalis and is another expression of the high chylomicron concentration. Patients with this type of hyperlipoproteinemia are not prone to vascular disease; the major threat to life is pancreatitis.

Type I hyperlipoproteinemia is inherited in an autosomal recessive fashion. Both sexes are equally affected, and it has been described in whites, blacks, and Japanese (12).

The diagnosis of type I hyperlipoproteinemia is made by collecting a sample of venous blood after a fast of 12 hours or more. The patient should have been eating the usual diet, should have a stable weight, and should have no recent history of febrile illness, other acute illness, trauma, or surgery. The patient should not be ingesting drugs that affect lipid levels, such as corticosteroids and estrogen containing medications.

An inexpensive aid to making this diagnosis is to look at the fasting blood sample after it has remained in the cold at 4 degrees centigrade overnight. It will be noticed that there is a creamy layer on top (chylomicron layer), with a clear or slightly turbid infranatant layer. This clear layer consists of endogenous triglycerides bound to very low density lipoproteins, which remain in suspension.

The diagnosis of type I hyperlipoproteinemia is made more definitively by measuring the concentrations of cholesterol and triglyceride and performing a lipoprotein electrophoresis. The total plasma cholesterol is normal to moderately elevated, since chylomicrons contain only 5-10% cholesterol. The total plasma triglyceride is markedly elevated, with values of 2000 mg/dl commonly seen. Chylomicrons are elevated. Very low density lipoproteins are normal or slightly increased with low density lipoproteins and high density lipoproteins being depressed.

The diagnosis of type I hyperlipoproteinemia must be confirmed by specific assays of lipoprotein lipase activity. Lipoprotein lipase activity is not normally detectable in plasma; however, the administration of heparin results in lipase activation which can then be definitively measured in plasma. Lipoprotein lipase can also be measured in adipose tissue (12).

It should be remembered that hypertriglyceridemia may also occur in pancreatitis, in uncontrolled type I and type II diabetes, and in chronic alcoholism.

Analphalipoproteinemia (Tangier Disease)

This rare disease is named after a family from Tangier Island in Chesapeake Bay (13) on the east coast of the USA. The disease may be accompanied by splenic enlargement and is characterized by severe deficiency or absence of normal high density lipoproteins (HDL). The role of high density lipoproteins in lipid metabolism is not well worked out, but they function in cholesterol transport and contribute to the modulation of chylomicron metabolism. The profound deficiency of HDL in analphalipoproteinemia may result in the generation of abnormal chylomicron remnants which accumulate as cholesteryl esters in histiocytes. The disease may involve a defect in the regulation of synthesis or catabolism of high density lipoproteins. The A apolipoproteins, apo A-I and apo A-II, which are the major apolipoprotein components of high density lipoproteins, are reduced below normal (14). Mechanisms important in the trancellular channelling of high density lipoproteins appear also to be faulty.

The histopathology in Tangier disease evolves from the increased concentrations of cholesteryl esters in macrophages in numerous organs, including the tonsils, lymph nodes, thymus, bone marrow, spleen, liver, rectal mucosa, and probably also in Schwann cells and cornea. Most of the cholesteryl esters are outside the lysosomes and are present in the cytoplasm of the histiocytes (15).

Analphalipoproteinemia is characterized clinically by hyperplastic orange tonsils, corneal opacities, and neuropathy. The neuropathy may be sensory, motor, mixed, transient, or permanent. Clinically evident cardiovascular abnormalities have not been seen in Tangier disease patients before the age of 40 (16).

Splenomegaly is a characteristic finding of this disorder while hepatomegaly is not always present. Mild thrombocytopenia and reticulocytosis secondary to the splenomegaly may be demonstrated. Hoffman, et al., reported a case of a 42 year old man with analphalipoproteinemia who presented with splenomegaly. He required splenectomy due to progressive anemia and thrombocytopenia. Histopathologic examination of the spleen revealed cytoplasmic droplets and clusters of cholesterol crystals (17).

Analphalipoproteinemia is a rare disorder inherited as an autosomal recessive trait. Approximately 25% of cases have resulted from consanguinous matings. Heterozygotes have plasma high density lipoprotein levels approximately half normal but do not develop neuropathy or cholesteryl ester storage (18).

The diagnosis may be made on clinical grounds by the appearance of the hyperplastic orange tonsils. If the tonsils were previously removed, the small remaining tags of tissue will remain recognizable. Proctoscopic examination of the rectal mucosa reveals discrete orange-brown spots.

The plasma cholesterol concentration is below 125 mg/dl, accompanied by normal or elevated triglyceride levels. Lipoprotein electrophoresis reveals no lipoproteins of the alpha-1 mobility, which indicates the absence of high density lipoproteins. The HDL concentration should be below 5 mg/dl. Patients may exhibit chylomicronemia after a 14 hour fast. Plasma very low density lipoproteins are normal or only mildly elevated (19).

DISORDERS OF SPHINGOLIPID METABOLISM

The sphingolipids comprise a group of chemically related compounds primarily localized in membranous elements of tissues throughout the body. Deficiencies in the enzymes that degrade these substances cause disorders in which excessive quantities of lipids accumulate in various organs and tissues. The accumulating lipids share a portion of their structure in common which is called ceramide.

Gaucher Disease

Gaucher disease is the most common disorder of sphingolipid metabolism. Splenomegaly is an essential feature in clinical diagnosis of this disorder, which is caused by a deficiency of glucocerebrosidase (20), an acid hydrolase found in lysosomes. Accumulation of glucocerebroside results. Glucocerebroside is a ubiquitous glycolipid resulting from the catabolism of a number of precursors found especially in membranes of neurons, red blood cells, and white blood cells.

Excessive lysosomal storage of glucocerebroside is found in the reticuloendothelial cells of the spleen, bone marrow, liver, and lymph nodes, and in perivas-

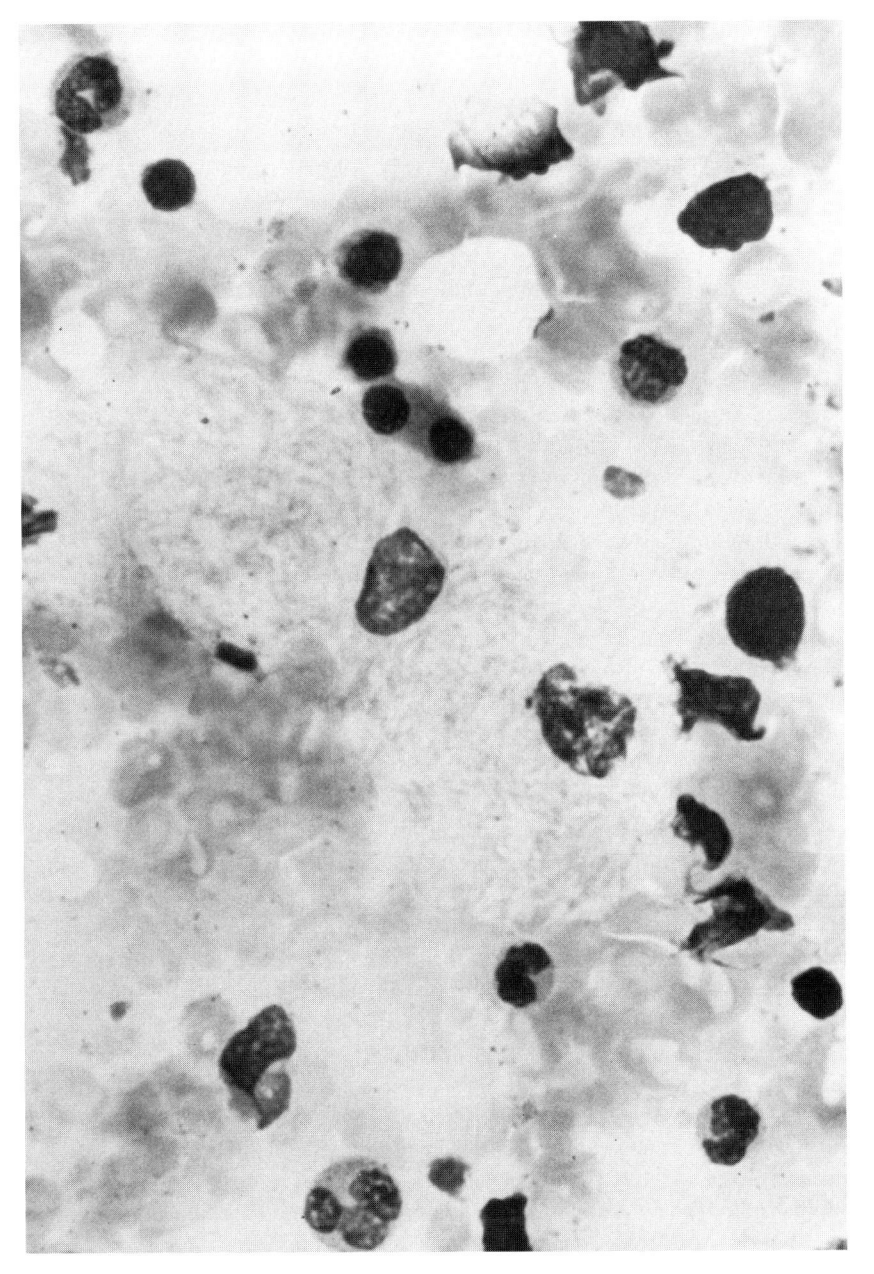

Figure 2 Gaucher cells. (Courtesy of Dr. Marvin L. Bloom.)

cular and endothelial cells of small blood vessels. Splenomegaly develops due to infiltration by the lipid storage cells in the red pulp.

The glucocerebroside storage cells have a distinct appearance and are called "Gaucher cells" (Figure 2). Gaucher cells are large with diameters of 20-100 μm. The nucleus is eccentric and the cytoplasm contains many fibrils of different lengths giving the characteristic "crumpled silk" appearance. The cytoplasm appears faintly blue in Wright's stained smears or in smears stained with Mallory's aniline blue and numerous fibrillae can be seen. The cells stain pale pink with hematoxylin and eosin. They are periodic acid Schiff positive and Sudan black B positive (21).

Three forms of Gaucher disease are recognized. Type I is the adult chronic non-neuropathic form. There are more than 4000 patients with this disorder in the United States. The disease usually presents in the first decade of life; survival may be into adult life.

The presenting symptom of type 1 Gaucher disease is often abdominal discomfort caused by an enlarging spleen. The spleen is usually firm, pale, and less filled with blood than normal which may explain its decreased tendency to rupture (22). Hepatomegaly and lymph node enlargement develop. Anemia is frequently encountered. This anemia may be secondary to bone marrow infiltration by Gaucher cells, due to hemorrhage associated with thrombocytopenia, due to hemodilution (from sequestration of red cells in the spleen) (23), or in rare cases it may be due to acquired autoimmune hemolytic anemia. Thrombocytopenia is present in about 50% of patients (24), and is related to hypersplenism and bone marrow infiltration by Gaucher cells. The bleeding tendency due to thrombocytopenia may present management problems. In addition, factor IX deficiency has been found in the plasma of Gaucher patients (25). Leukopenia is common but of little consequence, and resistance to infection is not impaired.

Splenectomy may be necessary for treatment of hypersplenism, to correct thrombocytopenia or to relieve abdominal discomfort due to the enlarging spleen. Following splenectomy there may be increase in the liver size and increase in bone lesions. These findings suggest that in the absence of the spleen the glucocerebroside can no longer be stored in the spleen and, to compensate, other storage sites must be increased. Partial splenectomy has been tried to reduce the incidence of postsplenectomy sepsis (26) and, theoretically, to protect against the development of bone lesions by retaining a splenic storage site for glucocerebroside.

Expansion of the marrow cavity, osteolytic lesions, and modeling deformities of bone are often seen and are accompanied by intermittent bone and joint pains. The femur is often the first bone to become symptomatic, and the distal femur may assume a characteristic "Erlenmeyer flask" configuration. There may be pathological fractures of the long bones, hips, and vertebral bodies which are major causes of morbidity (27).

Usually there is no nervous system involvement in type I Gaucher disease. Patients may exhibit a symmetrical yellow-brown pigmentation of the skin and mucous membranes. Pingueculae, yellowish spots of proliferation on the bulbar conjunctiva near the sclerocorneal junction may be noticed. Most patients have increased amounts of serum acid phosphatase that is not inhibited by tartarate, which is in contrast to the behavior of prostatic acid phosphatase. This form of Gaucher disease follows an autosomal recessive mode of inheritance and is common among Ashkenazi Jews.

The type 2 form of Gaucher disease is termed the acute infantile neuropathic variant. The prognosis for these patients is poor with survival generally less than two years. Both the nervous system and the viscera are involved in the disease. At about the third month of life infants with this disease present with failure to thrive, splenomegaly, and hepatomegaly. After the sixth month, neurological problems begin to dominate, with symptoms referable to the extrapyramidal tracts and cranial nerves. Characteristic signs are neck retroflexion, trismus, and stabismus. Feeding difficulties, choking attacks, and recurrent respiratory infections characterize the course of the disease. Muscular hypertonicity develops. Death before two years of age usually occurs from pulmonary infection or anoxia. Type 2 Gaucher disease is an autosomal recessive disorder with no known ethnic predilection (21).

Type 3 Gaucher disease is the least common type and is referred to as the subacute neuropathic juvenile form. The clinical course is prolonged and both visceral and neurological involvement occur. Hepatosplenomegaly is present in most cases. The presentation of the disease is the same as in type 1 but begins later in childhood and death occurs in the second decade. The disease has been reported in several interrelated families in Sweden (21).

The diagnosis of Gaucher disease is made on a presumptive basis by the finding of splenomegaly and the classic lipid-laden Gaucher cells in the bone marrow and other tissues. Gaucher cells are not pathognomonic for this disease, however, since similar cells are seen in patients with myeloproliferative disorders and hemolytic anemias. Increased rate of granulocyte and erythrocyte turnover increases the sphingolipid load; this may exceed the capability of the lysosomes to catabolize sphingolipid.

The diagnosis can now be made more readily and with greater certainty from measurement of beta-glucocerebrosidase activity in peripheral leukocytes (28) or in cultured skin fibroblasts, than from a microscopic examination of bone marrow. For a definitive diagnosis, the tissues must be shown to contain an excess of glucocerebroside and, in type 1, a reduction of glucocerebrosidase.

Niemann-Pick Disease

Niemann-Pick disease is due to a disorder of sphingomyelin metabolism which causes sphingomyelin accumulation. Sphingomyelin is a lipid constituent of the plasma membrane, subcellular organelles, endoplasmic reticulum, and mitochondria of all mammalian cells; it is also a major lipid of the myelin sheath. Accumulation of sphingomyelin in the spleen, liver, lymph nodes, and brain is due to decreased lysosomal spingomyelinase activity in some of the variants; but lysosomal sphingomyelinase activity is normal in other variants (29). There are 5 variants of Niemann-Pick disease designated by the letters A through E.

Accumulation of sphingomyelin, plus other phospholipids, and cholesterol occurs in the reticuloendothelial system where the characteristic foam cells may be seen (Figure 3). The foam cells are large, oval, or polyhedral in shape and are 20-90 μm in diameter. They are pale in appearance and contain droplets in the cytoplasm which in polarized light may be birefringent. The cytoplasmic droplets are well visualized under phase contrast microscopy. With Giemsa stain, the cytoplasm appears finely reticulated. More than one nucleus may be present. The cells may contain brown colored ceroid which is autofluorescent. Intracellular material may stain a shade of blue which has caused these cells to be called "sea blue histiocytes." The cells stain red with oil red O and black with Sudan black B stains. Periodic acid Schiff stain is variably positive. The cells are found in the bone marrow, rectal mucosa, liver, splenic pulp, lymph nodes, alveoli of the lungs, and ganglion cells.

The spleen is one of the most extensively affected organs in Niemann-Pick disease. The splenic pulp may be almost completely replaced by foam cells. The amount of sphingomyelin in the spleen of patients with the acute visceral and neurological variant of Niemann-Pick disease can be increased from a normal value of 15 mg per gram dry weight to 370 mg per gram dry weight (30). In addition, there may be increased amounts of unesterified cholesterol. In spite of the extensive involvement of the spleen, only moderate hematologic changes occur, usually as microcytic anemia and thrombocytopenia (30).

The first variant of Niemann-Pick disease classified type A, is the acute visceral and neurological variant. These patients are spingomyelinase deficient, they have decreased sphingomyelinase activity in leukocytes and cultured fibroblasts at about 4% of control activity (29).

The onset is in infancy with apathy, poor development, feeding difficulties, and failure to gain weight. Fever is prominent and lymphadenopathy and hepatosplenomegaly appear before the sixth month. Enlargement of the liver is more remarkable than in Gaucher disease. In the first year, brown-yellow pigmentation of the skin develops. Cherry red macular degeneration occurs in approximately 50% of cases. Spasticity, nerve deafness, and blindness ensue. Hyperplenism leads to anemia which is not as severe as in Gaucher disease. There is

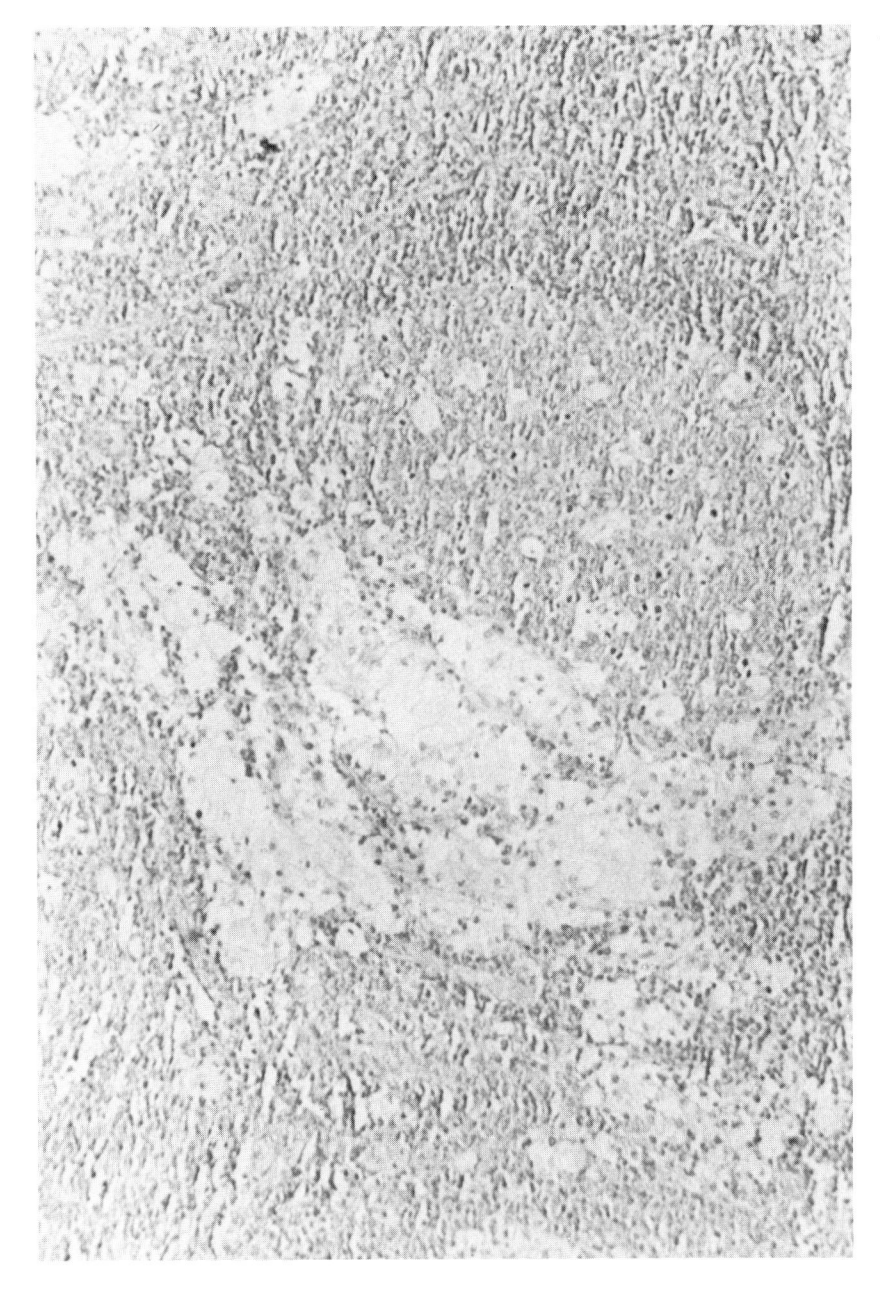

Figure 3 Foam cell infiltration in the tonsil of a patient with Niemann-Pick disease. (Courtesy of Dr. John Fisher.)

moderate thrombocytopenia and leukopenia or leukocytosis. The lungs become infiltrated and chest x-rays show a reticular pattern (31). Death usually occurs before the third year. Type A Niemann-Pick disease is an autosomal recessive disorder and the majority of affected persons are Ashkenazi Jews.

Type B Niemann-Pick disease is called chronic sphingomyelin lipoidosis without neurological involvement. In this form there is reduced sphingomyelinase activity (29). Initially, the nervous system is spared. The symptoms commence at birth, or during childhood, but progression is less rapid than in type A Niemann-Pick disease. Visceral changes may develop in the first six months. Enlargement of the spleen is usually the first manifestation, with hepatomegaly appearing later. Severe respiratory infections which develop are probably due to lung infiltrations (30). If the patient survives to the second or third decades, neurological involvement may ensue. The disease is acquired by autosomal recessive inheritance, and there is no predilection for Ashkenazi Jews.

Type C Niemann-Pick disease is the subacute neurological form. Sphingomyelin accumulation is less marked and sphingomyelinase activity in fibroblasts is only partially reduced (32). Sphingomyelinase activity in the liver and spleen is normal (30).

The patients appear to develop normally for the first one or two years of life. They gradually develop neurological abnormalities, such as ataxia, seizures, and loss of previously acquired speech. Hepatosplenomegaly is less severe. Patients live for 15 to 25 years (31). The disease follows an autosomal recessive mode of inheritance with no predilection for Ashkenazi Jews.

Type D Niemann-Pick disease is a variant of type C which was reported in a Nova Scotia family (33). There is no established enzymatic defect. Neurologic signs appear in childhood with slow progression; death occurs in adolescence.

Type E or the adult type of Niemann-Pick disease is extremely rare. Excess sphingomyelin storage occurs in the liver and spleen, but normal sphingomyelinase activity has been demonstrated. This form is diagnosed in adults who have visceral disease and the presence of foam cells in the marrow, but who have no neurological abnormalities. Type F Niemann-Pick disease is characterized by childhood onset of splenomegaly, lack of neurological involvement, and a temperature labile sphingomyelinase (34).

A presumptive diagnosis of type A Niemann-Pick disease may be based on the findings of hepatosplenomegaly, presence of lipid laden foamy histiocytes in the bone marrow, and the early development of mental retardation. The presence of macular degeneration in this disease will help distinguish it from Gaucher disease. Types B and C Niemann-Pick disease should be considered when lipid storage cells are found in bone marrow (30). The diagnosis of types A and B disease should be made by assessing sphingomyelinase activity in leukocytes from a sample of venous blood (28). Types A, B, and C may be diagnosed by measuring sphingomyelinase activity in extracts of cultured skin fibroblasts

(30). In type D Niemann-Pick disease, foam cells are seen in heterozygous carriers (33).

Sea-Blue Histiocyte Disease

Sea-blue histiocytes are seen in the bone marrow of patients with a variety of hematologic disorders. They are foam cells that appear blue-tinged when prepared with Giemsa stain or Wright stain. Neville et al. (35), described a progressive neurovisceral storage disorder in 9 patients who coincidentally had two rare findings: vertical supranuclear opthalmoplegia and infiltration of the bone marrow by sea-blue histiocytes. Eight of Neville's 9 patients had splenomegaly. The symptoms were usually manifested in the first or second decade. There was progression of the hepatosplenomegaly and cirrhosis, together with neurologic deterioration. No cherry-red macular deterioration accompanied this disease. In most of the cases sphingomyelinase activities were normal in spite of accumulation of sphingomyelin.

MUCOPOLYSACCHARIDOSES

The mucopolysaccharidoses are a class of lysosomal storage diseases. They are produced by an inherited deficiency of one or more of the lysosomal enzymes involved in degradation of acid mucopolysaccharides. Mucopolysaccharides are the major moiety present in the ground substance of connective tissue. They modify structural properties of connective tissue and affect molecular transport across cells, especially by trapping water (31). Mucopolysaccharides consist of a core polypeptide to which a number of polysaccharide chains are attached by a xylose link. The abnormal catabolism of mucopolysaccharides causes excessive intralysosomal accumulation of by-products, notably dermatan sulfate, heparan sulfate, and keratan sulfate. The accumulation of these substances occur especially in cartilage and bone. Progressive disability results from differing degrees of involvement of connective tissue, central nervous system, bones, and heart.

Hurler Syndrome

Hurler syndrome, with autosomal recessive inheritance, is the most common mucopolysaccharidosis. The disorder is caused by alpha-L-iduronidase deficiency (36). This enzyme is required for cleavage of L-iduronic acid residues which are present in both heparan sulfate and dermatan sulfate. In Hurler syndrome there is excess accumulation of dermatan sulfate and heparan sulfate with their subsequent increased urinary excretion.

Patients are normal during the first few months of life and then seek medical attention because of persistent rhinorrhea, frequent middle ear infections, and

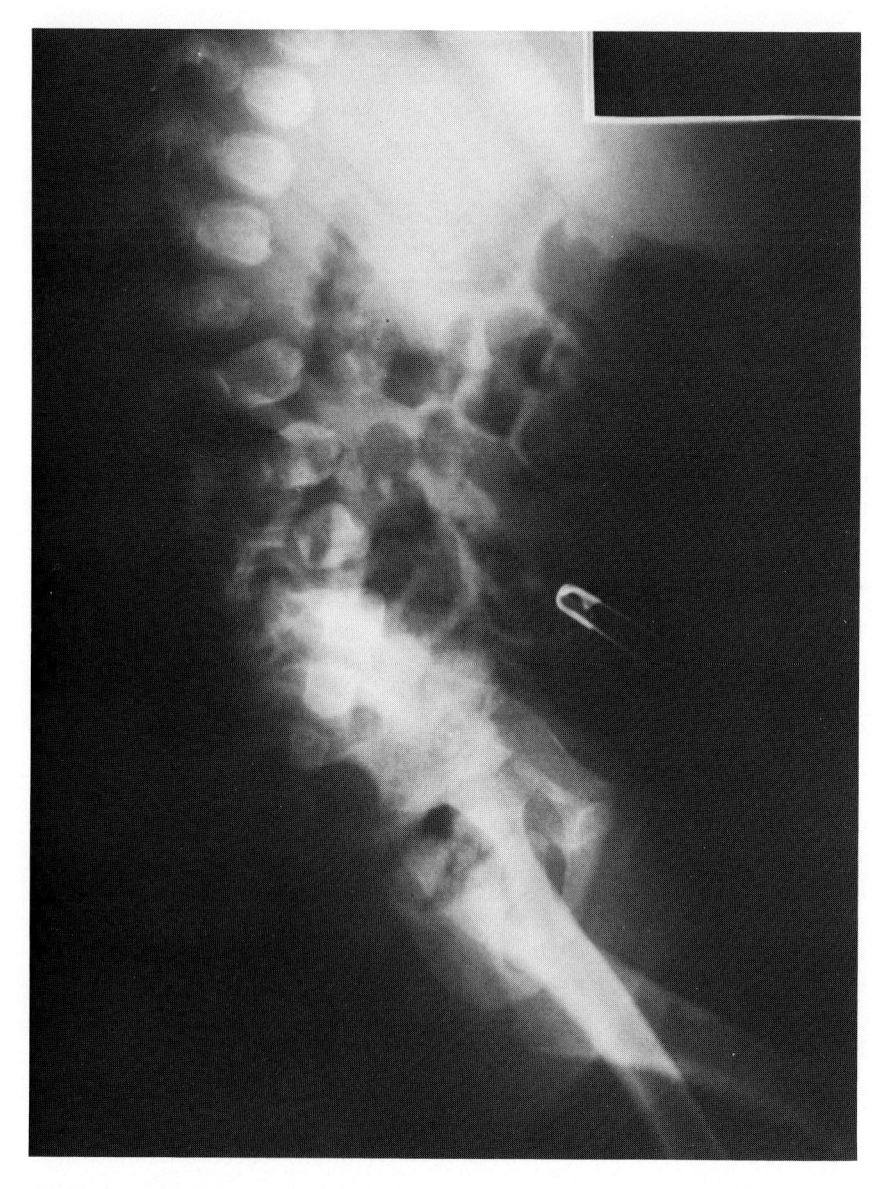

Figure 4 Spine x-ray in a 21-month-old patient with Hurler syndrome. Note vertebral deformity and spatulate ribs. (Courtesy of Department of Radiology, Children's Hospital of Buffalo.)

stertorous breathing. Feeding problems develop secondary to macroglossia and upper airway obstruction. Hepatosplenomegaly causes increasing prominence of the abdomen. Umbilical or inguinal hernias may be present. Later during the first year of life the facial features coarsen, joints stiffen, and alterations in bone structure occur, such as lumbar lordosis. The hands develop a claw-like appearance. Primary dentition may be splayed by gum infiltration. Corneal clouding, retinopathy, and optic atrophy appear. Growth is retarded. Deafness due to both neurosensory impairment and conduction defects ensue. Communicating hydrocephalus is commonly a result of infiltration in the leptomeninges. Arteriosclerosis of the coronary artery and aorta develop due to deposition of mucopolysaccharides in arterial smooth muscle cells. Heart valves may stiffen. Respiratory impairment develops due to limitation of motion of the thoracic cage, thickening of the airways, and upper airway obstruction. Death usually occurs at less than 10 years of age due to heart failure and respiratory failure.

The characteristic radiographic changes are important features in diagnosis of the mucopolysaccharidoses. These changes are called "dysostosis multiplex." There is a widening of the medial end of the clavicle. Premature closure of the sagittal suture, shallow orbits, and a J-shaped closure sella are seen on radiographs of the skull. The vertebral bodies are rounded. A gibbus is caused by a recessed, small vertebra in the low thoracic or upper lumbar spine. Anterior beaking and wedging of vertebral bodies develops at the site of the thoracolumbar gibbus. There is widening of ribs at the sternal end, giving rise to so-called "spatulate ribs," and proximal pointing of the metacarpal bones (Figure 4). There are modelling deformities of the pelvic bones which include flaring of the iliac wings (37).

Hunter Syndrome

The Hunter syndrome is due to sulfoiduronate sulfatase deficiency (38) which causes excess urinary excretion of dermatan sulfate and heparan sulfate. Hunter syndrome is an X-linked disorder that occurs in males in severe and mild forms.

Findings on physical examination include coarse facial features, growth failure, stiff joints with claw hands, deafness, and hepatosplenomegaly. Dysostosis multiplex is seen on x-ray examination. Pebbly, ivory-colored skin lesions on the back over the inferior angle of the scapulae are unique to this form of mucopolysaccharidosis. Atypical retinitis pigmentosa may lead to loss of vision. Progressive deafness occurs. Hunter syndrome may be differentiated from Hurler syndrome by differences in the primary enzyme deficiency and mode of inheritance. Also, corneal clouding is unusual and survival is longer in Hunter syndrome.

In the severe form of Hunter syndrome, mental retardation is progressive and survival beyond adolescence is rare. In the mild form, survival into adult life is possible. Patients have low intelligence, limitation in joint mobility and hepatosplenomegaly. The older patient with Hunter syndrome tends to have rosy cheeks and a hoarse voice. Degenerative arthritis occurs in the hips and heart disease may occur. Death is usually from heart disease due to abnormalities of the heart valves, myocardial pathology and ischemia (37).

Sanfilippo Disease

There are 4 clinically indistinguishable biochemical types in Sanfilippo disease. They are characterized by severe mental retardation and mild somatic abnormalities. Each has a different enzyme deficiency affecting heparan sulfate degradation.

The physical stigmata in Sanfilippo disease are milder than in Hurler syndrome or Hunter syndrome. However, there is more extreme mental retardation in Sanfilippo disease than in the other disorders. The diagnosis of Sanfilippo disease is easily missed if the mental retardation is not investigated. Neurological manifestations commence after the second year of life. As a toddler the child develops hyperactivity, gradually becomes a discipline problem, and loses the ability to speak. Some patients have mild hepatosplenomegaly. Corneal clouding is absent. Death usually occurs before the age of 14 years, but survival into adulthood is possible (37). The bone marrow contains a distinctive plasma cell (Bubot cells) that has an inclusion surrounded by a large halo (40).

Maroteaux-Lamy Disease

Maroteaux-Lamy disease is a rare autosomal recessive disease due to a deficiency of N-acetyl galactosamine-4-sulfatase, which has been recognized to be the same as arylsulfatase B. There is excessive accumulation and excretion of dermatan sulfate. Abnormal metachromatic inclusions in leukocytes are striking and help make the diagnosis.

The clinical findings resemble Hurler syndrome, but patients have normal intelligence. There is a classic form of Maroteaux-Lamy disease, but milder variants exist with the same enzyme deficiency. Children are not affected until 3 to 4 years of age. Growth retardation brings the patient to medical attention. Patients develop stiff joints, coarse facies, hepatosplenomegaly, corneal clouding, and optic atrophy. There is involvement of the heart valves. There is progressive genu valgum. Lumbar kyphosis develops, which is not usually accompanied by anterior vertebral beaking and anterior sternal protrusion. Hypoplasia of the odontoid process may be present, leaving the patient at risk for subsequent atlantoaxial subluxation with neurologic complications (37).

Sly Syndrome

The Sly syndrome was first described in 1973 (39). It is due to a primary beta-glucuronidase deficiency which leads to a block in the degradation of dermatan sulfate and heparan sulfate and mild mucopolysacchariduria. There is phenotypic variation in the patients reported. They may or may not have clouded corneas, coarse facies, heptasplenomegaly, or slow development. The original patient reported by Sly had short stature, hepatosplenomegaly, progressive skeletal deformities of the thorax and spine, and frequent symptomatic pulmonary infections. Beta-glucuronidase may be assayed in cultured skin fibroblasts and leukocytes.

The diagnosis of a mucopolysaccharidosis may be suspected by finding metachromatic granules in lymphocytes on the peripheral blood smear (40). In the bone marrow, all reticulum cells exhibit storage phenomena with inclusions that vary with regard to size, number, and shape (40).

The mucopolysaccharidoses have traditionally been screened for by examining for the presence of urinary heparan sulfate and/or dermatan sulfate. Various methods used have included measuring turbidity with acid-albumin, measuring a precipitate with cetylpyridinium chloride, or noting a metachromatic spot on paper impregnated with the toluidine blue paper test. Identification of the actual mucopolysaccharide excreted has been accomplished by electrophoresis or chromatography.

Emphasis on the diagnostic importance of urinary testing has diminished as the definitive enzyme assay for each of the mucopolysaccaride disorders has become available. Alpha-L-iduronidase (41), iduronate sulfatase (41), heparan N-sulfatase (41), aryl sulfatase B, and beta glucuronidase (42) may now be directly measured in cultured skin fibroblasts and in peripheral blood leukocytes.

SULFATIDE LIPIDOSIS

Multiple Sulfatase Deficiency Sulfatidosis

This disorder results from a single mutant gene affecting the expression of 9 distinct enzymes: including arylsulfatase A, B, and C, cholesterol sulfatase, dehydroepiandrosterone sulfatase, and iduronate sulfatase (43). There is consequent accumulation of sulfate-containing glycolipids, mucopolysaccharides, and steroids. Sulfatide concentrations are increased in the liver, gall bladder, kidney, and central nervous system. In addition, an increase in mucopolysaccharide levels has been demonstrated in the brain, liver, kidney, urine, and cultured skin fibroblasts (44).

This disorder presents in the first few months of life with developmental delay, weakness and hypotonia. The child never develops speech or the ability to walk. Mucopolysaccaridosis-like features such as coarse facies, deafness, hepatosplenomegaly, and skeletal anomalies like lumbar kyphosis appear. Ichthyosis is also present. The corneas are clear (44).

The diagnosis of multiple sulfatase deficiency sulfatidosis is suggested if the urine has increased quantities of dermatan and heparan sulfate. Peripheral blood smear shows dense granulation in neutrophils, eosinophils, and lymphocytes (40). Spinal fluid protein is elevated and nerve conduction velocity is slowed. The loss of arylsulfatase A, B, and C, 2 steroid sulfates, and 4 other sulfatases that help to degrade mucopolysaccarides may be demonstrated in cultured skin fibroblasts (44).

Gangliosidoses

Gangliosides are glycosphingolipids which contain sialic acid in their oligosaccharide chain. The brain has the highest content of gangliosides, but they are found in most cell types. There are two groups of defects of ganglioside catabolism, GM 1 and GM 2 gangliosidoses. In the GM 2 gangliosidoses, the retina and nervous system are affected and there is minimal or no visceral involvement, as seen in Tay-Sach's disease which is a GM 2 gangliosidosis. The GM 1 gangliosidoses involve both the viscera and the nervous system. They have the features of both a lipid storage disease and a mucopolysaccaridosis.

GM 1 gangliosidosis or generalized gangliosidosis is due to beta-galactosidase deficiency (45) with consequent accumulation of the ganglioside GM 1 in the brain, liver and spleen (46). Foamy histiocytes are found in the bone marrow, liver, spleen, lymph nodes, and in most visceral organs. Mucopolysaccharides also accumulate within the viscera, the most prominent being keratan sulfate. Clinically, there is a spectrum of severity with the infantile form being the most severe and the adult form being more slowly progressive. Splenomegaly is most commonly seen in the infantile form.

In infantile form of GM 1 gangliosidosis symptoms are present from birth, with delayed development, poor feeding and failure-to-thrive. The infants rarely progress in development beyond the stage of smiling. The facial appearance is dull with coarse features, a depressed nasal bridge, low-set ears, and presence of downy hirsutism. There may be macroglossia. There is hypotonia with hyperreflexia and the infant is hypoactive. Nystagmus and strabismus may be seen, and a cherry red macular spot is found in approximately 50% of patients. Hepatosplenomegaly is apparent after 6 months of age along with moderate lymphadenopathy. Dorsolumbar kyphoscoliosis and flexion contractures of the hands involving the fourth and fifth fingers become evident. Progressive neurologic involvement includes the presence of hyperacusis, blindness, deafness, and progressive loss of contact with the environment. Recurrent pneumonia is frequent and death occurs from respiratory infection or inanition by 2 years of age (31).

Radiologic changes are those of dysostosis multiplex and include deformities of the vertebral bodies with anterior beaking, spatulate ribs, and modeling deformities of the pelvic, hand and foot bones (47). The disease is inherited in autosomal recessive fashion.

In the peripheral blood 10-80% of the lymphocytes are vacuolated, and bone marrow examination may show vacuolation of histiocytes (40). Beta-galactosidase is reduced in leukocytes and in fibroblast cultures taken from biopsied skin where levels may be as low as 0.5% of normal (31).

MUCOLIPIDOSIS: I-CELL DISEASE

Mucolipidosis II (I-Cell Disease)

Mucolipidosis II is an autosomal recessive disorder caused by a defect in the post-translational processing, rather than a defect in the synthesis of multiple lysosomal enzymes. The abnormality is due to a defect in the production of a phosphomannosyl recognition residue on nearly all of the acid lysosomal hydrolases, including those involved in mucopolysaccharide degradation. Thus, these enzymes are secreted rather than targeted to lysosomes. The disease is called "I" cell disease because of the inclusions visible by phase contrast microscopy in fibroblasts (Figure 5). Hepatocytes, neurons, Kupffer cells, and granulocytes are not significantly affected in I-cell disease. Storage is more conspicuous in connective tissue (48).

This is a familial disorder which is clinically similar to Hurler syndrome, but the symptoms occur at an earlier age. At birth, coarse facial features, gum hyperplasia, hip dislocation, hernias, and pes equinovarus may be noticed (49). The characteristic skeletal changes of dysostosis multiplex are present, but the skull radiograph is normal. There is striking gingival hyperplasia as well as retardation of growth and psychomotor development (50). Affected children are unable to walk. Hepatosplenomegaly is often but not always present. There is no corneal infiltration. Joint contractures, skin thickening, and frequent respiratory infections are seen, with death occurring before 5 years of age (48).

Lymphocytes in this disorder also display the reddish coarse inclusions seen in the fibroblasts (40). Most serum lysosomal enzymes including beta-hexasaminidase, iduronate sulfatase, and arylsulfatase are elevated. Fibroblasts show generalized lysosomal deficiency of the enzymes beta-hexosaminidase, beta-galactosidase, beta-glucuronidase, arylsulfatase A and alpha-L-iduronidase. Mucopolysaccharide breakdown is abnormally slow. There is no excess urinary mucopolysaccharide excretion (48).

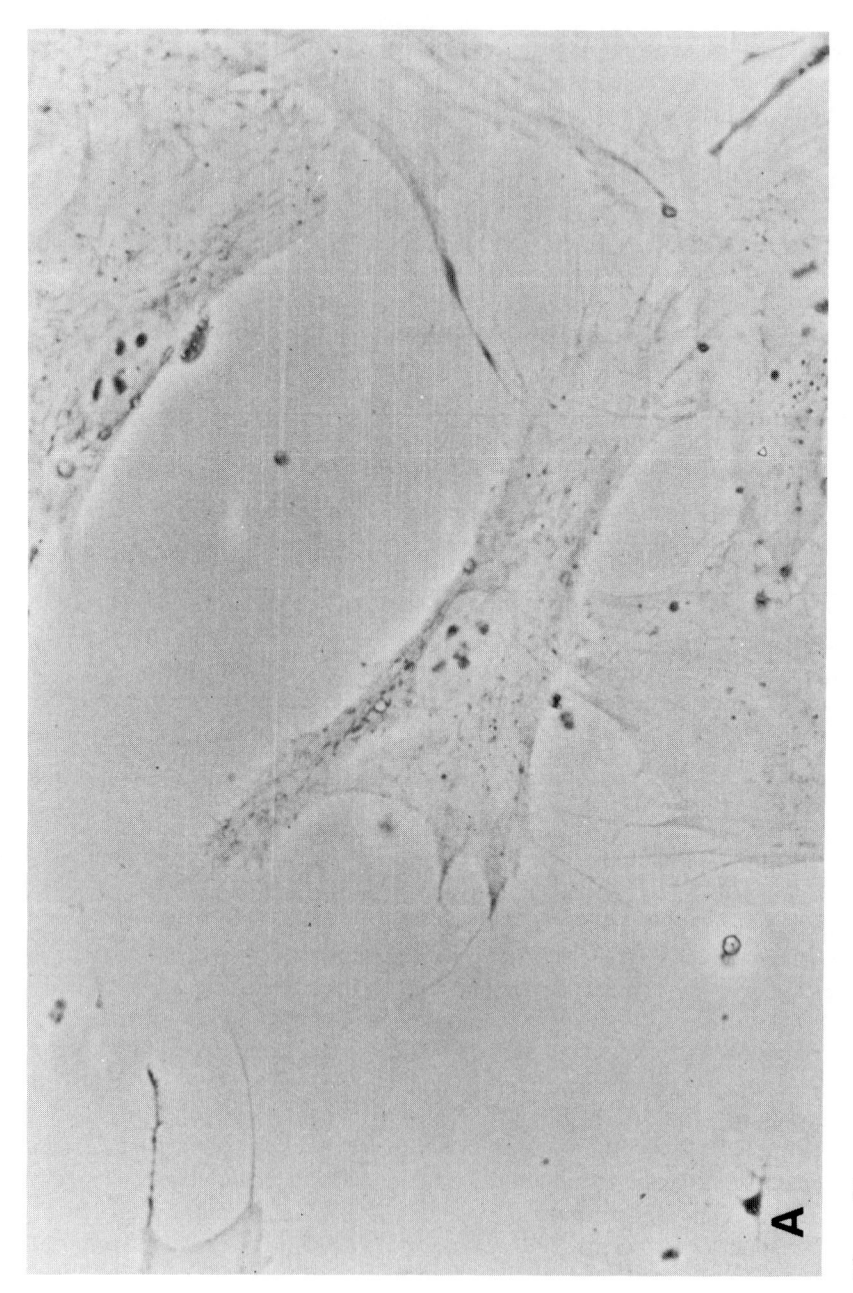

Figure 5A

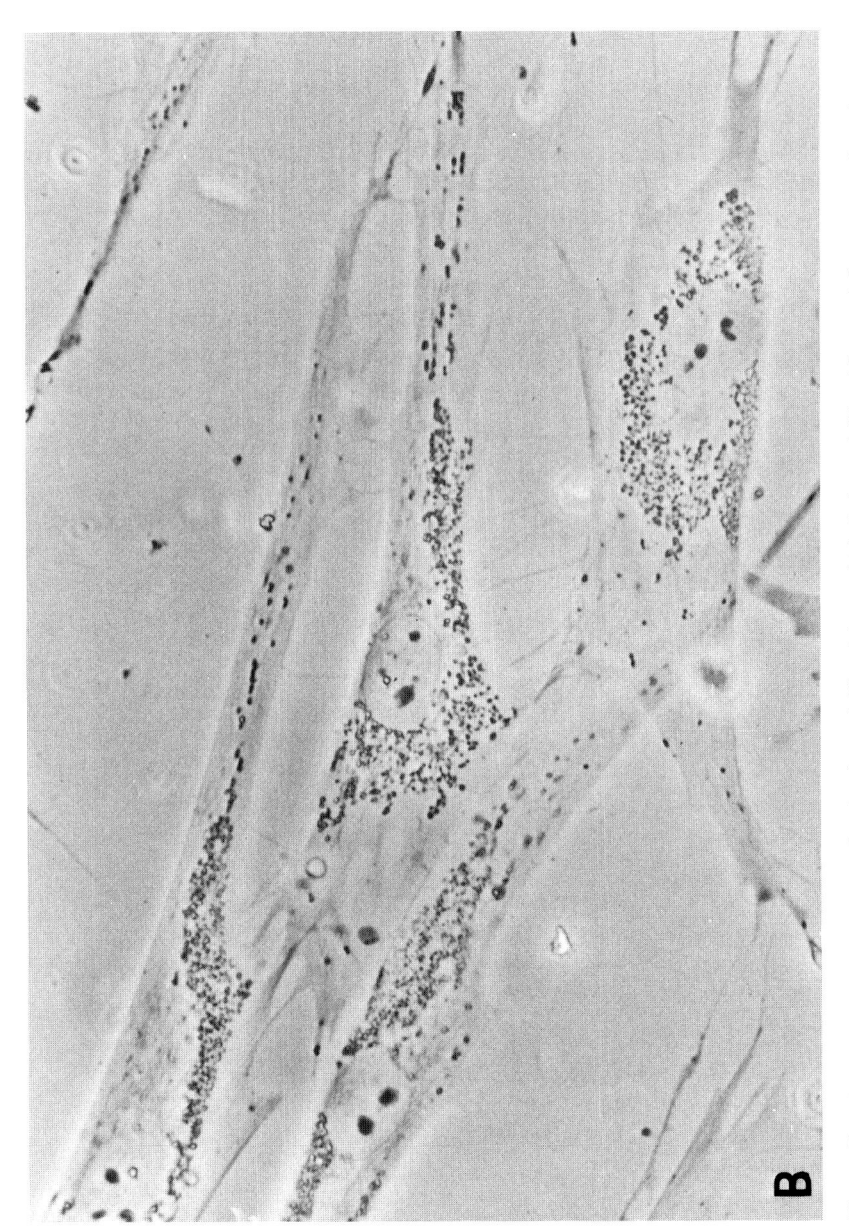

Figure 5 Phase-contrast photograph of cultured fibroblasts. (A) Cultured fibroblasts without cytoplasmic inclusions. (B) Cultured fibroblasts with multiple cytoplasmic inclusions of I-cell disease. (Reproduced with permission from Leroy, J. G., and DeMars, R. I. *Science* 157:804, 1967. © 1967 by the AAAS.)

DISORDERS OF GLYCOPROTEIN DEGRADATION

Glycoproteins are oligosaccharide chains attached to a peptide backbone. They are found widely in cells, on cell surfaces, and extracellularly. They are abundant in nervous tissue. Since the oligosaccharide linkages are not restricted to glycoproteins but may also be found in glycolipids and proteoglycans, an enzyme defect may result in accumulation of more than one class of molecules with oligosaccharides (51).

Mannosidosis

Mannosidosis is caused by deficiency of the enzyme alpha-mannosidase. The original description of this disorder was by Ockerman in 1967 (52). At least 50 cases have been reported (51). The enzyme deficiency causes the tissue accumulation of a mannose-containing compound in urine and in neural and visceral tissues.

There is clinical resemblance to Hurler's syndrome with mental retardation, deafness, hepatosplenomegaly, lumbar gibbus, gum infiltration, hernias, lenticular or corneal opacities, and some degree of dysotosis multiplex. Patients are susceptible to severe recurrent infections and have been found to be deficient in IgG (53). There is recognized clinical heterogeneity with a severe infantile type and a milder juvenile-adult phenotype. The more severe, infantile form is characterized by rapid progression of mental deterioration, hepatosplenomegaly, and death between 3 and 10 years of age. The disease is inherited in autosomal recessive fashion.

Mannosidosis is suspected in a patient who displays the mucopolysaccharidosis phenotype without excess mucopolysacchariduria. Vacuolated lymphocytes are present in the peripheral blood smear. In the bone marrow the plasma cells especially are densely filled with vacuoles (40). The diagnosis is made by measuring alpha-D-mannosidase activity in leukocytes and in cultured skin fibroblasts (53).

Fucosidosis

Fucosidosis is a disorder of glycoprotein degradation secondary to the absence of alpha-L-fucosidase (54) which has been reported in at least 30 patients (51). Fucose-containing H-isoantigenic lipids and a decasaccharide accumulate in the liver, skin, lungs, pancreas, spleen, and central nervous system (55).

There are two recognized clinical categories, the fatal infantile form which affects the majority of patients and a milder form with survival into adulthood. The infantile form has its onset in the first year with the finding of psychomotor retardation. The physical features of fucosidosis include coarse facies, dysostosis multiplex, hepatosplenomegaly, cardiomegaly, skin thickening, respiratory difficulties and infections, and progressive mental retardation. The sweat chloride concentration is increased. There is a loss of normal gall bladder function and fibrotic degeneration of pancreas. Death occurs by 10 years of age (55).

Patients with the milder phenotype of fucosidosis with survival into adulthood display slower progression of cerebral involvement, skeletal abnormalities, and angiokeratoma corporis diffusus. Hepatosplenomegaly is present. Inheritance in both types is in autosomal recessive fashion with a predilection for southern Italians (51).

The diagnosis of fucosidosis is suspected in a patient with a mucopolysaccharidosis phenotype without excess mucopolysacchariduria. Lymphocytes in the peripheral blood smear display more sparse, indistinct vacuoles as compared to mannosidosis. About half of the reticulum cells in the bone marrow have vacuoles and some granules (40). There is a deficiency of alpha fucosidase activity in leukocytes and fibroblasts.

Sialidosis

Sialidosis is an autosomal recessive disorder of glycoprotein degradation secondary to alpha-neuraminidase deficiency documented in cultured skin fibroblasts (56). The phenotype of this disorder without visceral involvement is called type I; type II has visceral involvement accompanied by coarse facies and dysostosis multiplex. Type II disease has been broken down into juvenile, infantile, and congenital forms. Splenomegaly has been reported in the congenital form which is associated with hydrops fetalis and stillbirth (56). Splenomegaly is also part of the visceromegaly found in the infantile form (51). Vacuolated lymphocytes are present in peripheral blood smear (40).

NEUTRAL LIPID STORAGE DISEASES

Low density lipoprotein (LDL) is the major cholesterol transport protein in human plasma. Low density lipoproteins are removed from plasma by tissues in the periphery through the process of LDL binding to a cell membrane receptor, which initiates its endocytosis and incorporation into the lysosome. The cholesteryl esters and triglycerides in low density lipoproteins are then hydrolysed by lysosomal acid lipase which is deficient in Wolman's disease and cholesteryl ester storage disease (CESD).

Wolman's Disease

The acid lipase deficiency in Wolman's disease was first described by Patrick in 1969 (57). Cholesteryl esters and triglycerides accumulate in many cells throughout the body, especially in the reticuloendothelial system. Cholesterol and neutral fat in foam cells infiltrate the liver, spleen, lymph nodes, bone marrow, thymus, and small intestinal mucosa. In addition, neutral fat deposits are seen in connective tissue cells, vascular endothelium, bile ducts, hepatic parenchymal cells, and adrenal cortical cells (58).

Wolman's disease presents in the first few weeks of life. The disease was first described in 1956 by Ambramov et al. (59), in an infant who had marked abdominal distension caused by hepatosplenomegaly and adrenal calcification. Severe failure to thrive and vomiting accompany the abdominal distension. The hepatosplenomegaly may become massive. Some infants have diarrhea and persistent fever or prolonged jaundice.

Anemia first appears during the second month of life and worsens as the disease progresses. Thrombocytopenia is not observed (60). After the first two months, delays in developmental milestones become evident. The infant becomes inert and hypotonic and clinical signs of malnutrition are seen. The clinical findings resemble Niemann-Pick disease, but adrenal calcification does not occur in Niemann-Pick disease. Death occurs between 3 and 6 months. The disease is inherited in autosomal recessive fashion.

Examination of the peripheral blood smear may reveal nuclear and cytoplasmic vacuoles in lymphocytes. The bone marrow shows lipid-laden histiocytes or foam cells (58). The acid lipase deficiency is demonstrated most conveniently by assay of acid p-nitrophenyl esterase activity in leukocytes (61). A plain radiograph of the abdomen reveals discrete calcification of the adrenal glands. Serum lipids are normal. Signs of adrencortical insufficiency are moderate (58).

Cholesteryl Ester Storage Disease (CESD)

CESD is a rare familial disorder due to deficiency of a lysosomal acid lipase (62) in the liver, intestine, spleen, lymph nodes, and aorta (60). It is characterized by the excessive accumulation of cholesteryl esters. There is excessive lipid deposition in the liver and also in the lacteals of the lamina propria of the small intestine and in the macrophages of bone marrow and spleen. Tissue triglycerides are not as elevated as in Wolman's disease. CESD is not as severe as Wolman's disease.

Cholesteryl ester storage disease may present in infancy or in childhood, or may not be detected until adulthood. Hepatomegaly is prominent and often progresses to hepatic fibrosis and cirrhosis. Esophageal varices are sometimes detected. Splenomegaly is common and may reflect the degree of cirrhosis and portal hypertension, since increased lipid in the spleen cannot totally explain the splenic enlargement (63). Premature atherosclerosis has been found (63). The inheritance pattern has not been established.

The disease is suspected in a patient with hepatomegaly who has foam cells in the bone marrow. Lipid storage vacuoles are found in lymphocytes. Hypercholesterolemia and sometimes hypertriglyceridemia is present (60). Definitive diagnosis is made by detection of acid lipase deficiency in cultured skin fibroblasts and leukocytes. CESD may be confused clinically with glycogen storage disease where hepatomegaly and hyperlipemia predominate in an otherwise normal child. Thus, glycogen storage disease needs to be ruled out in the diagnostic evaluation.

AMYLOIDOSIS

The systemic amyloidoses are a group of diseases caused by the extracellular deposition of characteristic beta-pleated protein fibrils (64). These inert amyloid fibrils are formed from various proteins by several different pathogenic mechanisms. Their accumulation in tissue leads to pressure atrophy and cellular death, causing interference with the normal metabolic functions of affected viral organs such as the heart and kidney.

The systemic amyloidoses occur in both acquired and genetic forms. The acquired forms may be primary or secondary. Primary acquired amyloidosis is associated with plasma cell and lymphocyte neoplasms. The secondary acquired forms may be due to chronic inflammatory processes or infectious diseases, notably osteomyelititis, tuberculosis, leprosy, ulcerative colitis, and rheumatoid arthritis. Amyloidosis is a rare disease in childhood. It is most often secondary to juvenile rheumatoid arthritis, familial Mediterranean fever, and chronic suppurative diseases (65).

The genetic forms of amyloidosis constitute a collection of familial diseases that have in common the systemic deposition of amyloid. There are varying degrees of involvement of the nervous system, kidney and heart.

The most common kidney involvement by amyloidosis is in familial Mediterranean fever which is an autosomal recessive disease, more commonly diagnosed in boys, and mainly found in Jewish people of Mediterranean descent. The disease is characterized by brief, spontaneous, recurrent bouts of fever and peritonitis, pleuritis, or synovitis. Onset is usually in late childhood or adolescence. The initial manifestation of amyloidosis is proteinuria. Hepatosplenomegaly may be present (66).

Amyloidosis is suspected in patients who have proteinuria and hepatosplenomegaly. It has also been reported in a patient who was presented with fulminant sepsis due to hyposplenism (67). There are no specific biochemical tests that allow differentiation of one type of genetic amyloidosis from another. Diagnosis rests on the specific clinical pattern together with the demonstration of amyloid infiltration on biopsy specimens and a history of familial involvement. Biopsies may be done of the gingiva, rectal mucosa, liver, or kidney. Amyloid is recognized by its homogeneous eosinophilic appearance when viewed by light microscopy and by its staining properties with congo red and certain metachromatic dyes.

CYSTINOSIS

Cystinosis is the only metabolic disorder known where there is excessive lysosomal storage of a free amino acid. The disease was originally recognized by Aberhalden in 1903 who first noted the crystals in the liver and spleen at autopsy of a child 21 months of age. Current evidence suggests that the basic metabolic error is an abnormality of the lysosomal enzymes which normally transport disulfide amino acids.

Most tissues of the body are affected, including the kidney, the liver, the intestinal mucosa, the cornea, the conjuctivae, bone marrow (leukocytes), and the reticulendothelial system. There is a high intracellular content of free cystine which is compartmentalized within lysosomes.

There are both severe and benign forms of cystinosis. The most severe is nephropathic cystinosis. In this form, children are normal at birth and for the first 6 months of life. The first overt signs are secondary to a renal tubular defect in water reabsorption, leading to dehydration, and recurrent fevers. By one year there is growth retardation, rickets, acidosis and evidence of renal tubular abnormalities. Glomerular damage occurs as well, and it is progressive. Splenomegaly, although present, is not a prominent feature. The disease is progressive and renal failure occurs which may become sufficiently severe to require renal transplantation before 10 years of age. The children are fair-complexioned and have blonde hair (67).

There are patients with a milder form of cytinosis with later onset of renal disease and renal failure (68). In addition, there is a benign cystinosis usually discovered on an ophthalmologic examination which reveals characteristic crystalline opacities in the cornea and conjunctiva (69). The disease is inherited in an autosomal recessive fashion with genetic heterogeneity suggested by the variations in severity among families.

Diagnosis may be made by finding a combination of glycosuria, acidosis, hypokalemia, hypophosphatemia, and hyperaminoaciduria. Cystine excretion is increased in the same proportion as other amino acids. Slit-lamp exam may reveal characteristic irridescent crystalline particles in the cornea which are virtually pathognomonic. In the bone marrow, reticulum cells with crystals are detectable and are observed easily under a polarization microscope (40).

HEMOCHROMATOSIS

Hemochromatosis is a systemic disease of the liver, heart, pancreas, endocrine tissue, skin, and joints in which tissue iron overload is associated with skin pigmentation, liver cirrhosis, diabetes, cardiomyopathy, hypogonadism, and arthritis.

There are two types of hemochromatosis with the first being idiopathic hemochromatosis which is secondary to a regulatory abnormality in iron absorption. The second type of hemochromatosis is due to disorders of erythropoiesis, especially in the forms of hemolytic anemia and ineffective erythropoiesis.

Idiopathic hemochromatosis is an hereditary disease. Usually the disease is latent and its course depends on sex, dietary intake, and presence of hepatotoxins such as alcohol. Males are 5 times as likely to have clinical manifestations than females. The symptoms and signs rarely appear before 20 years of age with a peak in the fifth decade. The cardinal manifestations are skin pigmentation, cirrhosis, hepatomegaly, diabetes, and cardiac dysfunction. The spleen is usually enlarged. However, the storage of iron in the reticuloendothelial system is innocuous and is not of much clinical consequence.

The diagnosis of hemochromatosis is screened for by measuring plasma iron, iron-building capacity and plasma ferritin. The 24 hour urinary iron excretion after intramuscular injection of desferroxamine is measured as a step toward a more definitive diagnosis (70). If the urinary iron is positive, liver biopsy is performed (71). Evaluation should be made of the extent of the tissue damage by measuring liver function, testing for diabetes, and performing an electrocardiogram. A peripheral blood smear should be evaluated for evidence of disturbed erythropoiesis.

SUMMARY

The storage disorders that cause splenomegaly are rare diseases. Many, but not all, are due to lysosomal enzyme deficiencies. Clues to diagnosis may be found on physical exam (e.g., dysmorphism in the mucopolysaccharidoses, sulfatide lipidosis, and mannosidosis) and from the history (e.g., failure-to-thrive in type IV glycogenosis, type 2 Gaucher disease, and Wolman's disease). Examination of peripheral blood smears and bone marrow aspirates where changes like Gaucher cells, I-cells, foam cells, and vacuolated lymphocytes may be seen also provides diagnostic assistance. Confirmation of the specific storage disorder may be made in many cases by assay of the particular deficient enzyme like brancher enzyme in type IV glycogenosis, betaglucocerebrosidase in Gaucher disease, and sphingomyelinase in Niemann-Pick disease. Although these disorders are not common, familiarity with them is necessary in the evaluation of a patient at any age with splenomegaly.

REFERENCES

1. Andersen DH: Familial cirrhosis of the liver with storage of abnormal glycogen. *Lab Invest* 1956;5:11-20.
2. Howell RR, Williams JC: The glycogen diseases; In, Stanbury JB, Wyngaarden JB, Fredrickson DS, Goldstein JL, Brown BS (eds): *The Metabolic Basis of Inherited Disease*, 5th ed. New York, McGraw-Hill, 1983, p. 141.
3. Howell RR, Kaback MM, Brown BI: Type IV glycogen storage diseases, branching enzyme deficiency in skin fibroblasts and possible heterozygote detection. *J Pediatr* 1971;78:638-642.
4. Sidbury JB, Mason J, Burns WB, Ruebner BH: Type IV glycogenosis; report of a case proven by characterization of glycogen and studied at necropsy. *Bull John Hopkins Hosp* 1962;111:157-181.
5. McMaster KR, Powers JM, Hennigar GR, et al: Nervous system involvement in type IV glycogenosis. *Arch Pathol Lab Med* 1979;103:105-111.
6. Brown BI, Brown DH: Lack of an alpha-1,4-glucan: alpha1,4-glucan 6 glycosyl transferase in a case of type IV glycogenosis. *Proc Natl Acad Sci USA* 1966;56:725-729.
7. Warren S, Root HG: Lipoid-containing cells in the spleen in diabetes with lipemia. *Am J Pathol* 1926;2:69-80.
8. Dunn FL: Hyperlipidemia and diabetes. *Med Clin N Am* 1982;66:1347-1360.
9. Ferrans VJ, Biya M, Roberts WC, Frederickson DS: The spleen in type I hyperlipoproteinemia. *Am J Pathol* 1971;64:67-96.
10. Ferrans VJ, Roberts WC, Levy RI, Frederickson DS: Chylomicrons and the formation of foam cells in type I hyperlipoproteinemia. A morphologic study. *Am J Pathol* 1973;70:253-272.
11. Frederickson DS, Levy RI: Familial hyperlipoproteinemia. In Stanbury JB, Wyngaarden JB, Frederickson DS (eds): *The Metabolic Basis of Inherited Disease*, 3rd ed. New York, McGraw-Hill, 1972, p. 545.
12. Nikkila EA: Familial lipoprotein lipase deficiency and related disorders of chylomicron metabolism. In, Stanbury JB, Wyngaarden JB, Frederickson DS, Goldstein JL, Brown BS (eds): *The Metabolic Basis of Inherited Disease*, 5th ed. New York, McGraw-Hill, 1983, p. 622.
13. Frederickson DS, Altrocchi PH, Avioli LV, et al: Tangier disease. *Ann Int Med* 1961;55:1016.
14. Assmann G, Smootz E, Adler K, et al: The lipoprotein abnormality in Tangier disease. Quantitation of A apoproteins. *J Clin Invest* 1977;59:565-575.
15. Herbert PN, Assmann G, Gotto AM, Frederickson DS: Familial lipoprotein deficiency; abetalipoproteinemia, hypobetalipoproteinemia, and Tangier disease. In: Stanbury JB, Wyngaarden JB, Frederickson DS, Goldstein JL, Brown MS (eds); *The Metabolic Basis of Inherited Disease*, 5th ed. New York, McGraw-Hill, 1983, p. 589.
16. Schaefer EJ, Zech LA, Schwartz DE, Brewer HB: Coronary heart disease prevalence and other clinical features in familial high-density lipoprotein deficiency (Tangier disease). *Ann Intern Med* 1980;93:261-266.

17. Hoffman HN, Fredrickson DS: Tangier disease (familial high density lipoprotein deficiency); clinical and genetic features in two adults. *Am J Med* 1965;39:582-593.
18. Fredrickson DS: The inheritance of high density lipoprotein deficiency (Tangier disease). *J Clin Invest* 1964;43:228-236.
19. Fredrickson DS, Gotto AM, Levy RI: Familial lipoprotein deficiency (abetalipoproteinemia, hypobetalipoprotenemia, and Tangier disease). In, Stanbury JB, Wyngaarden JB, Fredrickson DS (eds): *The Metabolic Basis of Inherited Disease*, 3rd ed. New York, McGraw-Hill, 1972, p. 493.
20. Brady RO, Kanfer JN, Shapiro D: Metabolism of glucocerebrosides II. Evidence of an enzymatic deficiency in Gaucher's disease. Biochem *Biophys Res Commun* 1965;18:221-225.
21. Brady RO, Barranger JA: Glucosylceramide lipidosis: Gaucher's disease, In, Stanbury JB, Wyngaarden JB, Fredrickson DS, Goldstein JL, Brown BS (eds): *The Metabolic Basis of Inherited Disease*, 5th ed. New York, McGraw-Hill, 1983, p. 842.
22. Salky B, Kreel I, Gelernt, et al: Splenectomy for Gaucher's disease. *Ann Surg* 1979;190:592-594.
23. Bowdler AJ: Dilution anemia corrected by splenectomy in Gaucher's disease. *Ann Intern Med* 1963;58:664-669.
24. Medoff AS, Bayrd ED: Gaucher's disease in 29 cases; hematologic complications and effect of splenectomy. *Ann Intern Med* 1954;40:481-492.
25. Boklan BF, Sawitsky A: Factor IX deficiency in Gaucher disease. *Arch Intern Med* 1976;136:489.
26. Bar-Moar JA, Govrin-Yehudain J: Partial splenectomy in children with Gaucher's disease. *Pediatrics* 1985;76:398-401.
27. Lachiewicz PE: Gaucher's disease. *Orthoped Clin N Am* 1985;15:765-774.
28. Kampine JP, Brady RO, Kanfer JN, et al: Diagnosis of Gaucher's disease and Niemann-Pick disease with small samples of venous blood. *Science* 1967;155:86-88.
29. Sloan HR, Uhlendorf BW, Kanfer JN, et al: Deficiency of sphingomyelin clearing enzyme activity in tissue cultures derived from patients with Niemann-Pick disease. *Biochem Biophys Res Commun* 1969;34:582-588.
30. Brady RO: Sphingomyelin lipidoses: Nieman-Pick disease. In, Stanbury JB, Wyngaarden JB, Fredrickson DS, Goldstein, JL, Brown BS (ed). *The Metabolic Basis of Inherited Diseases*, 5th ed. New York, McGraw-Hill, 1983, p. 831.
31. Sinclair L: Disorders characterized by excessive storage or accumulation. In, Sinclair L: *Metabolic Disease in Childhood*. Oxford, Blackwell, 1979, p. 251.
32. Besley GTN: Sphingomyelinase defect in Niemann-Pick disease, type C, fibroblasts. Federation of Experimental Biology Societies. Letters. 1977; 80:71-74.
33. Winsor EJT, Welch JP: Genetic and demographic aspects of Nova Scotia Niemann-Pick disease (Type D). *Am J Hum Genet* 1978;30:530-538.

34. Schneider EL, Pencher PG, Hibbert SR, et al: A new form of Niemann-Pick disease characterized by temperature-labile sphingomyelinase. *J Med Genet* 1978;15:370-374.
35. Neville BGR, Lake BD, Stephen R, Sanders MD: A neurovisceral storage disease with vertical supranuclear opthalmoplegia and its relationship to Niemann-Pick disease. *Brain* 1973;96:97-120.
36. Matalon R, Dorfman A: Hunter's syndrome, an alpha-L-iduronidase deficiency. *Biochem Biophys Res Commun* 1972;47:959-964.
37. McKusick VA, Neufeld EF: The mucopolysaccharide storage disease. In, Stanbury JB, Wyngaarden JB, Fredrickson DS, Goldstein JL, Brown BS (eds): *The Metabolic Basis of Inherited Disease*, 5th ed. New York, McGraw-Hill, 1983, p. 751.
38. Sjoberg I, Fransson LA, Matalon R, Dorfman A: Hunter's syndrome; deficiency of L-idurono-sulfatase. *Biochem Biophys Res Comm* 1973;54:1125-1132.
39. Sly WS, Quinton BA, McAlister WH, Rimoin DL: Beta-glucuronidase deficiency; report of clinical, radiologic and biochemical features of a new mucopolysaccharidosis. *J Pediatr* 1973;82:249-257.
40. Hansen HG, Graucob E: *Hematologic Cytology of Storage Diseases*. Berlin, Springer-Verlag, 1985.
41. Hall CW, Liebaers I, Dinatate P, Neufeld EF: Enzymatic diagnosis of the genetic mucopolysaccharide storage disorders. *Meth Enzymol* 1978;50:439-556.
42. Glaser JH, Sly WS: Betaglucuronidase deficiency mucopolysaccharidosis; methods for enzymatic diagnosis. *J Lab Clin Med* 1973;82:969-977.
43. Basner R, Von Figura K, Glossl J, et al: Multiple deficiency of mucopolysaccharide sulfatases in nucosulfatidosis. *Pediat Res* 1979;13:1316-1318.
44. Kolodny EH, Moser HW: Sulfatide lipidosis; metachromatic leukodystrophy. In, Stanbury JB, Wyngaarden JB, Fredrickson DS, Goldstein JL, Brown BS (eds): *The Metabolic Basis of Inherited Disease*, 5th ed. New York, McGraw-Hill, 1983, p. 881.
45. Okada S, O'Brien JS: Generalized gangliosidosis; beta-galactosidase deficiency. *Science* 1968;160:1002-1004.
46. O'Brien JS, Stern MB, Landing BH, et al: Generalized gangliosidosis. *Am J Dis Child* 1965;109:338-346.
47. O'Brien JS: The gangliosidoses, In, Stanbury JB, Wyngaarden JB, Fredrickson DS, Goldstein JL, Brown BS (eds): *The Metabolic Basis of Inherited Disease*, 5th ed. New York, McGraw-Hill, 1983, p. 945.
48. Neufeld EF, McKusick VA: Disorders of lysosomal enzyme synthesis and localization: I-cell disease and pseudo-hurler polydystrophy. In, Stanbury JB, Wyngaarden JB, Fredrickson DS, Goldstein JL, Brown BS (eds): *The Metabolic Basis of Inherited Disease*, 5th ed. New York, McGraw-Hill, 1983, p. 778.
49. Cipolloni C, Boldrini A, Donti E, et al: Neonatal mucolipidosis II (I-cell disease); clinical, radiological and biochemical studies in a case. *Helv Paediatr Acta* 1980;35:85-95.

50. Leroy JG, Spranger JW, Feingold M, et al: I-cell disease; a clinical picture. *J Pediatr* 1971;79:360-365.
51. Beaudet AL: Disorders of glycoprotein degradation; mannosidosis, fucosidosis, sialidosis, and aspartylglycosaminuria. In, Stanbury JB, Wyngaarden JB, Fredrickson DS, Goldstein JL, Brown BS (eds): *The Metabolic Basis of Inherited Disease*, 5th ed. New York, McGraw-Hill, 1983, p. 788.
52. Ockerman PA: A generalized storage disorder resembling Hunter's syndrome. *Lancet* 1967;2:239-241.
53. Desnick RJ, Sharp HL, Grabowski GA, et al: Mannosidosis; clinical, morphologic, immunologic, and biochemical studies. *Pediatr Res* 1976;10:985-996.
54. Van Hoof F, Hers HG: Mucopolysaccharidosis by absence of α-fucosidase. *Lancet* 1968;1:1198.
55. Durand P, Borrone C, Della Cella G: Fucosidosis. *J Pediatr* 1969;75:665-674.
56. Kleijer WJ, Hoogeveen A, Verheijen FW, et al: Prenatal diagnosis of sialidosis with combined neuraminidase and beta-galactosidase deficiency. *Clin Genet* 1979;16:60-61.
57. Patrick AD, Lake BD: Deficiency of an acid lipase in Wolman's disease. *Nature* 1969;222:1067-1068.
58. Crocker AC, Vawter GF, Neuhauser EBD, Rosowsky A: Wolman's disease; three new patients with a recently described lipidosis. *Pediatrics* 1965;35:627-640.
59. Abramov A, Schorr S, Wolman M: Generalized xanthomatosis with calcified adrenals. *Am J Dis Child* 1956;91:282-286.
60. Assman G, Fredrickson DS: Acid lipase deficiency; Wolman's disease. In, Stanbury JB, Wyngaarden JB, Fredrickson DS, Goldstein JL, Brown BS (eds): *The Metabolic Basis of Inherited Disease*, 5th ed. New York, McGraw-Hill, 1983, p. 803.
61. Young EP, Patrick AD: Deficiency of acid esterase activity in Wolman's disease. *Arch Dis Child* 1970;45:664-668.
62. Sloan HR, Fredrickson DS: Enzyme deficiency in cholesteryl ester storage disease. *J Clin Invest* 1972;51:1923-1926.
63. Beaudet AL, Ferry GD, Nichols BL, Rosenberg HS: Cholesterol ester storage disease; clinical, biochemical and pathological studies. *J Pediatr* 1977;90:910-914.
64. Eanes ED, Glenner GG: X-ray diffraction studies on amyloid filaments. *J Histochem Cytochem* 1968;16:673-677.
65. Strauss RG, Schubert WK, McAdams AJ: Amyloidosis in childhood. *J Pediatr* 1969;74:272-282.
66. Sohar E, Gafni J, Pras M, Heller H: Familial Mediterranean fever; a survey of 470 cases. A review of the literature. *Am J Med* 1967;43:227-253.
67. Schneider JA, Schulman JD: Cystinosis, In Stanbury JB, Wyngaarden JB, Fredrickson DS, Goldstein JL, Brown BS. *The Metabolic Basis of Inherited Disease*. McGraw-Hill, New York, 1983, p. 1844.

68. Pittman G, Deodhar S, Schulman JD, Lando JB: Nephropathic cystinosis in a young adult; report of a case. *Lab Invest* 1971;24:442.
69. Yamamoto GK, Schulman JD, Schneider JA, Wong VG: Long-term ocular changes in cystinosis; observations in renal transplant recipients. *J Pediatr Opthalmol Strabis* 1979;16:21-25.
70. Harker LA, Funk DD, Finch CA: Evaluation of storage iron by chelates. *Am J Med* 1968;45:105-115.
71. Kent G, Popper H: Liver biopsy in diagnosis of hemochromatosis. *Am J Med* 1968;44:837-841.

Part IV

Imaging and Surgery

12
Imaging the Spleen

JOHN R. STY and ROBERT G. WELLS
Children's Hospital of Wisconsin, Milwaukee

The spleen has interested physicians since the time of Hippocrates and Aristotle. In these early works, the anatomic relationships of this organ were described with a mixture of fact and fantasy. Galen said it was an organ of mystery. He thought that the spleen extracted melancholic humors from the circulatory system and consequently could be associated with humor or levity. Later investigations have shown that, although the spleen has many dissimilar functions, none of these functions are absolute requirements for life (Table 1). Today many of these functions and anatomic relationships can be studied in vivo with imaging techniques. Radionuclide imaging, computed tomography, and ultrasound represent the most direct diagnostic techniques presently available for evaluation of the spleen.

Two splenic functions can be utilized for radionuclide imaging: phagocytosis and red-blood cell sequestration. Phagocytosis is present in the newborn (1,2). The importance of this function is indicated by the increased incidence of sepsis which occurs when the spleen is absent. The reticuloendothelial components of the spleen remove foreign material, including bacteria, from the circulation (3,4). Radionuclides such as 99m-technetium sulfur colloid are also phagocytized by the reticuloendothelial cells within the spleen. Because of the uniform distribution of these cells, a technetium scan depicts splenic morphology.

Senescent red blood cells, as well as those which contain intracellular inclusions, are sequestered in the red pulp area of the spleen (5). The plasma clearance rate of labeled damaged red blood cells can be used to assess red cell seques-

Table 1 Functions of the Spleen

1. Erythrocyte destruction
2. Immunologic functions
3. Phagocytosis
4. "Pitting" of red blood cells
5. Platelet destruction
6. Reservoir (for platelets, factor VII)
7. Sites of hematpoiesis and control of hematopoiesis

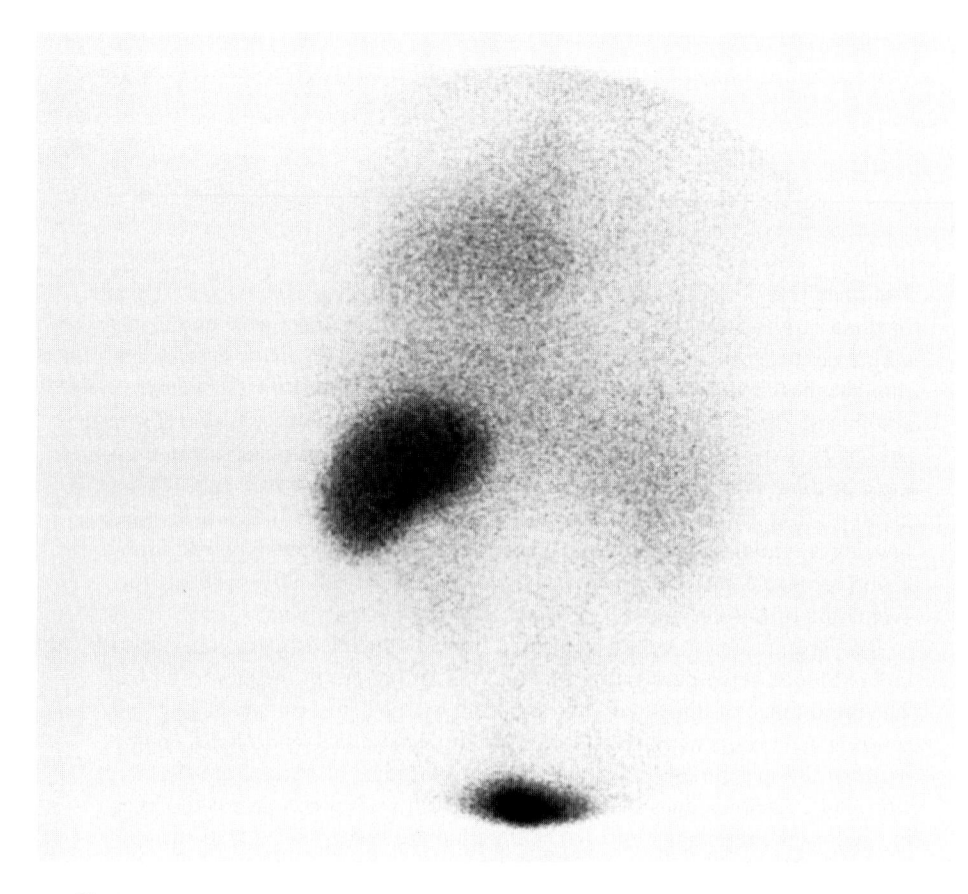

Figure 1 99m-technetium sulfur colloid labeled heat-damaged red blood cell scan. Normal. Scan demonstrates intense accumulation of tracer in the spleen. There is no evidence of accessory spleen. The spleen is readily visualized in comparison to the liver.

tration in the spleen. Also, since there is no significant hepatic uptake of this isotope, radio-labeled damaged red blood cells may be used for spleen-specific scintigraphy (Figure 1). Schnitzer et al. (6), showed that plasmodium-laden erythrocytes do not clear the venous sinusoids of the spleen whereas normal red blood cells readily pass through this filter. Electron microscopy demonstrates the trapping of plasmodium-containing erythrocytes at the sinusoid interface where they eventually undergo fragmentation. The nonphagocytized portion of the cell is transferred into the sinusoid. This process is called the "pitting" function of the spleen. Characteristic inclusion bodies, Howell-Jolly bodies, are present in the red cells of patients who lack a functioning spleen (1).

Use of gray scale ultrasonography as a diagnostic modality in pediatrics has greatly increased in the last 5 years. This increased use is due to the greater sophistication of ultrasound equipment and the acceptance of this imaging modality by clinicians. Diagnostic ultrasonography in children allows excellent depiction of splenic morphology, without the risks of injecting radiographic contrast material and the adverse biological effects of ionizing radiation. Ultrasonography is an anatomic diagnostic study; thus, organ function (physiology) can only be inferred. Relationships among various organs may be accurately defined with ultrasonography, and internal tissue consistency of individual organs often reflecting true pathologic states, may be demonstrated. However, intestinal gas, ribs and patient motion interfere with diagnostic accuracy of ultrasonography.

Like other newer imaging modalities, ultrasonic findings have relatively specific implications (Figure 2). The specificity of these terms must be understood by the clinician. The term *anechoic* indicates the absence of internal echoes. An area that is anechoic may indicate the presence of a totally homogeneous lesion, such as a lymphoma, or it may be a cystic structure filled with a medium of low echogenicity. True cystic structures are anechoic. They are characterized by a sharply defined posterior wall and through-transmission which enhances tissue deep to the cyst. These latter findings are not present in a homogeneous lesion that is not purely cystic.

The term *hypoechoic* indicates a structure of somewhat reduced echogenicity, but not sonolucent or anechoic. A hypoechoic structure would be typified by a soft tissue mass with tissue texture similar to skeletal muscle.

Hyperechoic abnormalities are characterized by an increased number of echoes. Hyperechoic lesions appear bright on images and may produce acoustic shadowing. This finding is usually indicative of fibrous or collagenous tissue, such as dense supporting stroma, or lipomatous tissue.

Sonography is 80 to 90% accurate in the detection of focal malignancy, either primary or secondary, in the liver. Similar degrees of accuracy can be ob-

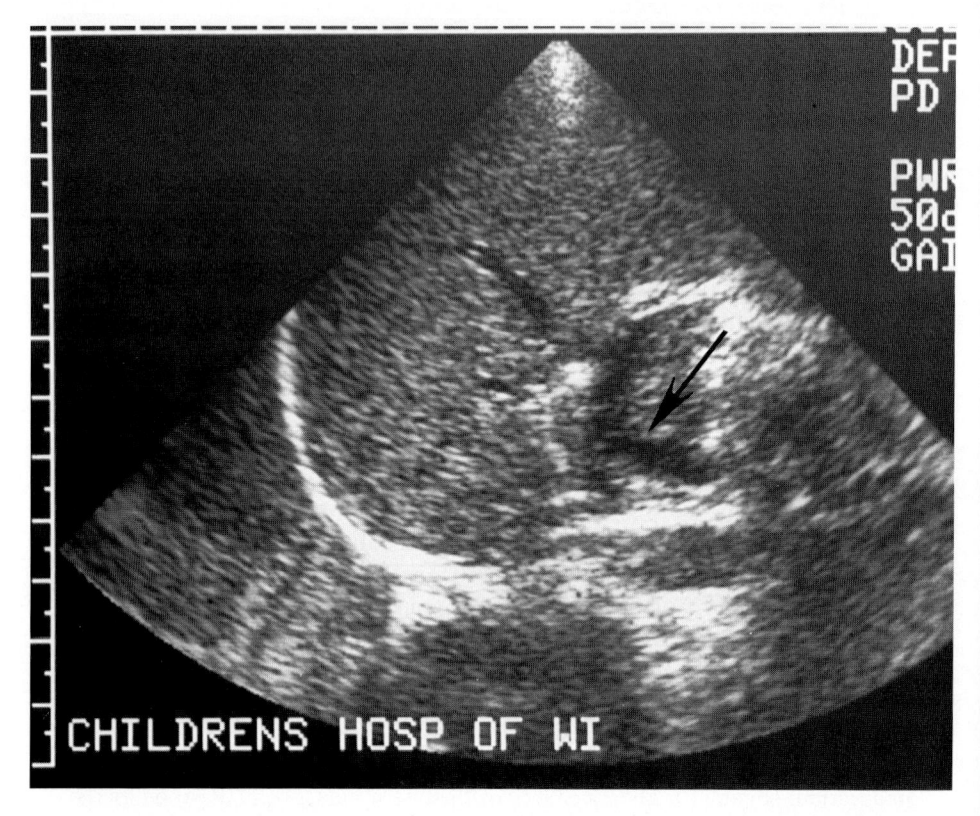

Figure 2 Normal longitudinal image of the spleen. The image identifies normal internal echoes without focal abnormalities. The curvilinear hypoechoic structures (arrow) represent splenic vessels in the region of the hilum.

tained for assessing malignant diseases that involve the spleen. This method of evaluation displays anatomy based on the acoustic characteristics of various tissues. The perisplenic regions can also be assessed. This is a distinct advantage over 99m-technetium sulfur colloid imaging for some disease processes. At times, sonography can demonstrate abnormalities in children which are not normally apparent on CT or 99m-technetium sulfur colloid imaging.

A broad spectrum of pathological conditions may be evaluated with sonography. The most frequently encountered abnormality is splenomegaly. Metastatic disease, primary tumors, and abscesses may be detected. Although solid and cystic lesions may be distinguished with sonography, specific histologic diagnoses are usually not possible based only on sonographic findings.

SPLEEN IMAGING

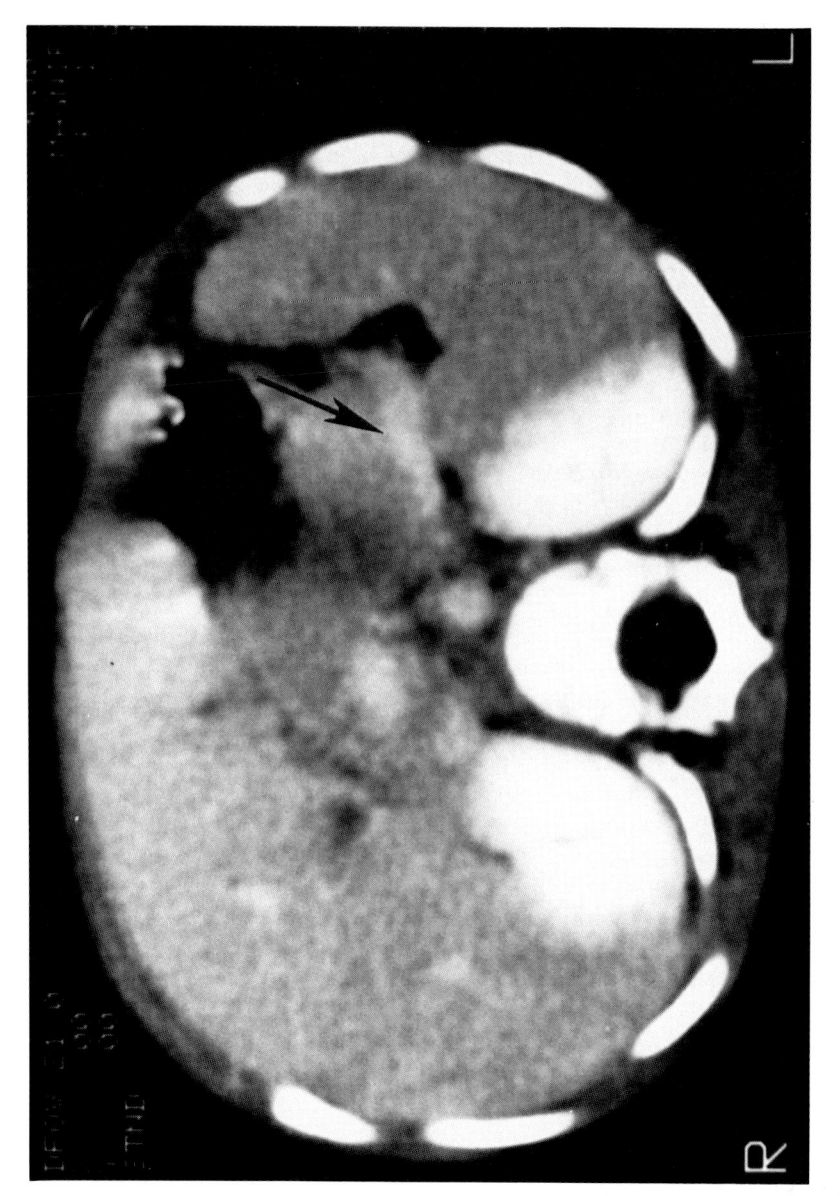

Figure 3 Normal contrast-enhanced computed tomographic image of the midportion of the spleen. This study identifies the spleen in the left upper quadrant lateral to the kidney and adjacent to the ribs. The enhanced linear structure anterior to the spleen represents the splenic vein (V).

Demonstration of anatomic detail with computed tomography is less satisfactory in infants and small children than in older children and adults. Many factors contribute to the difficulty in defining organs and visualizing tissue interfaces in small children. Small size of anatomical structures in children is one factor, but this can be partially compensated for by magnification. Patient motion, especially respiratory motion, may be overcome with the new fast scanners. Because children have less body fat than older patients, delineation of organs and fascial planes is more difficult.

Usually the spleen is evaluated as part of an examination of the upper abdomen; only in rare instances is computed tomography of the spleen specifically requested. Like ultrasonography, computed tomography is an anatomic study. Information regarding splenic function is only inferred from the anatomic findings. Also like ultrasonography, CT provides information about all upper abdominl structures including the peritoneum. Computed tomography provides axial projection imaging without interference from artifacts, such as the ribs. This capability represents an advantage over ultrasonography in assessing many disease processes (Figure 3).

ANATOMY AND EMBRYOLOGY

The spleen arises from mesenchymal cells in the dorsal mesogastrium during the fifth week of gestation. Its characteristic adult shape is usually attained by the third month. Failure of fusion of these primordial clusters of mesenchymal cells results in the formation of accessory spleens, surface notches, clefts, and lobulation. These normal variations in splenic structure must be recognized for proper interpretation of diagnostic imaging procedures. By 4 months of age, the spleen is an active center of hematopoiesis; however, the germinal cells are not fully developed during fetal life.

The spleen is fixed in the left upper quadrant of the abdomen by the lienorenal ligament, which contains the splenic vessels. The spleen is also held in place by the lienogastric ligament, which connects the ventral aspect of the spleen to the greater curvature of the stomach. The phrenocolic ligament forms a sling between the splenic flexure of the colon and the left hemidiaphragm, in which the caudal end of the spleen rests. A so-called "wandering spleen" results from laxity or absence of these structures (7-9).

VARIATIONS IN SPLEEN SIZE

During growth and development, the weight of the spleen is almost a linear function of body weight. At birth, it weighs approximately 15 to 20 grams. At about 6 years of age, the spleen weighs approximately 60 grams and at puberty, it weighs nearly 150 grams (10-12). Splenic weight is characterized by an allometric relationship (13). Spleen weight = $3.5 \times 10^{-3} \times 0.97 \times$ body weight. At puberty, the spleen achieves its maximum weight, and thereafter the weight decreases with age. As with other abdominal organs, several formulas are available for calculating size of the spleen as related to patient age (14). Approximate splenic size can be calculated from the formula: Length of the spleen (in centimeters) = 5.7 + 0.31 × child's age (in years).

In adults, the spleen must be one and one-half to two times larger than normal in order to be palpable. This rule does not apply to children. Spleens are more often palpable in infants and children because of the thinness of the abdominal wall. The spleen is palpable in as many as 10% of normal children.

Many conditions are associated with a small spleen. Familial splenic hypoplasia was observed in 3 offspring of consanguineous parents (15). These children were reported to have multiple and recurrent severe bacterial infections. A small spleen is found in children with Fanconi's aplastic anemia (16). Splenic atrophy has also been noted in a variety of diseases in adults (17-22). These include celiac disease, dermatitis herpetiformis, Fanconi's anemia, sickle cell disease, thyrotoxicosis, and ulcerative colitis.

Technetium sulfur colloid imaging or sonography can be used to confirm a clinical impression of splenomegaly (Figure 4). Computed tomography is not usually needed in confirming splenic size. The various possible causes of splenomegaly in children are listed in Table 2. Spleen imaging is not useful in obtaining a specific diagnosis as to the cause of enlargement. However, imaging is indispensable in determining size and in following, over time, the course of a disease associated with splenomegaly.

Radionuclide imaging may show increased splenic uptake or augmentation in many conditions in addition to splenomegaly (Table 3). The mechanisms for splenic augmentation (diffuse increased uptake of isotope) are poorly understood; because of the diversity of conditions in which it occurs, the finding is usually of little clinical value.

TECHNIQUES FOR IMAGING THE SPLEEN

Sonography

Sonography in pediatrics is usually performed with real-time or dynamic imaging. Real-time ultrasound functions by repeated generation and decay of images at a high enough frequency to provide a continuous image; at 10 to 30 frames/ second. Images are conventionally obtained in longitudinal (parasagittal) and transverse (axial) sections. However, in practice, coronal and oblique scanning is often utilized.

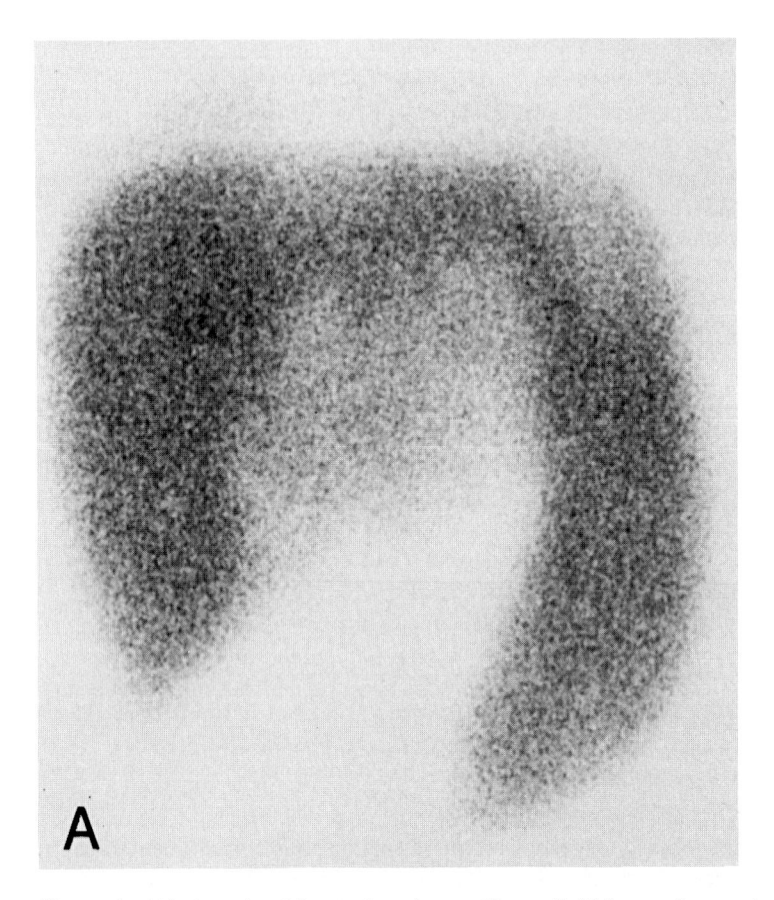

Figure 4 (A) Anterior 99m-technetium sulfur colloid image demonstrates marked splenomegaly. No focal defects are identified. The overall length of the spleen is greater than the liver. The child had infectious mononucleosis. (B) Longitudinal ultrasonic image of the spleen (S) in the same child demonstrates splenic enlargement with compression of the kidney (K). The caudal extent of the spleen is greater than the lower pole of the kidney.

An advantage of sonography is that images are obtained directly without significant reconstruction by computer techniques. Relationships between organs and anatomy of blood vessels are accurately demonstrated. Transducers used in a particular patient are selected according to the depth of the organ under evaluation. The highest frequency transducers provide the best resolution, but

SPLEEN IMAGING 363

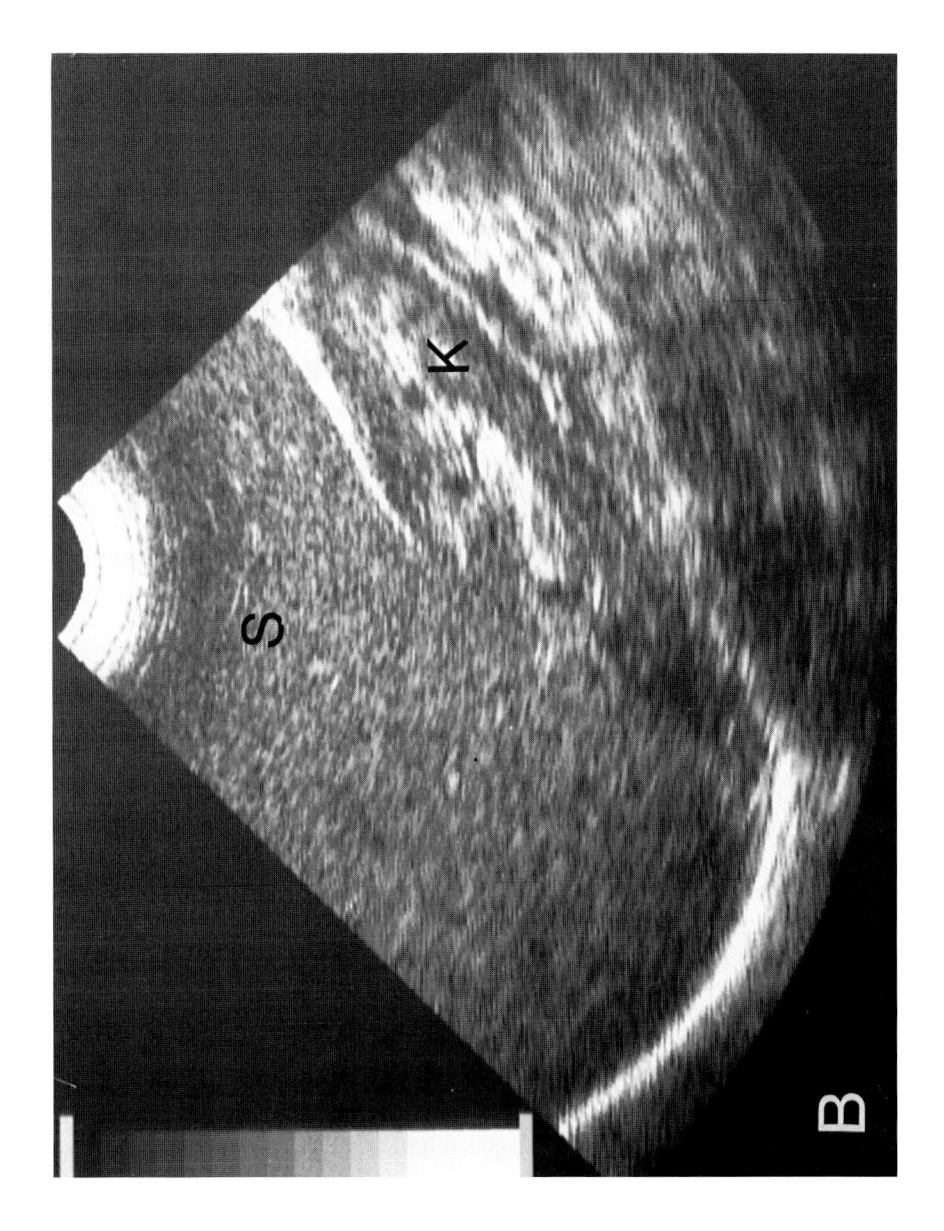

Table 2 Causes of Splenomegaly

1. Congestive disorders
   Cirrhosis
   Hepatic fibrosis
   Cystic fibrosis
   Portal hypertension
   Banti syndrome
   Chronic congestive heart failure
2. Cysts
   True
   Pseudocyst
   Parasitic
3. Extramedullary hematopoiesis
   Thalassemia major
   Osteopetrosis
   Myelofibrosis
4. Hemolytic anemias
   Hereditary spherocytosis
   Nonspherocytic hemolytic anemia
   Hemoglobinopathic
   Thalassemia major
5. Infections
   Hepatitis
   Endocarditis
   Malaria
   Infectious mononucleosis
   Sarcoidcsis
   Tuberculous peritonitis
6. Tumors
   Leukemia
   Hodgkin's disease
   Lymphoma
   Metastatic
   Hemangioma
   Hamartoma
7. Storage disorders
   Lipidosis
   Mucopolysaccharidosis
   Glycogen-storage disease (type 1)

allow less tissue penetration. Real-time imaging systems typically have a small field of view. The viewing field is often wedge-shaped or rectangular, ranging from 5 to 15 cm in maximal diameter. Active participation by the physician is required in a manner analogous to the technique in fluorscopic radiology.

SPLEEN IMAGING

Table 3 Causes of Increased Splenic Uptake

1. Cardiovascular abnormalities
    Heart failure
2. Diffuse liver disease
    Cirrhosis
    Fatty infiltration
    Hepatitis
    Metastatic disease
3. Hematologic abnormalities
    Anemia
4. Neoplastic diseases
    Malignant melanoma
    Sarcoma botryoides
5. RES stimulation
    Chronic granulomatous disease
    Septicemia

Radionuclide Scans

After the intravenous injection of 99m-technetium sulfur colloid (which has a particle size of 1 micron), about 10% of the administered radionuclide localizes in the spleen. The remainder of the technetium colloid accumulates within the liver and the balance is taken up in the bone marrow and lungs. The gamma camera is positioned to view the posterior left upper quadrant of the abdomen. The choice of collimator depends on the avialable equipment and the size of the organ that is being investigated.

After bolus injection of a dose of 4 millicuries/$1.7m^2$ of 99m-technetium sulfur colloid, images are obtained at 1 to 5 second intervals for a dynamic evaluation. If it is injected into a foot vein, the radionuclide is first visualized in the inferior vena cava or collateral abdominal venous vessels. Then the radionuclide is seen in the aorta, and within 3 to 5 seconds there is simultaneous perfusion of the kidneys and the spleen. The liver is visualized later during the sequence because the majority of hepatic blood flow originates from the portal venous system. In general, dynamic imaging following bolus infection of radionuclide is most useful in evaluating the gross anatomic configuration of the abdominal venous channels, as in assessing patients with asplenia-polysplenia syndromes (Figures 5 and 6). This technique is also useful for evaluating the vascularity of mass lesions. Dynamic imaging has limited usefulness in other clinical circumstances.

About 15 minutes after intravenous injection of the radionuclide, static images are obtained in the posterior, anterior, lateral, and left anterior oblique projections, with 400,000 to 500,000 counts/view. Other oblique projections can be obtained if desired, following a review of the initial images.

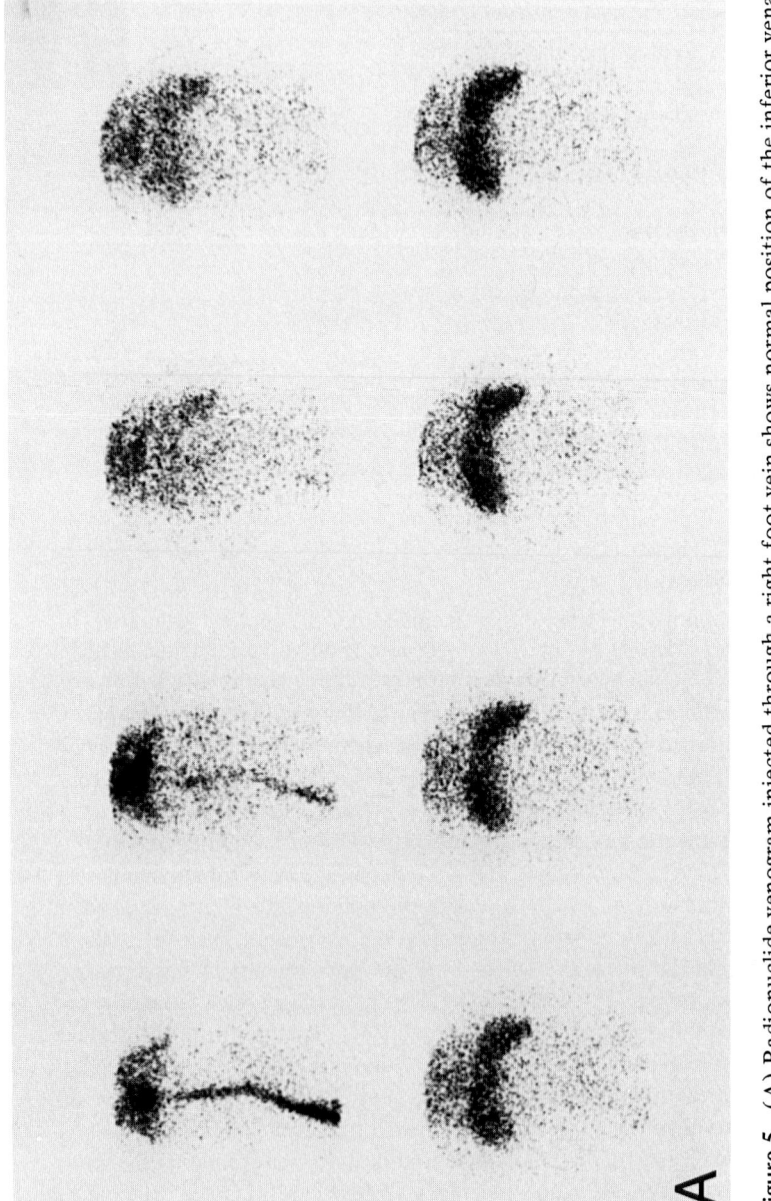

Figure 5 (A) Radionuclide venogram injected through a right foot vein shows normal position of the inferior vena cava. No spleen is identified. (B) Same patient, delayed image following the 99m-technetium sulfur colloid venogram in the posterior projection shows an indentation due to the spine without evidence of a spleen. Diagnosis: transverse liver with asplenia.

B

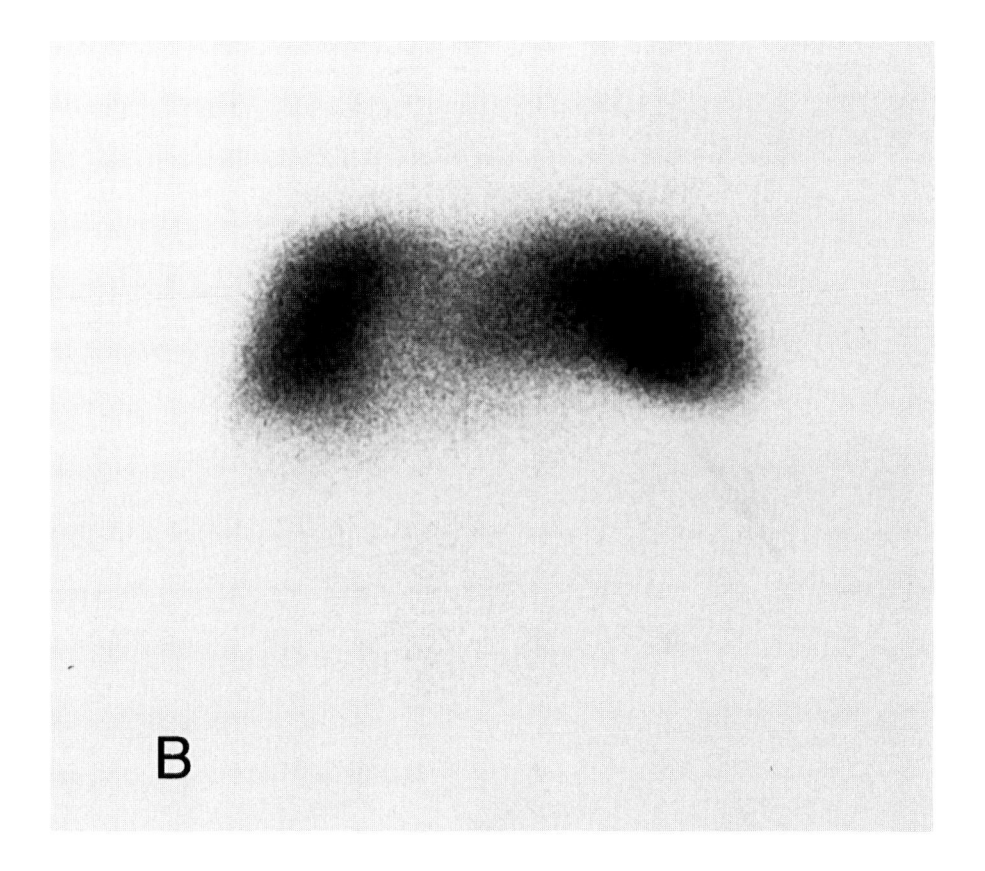

Several features of splenic anatomy are important for accurate interpretation of radionuclide scans of the spleen. First, the spleen is oriented such that the upper pole lies posterior to the lower pole. Second, the left lobe of the liver often overlaps the spleen. Visual separation of the two organs requires appropriate positioning of the patient; that is, placing the patient in the left anterior oblique position with respect to the xray film. A helpful additional view is the posterior view with caudal angulation. A third significant feature of splenic anatomy is the fact that a wide spacing between the liver and spleen may simulate presence of a mass. Technetium-99m pertechnetate can be given by mouth to visualize the stomach (23). The fundus of the stomach normally is interposed between the left lobe of the liver and the spleen when viewed in the left anterior oblique projection.

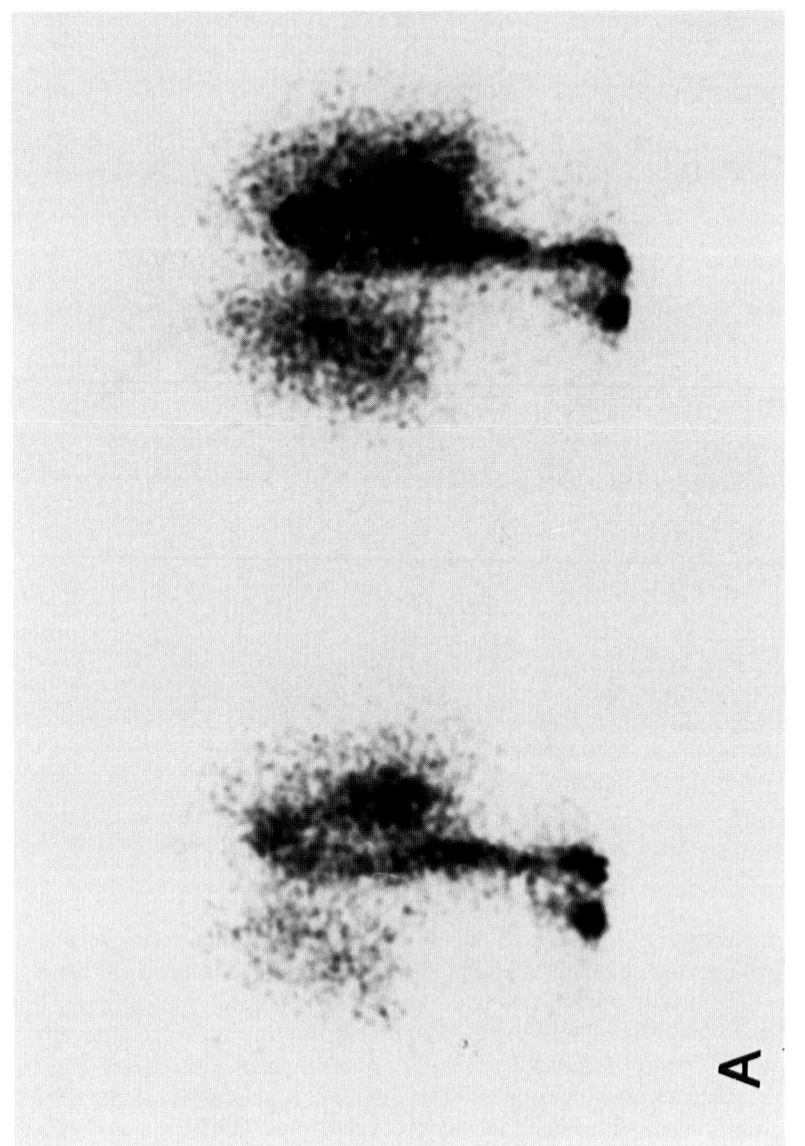

Figure 6 (A) The radionuclide venogram demonstrates azygos continuation of the inferior vena cava. (B) Delayed posterior image shows polysplenia.

B

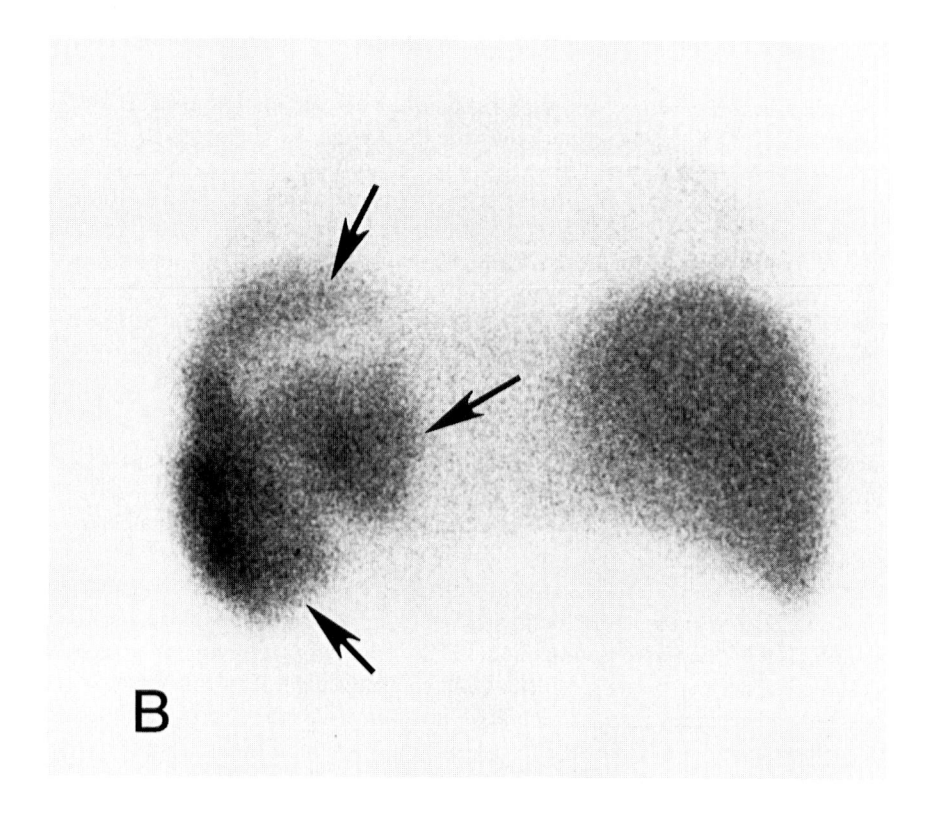

Occasionally, despite multiple views, superposition of the left lobe of the liver over the spleen will preclude adequate splenic visualization. In this circumstance, the spleen can be imaged with labeled damaged red blood cells (24). This technique may be clinically important in patients after splenectomy for hypersplenism. It may also be useful in the occasional patient in which scans following injection of technetium sulfur colloid for suspected asplenia or polysplenia give inconclusive findings. Another imaging technique that may be helpful in these circumstances is the use of comparative imaging with 99m-technetium hepatobiliary radiopharmaceuticals. Discrepancies between the organ morphology seen with technetium sulfur colloid imaging and with hepatobiliary imaging indicates the spleen is present, whereas similarity of the two images suggests the spleen is absent (25).

Dosage of radiation is an important consideration especially in diagnostic imaging of children. The radiation dose to the spleen in pediatric patients undergoing 99m-technetium sulfur colloid imaging is safe when considered with respect to the benefits it provides. The effective half-life of 99m-technetium sulfur colloid in the spleen is 5.2 ± 0.68 hours. The dose per administered activity ranges from 0.35 to 1.96 cGy per millicurie for the spleen. The doses of radiation extrapolated from observed values in adults are comparable to those seen in children. The radiation dose to the spleen from radiolabelled heat-denatured red blood cell varies from 4 cGy/100 microcuries of 99m-technetium in the newborn to 2 cGy/500 microcuries of 99m-technetium in a 15 year old adolescent (26,27).

Computed Tomography

Computed tomographic scans, 1 cm thick and taken at intervals of 1 or 2 cm, are usually adequate to evaluate the spleen. Precontrast images add very little information; thus, splenic CT scans are usually performed only after intravenous administration of contrast.

In examining the spleen by computed tomography, a number of parameters are assessed. These include size, parenchymal character, attenuation values, contour, and position. Differences in contrast-enhancement between normal and abnormal regions aid in the detection and differential diagnosis of focal splenic abnormalities. Associated findings may aid in determining the cause of splenic abnormalities. Thus, presence of liver disease, enlargement of splenic vessels disease in adjacent organs with secondary involvement of the spleen, or presence of similar abnormalities in other organs (such as cysts or metastases), may be useful in identifying disease in the spleen. For these reasons, computed tomography and ultrasonography provide a more complete examination than radionuclide scans.

Focal areas of low attenuation on the CT scan, as compared to normal splenic tissue, may be produced by artifacts from adjacent ribs, breathing, or contrast agents present in the gastrointestinal tract. These artifacts must be appreciated in order to distinguish them from true splenic pathology. These artifacts are usually flame-shaped, have ill-defined margins, and radiate directly from the structure causing the artifact. Low-attenuation regions that do not radiate directly from high attenuation structures most often represent a pathologic lesion. If the appearance is equivocal, repeat scanning through the area of concern after change in the patient's position usually produces a definitive image. The spleen normally shows homogeneous enhancement. Non-homogeneity of the spleen may be caused by patient motion or respiration. In children, sedation may be required to avoid or eliminate this artifact. The attenuation value of a small mass may be artificially raised by partial volume effect when the mass only partially fills the slice.

The absolute attenuation value of the spleen is variable with different equipment and varies among individuals within any patient population. However, the attenuation value of the spleen is stable and reproducible within a given individual. A mean CT number of 42 HU with a range of 30 to 68 has been reported. The wide range of CT numbers is due to technical factors such as beam-hardening artifacts, patient size and shape, varying kilovolt peak of the anode, and intermittent software revisions in scanner systems.

However, in the normal patient, the liver and spleen maintain constant relationship in attenuation values. The liver is almost always slightly more dense than the spleen. Since the spleen has a relatively low rate of metabolic activity, large fluctuations of chemical content to not occur. Therefore, alterations in the relationship between liver and spleen CT numbers are usually due to changes in liver composition rather than changes in attenuation values of the spleen. The spleen, however, may demonstrate increased attenuation as a result of hemosiderin deposition in patients with beta-thalassemia following multiple blood transfusions. The spleen is usually of normal density in primary hemochromatosis.

CLINICAL APPLICATIONS OF IMAGING IN DIAGNOSING SPLENIC ABNORMALITIES

Herniation of the Spleen Through the Diaphragm

A chest xray showing a mass at the base of the lung contiguous with the hemidiaphragm can represent a difficult diagnostic problem. The mass may originate from the lung, the pleura or the diaphragm. Lesions of the lung include pulmonary sequestration and primary or metastatic neoplasms. The pleura may be the origin of loculated fluid. The hemidiaphragm may be the source of a "mass" because of diaphragmatic eventration, or an abdominal hernia. Occasionally, the spleen may present as a mass at the base of the lung through herniation or eventration.

Herniation of the spleen through the diaphragm is readily identified by imaging with 99m-technetium sulfur colloid. Sonography and computed tomography may then show that the soft tissue mass demonstrated on the chest xray is of the same character as the spleen. They will also demonstrate the abnormal position of the spleen.

Hypersplenism and Accessory Spleens

Sequestration and phagocytosis of erythrocytes with removal of senescent red cells is an important function of the spleen. The spleen also acts to remove abnormal neutrophils and platelets as well as particulate matter from the circulation. An abnormal increase in these functions of sequestration and phagocytosis by the spleen is called hypersplenism. At times, surgical removal of the spleen is performed as treatment for this condition.

Accessory spleens are present in 10 to 30% of patients with hypersplenism. Accessory spleens may be microscopic in size or up to several centimeters in diameter. Most often, they are multiple, but usually less than 6 in number. They are most frequently located in the region of the splenic hilum. However, they may also be encountered in the tail of the pancreas or in the suspensory ligaments of the spleen. They may originate, or develop following implantation, in the wall of the stomach, greater omentum, mesentery, bowel wall, pelvis or even in the scrotum.

Accessory spleens may attain large size after removal of the spleen itself, particularly in hypersplenic conditions. If the diagnosis of accessory spleen is considered after splenectomy, a 99m-technetium sulfur colloid spleen scan will usually demonstrate an accessory spleen if it is at least 2 cm in diameter. Upon removal of the spleen, the left lobe of the liver often protrudes into the splenic fossa (28). This unusual configuration of the left lobe of the liver has been termed the liver tail. An accessory spleen situated adjacent to the left lobe of the liver may be difficult to differentiate from the liver tail. A hepatobiliary scan will define the contours of the liver. Comparison of the hepatobiliary scan with the technetium sulfur colloid scan will differentiate an accessory spleen from the left lobe of the liver. Splenectomy in childhood is most often indicated in hematologic diseases such as spherocytosis or idiopathic thrombocytopenic purpura (Figure 7).

Computed tomography is another accurate method of diagnosing both symptomatic and asymptomatic accessory spleens. An accessory spleen usually appears as a round or oval mass located in or near the hilum, and having the same attenuation as a normal spleen both before and after intravenous contrast administration. Comparing the pre-contrast and post-contrast images is necessary when trying to differentiate lymph nodes from accessory spleens. Ultrasonography may have difficulty in distinguishing lymph nodes from accessory spleens (Figures 8 and 9).

Splenic-Gonadal Fusion

Splenic-gonadal fusion is an embryopathy resulting from fusion of the splenic and gonadal anlages. The diagnosis is rarely considered pre-operatively because of the rarity of this condition. The diagnosis is usually established during surgical exploration of the scrotum or abdomen, when splenic tissue is found together with associated gonadal tissue in a site where a tumor mass was palpated.

The splenic anlage forms in the left dorsal mesogastrium at the sixth or seventh week of gestation. The splenic anlage is in close proximity to the mesonephros of the left gonadal anlage until the initiation of gonadal descent, at about the eighth week of gestation (29,30). As the developing organs migrate, abnormal fusion results in either drawing out of splenic tissue into a long con-

SPLEEN IMAGING 373

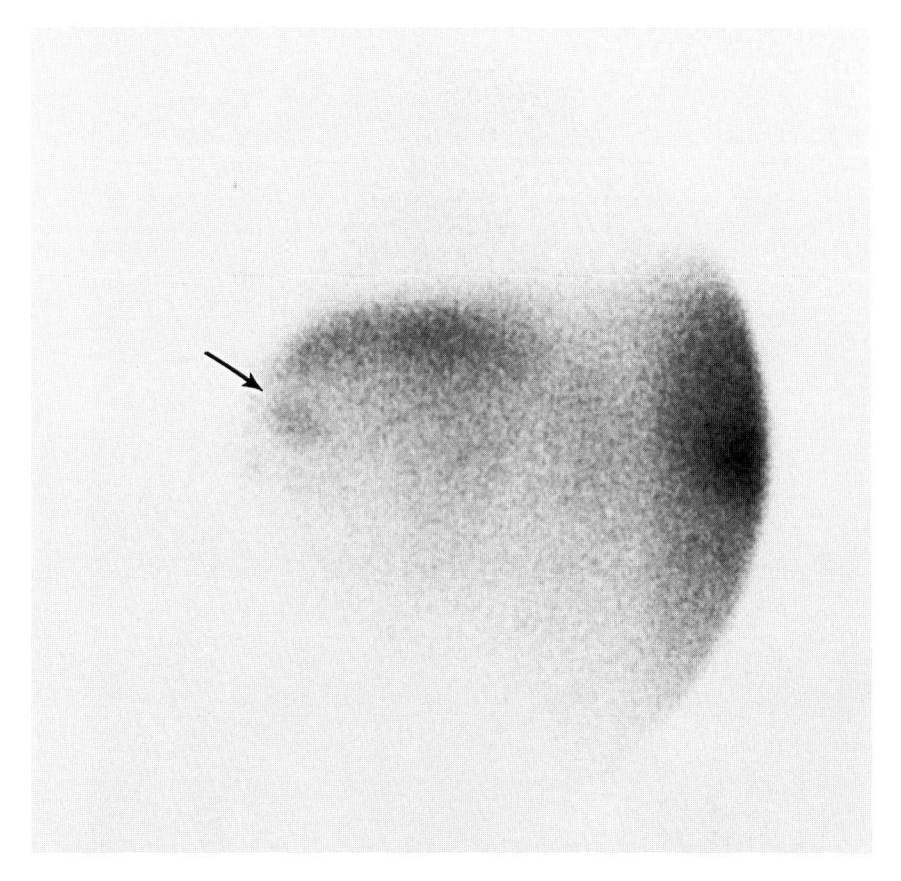

Figure 7 99m-technetium sulfur colloid image of the left upper quadrant posterior view in a splenectomized patient, shows a small area of accumulation of tracer. This proved to be a hypertrophy accessory spleen.

tiguous connecting cord or separation of part of the spleen which then descends with the gonad. The anomaly, therefore, can be divided into two types: continuous and discontinuous. In the continuous variety, a band of tissue connects a normally located spleen with the testis, epididymis, ovary, or mesovarium. This band may be composed of splenic or fibrous tissue or an admixture of the two tissues. Cryptochism is associated with the continuous variety. In the discontinuous type, there is no connection between the orthotopic and the heterotopic splenic tissue. This variety is most often found in the adult, but this type of splenic-gonadal fusion also is seen in children (31,32). Intra-abdom-

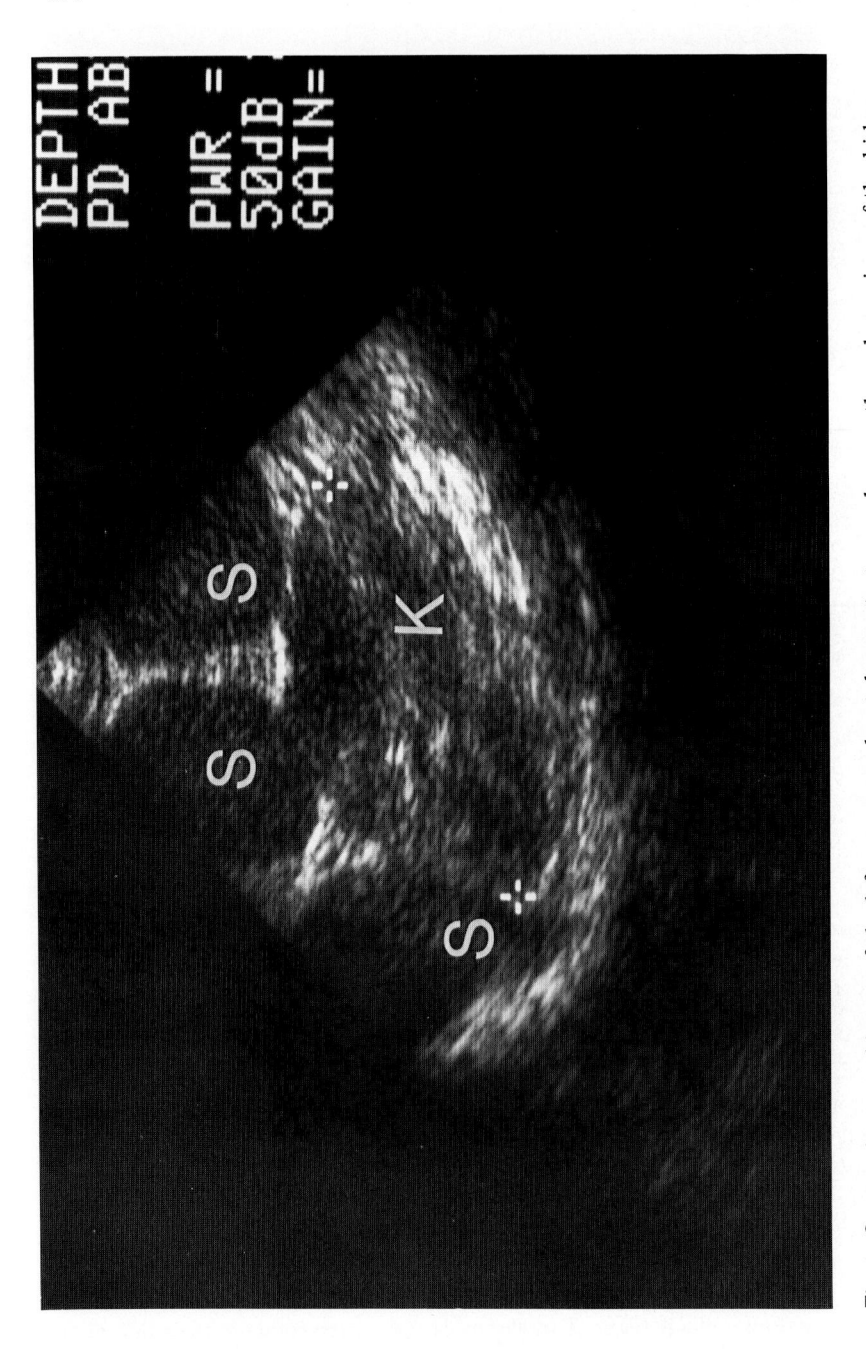

Figure 8 An ultrasound image of the left upper quadrant demonstrates markers on the polar regions of the kidney. Immediately adjacent of the kidney are three hypertrophied accessory spleens.

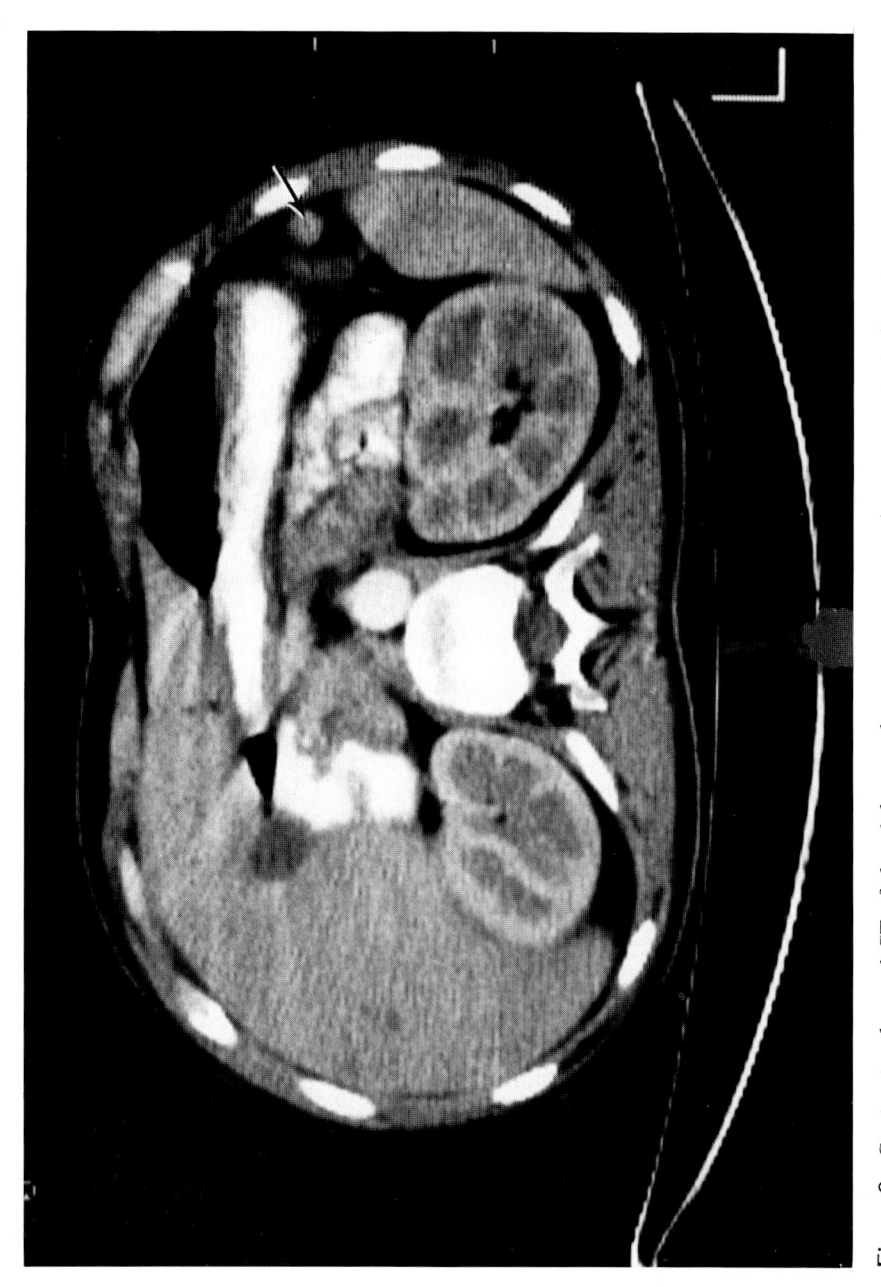

Figure 9 Contrast-enhanced CT of the abdomen demonstrates normal structures including the spleen. Immediately anterior to the spleen, a small region of enhancement is identified (arrow). This has the same contrast characteristics as the spleen, and represents a small accessory spleen.

inal splenic tissue other than that forming the connecting cord is not a common feature of this condition: the othotopic spleen is usually single.

Exploratory laparotomy, therefore, is not recommended to confirm the diagnosis of splenic-gonadal fusion. Laparotomy is also not indicated as a routine prophylactic measure once the diagnosis has been made. If information about the intra-abdominal extent of the process is needed, a radionuclide technetium sulfur colloid scan of the left half of the abdomen should be performed (33). This diagnosis relies more on radionuclide imaging than on findings from computed tomography or sonography.

Asplenia and Polysplenia Syndromes

Technetium-99m sulfur colloid imaging, CT, and ultrasound are all useful for evaluating children with severe congenital heart disease and associated asplenia or polysplenia. A particularly severe form of congenital heart disease has been reported in which there is associated midline positioning of the liver and presence of asplenia (34). It is important to differentiate this condition from functional hyposplenia, which may be associated with certain types of cyanotic congenital heart disease in the newborn (35).

Specific types of cardiovascular abnormalities are sometimes associated with abnormalities of the spleen and malposition and malformation of other organs. The complexity of the cardiac malformation determines the clinical course and prognosis. Consequently, it is important to identify the child who has asplenia or polysplenia syndromes in order to anticipate potential complications. X rays of the chest and abdomen plus an abdominal radionuclide angiogram and liver-spleen scan provide important information in patients who may have multiple malformations associated with asplenia or polysplenia.

A radionuclide angiogram performed by injection through a foot vein will demonstrate a normal inferior vena cava or azygos continuation of the inferior vena cava. Delayed static images indicate the positions of the liver and spleen, as well as absence of the spleen or the presence of multiple foci of splenic tissue. Likewise, computed tomography and sonography provide noninvasive means for evaluating several components of these syndromes. These imaging modalities will demonstrate multiple spleens, situs inversus, configuration of the liver, absence of the suprarenal inferior vena cava, and enlarged azygos and hemiazygos veins adjacent to the aorta. Sonography is also the imaging procedure best suited to assess the cardiac defects.

Rose et al. (36), reviewed patients with asplenia and polysplenia in 60 cases of cardiac and noncardiac malformations. They gave special attention to diagnosis and prognosis. It was noted that patients with asplenia were usually boys and presented with marked cyanosis. Frequently, these patients had transposition of the great vessels with pulmonary stenosis or atresia and total anomalous venous drainage. Most patients died within the first year of life. Patients with polysplenia were usually girls, they showed longer survival, and the clinical findings were usually less severe. Azygos continuation of the inferior vena cava often occurred in patients with polysplenia. Aortic-caval juxtaposition was commonly associated with asplenia, but on occasion this abnormality was also seen with polysplenia.

The asplenia and polysplenia syndromes both show a striking tendency for symmetrical development of normally asymmetric organs or organ systems. It is well established that in the asplenia syndrome the left lung and left lobe of the liver anatomically resemble their right counterparts in a mirror-image configuration. More recently, it has been shown that morphologically the left atrium resembles the right atrium, and in a few cases a bilateral sino-atrial node has been demonstrated. Because patients with asplenia appear to have two right sides, congenital asplenia has been referred to as a syndrome of bilateral right-sidedness. Likewise, the right lung and bronchial tree in the polysplenia syndrome morphologically mirror-image those on the left, and frequently the hepatic segment of the inferior vena cava is absent resulting in azygos continuation of the inferior vena cava. Thus, congenital polysplenia has been termed the syndrome of bilateral left-sidedness. Radionuclide imaging is very useful for identification of the position of the liver and for detecting the presence of asplenia or polysplenia. In addition, if the tracer is injected through a foot vein, the inferior vena cava, the azygos continuation, or both, can be readily observed.

Abnormalities associated with congenital asplenia other than those in the cardiopulmonary system have received little attention. However, Freedman (37) and Putschar and Manion (38) have brought to light some of the gastrointestinal, genitourinary, and neuromuscular abnormalities that may be found in asplenia. Mishalany (39) retrospectively reviewed 36 patients with gastrointestinal anomalies who died with this disease. A significant number were found to have situs inversus, malrotation of the gastrointestinal tract, esophageal varices, duplication and hypoplasia of the stomach, Hirschprung disease, imperforate anus, and duplication of the gastrointestinal tract. These patients presented with symptoms of gastrointestinal anomalies and did not appear to have cardiopulmonary abnormalities or absence of the spleen. Therefore, it is important to establish the presence of the spleen in an infant in whom there are various anomalies of the gastrointestinal tract because overwhelming septicemia can occur if the spleen is absent.

It is also interesting to note that all children in the series who presented with gastrointestinal obstructions or hematemesis had no initial symptoms suggesting congenital asplenia. As many as 86% of the patients in their series died of overwhelming sepsis. It was concluded that many patients with congenital asplenia have concomitant gastrointestinal anomalies. Cardiac and pulmonary symptoms may not always be evident initially in these patients. Determining presence or absence of the spleen is important in patients with gastrointestinal anomalies because of the severe morbidity associated with overwhelming sepsis.

Wandering Spleen

The wandering spleen occurs in association with other abnormal congenital anomalies. The spleen and colon develop in the dorsal mesogastrium. When there is abnormal development of the mesogastrium, the lienorenal and lienogastric ligaments are defective, and the phrenicolic ligament that forms a sling to support the spleen fails to develop appropriately. A wandering spleen is rarely found in patients subjected to splenectomy. The majority of patients with this abnormality are women between the ages of 20 and 40. The wandering spleen occurs in association with prune-belly syndrome and in agenesis of the left kidney. The spleen may migrate into the left renal fossa in congenital absence of the kidney and may be mistaken for a kidney on radionuclide flow studies (8,40).

Symptoms associated with wandering spleen are variable and may result from splenic congestion or ligamentous pressure. Occasionally, there may be symptoms of an acute abdomen due to torsion of the splenic pedicle. Mistaken diagnoses include a variety of abnormalities. In children, the most common misinterpreted disease is appendicitis (9). Major complications of splenic torsion include abscess, gangrene and infarction. There is relatively high mortality rate associated with these major complications (Figure 10).

Plain radiographs of the abdomen in cases of wandering spleen show absence of a spleen in the left upper quadrant and the presence of a soft tissue mass elsewhere in the abdomen or in the pelvis. Barium enema and IVP produce variable findings and thus are not the examinations of choice. 99m-technetium sulfur colloid scan demonstrates inferomedial position of the spleen and allows a specific diagnosis. Computed tomography and sonography demonstrate the normal splenic architecture and vascular pedicle. These findings establish presence of the spleen in the abnormal location.

Functional Asplenia

Imaging the spleen with 99m-technetium sulfur colloid depends on phagocytosis of the radiocolloid. Therefore, any disease that interferes with function of the reticuloendothelial system will result in photopenic areas in the spleen. Functional asplenia has been described by Pearson in children with sickle cell disease. The spleen is present, but phagocytic function is diminished. The diminished phagocytic function has been shown to be reversible following transfusion of normal red blood cells. In addition, various disorders may cause functional asplenia (41).

There are many known or suspected causes of functional asplenia. Asplenia may be caused by disturbance of splenic vascular supply. Vascular supply may be disturbed by (1) blockade of major splenic vessels (arteries, veins, or both), or (2) blockade of capillaries (as in hemoglobin SS or SC disease).

Also functional asplenia may be caused by alterations in splenic reticuloendothelial activity. These alterations in reticuloendothelial activity may be due to (1) damage from vascular obstruction and irradiation, (2) combined effects of irradiation plus chemotherapy, (3) reticuloendothelial cell replacement by infiltrating tumor, (4) damage to reticuloendothelial cells, as in celiac-sprue disease (nutritional or immune compromise), (5) anoxia of the spleen (as in congenital cyanotic heart disease), and (6) immunosuppression associated with bone marrow transplantation.

If splenic vascular occlusion is acute, Howell-Jolly bodies may not initially be seen in the peripheral blood, despite the finding of functional asplenia by spleen scan. In severe hematopoietic stress, the reverse is true, that is, Howell-Jolly bodies are present but the spleen scan shows normal function.

Vascular occlusions of the spleen can also be detected with computed tomography. Infarcts may be silent clinically, or at times they may be associated with left upper quadrant pain. Infarcts may be single, multiple, or involve the whole spleen. With CT imaging, infarcts are usually wedge-shaped or round, and they are often located in peripheral areas of of the spleen. Infarcts usually have a lower attenuation value than normal spleen and do not enhance. Therefore, there is a greater chance to detect infarcts after injecting intravenous contrast media. Unless infarcts are wedge-shaped on CT, their appearance is not specific (Figure 11).

Trauma

The role of radionuclide imaging in assessing trauma of the spleen is well established (22,42-48). The clinical findings of left upper quadrant tenderness and abdominal pain, in addition to signs of hypovolemia, suggest a diagnosis of splenic rupture. Unstable patients with these findings require immediate surgery. However, in cases in which the diagnosis is questionable and the patient is stable, radiologic imaging is useful in documenting the presence of splenic injury. Radionuclide imaging is as useful as computed tomography and contrast angiography, and all three are more sensitive than ultrasound (49,50). The major limitation of spleen scintigraphy is the lower limit of resolution of approximately 2 cm for identification of anatomical structures. Rarely, the presence of polysplenia may mimic splenic trauma. Injury to the lower pole of the spleen is most difficult to detect by spleen scan, particularly when the lesion is located superficially. A scan showing decreased localization of radionuclide in the lower pole, without demonstrating a clear-cut laceration, should be interpreted with

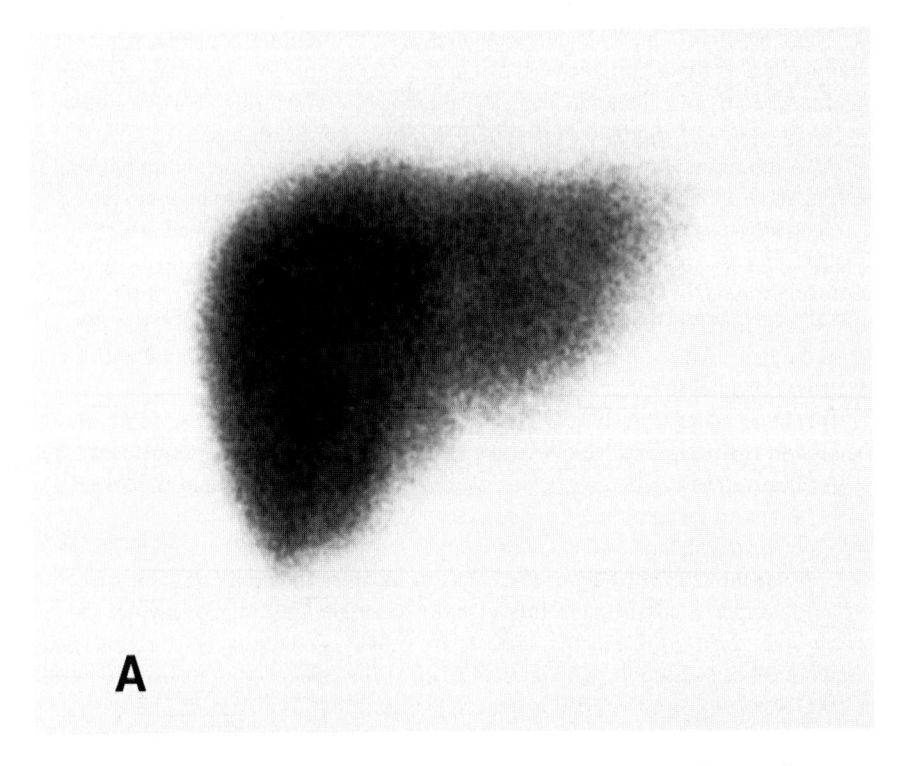

Figure 10 (A) A 99m-technetium sulfur colloid spleen scan in the anterior projection shows a normal liver. No spleen is identified. (B) Same patient as in A. Contrast-enhanced computed tomographic study of the mid-abdomen. This study identifies a necrotic spleen in a lower position than normal. At surgery, an infarcted wandering spleen was identified.

caution. In such cases, CT scan or follow-up radionuclide examinations are useful (Figure 12).

In a series of children with suspected splenic trauma, the incidence of false-negative results on spleen scans was about 1.5% (22). In patients who are stable, serial radionuclide spleen scans may be necessary to distinguish trauma from a normal variation of splenic contour. These additional studies will help prevent false-diagnosis of splenic trauma in children whose intact spleens have an atypical contour.

Computed tomography is used more frequently than liver-spleen scintigraphy in evaluating blunt trauma to the abdomen. CT is more useful because it allows evaluation of the urinary tract, peritoneal cavity and retroperitoneal structures, in addition to imaging of the liver and spleen. The spleen is the intra-

SPLEEN IMAGING 381

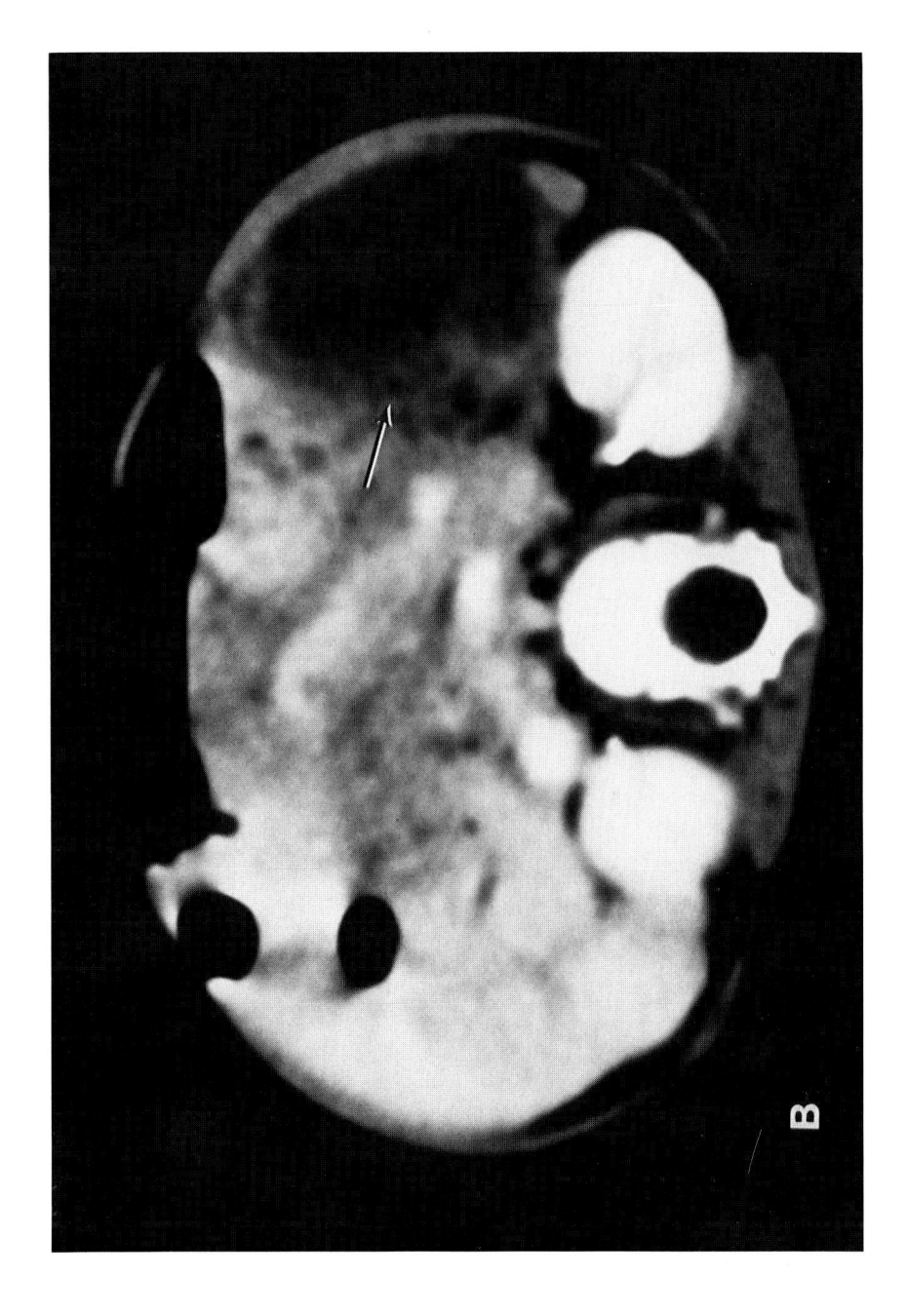

A

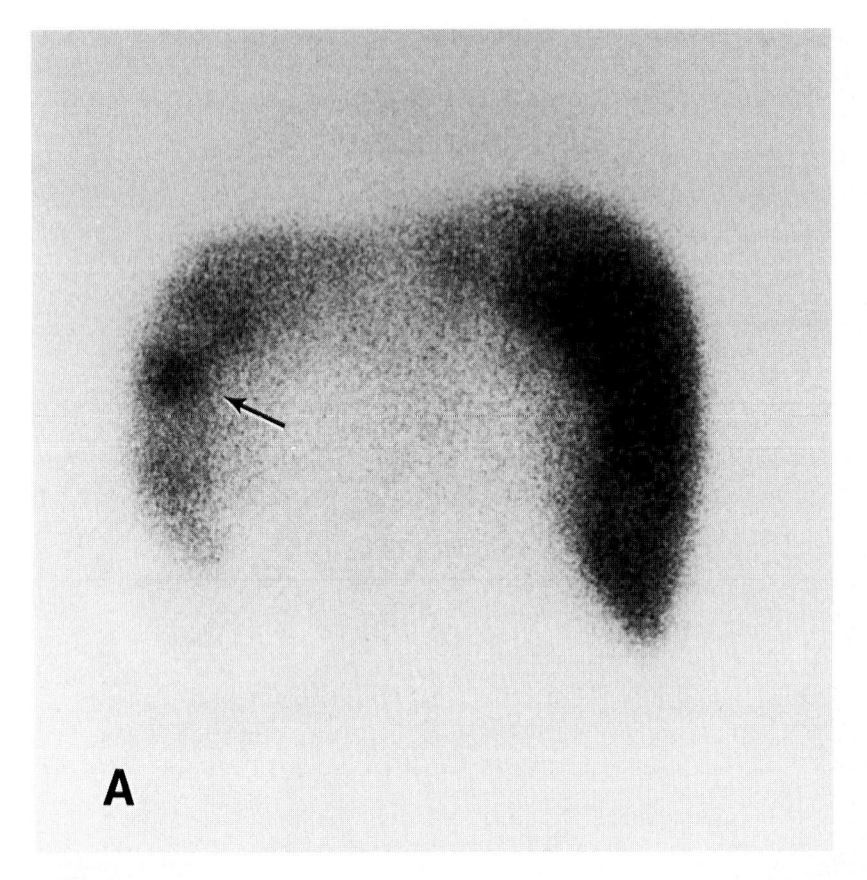

Figure 11 A 99m-technetium sulfur colloid scan in the posterior projection shows multiple areas of decreased activity confined to the splenic tissue. The liver is normal. (B) A contrast-enhanced computed tomographic study of the upper abdomen demonstrates patchy enhancement of the spleen (S). Peripheral regions of nonperfusion are identified. This abnormality was due to splenic infarctions in a patient with sickle cell disease.

peritoneal organ most frequently injured by blunt trauma of the abdomen. In children, blunt trauma is more common than penetrating injury. Abdominal trauma can result in frank splenic laceration or a hematoma that is confined within the splenic capsule. Most subcapsular hematomas have a characteristic appearance on CT scan. This appearance consists of a crescentic peripheral low attenuation area along the margin of the spleen, which flattens or indents the normally convex margin. The size and margins of the subcapsular hematoma are best appreciated when intravenous contrast material is used. When a CT

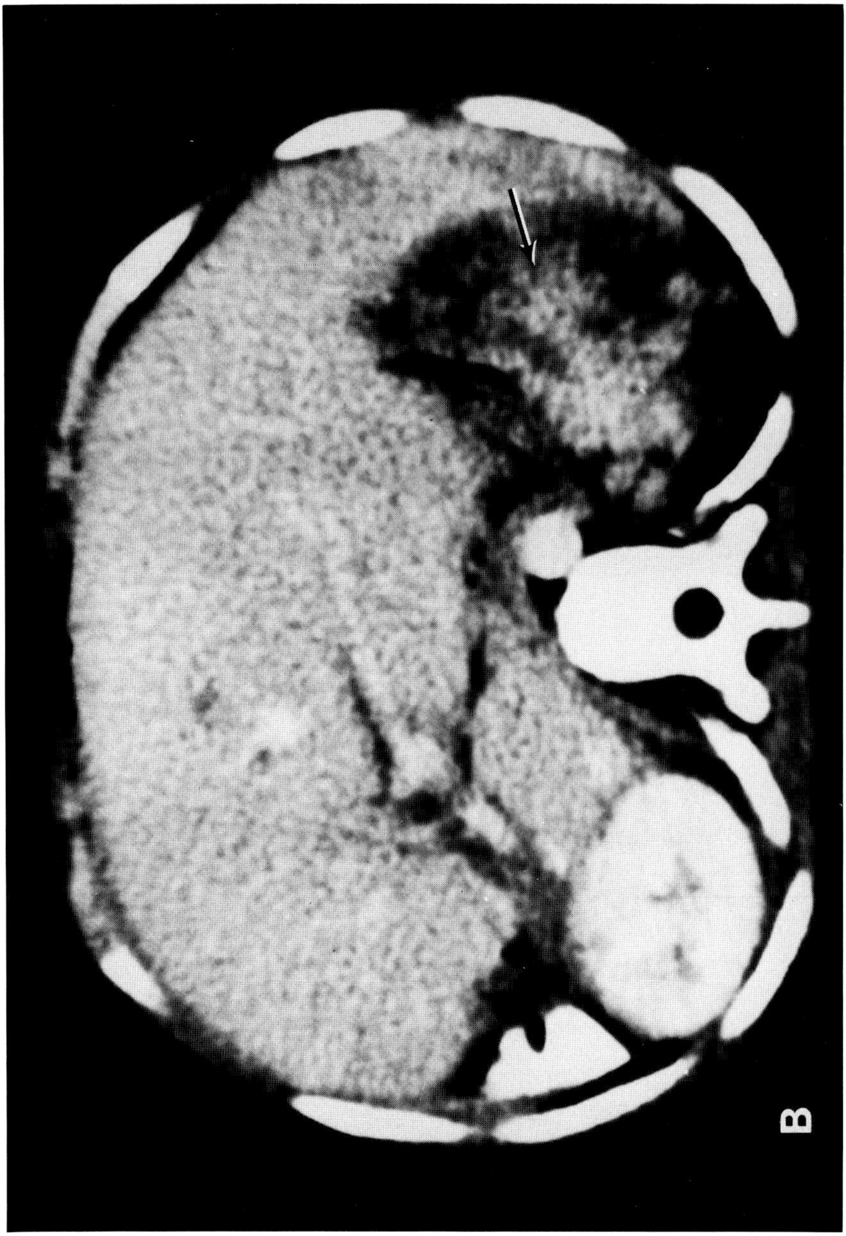
B

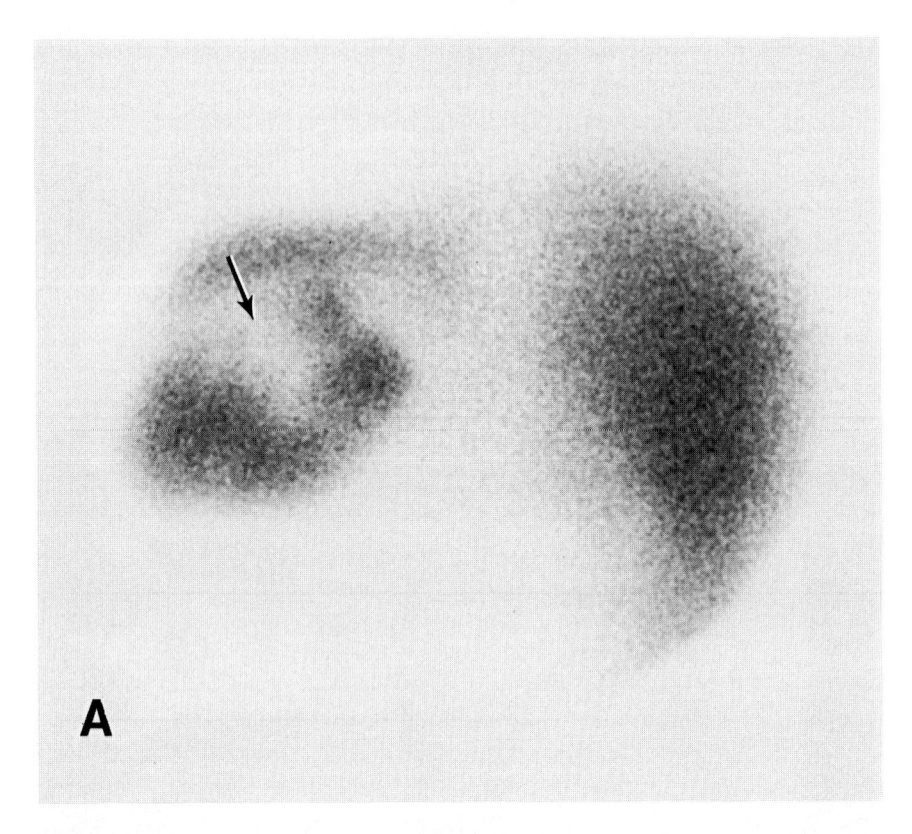

Figure 12 (A) 11 year old boy with trauma to the spleen. The posterior 99m-technetium sulfur colloid scan demonstrates multiple defects within the spleen. (B) A computed tomographic study of the same child demonstrates a linear laceration (arrow) through the midportion of the spleen, and patchy accumulation of the contrast medium in the dorsal aspect of the spleen. These findings are typical of a factured spleen.

scan is performed immediately after splenic injury, without intravenous contrast material, subcapsular intrasplenic hematomas appear isodense or even slightly hyperdense when compared to the normal spleen. Thus, splenic injury may not be detected if intravenous contrast is not used.

As a splenic subcapsular hematoma matures, the density of the hematoma increases as a result of a decrease in hemoglobin and an increase in water content of the lesion.

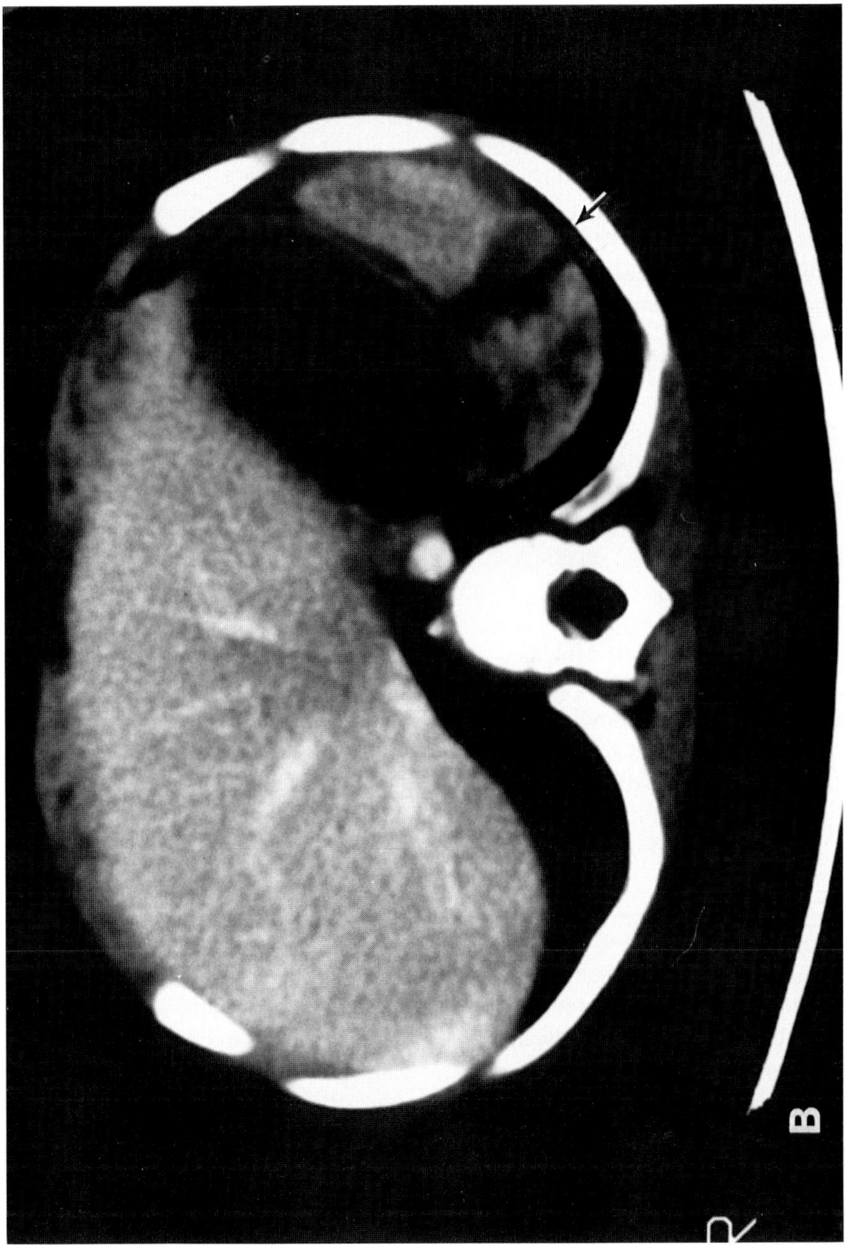
B

Splenic lacerations can be diagnosed by computed tomography, although the findings are more subtle and variable than those with subcapsular hematoma. Splenic lacerations usually produce indistinct margins of the spleen, plus irregular low density bands or clefts through the splenic parenchyma. Lacerations virtually always involve part of the lateral contour of the spleen and are associated with perisplenic bleeding or presence of blood in the peritoneal cavity. It is important to differentiate these defects indicating splenic laceration from congenital splenic clefts. Also, a prominent left lobe of the liver extending across the midline to a point near the spleen must not be mistaken for a splenic laceration. These types of anatomic variation also pose problems in interpreting radionuclide spleen scans.

An interesting sequela of trauma to the spleen is splenosis. Splenosis is defined as heterotopic autotransplantation of splenic tissue. It is thought that disruption of the splenic capsule with fragmentation of the spleen allows spillage of fragments of red pulp into the peritoneal cavity. Because these splenic fragments can derive their blood supply from any tissue to which they attach, they may occur anywhere throughout the peritoneal cavity. Splenic cell rests have been found on serosal surfaces of the small intestine, the greater omentum, the parietal peritoneum, the large intestinal surface, the mesentery, and on the under surface of the diaphragm. Rarely these splenic fragments simulate a gastric mass. Auto transplanted fragments of spleen may range in number from a few to hundreds and their size is variable, from several millimeters to as large as 10 cm (50). Splenic rupture may also be associated with rupture of the left diaphragm. In this way, splenic tissue may be transplanted into the lung and pleural space and simulate pulmonary or pleural nodules (51).

The clinical significance of splenosis is twofold. First, recurrence of hematologic disorders such as hemolytic anemia, Felty's syndrome, and idiopathic thrombocytopenic purpura have been reported in patients following splenectomy (50). Second, according to Pearson, splenosis is not uncommon after splenic trauma (52).

In addition to its value in detection and recognition of splenic trauma, radionuclide scanning is useful for nonoperative follow up of ruptured spleen (56, 57). Radionuclide scans show delayed splenic rupture. Delayed splenic rupture may be the cause for some false negative findings in cases of splenic trauma. Pseudocyst formation is another complication after trauma that can readily be identified with scintigraphy. In patients with subcapsular hematoma or frank rupture of the spleen, follow-up studies are recommended immediately before discharge from the hospital and again about two months later (56,57).

Postsplenectomy Sepsis

Postsplenectomy sepsis can be defined as septicemia, meningitis, or pneumonia, usually fulminant, occurring at anytime up to many years following removal of the spleen. The disease is typically abrupt in onset and rapidly reaches a critical state within hours or a few days. In fatal cases, adrenal hemorrhage (as in the Waterhouse-Friderichsen syndrome) may occur, regardless of the microbial etiology of sepsis. Repeated episodes of severe infection can also occur.

In an analysis by Singer of 2,796 splenectomy patients, sepsis occurred in 119 (4.5%), and 71 patients (2.52%) died of infection. Death from sepsis is 200 times more common in persons following splenectomy than death due to sepsis in the general population (58). Death due to infection occurs in 0.3% of infants less than one year of age (59). In children age 1 to 7 years, the incidence of mortality due to infection is only 0.02%. In the general population of individuals with normal spleens and including all ages, the incidence of mortality due to sepsis is as low as 0.01%.

The disease for which splenectomy is performed is an additional factor that influences the incidence of postsplenectomy sepsis. In patients who have splenectomy because of traumatic splenic rupture, mortality due to sepsis is 0.58%. In other diseases requiring splenectomy, the mortality rate due to sepsis in asplenic individuals is as follows: splenectomy performed incidental to other operations 0.85%, splenectomy for idiopathic thrombocytopenia 1.43%, for congenital spherocytosis 2.23%, for acquired hemolytic anemia 2.9%, for portal hypertension 5.9%, for primary anemia 7.01%, for reticuloendothelial disease 10.1%, and for splenectomy for thalassemia major 11.0%.

The infecting organism most often recovered from patients with postsplenectomy sepsis is the pneumococcus, *Streptococcus pneumonae*. In decreasing numbers, meningococcus, *Escherichia coli*, *Hemophilus influenzae*, staphylococcus, *Mycobacterium tuberculosis*, varicella, and the parasite of *Babesia microtie* have been responsible for fatal sepsis following splenectomy (58). From experimental observations and practical experience it has been concluded that asplenic individuals are most likely to develop infection from blood-born innoculae of pneumococcus, meningococcus, E. *coli*, and H. *influenzae*. The spleen serves as the primary site for removal of these micro-organisms from the circulation. Splenic function is especially important when a microbial organism has a polysaccharide capsule. Splenic antibody production against these organisms is yet another factor in determining the risk of postsplenectomy sepsis.

When the spleen is absent, the phagocytic and antibody producing functions are lost or disturbed and postsplenectomy sepsis may result. If the volume of the spleen is reduced to less than 25% of normal, or if the blood supply to the spleen is significantly altered, (as may be the case with splenosis), sepsis is more common. Similarly, if splenic function is impaired, such as in sickle cell anemia, sepsis occurs more frequently. Non-hematogenous infections probably do not occur more commonly in asplenic persons than in normal individuals (58,61).

Although splenosis is generally believed to occur infrequently, interference-phase microscopy of red blood cells of persons who have had splenectomy for trauma has shown evidence of return of splenic function in over half of these individuals (52,62,63). This may be the reason for the difference in mortality rate between splenectomy for trauma and splenectomy performed as incidental to other operations. 99m-technetium sulfur colloid scans of the abdomen have shown multiple splenic nodules in some of these patients. The regrowth of splenic tissue after splenectomy has been attributed to work hypertrophy. In one study, following splenectomy, remaining splenic tissue showed a growth rate of 0.24 to 0.32 grams/day.

It has been suggested that regenerated splenic tissue due to splenosis may offer some degree of protection against bacterial infections and may, in part, account for the lower frequency of sepsis after splenectomy for trauma. However, bacterial sepsis has occurred in individuals with proven splenosis. It is not known whether a critical mass of splenic tissue is necessary for complete protection against bacterial infections. Experimental studies in animals have actually yielded conflicting results. One study involving induced transepithelial infection indicated that transplanted splenic tissue does not significantly reduce mortality. Nonetheless, successful autotransplantation of splenic tissue has been achieved in patients undergoing splenectomy for trauma. Splenic function returned to normal shortly after autotransplantation (65).

Splenic Cysts and Abscesses

Primary masses of the spleen in children are rare, but include cysts, abscesses, hemangiomas, lymphangiomas, and hamartomas. All appear as focal defects on radionuclide spleen scans and their appearance is nonspecific. Some splenic neoplasms such as lymphangiomas, hemangiomas, hamartomas, and desmoids, can produce lesions of the spleen that are predominantly cystic in nature. Although the CT appearance of these tumors has not been fully characterized in children, computed tomography eventually will probably be able to identify these benign splenic masses. However, it is likely that differentiation between the various neoplasms will be difficult. This principle also applies to the use of sonography to discriminate between these various tumors.

Cysts are the most common primary lesions of the spleen in children. Worldwide, the majority of cysts in the spleen are due to parasites. In the United States, hydatid cysts are rare and congenital cysts and pseudocysts of the spleen are more common (71).

Primary nonparasitic cysts of the spleen are most often classified histologically as epidermoid on the basis of their epithelial lining. These cysts usually present clinically as a left upper quadrant mass, and they are readily documented with radionuclide imaging or by other diagnostic imaging. Nonparasitic cysts appear to be more common in females. Although splenic cysts in general are most often seen in the age group from 20 to 40 years, epidermoid cysts occur more frequently in persons younger than 20 years (72). Symptoms are usually absent or minimal. Left upper quadrant pain and fullness, which can radiate to the shoulders, chest or back, may be present. Because the early symptoms are minimal, splenic cysts are usually large by the time they are discovered. Most often the cysts are solitary and unilocular. Occasionally, multiple primary splenic cysts may occur as an isolated abnormality, but usually multiple cysts are associated with polycystic disease of the liver and kidneys (72). Pseudocysts of the spleen are cysts occurring as a result of intrasplenic hematoma. These have been reported in children and may occur after trivial trauma with or without enlargement of the spleen.

Scintigraphy, computed tomography, and sonography usually cannot differentiate between these two types of cysts: primary cysts and pseudocysts. Technetium-99m sulfur colloid imaging shows the photopenic areas in the spleen, although if the defects are located in a peripheral region they may be mistaken for an extrinsic mass with splenic displacement (Figure 13).

Primary splenic cysts and pseudocysts appear identical on computed tomography. Both varieties are typically unilocular, homogeneous, water-density lesions having sharp, thin margins. Parasitic splenic cysts are almost always due to echinococcus. The most common organism is *E. granulosis*, which tends to produce a round or oval mass with nearly the density of water, and having sharp margins. CT scan reveals a homogeneous mass with sharp margins that may have foci of small calcifications. The cyst wall may or may not contain foci of calcification. Non-calcified portions of the cyst wall will enhance after contrast, and daughter cells budding from the outer cyst wall will give a multi-oculated appearance.

Primary infections with abscess formation in the spleen are unusual in an otherwise healthy child. Most splenic infections occur in immunocompromised individuals or in conjunction with bacterial endocarditis. Certain infections are known to be complicated by splenic abscesses with unusual frequency. In the pre-antibiotic era, 10% of the patients who died of bacterial endocarditis had suppurative lesions within the spleen. But even now, splenic infection occasionally causes persistent bacteremia, despite appropriate antibiotic therapy for endocarditis. Splenic abscesses also may be associated with amebic dysentery, otitis media, mastoiditis, peritonsillar abscess, cutaneous infections of various types, pneumonia, empyema, appendicitis, osteomyelitis, and intravenous drug abuse (73,74).

Various hemoglobinopathies also predispose to the development of splenic abscesses. In Nigeria, 75% of patients with splenic abscesses have sickle cell disease. In the United States, the most common hemoglobinopathies associated with splenic abscesses are sickle trait and hemoglobin SC disease and, rarely, sickle-beta-thalassemia and hemoglobin AC. The absence of splenic abscesses in patients with hemoglobin SS disease may be related to the functional asplenia that begins in early childhood (75-78). With functional asplenia there is less phagocytosis of microorganisms in the spleen and less likelihood to have localized infections in the spleen.

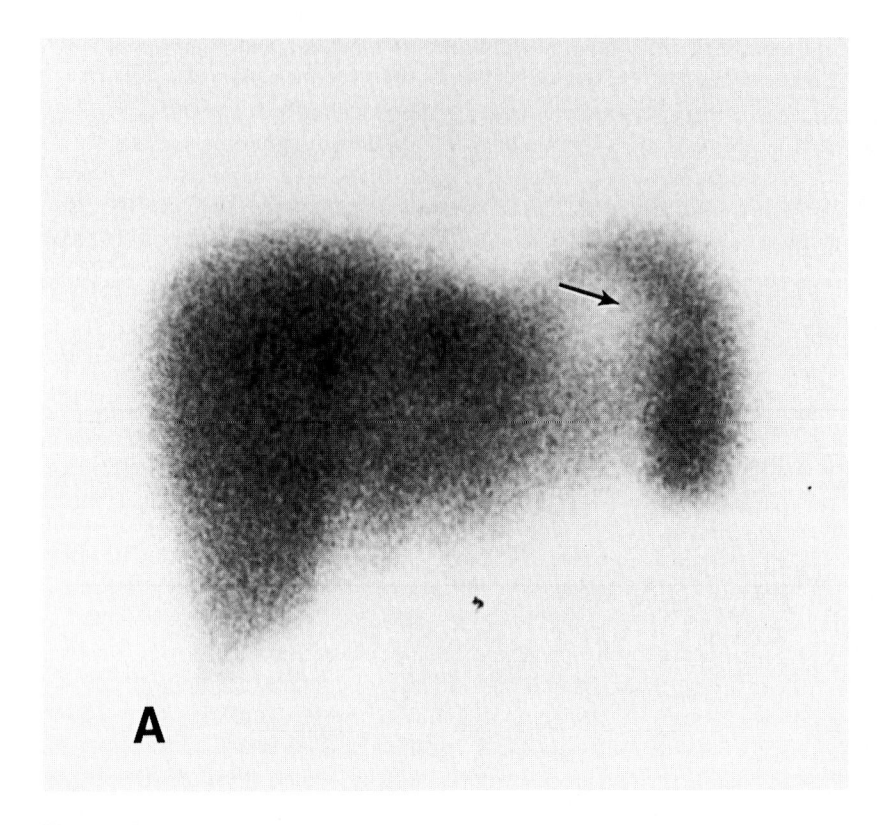

Figure 13 A 99m-technetium sulfur colloid scan demonstrates a photopenic area in the upper medial aspect of the spleen (arrow). The remainder of the spleen and liver appear normal. (B) A computed tomographic study after intravenous contrast demonstrates a cystic region in the anterior aspect of the spleen. This is immediately anterior to the splenic hilum. (C) An ultrasound of the upper abdomen in the transverse projection shows a fluid level in the splenic mass. This examination is an example of an epithelial cyst of the spleen with hemorrhage.

About 75% of patients with splenic abscess have multiple small abscesses that are usually less than 2 cm in diameter. Standard radiography and findings on physical examination are usually normal or nonspecific in these patients. The remaining 25% with solitary large splenic abscesses show enlargement of the spleen and abnormal findings near the left hemidiaphragm on chest xray. Radionuclide scan of the spleen in patients with multiple small abscesses will show nonhomogeneous splenic uptake or multiple defects if the lesions are larger than

SPLEEN IMAGING

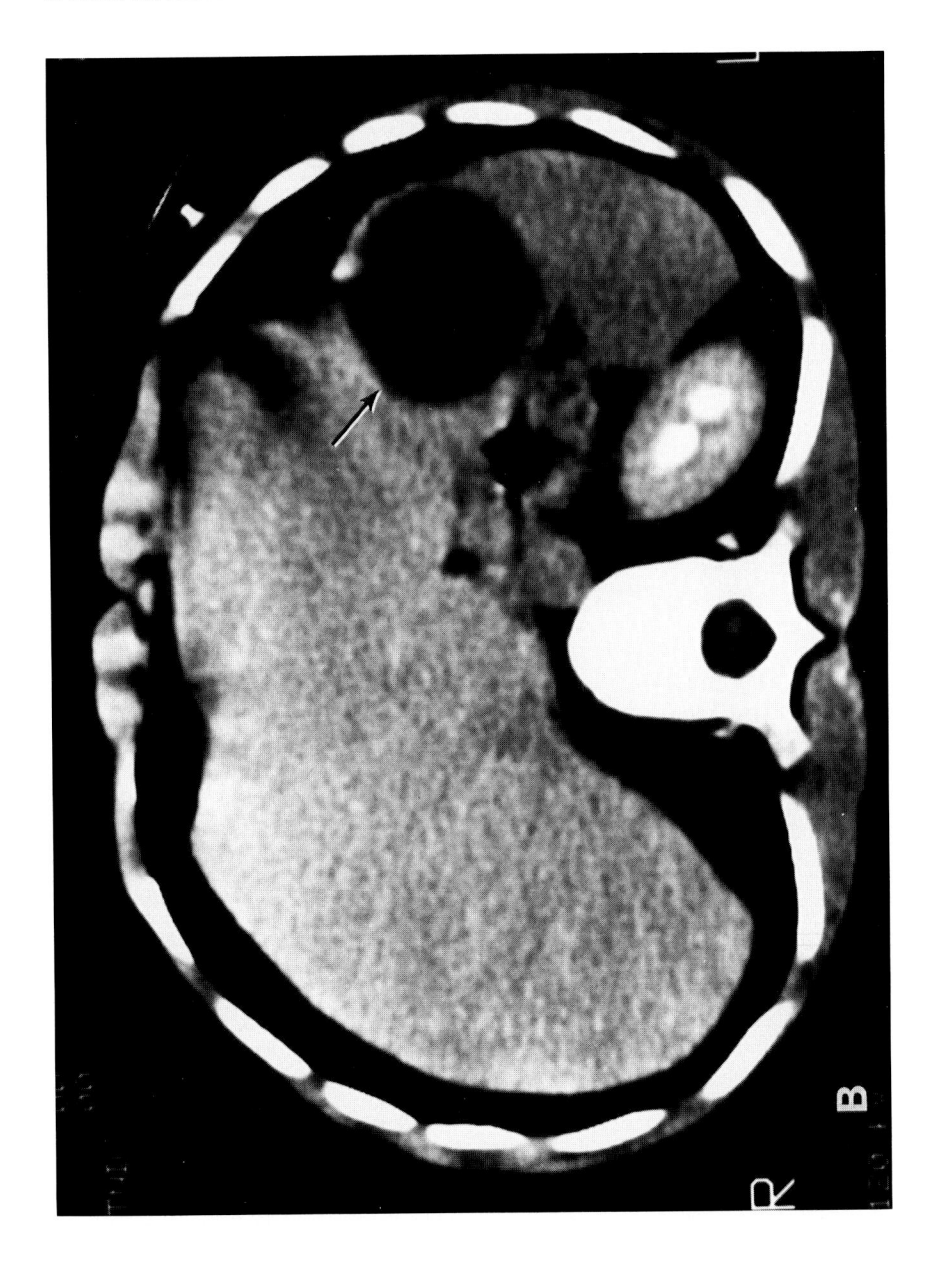

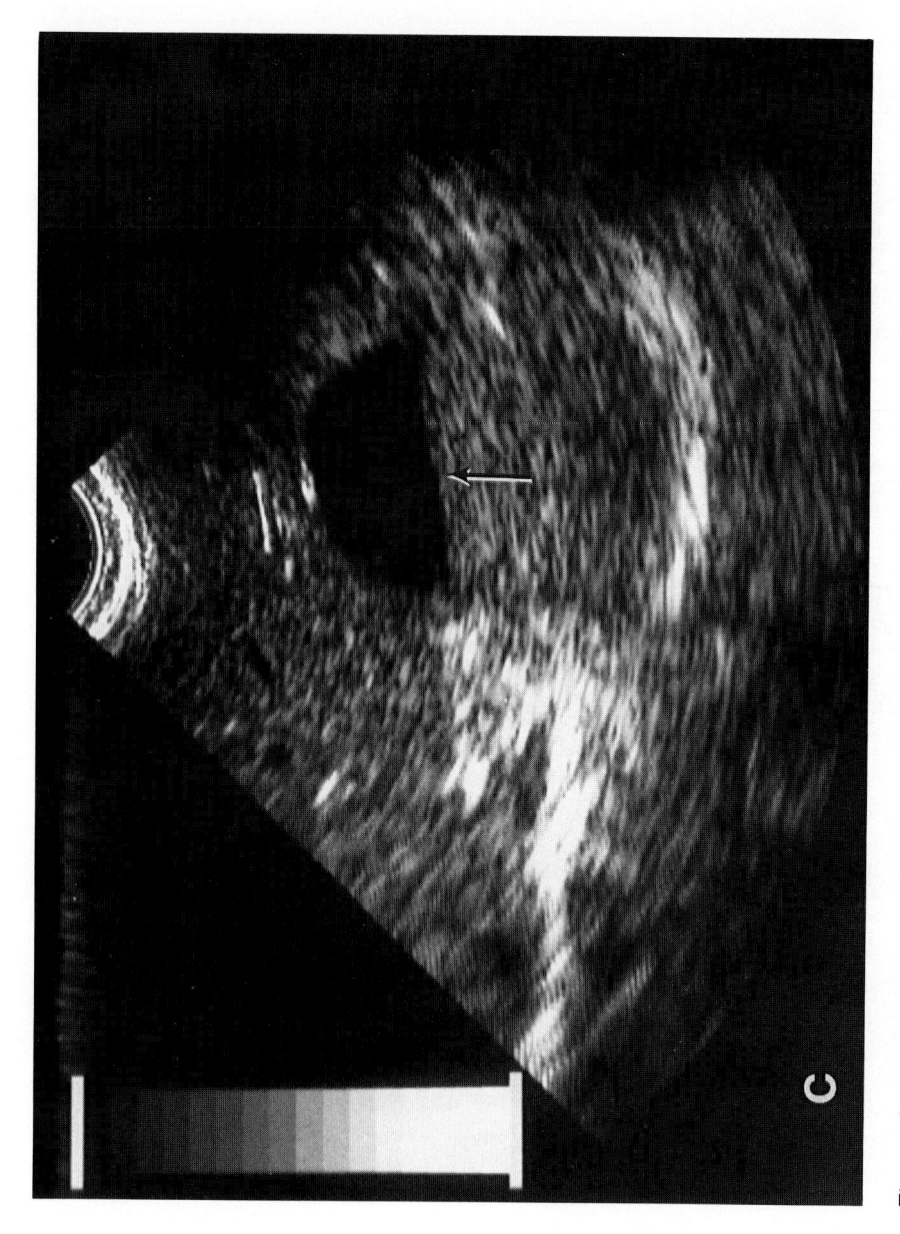

Figure 13 (Continued)

SPLEEN IMAGING 393

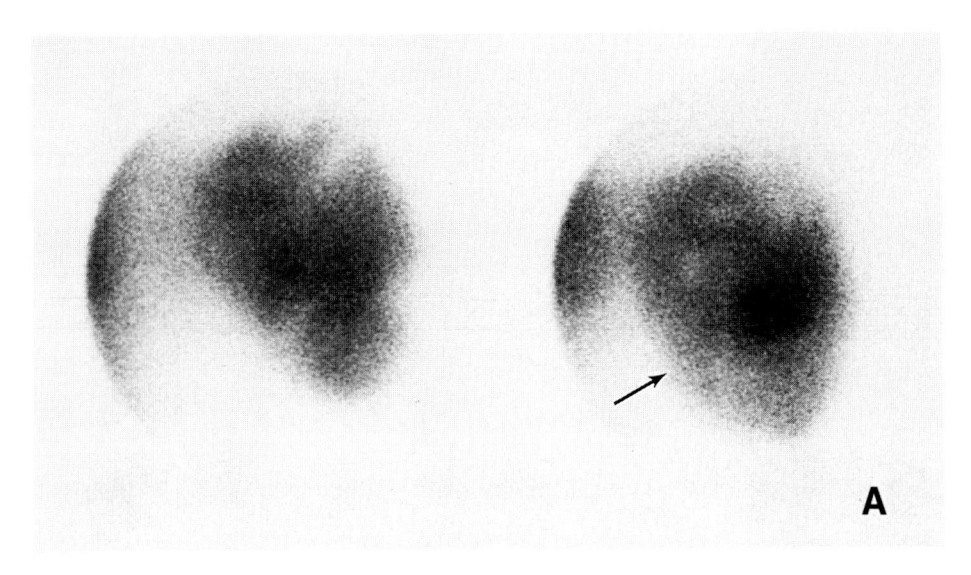

Figure 14 (A) Posterior view of a 99m-technetium sulfur colloid scan shows marked splenic enlargement with mulitfocal defects throughout the spleen. (B) A computed tomographic scan of the same patient demonstrates marked splenomegaly with multifocal low density regions within the spleen. (C) An ultrasound of the same patient demonstrates hypoechoic target or bulls-eye type lesions within the spleen. All these abnormalities represented splenic abscesses.

2 to 3 cm in diameter. In cases with solitary large splenic abscesses, a photopenic defect is identified on the scan and, together with the characteristic clinical history, make the diagnosis fairly specific.

CT has proven to be the most effective means for early diagnosis of both isolated and multiple splenic abscesses. Also, CT is extremely valuable in the search for intraabdominal abscesses in the immunocompromised patient. CT scans show multiple, small, rounded hypodense or cystic lesions that may have a central region of higher density. Frequently, the abscess lacks a well-defined wall and does not enhance significantly following injection of intravenous contrast. The spleen is usually enlarged as a result of the abscess formation. Similar small abscesses are frequently also seen in the liver and kidney. Because of multiple organ involvement, both ultrasound and computed tomography are more valuable than 99m-technetium sulfur colloid scans. Although gram-negative bacilli are generally the most common infectious agents in splenic abscesses, fungi are the most common causes of splenic abscess in immunosuppressed patients. CT-guided aspiration and fungal stain of the contents of abscesses may quickly establish the microbial etiology (Figures 14 and 15).

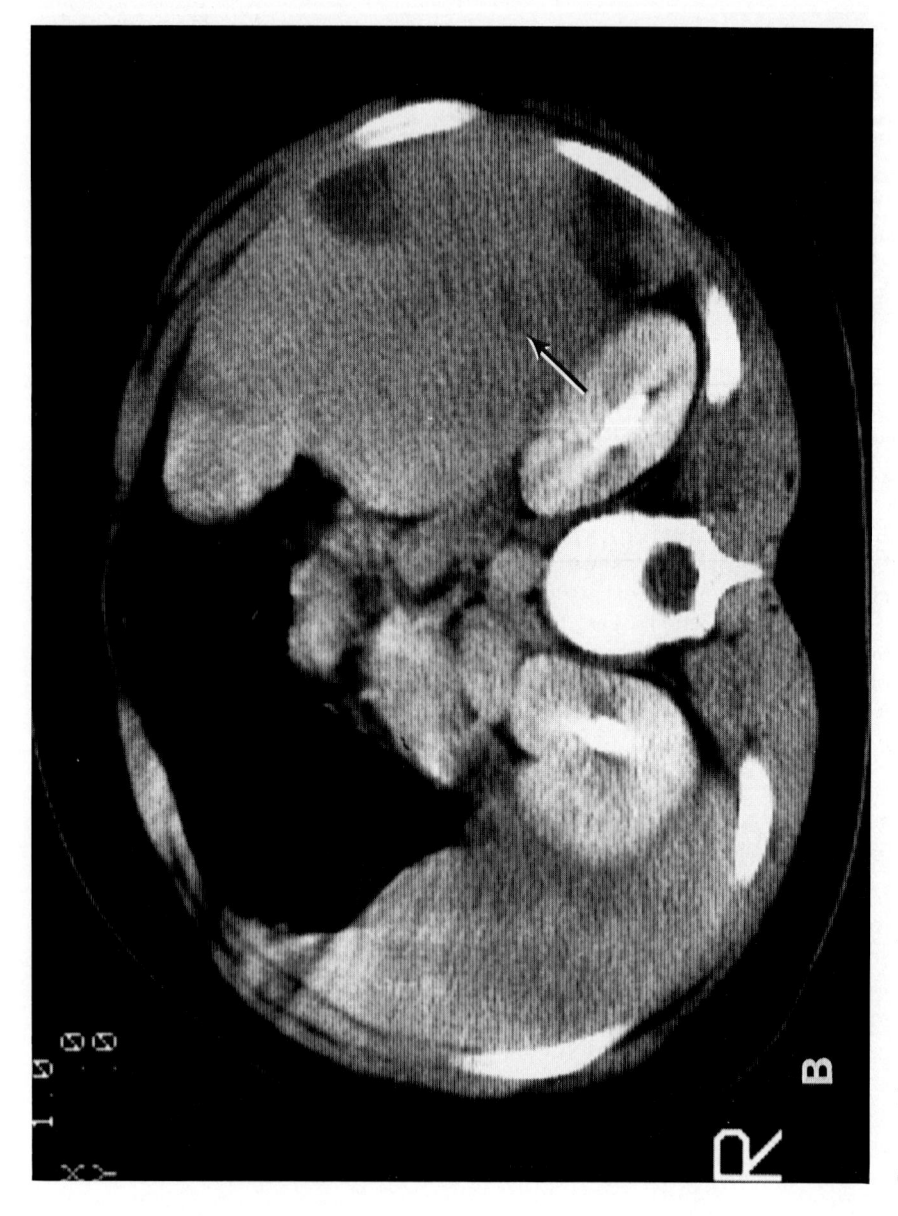

Figure 14 (Continued)

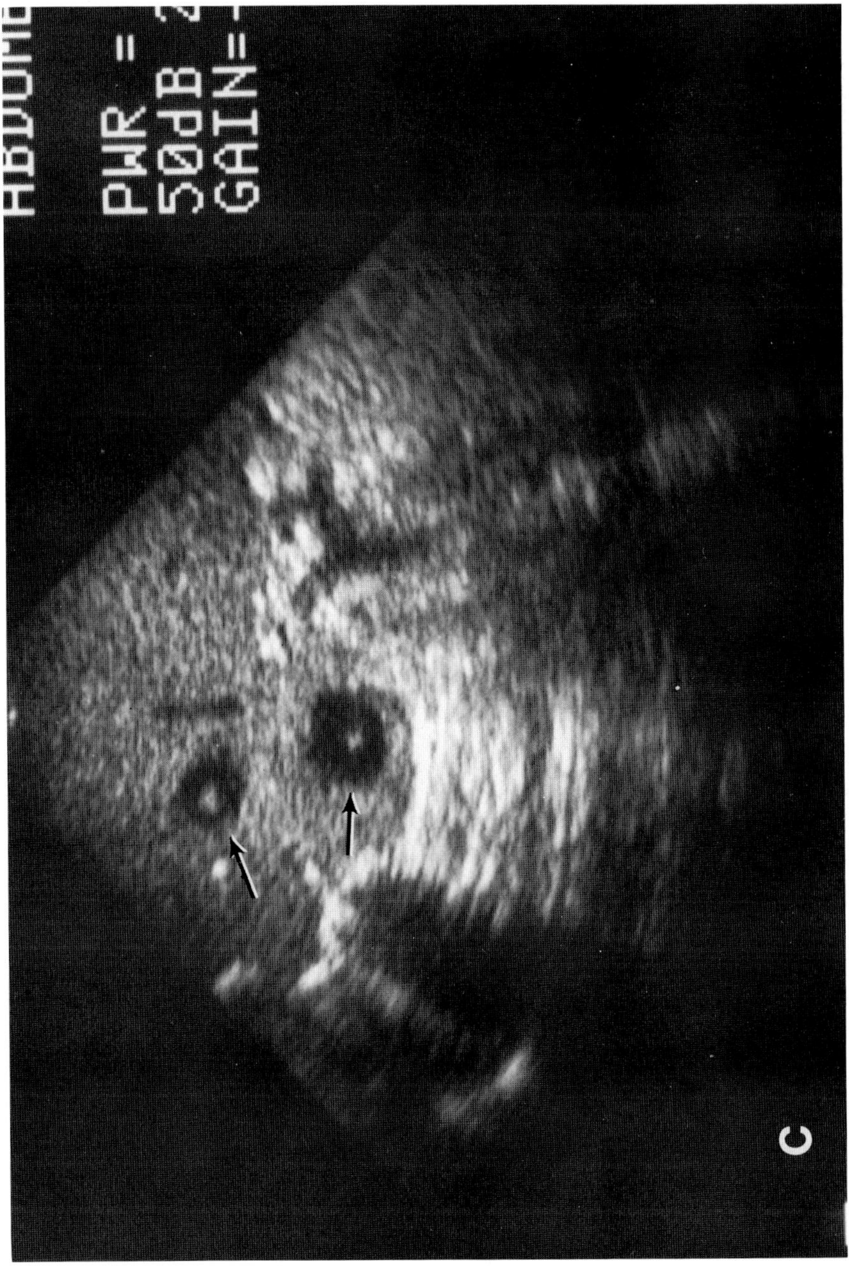
C

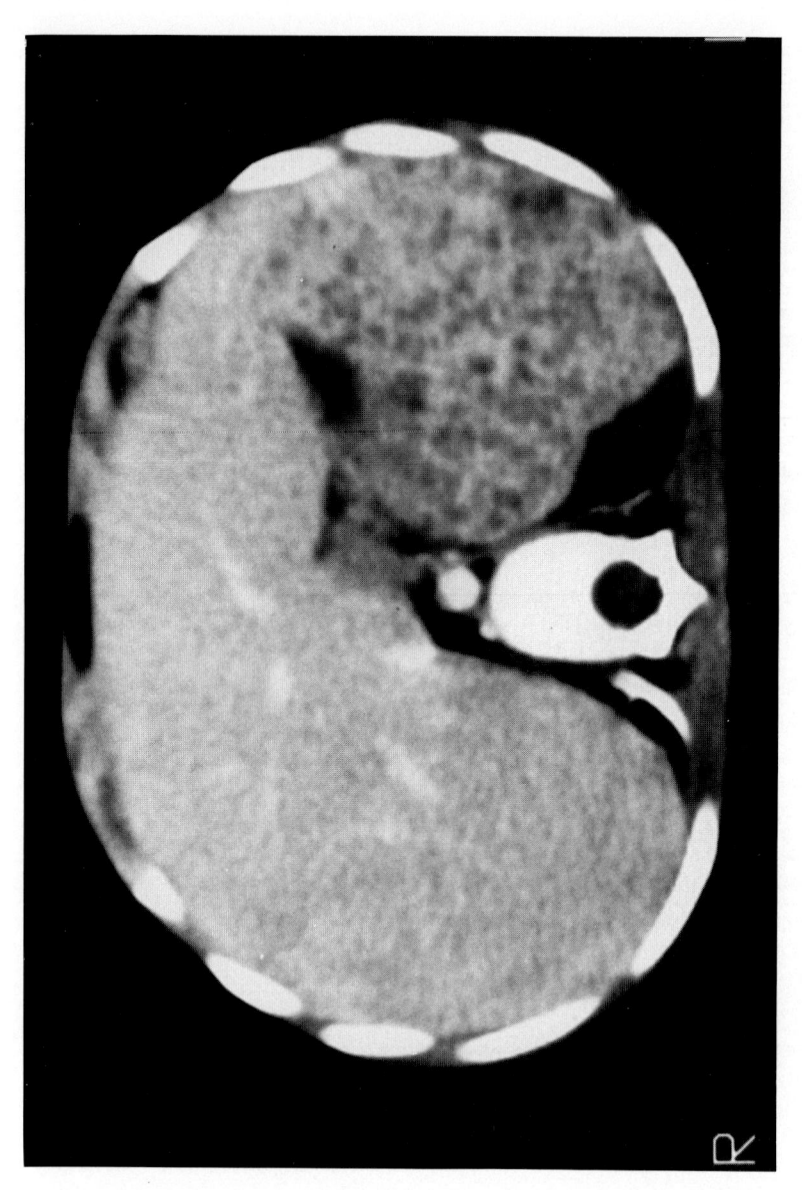

Figure 15 An enhanced computed tomographic image of the spleen in a child with leukemia. Examination shows marked splenomegaly with multifocal small nonenhancing lesions within the spleen. On histopathological examination these lesions proved to be monilial abscesses.

Certain systemic diseases of viral or bacterial etiology, such as infectious mononucleosis, typhoid fever, and bacterial endocarditis, can produce splenomegaly without the presence of abscesses. Computed tomography in such patients usually shows only nonspecific splenomegaly. Occasionally, there are multiple small intrasplenic hemorrhages or the associated finding of enlarged retroperitoneal lymph nodes.

Benign and Malignant Tumors

Hamartoma of the spleen is an unusual and rare tumor. Only 3 cases of splenic hamartoma have been reported in children (79,80). However, it is the most common benign splenic neoplasm and constitutes a significant proportion of all primary splenic masses. A multimodality approach to diagnosis is needed. Appearance of splenic hamartomas on radionuclide scans is not consistent (81). Both sequestration of damaged red cells and lack of sequestration of damaged red cells have been reported. 99m-technetium sulfur colloid scans show similar results, i.e., areas of increased uptake, or a region of decreased tracer accumulation. Nonetheless, both scintigraphic techniques are valuable in determining the presence of a lesion. Furthermore, sequestration of labeled red cells and increased uptake of 99m-technetium sulfur colloid are important differential findings since hamartomas are the only primary splenic tumors that contain functioning splenic tissue.

Cystic lymphangioma is a benign lymphatic malformation of undetermined etiology. Cystic lymphangioma of the spleen is rare. Ultrasound imaging shows multi-loculated cystic lesions in the intra-abdominal mass. These cystic lesions are identified on radionuclide scans as areas of decreased uptake. When the spleen is massively enlarged and has a multicystic appearance, the scintigraphic and sonographic findings can aid in noninvasive preoperative recognition of cystic lymphangioma. In general, splenic lymphangioma is a localized abnormality and other organ systems are not involved (82,83).

Presence of malignant tumors in the spleen is unusual in children except in the lymphoproliferative disorders (Figure 16). Most solid tumors metastasize to many other organs before involving the spleen. The earlier studies suggested that sulfur colloid imaging is insensitive in detecting lymphomatous involvement of the spleen (84). This lack of sensitivity is probably due to the infiltrative nature of the splenic involvement in lymphomas, as well as the tendency of lymphomas to form numerous small nodules that are below the limits of resolution of gamma cameras. However, unexplained splenomegaly must be considered to indicate lymphomatous involvement until proven otherwise in patients with documented lymphomas.

In children with non-Hodgkin's lymphoma, presence of micrometastases in the spleen and other reticuloendothelial organs is generally assumed to be part of the hematogeneous nature of the disease. The approach to treatment, there-

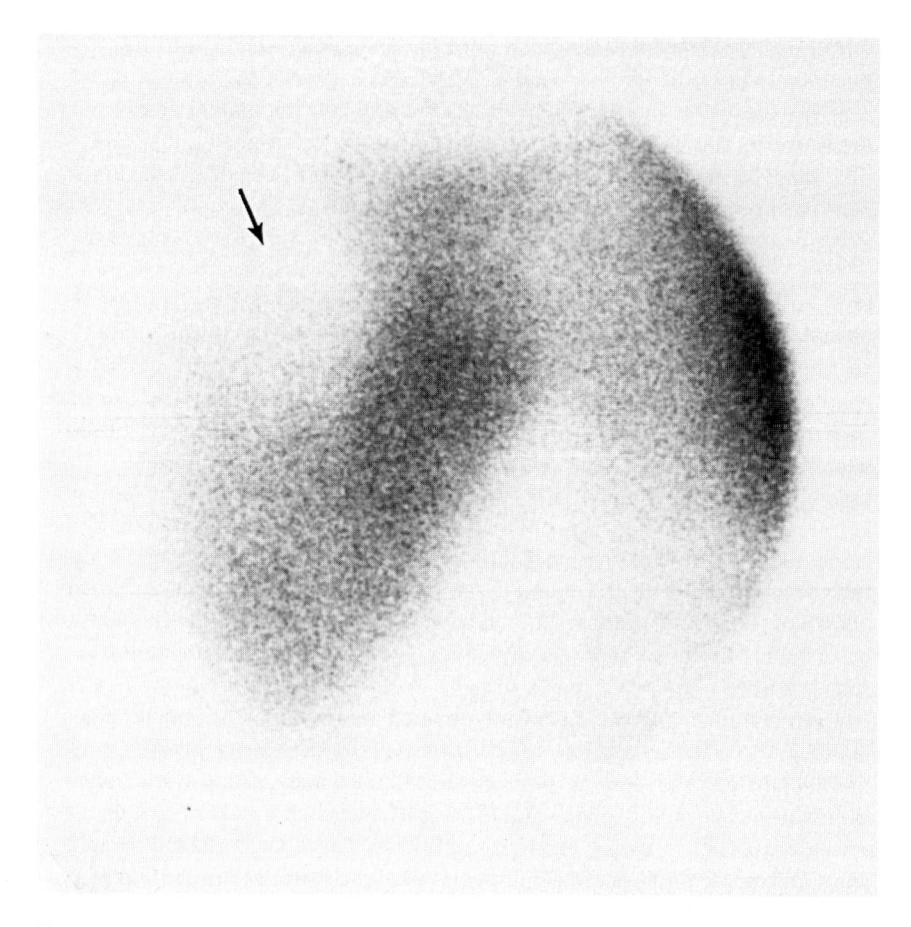

Figure 16 Posterior view of the left upper quadrant in a child with Hodgkin's disease. Examination showed a large lesion in the upper aspect of the spleen. At surgery, this proved to be Hodgkin's disease. This is an unusual finding in a patient presenting with Hodgkin's disease.

fore, is designed to include a period of systemic chemotherapy in all patients. Presence of marked splenomegaly suggests extensive involvement by lymphoma and probably indicates that there is a large tumor load.

Conversely, precise determination of abdominal involvement, especially invasion of the spleen, is vital for staging as a basis for prescribing treatment of Hodgkin's disease. Findings from clinical examination and diagnostic imaging cannot reliably detect the presence of Hodgkin's disease in the spleen. Moreover, the spleen may be the only site of disease below the diaphragm in up to 15% of the cases with abdominan involvement.

Some observers claim that sonography can discriminate between splenomegaly due to neoplastic infiltration and splenomegaly due to other causes (85, 86). This observation has not been confirmed by others (87,88). Gallium-67 imaging has a true positive rate of about 52% for detecting splenic involvement, with a false negative rate of about 12% (89-95).

Sonographic demonstration of spleen size correlates poorly with infiltration of the spleen by lymphoma. Although splenic involvement is usually not demonstrable by ultrasound, focal hypoechoic areas, similar to those in the liver, are occasionally seen. These lesions may be single or multiple and vary in size ranging from large confluent regions to small discrete nodules that are hypoechoic or nearly anechoic. Abnormal echogenicity of the spleen relative to the liver, but without focal defects, has been observed in individuals with proven splenic involvement by lymphoma. A focal area of sonographic abnormality in the spleen of a child with lymphoma is most likely to represent lymphomatous involvement, but early inflammatory processes such as fungal infections may rarely occur. Sonographic evidence of lymphadenopathy in the splenic hilum is often associated with lymphoma of the spleen (96,97).

Demonstration of splenic lymphoma by CT is very difficult, since focal lesions are found only in a minority of cases. Enlargement of the spleen as seen on the CT scan is common, but this finding must be interpreted with caution. Diffuse lymphomatous lesions are usually isodense with the surrounding splenic parenchyma. Focal involvement by lymphoma may be seen as single or multiple areas of reduced attenuation. These may be multiple, discrete, and well-defined but, more frequently large, confluent, poorly defined areas are observed. Varying window width should be used in an attempt to identify lesions which may be further accentuated following administration of contrast material.

We may now compare the usefulness of scintigraphy, CT scans, and ultrasound imaging of the spleen in patients with both Hodgkin's disease and non-Hodgkin's lymphoma. Experience indicates that CT has the overall highest sensitivity, specificity, and accuracy for detection of local involvement by lymphoma. However, in most cases lymphomatous infiltration of the spleen is not detectable by any of these imaging modalities. The CT demonstration of lymphadenopathy in the splenic hilum is a strong indication of splenic invasion by lymphoma. These nodes may be seen as low density masses adjacent to the splenic parenchyma. Dynamic scanning following a bolus administration of contrast may be helpful in differentiating accessory spleens from lymph nodes.

SUMMARY

Despite the fact that the spleen has multiple functions, none are an absolute requirement for life. One of these functions has been utilized by radionuclide techniques for evaluation of splenic morphology. The usual splenic uptake of 99m-technetium sulfur colloid can be used to determine size, location and integrity of the organ. The major use of radiocolloid imaging has been in the study of congenital defects, thus eventration of the diaphragm, accessory spleens, splenogonadal fusion, the asplenia and polysplenia syndromes, and the wandering spleen are amenable to study by means of intravenously administered radiocolloid. Interference with splenic uptake of radiocolloid can be either focal or generalized, as in functional asplenia.

Imaging of the spleen has a major role in evaluating suspected trauma of the organ and following its clinical course. In this regard computed tomography has replaced the radionuclide technique. The major reason for its use in trauma is because the technique can evaluate the solid abdominal organs. The return of splenic function after splenectomy (splenosis or accessory spleen) can be documented with radionuclide imaging. Rebirth of the spleen may also be shown by hematologic techniques when the volume of splenic tissue is sufficiently large. The detection of intrasplenic lesion is important in evaluating both benign and malignant disease. In this respect ultrasonography and computed tomography represent the most reliable techniques.

REFERENCES

1. Johnson PM, Spencer RP: The spleen. In, Freeman LM, Johnson PM (eds): *Clinical Scintillation Imaging* (ed 2). Orlando, Florida, Grune & Stratton, 1975, p. 639.
2. Schulkind ML, Ellis EF, Smith RT: Effect of antibody upon clearance of I-125 labeled pneumococci by the spleen and liver. *Pediatr Res* 1967;1: 178.
3. Horan M, Colebratch JH: Relation between splenectomy and subsequent infection. A clinical study. *Arch Dis Child* 1962;37:398.
4. Gates GF: Sepsis in children following splenectomy. *J Nucl Med* 1978; 19:113,
5. Crosby WH: Hyposplenism; an inquiry into the normal functions of the spleen. *Ann Rev Med* 1963;14:349.
6. Schnitzer B, Sodeman T, Mead ML, et al: Pitting function of the spleen in malaria; ultrastructural observations. *Science* 1972;177:175.
7. Smulewicz JJ, Clemett AR: Torsion of the wandering spleen. *Digest Dis Sci* 1979;20:274.
8. Gordon DH, Burrell MI, Levin DC, et al: Wandering spleen—the radiological and clinical spectrum. *Radiology* 1977;125:39.
9. Broker FHL, Fellows K, Treves S: Wandering spleen in three children. *Pediatr Radiol* 1978;6:211.
10. Schulz DM, Giordano DA, et al: Weights of organ of fetuses and infants. *Arch Pathol* 1962;74:244.
11. DeLand FH: Normal spleen size. *Radiology* 1970;97:589.

12. Krumbhaar EB, Lippincott SW: The postmortem weight of the "normal" spleen at different ages. *Am J Med Sci* 1939;197:344.
13. Spencer RP, Chaundhuri TK: Quantitative estimates of changes in splenic size during life. *Yale J Biol Med* 1969;41:333.
14. Spencer RP, Pearson HA, Lange RC: Human spleen; scan studies on growth and response to medications. *J Nucl Med* 1971;12:466.
15. Kevy SV, Tefft M, Vawter GF, et al: Hereditary splenic hypoplasia. *Pediatrics* 1968;42:752.
16. Garega S, Crosby WH: The incidence of leukemia in families of patients with hypoplasia of the marrow. *Blood* 1959;14:1008.
17. Marsh GW, Stewart JS: Splenic function in adult coeliac disease. *Br J Haematol* 1970;19:445.
18. Martin JB, Bell HE: The association of splenic atrophy and intestinal malabsorption; report of a case and review of the literature. *Can Med Assoc J* 1965;92:875.
19. Ryan FP, Smart RC, Holdsworth CD, et al: Hyposplenism in inflammatory bowel disease. *Gut* 1978;19:50.
20. Pettit JE, Hoffbrand AV, Sea PP, et al: Splenic atrophy in dermatitis herpetiformis. *Br Med J* 1972;2:438.
21. Brownlie BE, Hamer JW, Cook HB, et al: Thyrotoxicosis associated with splenic atrophy. *Lancet* 1975;2:1046.
22. Gilday DL, Alderson PO: Scintigraphic evaluation of liver and spleen injury. *Semin Nucl Med* 1974;4:357.
23. Weiss S, Conway JJ: Oral 99m-Tc pertechnetate; an aid in the differentiation of epigastric lesions. *J Nucl Med Tech* 1974;2:146.
24. Ehrlich CP, Papanicolaou N, Treves S, et al: Splenic scintigraphy using 99m-Tc labeled heat denatured red blood cells in pediatric patients: Concise communication. *J Nucl Med* 1982;23:209.
25. Rao BK, Shore RM, Lieberman LM, et al: Dual radiopharmaceutical imaging in congenital asplenia syndrome. *Radiology* 1982;145:805.
26. Thomas SR, Purdom RC, Kereiakes JG, et al: Dose to the liver and spleen in pediatric patients undergoing technetium-99m sulfur colloid scans. *Radiology* 1979;133:465.
27. Gonzalez G: Isotope scanning for diagnosing lesions projecting into the lower chest. *JAMA* 1971;218:590.
28. Custer JR, Shafer RB: Changes in liver scan following splenectomy. *J Nucl Med* 1975;16:194.
29. Putschar WGJ, Manion WC: Splenic-gonadal fusion. *Am J Pathol* 1956;32:15.
30. Gray SW, Skansalakis JE: Body asymmetry and splenic anomalies. In: *Embrylogy to Surgeons: The Embryological Basis for the Therapy of Congenital Defects*. Philadelphia, W. B. Saunders, 1972, p. 891.
31. Bennett-Jones MJ, St Hill CA: Accessory spleen in the scrotum. *Br J Surg* 1952;40:259.
32. Grossman SI, Goldberg MM, Hermann HB: A case report of ectopic splenic tissue in the scrotum. *J Urol* 1959;81:294.

33. McLean GK, Alavi A, Ziegler MM: Splenic-gonadal fusion. Identification by radionuclide scanning. *J Pediatr Surg* 1981;16:649.
34. Ivemark RI: Implications of agenesis of the spleen on the pathogenesis of cono-truncal anomalies in childhood; an analysis of heart malformation in splenic agenesis syndrome, with 14 new cases. *Acta Pediatr* 1955 (suppl 104);44:1.
35. Pearson HA, Schiebler GL, Spencer RP: Functional hyposplenia in cyanotic heart disease. *Pediatrics* 1971;48:277.
36. Rose V, Izukawa T, Moes CAF: Syndromes of asplenia and polysplenia. A review of cardica and noncardiac malformations in 60 cases with special reference to diagnosis and prognosis. *Br Heart J* 1975;37:840.
37. Freedom R: The heterotaxy syndrome. *Circulation* 1971(suppl 2);44:113.
38. Putschar W, Manion W: Congenital absence of the spleen and associated anomalies. *Am J Clin Pathol* 1956;26:429.
39. Mishalany H, Mahnovshi V, Woolley M: Congenital asplenia and anomalies of the gastrointestinal tract. *Surgery* 1982;91:38.
40. Teramoto R, Opas LM, Andrassy R: Splenic torsion with prune belly syndrome. *J Pediatr* 1981;98:91.
41. Spencer RP. Spleen imaging. In, Alvai A, Arger PH, (eds): *Multiple Imaging Procedures: Abdomen* (ed 1). Orlando, Grune & Stratton, 1980, p. 73.
42. Lutzker L, Koenigsberg M, Meng CH, et al: The role of radionuclide imaging in spleen trauma. *Radiology* 1974;110:419.
43. Nebesar RA, Rabinov KR, Potsaid MS: Radionuclide imaging of the spleen in suspected splenic injury. *Radiology* 1974;110:609.
44. Griffin LH Jr, Garrison AF, Ihnen M: The influence of radioisotope imaging on current treatment of blunt spleen trauma. *Am Surg* 1978;44:318.
45. Messina S, Goodman M, Van Der Schaaf A, et al: The radioisotope spleen scan in the assessment of patients with suspected spleen trauma. *Med J Aust* 1979;1:144.
46. Gold RE, Redman HC: Splenic trauma; assessment of problems in diagnosis. *AJR* 1972;116:413.
47. Lepasoon J, Olin T: Angiographic diagnosis of splenic lesions following blunt abdominal trauma. *Acta Radiol Diagnos* 1971;11:257.
48. Jeffrey RB, Laing FC, Federle MP, et al: Computed tomography of splenic trauma. *Radiology* 1981;141:729.
49. Froelich JW, Simeone JF, McKusick KA, et al: Radionuclide imaging and ultrasound in liver/spleen trauma: A prospective comparison. *Radiology* 1982;145:457.
50. Fleming CR, Dickson ER, Harrison EG Jr: Splenosis: Autotransplantation of splenic tissue. *Am J Med* 1976;61:414.
51. Jariwalla AG, Al-Nasiri NK: Splenosis pleurae. *Thorax* 1979;34:123.
52. Pearson HA, Johnston D, et al: The born again spleen; return of splenic function after splenectomy for trauma. *N Engl J Med* 1978;298:1389.
53. Fischer KC, Eraklis A, Rossello P, et al: Scintigraphy in the follow-up of pediatric splenic trauma treated without surgery. *J Nucl Med* 1978;19:3.

54. Solheim H, Nerdrum HJ: Radionuclide imaging of splenic laceration and trauma. *Clin Nucl Med* 1979;4:528.
55. Mishalany HG, Miller JH, Woolley MM: Radioisotope spleen scans in patients with splenic injury. *Arch Surg* 1982;117:1147.
56. Flickinger FW, Jackson GL: Radionuclide scan findings in delayed splenic rupture. *Radiology* 1978;129:763.
57. Slavin JD Jr, Minehan TF, Spencer RP: Scan demonstration of delayed splenic rupture. *J Nucl Med* 1974;15:632.
58. Singer DB: Post splenectomy sepsis. *Perspect Pediatr Pathol* 1973;1:285.
59. Shapero S, Schlesinger ER, Nesbitt REL: Infant, perinatal, maternal and childhood mortality in the United States. Cambridge, Mass, Harvard University, 1968, pp. 18, 341.
60. Dauer CC, Korns RF, Schuman LM: *Infectious Disease*. Cambridge, Mass, Harvard University Press, 1968, p. 134.
61. Schwartz AD, Dadash-Zedah M, Goldstein R, et al: Antibody response in intravenous immunization following splenic tissue autotransplantation in Sprague Dowley rats. *Blood* 1977;49:779.
62. Ritchy K, Pearson HA, Smith KA, et al: Splenosis following splenectomy for trauma in adults. *Blood* 1978(suppl 1);52:88.
63. Messmore HL: Autotransplantation of spleen tissue after trauma; encouraging evidence. *JAMA* 1979;241:437.
64. Spencer RP, Dhawan V, Sziklas JJ: Rate and characteristics of regrowth of splenic tissue. *Clin Nucl Med* 1977;2:442.
65. Singer DB: Post splenectomy sepsis. Perspect Pediatr Path 1973;1:285.
66. Hyslop NE: Fever and circulatory collapse in an asplenic man. *N Engl J Med* 1975;293:547.
67. Schwartz AD, Goldthorn JF, Winkelstein JA, et al: Lack of protective effect of autotransplanted splenic tissue to pneumococcal challenge. *Blood* 1978; 51:475.
68. Schwartz AD, Moxon ER: Prevention of Haemophilus influenzae meningitis and fatal sepsis by splenic autotransplantation. *Pediatr Res* 1980; 14:539.
69. Patel J, Williams JS, Shmigel B, et al: Preservation of splenic function by autotransplantation of traumatized spleen in man. *Surgery* 1981;90:683.
70. Cullingford GL, Surveyor I, Edis AJ: Demonstration of functioning heterotopic splenic autografts by scintigraphy. *Aust NZ J Surg* 1983;53:343.
71. Clyne C: Cysts of the spleen. *J R Coll Surg Edinb* 1978;23:234.
72. Griscom NT, Hargreaves H, Schwartz M: Huge splenic cyst in a newborn: Comparison with 10 cases in later childhood and adolescence. *AJR* 1977; 129:889.
73. Lingeman CJ, Smith EB, Battersby S, et al: Subacute bacterial endocarditis. Splenectomy in cases refractory to antibiotic therapy. *Arch Intern Med* 1956;97:309.
74. McSherry CK, Dineen P: The significance of splenic abscess. *Am J Surg* 1962;103:618.
75. Chulay JD, Lankerani MR: Splenic abscess. *Am J Med* 1976;61:513.

76. Anand SV, Davey WW: Surgery of the spleen in Nigeria. *Br J Surg* 1965; 52:335.
77. Cockshott WP, Weaver EJM: Primary tropical splenic abscess; a misnomer. *Br J Surg* 1962;49:665.
78. Kolawole TM, Bohrer SP: Splenic and the gene for hemoglobin S. *AJR* 1973;119:175.
79. Grahm JC, Weidner WA, Vinik M: The angiographic features of organizing splenic hematoma. *AJR* 1969;107:430.
80. Wexler L, Alramo HL: Hamartoma of the spleen. Angiographic observations. *AJR* 1964;92:1150.
81. Kuykendall JD, Shanser JD, Sumner TE, Goodman LR: Multimodal approach to diagnosis of hamartoma of the spleen. *Pediatr Radiol* 1977;5:239.
82. Rao BK, AuBuchon J, Liberman LM, Polcyn RE: Cystic lymphangioma of the spleen. A radiologic-pathologic correlation. *Radiology* 1981;141:781.
83. Tuttle RJ, Minielly JA: Splenic cyst lymphangiomatosis. *Radiology* 1978; 126:47.
84. Silverman S, DeNardo GL, Glatstein E, et al: Evaluation of the liver and spleen in Hodgkin's disease: II. The value of splenic scintigraphy. *Am J Med* 1972;52:362.
85. Taylor KJW, McCready VR: A clinical evaluation of gray-scale ultrasonography. *Br J Radiol* 1975;49:244.
86. Taylor KJW, Milan J: Differential diagnosis of chronic splenomegaly by gray-scale ultrasonography: Clinical observations and digital A-scan analysis. *Br J Radiol* 1976;49:519.
87. Rochester D, Bowle JD, Kunzman A, et al: Ultrasound in the staging of lymphoma. *Radiology* 1977;124:483.
88. Filly RA, Marglen S, Costellino RA: The ultrasonographic spectrum of abdominal and pelvic Hodgkin's disease and nonHodgkin's lymphoma. *Cancer* 1976;38:2143.
89. Johnston GS, Go MF, Benua RS, et al: Gallium 67 citrate imaging in Hodgkin's disease; final report of cooperative group. *J Nucl Med* 1977;18:692.
90. Greenlow RH, Weinstein MB, Brell AB: 67 Ga-citrate imaging in untreated malignant lymphoma; preliminary report of cooperative group. *J Nucl Med* 1974;15:404.
91. Levi JA, O'Connell MJ, Murphy WC, et al: Role of 67 gallium citrate in scanning in the management of nonHodgkin's lymphoma. *Cancer* 1975; 36:1690.
92. Horn NL, Ray GR, Kriss JP: Gallium-67 citrate scanning in Hodgkin's disease. *Cancer* 1976;37:250.
93. Kay DN, McCready VR: Clinical isotope scanning using 67 Ga citrate in the management of Hodgkin's disease. *Br J Radiol* 1972;45:437.
94. McCaffrey JA, Rudders RA, Kahn PC, et al: Clinical usefulness of 67-gallium scanning in malignant lymphomas. *Am J Med* 1976;60:522.
95. Gottschalk A: Tumor scanning of lymphomas. In: Gottschalk A, Potchen EJ (eds): *Diagnostic Nuclear Medicine*. Baltimore, Williams & Wilkins, 1976, p. 544.

96. Wafula JMC: Ultrasound and CT demonstration of primary angiosarcoma of the spleen. *Br J Radiol* 1985;58:903-907.
97. King DJ, Dawson AA, Bayliss: The value of ultrasonic scanning of the spleen in lymphoma. *Clin Radiol* 1985;36:473-474.

13
Splenectomy
Indications in Childhood

DEBORAH HURST and ELLIOTT P. VICHINSKY
Children's Hospital Oakland, Oakland, California

Increased awareness of the dangers of overwhelming postsplenectomy infection has prompted a more conservative approach to splenectomy in the 1980s compared with previous decades. Previously, the spleen was considered a nonessential organ. Now even with the availability of pneumococcal vaccine and prophylactic penicillin, splenectomy cannot be recommended without weighing the risk of possible overwhelming sepsis in each case.

Fortunately, medical advances have also increased the number of therapeutic alternatives to splenectomy. Patients today have available diagnostic CT scans and radio-isotope scans, surgical techniques of splenic salvage, and re-implantation and splenic embolization. There is also therapy with new pharmaceutical preparations, such as high-dose gammaglobulin, immunosuppressive and chemotherapeutic agents. In many clinical situations where splenectomy had previously been accepted therapy (Table 1) indications for the operation are being reassessed. We will review the most common indications for splenectomy in childhood and discuss current approaches to management.

SPLENECTOMY FOR TRAUMATIC RUPTURE

Prior to the 1970s, suspected splenic rupture was an accepted indication for laparotomy, and removal of the spleen in toto was considered the safest approach to treating a partially damaged organ. A surgical text from this period states, "The minimal importance of the spleen and the ability of the body to

Table 1 Conditions Frequently Associated with Splenectomy in Childhood

I. Surgical—post-traumatic
II. Hematologic conditions
   A. Red cell disorders
      1. Membrane disorders (hereditary spherocytosis, pyropoikilocytosis, severe elliptocytosis)
      2. Hemoglobinopathies (sickle cell disease, thalassemias)
      3. Enzymopathies
      4. Chronic autoimmune hemolytic anemias
   B. Idiopathic thrombocytopenia (acute, chronic)
III. Hypersplenism due to underlying disease (biliary atresia, cirrhosis, Gaucher's disease, Wiscott-Aldrich syndrome, skeletal and splenic hemangiomatosis, congenital and erythropoietic porphyria, osteopetrosis, etc.)
IV. Oncologic conditions (Hodgkin's disease staging, chronic myeloid leukemia, splenic tumors)
V. Infections (splenic abscess)

adjust to its loss with no apparent ill effects are additional reasons for removing the spleen in all cases of trauma . . . The institution of early splenectomy in suspected cases is essential to successful treatment (1)."

In the following decade, increased understanding of the risk of overwhelming bacterial infection in splenectomized patients led to a radical change in the surgeon's approach to a traumatized spleen. Surgeons began to advocate a period of observation and a conservative surgical technique. Laparotomy was now performed only when there was evidence of significant continued bleeding, when there was evidence of possible peritonitis from associated gastrointestinal injuries, or when a nuclear scan showed loss of vascularization or severe fragmentation of a major portion of the spleen (2).

In a series of 49 patients with splenic injuries managed with an initial period of medical support and observation, total splenectomy was required in only 6 patients, 2 of whom had penetrating wounds of the abdomen (3). In 15 patients, the spleen was salvaged by surgical repair. The remaining 28 were managed by observation alone. In another series, splenectomy was necessary in only one of 46 cases (4). Studies of splenic function after healing of traumatic rupture indicated no signs of decreased splenic function. In comparison, a group of patients splenectomized for trauma showed significantly higher platelet counts, a higher percentage of "pitted" red cell cells, and the presence of Howell-Jolly bodies. All of these findings are indicators of hyposplenism.

Despite these optimistic reports of splenic salvage, it is important not to become casual in the management of suspected splenic trauma. Prompt laparotomy and splenic repair are still indicated if intensive care facilities and modern diagnostic equipment are not available during the period when the patient must be closely observed. Assessment of possible splenic injury on clinical grounds alone can be difficult, since the majority of patients will have multiple injuries in other organ systems which may mask the classical findings of abdominal tenderness and guarding in the left upper quadrant. In such cases, computerized axial tomography, angiography, and technetium-99^m sulfur colloid liver/spleen scans can help establish the diagnosis. The radionuclide scan is particularly valuable. It provides an accurate picture of spleen size and blood supply at the ICU bedside before the patient is stable enough for transport to the x-ray department.

Hypovolemia with hypotension and tachycardia are common and should be treated at once with fluids and transfusion. The patient should then be followed with examinations and spleen scans until the condition either stabilizes or deteriorates. Generally, operations performed after a period of 12-24 hours observation reveal a single splenic laceration which has stopped bleeding (5,6). Such experience has led surgeons to avoid laparotomy completely in patients who have been stable for this period of time. If surgery is necessary, ruptured spleens are repaired to the extent possible.

For patients whose spleens are damaged beyond repair, some surgeons have tried implanting splenic tissue in the abdomen at the time of splenectomy in hopes of preserving splenic function. This technique was based on the observation that some splenectomized patients developed small nodules of splenic tissue in their abdomen, a phenomenon known as "splenosis." Pearson studied this phenomenon in a group of splenectomized children by determining the percentage of pitted red blood cells and measuring the extra-hepatic uptake of technetium on liver/spleen scan (8). Partial return of splenic function was found in more than half of children splenectomized for trauma. In contrast, no recovery of splenic function was seen in those children splenectomized for hematologic or oncologic indications, whose spleens had been removed with intact capsules (without rupture). The partial return of splenic function due to splenosis may exlain why patients splenectomized for trauma have shown a lower rate of fatal infection than those splenectomized electively for hematologic disorders (9). But the degree of return of splenic function from splenosis is variable, as indicated by the considerable variability in the numbers of pitted red cells seen in these patients. Moreover, several splenectomized patients who died from overwhelming bacterial infections were found to have splenosis on autopsy (10). Only small amounts of splenic tissue were present in these cases, leading to the speculation that volume and blood supply of the splenic implant may determine its immunologic competence (11).

In an effort to simulate the natural phenomena of splenosis, various surgical teams have experimentally implanted splenic tissue into the omentum at the time of splenectomy. This technique offers hope of preserving some degree of immune function (12,13). However, it remains to be shown whether such splenic implants can reduce the incidence of post-splenectomy sepsis. Studies in animals have given contradictory results, possibly due to differences in implantation techniques and experimental design (14,15). Only a small number of patients have received implants so far. Follow-up of a much larger number would be necessary to demonstrate a protective effect against post-splenectomy sepsis.

For the present, patients with reimplanted splenic tissue or spontaneous splenosis should be counseled and treated in the same manner as splenectomized patients; that is, they should be given prophylactic antibiotics, pneumococcal vaccine, and prompt antibiotic treatment for any febrile episodes. Surgeons should continue to avoid performing splenectomies whenever possible; they should attempt to repair lacerated spleens rather than remove them.

HEMATOLOGIC INDICATIONS FOR SPLENECTOMY: RED CELL DISORDERS

Hereditary Spherocytosis

The majority of elective splenectomies in childhood are performed for hereditary spherocytosis (HS). In this disorder, a deficiency in the red cell membrane protein spectrin increases the cell's fragility to mechanical and osmotic stresses. Red cells gradually lose surface area and become relatively rigid spherocytes, which are then easily trapped in the splenic pulp and destroyed. Removal of the spleen allows the abnormal cells to continue to circulate. This increases red cell survival to near normal, essentially "curing" the hemolytic anemia (16).

In the 1970s splenectomy was felt to be indicated in virtually all children with spherocytosis in order to prevent the complications of acute anemic crises and gallstones (17,18). Ideally, the operation was delayed until the age of five or six years, an age before gallstones were likely but after some resistance to infection had developed. Younger children had splenectomy only if their anemia was associated with significant symptoms, such as delayed growth, acute hemolytic crises, or the need for periodic red cell transfusions. Hereditary spherocytosis was one condition in which splenectomy seemed unequivocally beneficial, and the indications for the operation at different ages were relatively well defined. Recently, however, concern about the risks of overwhelming post-splenectomy sepsis has called this therapeutic dogma into question for selected cases.

Many patients with hereditary spherocytosis are asymptomatic, with little or no anemia and only minimal elevation of the reticulocyte count. Splenectomy offers no immediate benefit to such patients, but exposes them to the risks of overwhelming sepsis. To justify splenectomy in such cases, the risk of future morbidity and mortality from gallstones or from sudden severe anemia must be shown to be greater than the risk of sepsis. In the absence of a large follow-up study of patients, therapeutic recommendations can be based only on incomplete historical data.

The best estimate of the incidence of gallstones in hereditary spherocytosis comes from a report in 1952 on 152 patients. This study clearly showed an increased incidence of gallstones with age. Gallstones were rare in any patient under the age of 10 years, but they were found in 30-50% of adults with hereditary spherocytosis (19). A more recent review of 58 patients reported a similar incidence. Only one out of 31 children under the age of 10 years, or 3%, had cholelithiasis, as opposed to the occurrence of gallstones in 41% of patients over 10 (20).

What proportion of patients with gallstones will have significant complications is another question. In the general population, earlier studies suggested that 50% of patients with gallstones develop symptoms and 20% develop complications (21). A recent study reported a much lower incidence of problems, with only 18% of patients having symptoms or complications after a 15-year follow-up (22). Operative mortality is reported to be about 2.5% for emergency surgery, while elective cholecystectomy is associated with a mortality rate of only 0.1% to 0.5%, depending on the age of the patient (23). Such figures have led to the general practice of removing symptomatic gallstones electively, but leaving silent gallstones alone.

The incidence of symptoms and complications from gallstones in hereditary spherocytosis is not known, but it is probably similar to that seen with other types of gallstones. Operative mortality should also not differ from the general population, once anemia is corrected by red cell transfusion. This means that the highest estimated mortality from gallstones in hereditary spherocytosis would be the 2.5% fatality rate reported in cases requiring emergency surgery. For elective cholecystectomies, the highest reported mortality rate is 0.5% of cases with symptomatic gallstones. If all patients had cholecystectomy soon after symptoms developed, the chance of requiring emergency surgery would be minimized and the mortality related to gallstones should be well below 1%.

Splenectomy for hereditary spherocytosis, on the other hand, has been associated with a 3.3% incidence of sepsis and a 2.1% mortality rate from overwhelming infection (9). These figures are from a 1973 review of 16 different reports on a total of 850 patients whose ages were not all recorded. The author stated that many patients had splenectomy as infants. The mortality in a group of patients with hereditary spherocytosis who were splenectomized after age 5 years would be expected to be lower than the often quoted rate of 2.1%. Nonetheless, the risk of fatal sepsis would have to be reduced to well below 1% before splenectomy would seem justified for gallstone prevention alone (24).

In addition to reducing the incidence of gallstones, splenectomy prevents acute life-threatening anemic crises. These anemic crises may be due to increased hemolysis or bone marrow depression associated with infection. While the incidence of sudden severe anemia is probably quite low, even HS patients with mild hemolysis may be susceptible to this complication. For example, one report describes an 8 year old boy with mild, asymptomatic hereditary spherocytosis (baseline hemoglobin level over 11 g/dl, reticulocyte count of 5 to 7%) whose hemoglobin fell to 5.5 gm/dl on the eighth day of a parvovirus infection (25). While parovirus epidemics are rare, similar effects on the blood can occur with other infections. Many children with hereditary spherocytosis become jaundiced and show a fall of hemoglobin level of several grams during common febrile illnesses. While the hemoglobin level may not fall low enough to require transfusion, these periods of increased anemia could be expected to cause increased symptoms and a longer convalescence associated with otherwise mild illnesses.

A prudent recommendation for the child with mild hereditary spherocytosis, based on the incomplete data available, would be to delay splenectomy until the child is at least 10 years old. If jaundice and anemia were shown to occur with mild infections or if a severe anemic crisis occurred, splenectomy should be done earlier. If splenectomy is refused, the patient should be carefully observed for development of symptomatic gallstones, then cholecystectomy would be recommended before serious complications occur.

Children who are significantly anemic, (that is, with a hemoglobin level of 8-10 gm/dl), but who are otherwise asymptomatic, should probably have splenectomy at the conventional age of five or six years. The significant hemolysis of these children puts them at increased risk of earlier complications. In addition, they may derive some immediate benefit from an increased hemoglobin level. Even patients considered asymptomatic prior to splenectomy may report an increased sense of well-being and increased energy following the operation (26).

The small group of severely affected children who are symptomatic or who require frequent red cell transfusions may require splenectomy earlier than age five. Some of these patients may actually have a homozygous form of hereditary spherocytosis, inherited in an autosomal recessive fashion from both parens. Patients with extremely severe variants of hereditary spherocytosis may continue to have increased hemolysis even after splenectomy.

Prior to splenectomy, an ultrasound examination of the gallbladder should be done. If stones are found, the surgeon can then remove the gallbladder at the same operation. The surgeon should search the abdomen carefully for any accessory spleens which could hypertrophy if left in place and cause recurrent hemolysis (27).

Perhaps if splenectomy is delayed in patients who have a very mild form of hereditary spherocytosis, follow-up studies would more clearly determine the incidence of complications in the unsplenectomized patient. Future studies should also show to what extent modern treatment has decreased mortality from overwhelming post-splenectomy sepsis. Recommendations for or against splenectomy could then be made on a more rational basis.

Other Membrane Disorders

Hereditary elliptocytosis is another red cell membrane disorder which responds to splenectomy. Only patients with evidence of significant hemolysis should be splenectomized, since most patients do not have a significant decrease in red cell lifespan. Hereditary stomatocytosis has also been treated by splenectomy, but failure to decrease hemolysis or only partial improvement following the operation has been reported.

Enzyme Deficiencies

Red cell enzyme deficiencies may impair the generation of ATP, resulting in levels of ATP insufficient to maintain the red cell membrane pump. Osmotic water loss results in dehydrated, distorted and rigid red cells which are prematurely destroyed in the splenic pulp. Deficiencies of pyruvate kinase, glucose phosphate isomerase, phosphopyruvate kinase, and hexokinase all result in hemolysis which improves somewhat, but not completely, following splenectomy. In contrast, there is little improvement after splenectomy in pyrimadine-5-nucleotidase deficiency and in congenital non-spherocytic anemia due to glucose-6-phosphate dehydrogenase deficiency (28).

Hemoglobinopathies

Splenectomy is also considered in certain hemoglobinopathies, namely, sickle cell anemia and thalassemia.

The spleen in sickle cell anemia shows progressive loss of function starting in the early months of life. Repeated intrasplenic sickling results in tissue infarction and the occurrence of functional asplenia some time between the ages of 5 and 36 months (29). Studies of splenic function in over 2,000 babies followed in the National Cooperative Study of Sickle Cell Disease showed that splenic dysfunction first appeared when the hemoglobin F level fell below 15-20% in patients with homozygous sickle cell anemia (30). As many as 70% of patients had functional asplenia by the age of 4 years. Patients with hemoglobin SC disease and those with sickle-beta-thalassemia also showed progressive splenic dysfunction, although the dysfunction was less severe than that of the patients with hemoglobin SS. In young children, splenic function may return following red cell transfusion, but after the age of about 4 to 6 years the splenic dysfunction is generally irreversible (31). The high incidence of fatal bacterial sepsis reported in young children with sickle cell disease is largely due to this unavoidable loss of spleen function.

It is desirable to preserve splenic function as long as possible in children with sickle cell disease. Nonetheless, splenectomy may become necessary because of acute splenic sequestration, which is the second most common cause of death in children with sickle cell anemia under the age of 5 years (32). In a sequestration crisis, the spleen can become enormously enlarged over several hours. There is trapping of red cells and the hemoglobin level drops precipitously, resulting in hypovolemic shock and death. Minor episodes of splenic sequestration may also occur, associated with a moderate increase in spleen size and a drop in hemoglobin level of only 2 to 3 g/dl.

All sequestration crises must be managed carefully and followed up closely because of the high mortality rate and the frequency of recurrence. A study of over 200 Jamaican children with acute sequestration crises showed a 12% mortality rate from the first episode of sequestration (33). In 27% of these children there was a second episode of sequestration, and in about 30% there was a third sequestration crisis. The mortality rate from the second sequestration was 21% and the mortality rate from the third sequestration crisis was 20%. One death from severe sequestration occurred in a child with a history of two previous episodes of sequestration which had been asymptomatic and showed spontaneous recovery.

Splenic sequestration is quickly reversible by red cell transfusion. Because of the high recurrence rate, transfusion should be continued until splenectomy is performed to prevent a fatal episode. One approach to management of the young child with splenic sequestration is to continue transfusions until the age of two years before splenectomy is performed (34). In this way, the child is protected from repeat sequestration crises, and splenic function is maintained during the period of highest vulnerability to overwhelming infection. The spleen can then be removed when the child is more immunologically mature and is able to mount a more effective antibody response to the pneumococcal and *Hemophilus influenzae* vaccines. Before embarking on such a transfusion program, splenic function should be assessed by technetium scan. If normal splenic function does not return after transfusion, splenectomy can be done at once, avoiding unnecessary future exposure to blood products.

The decision to undertake transfusion and splenectomy in a child who has only mild episodes of splenic sequestration is not always easy. When a moderate increase in spleen size and drop in hemoglobin level of 2 to 3 g/dl occurs at the time of infection, the diagnosis of splenic sequestration may not be clear-cut. In our experience such a child needs to be followed extremely closely, and if repeated "suspicious" episodes occur, suggesting the occurrence of splenic sequestration, splenectomy is indicated.

Splenic sequestration can also occur in older children and adults with hemoglobin SC disease or sickle-beta-thalassemia. In these patients the spleen may remain enlarged and only partially functional. Splenic sequestration in such patients is generally mild, self-limited, and does not require to be treated with blood transfusion or splenectomy. However, these patients may require splenectomy for hypersplenism, which is manifested by an increase in spleen size accompanied by a fall in the hemoglobin level. In addition, a massively enlarged spleen may become painful or arouse concern about the danger of traumatic rupture. In the absence of these specific indications for splenectomy, an enlarged spleen in a patient with sickle cell disease should be left intact.

Patients with thalassemia major who are being treated with chronic transfusion programs must be kept in negative iron balance through an effective chelation program. At the same time, the amount of blood transfused must be minimized since each unit of red cells contributes another 167 mg of iron to the total body iron burden. Blood requirements must be scrutinized and splenectomy considered when transfusion requirements increase.

Even on hypertransfusion regimens where the hemoglobin has been kept above 10 g/dl, splenomegaly develops by the age of about 6 to 8 years (35). One study reviewed the blood requirements of 65 thalassemia patients who had been transfused to keep their hemoglobin levels above 8 g/dl. Splenectomy in these patients was associated with a decrease in transfusion requirement from a mean of 272 (+/- 62) ml packed RBC/kg/year pre-splenectomy to 127 (+/- 16) ml packed RBC/kg/year postsplenectomy (36). These authors suggest that splenectomy should be considered when transfusion requirements exceed 200 ml of packed RBC/kg/year. On a transfusion regimen in which the hemoglobin level is maintained above 11.5 g/dl, the transfusion requirement is slightly higher and splenectomy is recommended for a requirement of packed RBC of more than 220 ml/kg/year (37).

The decision to recommend surgery should be made on an individual basis, taking into account the patient's age and the size of the iron burden. In young children, splenectomy should be postponed if possible until after the age of 5 years to decrease the risk of sepsis. Children presenting with large spleens who have been under-transfused or who have not previously required transfusion, should be adequately transfused for a period of at least 6 months to assess whether spleen size and transfusion requirements fall into an acceptable range. Splenectomy can be safely delayed if ferritin levels remain under 1,000 ng/l, and if calculations of iron excretion indicate maintenance of a negative iron balance despite the high transfusional iron load. On the other hand, if compliance with prescribed subcutaneous administration of desferioxamine is less than ideal, or if the drug is tolerated only at low doses, the risk of irreversible organ damage from iron deposition increases. Splenectomy then becomes more clearly indicated. In children over 5 years, transfusion requirements should be assessed every 6 months and splenectomy recommended when the amount of blood needed increases over the acceptable range.

In thalassemia intermedia, transfusion requirements are not an issue since most patients are not chronically transfused. Nevertheless, most patients eventually require splenectomy because of hypersplenism or because of abdominal discomfort from the enlarged spleen. Sometimes a patient's hemoglobin level which has been stable for years will begin to decline. Splenectomy may then be followed by an increase in the baseline hemoglobin from 6 g/dl to 7 or 8 g/dl, accompanied by increased energy and a sense of well-being. Of course, the presence of other causes for a fall in hemoglobin should be ruled out before splenectomy is recommended.

It can be difficult to determine at what point a patient with thalassemia intermedia may benefit from splenectomy. The decision is best made on clinical grounds. Splenectomy should be recommended to a patient whose condition seems to be deteriorating, as shown by decreased rate of growth, increased symptomatology, increasing iron overload, or a fall in hemoglobin level (38). If splenectomy alone is not followed by the desired improvement, the patient should be started on a chronic transfusion program coupled with effective chelation. Splenectomy then has the added beneficial effect of minimizing transfusion requirements.

Other patients with thalassemia intermedia may not benefit from splenectomy. A truly asymptomatic patient who appears to be leading a normal, active life, and who denies any symptoms that could be due to increased splenic bulk, can be followed without surgical intervention. Splenectomy can then be reconsidered if symptoms appear, blood counts decrease, or spleen size increases.

Several special considerations arise when considering splenectomy in the patient with iron overload. It is argued that removal of the spleen may increase iron toxicity to vital organs by removing the splenic reticuloendothelial cell reservoir (39). This removal of the RE cell reservoir may be a real danger in a patient who is not being effectively chelated. However, in patients on regular transfusion and chelation programs, the expected improvement in iron balance has been documented by iron excretion studies both pre-splenectomy and post-splenectomy, and no clinical deterioration has been seen (37).

Another special problem in iron overloaded thalassemia patients is a decreased resistance to infection due to reticuloendothelial phagocytosis of iron. In reported studies, patients with thalssemia showed a 25% incidence of post-splenectomy sepsis and an 11% mortality rate, rates much higher than those seen in patients splenectomized for other hematologic diseases (9,40,41). In a recent review of splenectomized thalassemia patients, however, the only bacterial sepsis documented in 61 patient-years was from Yersinia enterocolitis, an infection associated with iron overload rather than splenectomy (37). It is possible that high fatality rates reported in the past were related to the poor general health of the patients, who were chronically anemic and iron overloaded. With modern management using hypertransfusion regimens and aggressive chelation, patients are healthier and less susceptible to infections.

An alternative to splenectomy is partial splenic embolization, a technique which has been used in thalassemia patients to alleviate hypersplenism while maintaining partial splenic function (42). Follow-up studies have not yet determined the length of time before relapse of hypersplenism will occur, or the extent of difficulties to be encountered with repeat embolization or subsequent splenectomy.

If larger long-term studies confirm that the rate of post-splenectomy sepsis in splenectomized thalassemia patients is now acceptably low, the decision for splenectomy may become easier in the future. For the time being, however, splenectomy remains a controversial recommendation, calling for thoughtful clinical judgment and participation of the patient and family in the decision.

HEMATOLOGIC INDICATIONS FOR SPLENECTOMY: IMMUNE CYTOPENIAS

Idiopathic Thrombocytopenic Purpura (ITP)

Splenectomy for idiopathic thrombocytopenic purpura (ITP) is traditionally recommended in two situations: (1) in acute ITP as an emergency treatment of life-threatening hemorrhage, and (2) in chronic ITP as a treatment of last resort for patients who are felt to be at high risk of bleeding or who are steroid dependent. In children under the age of 10 years, most hematologists familiar with the benign natural course of childhood ITP tend to delay splenectomy as long as possible. Follow-up studies have shown late recovery of near-normal platelet counts in as many as 9 out of 15 patients in whom splenectomy was delayed for one to four years (43). Nonetheless, there are some patients for whom watchful waiting during this long a period seems unsafe (44). These are the patients with persistently low platelet counts, below 10,000/mm^3; those with recurrent purpura or bleeding; or those with a dangerously high activity level due to age, temperament, or psychosocial factors.

The dramatic effectiveness of high-dose gammaglobulin in raising platelet counts now offers an alternative to early splenectomy for high-risk patients (45, 46). The platelet count usually doubles by 24 hours after the first day's infusion of 500 to 1,000 mg/kg of gammaglobulin. By the completion of a 3 to 5 day course, the count generally rises well into the normal range (47,48). Gammaglobulin is thought to work by blocking uptake and destruction of the antibody/

platelet complex in the reticuloendothelial cells. It does not appear to decrease antiplatelet antibody production or have any known effect on shortening the course of the disease. Therefore, unless the ITP spontaneously resolves, patients require "booster" gammaglobulin infusions periodically to maintain adequate platelet counts. At some point, splenectomy becomes a more attractive alternative than recurrent hospital admissions for gammaglobulin infusions, but the operation should be postponed if possible until a child is over 5 or 6 years old. In teenagers, splenectomy might be considered sooner than in the younger age group, since older children more commonly have a chronic course and are at less risk of overwhelming infection.

At present, experience with the use of high-dose gammaglobulin is accumulating, and patients are being followed longer without splenectomy. In the future, we may find that splenectomy is almost never necessary in childhood ITP because of a higher incidence of late resolution than was previously observed. However, splenectomy will most likely continue to have a prominent role in the treatment of adults and teenagers with chronic ITP.

Splenectomy results in prolonged remission in about 70% of otherwise refractory patients, or in about 90% of steroid-responsive patients (49). When splenectomy is recommended for steroid-treated patients, it is important to give hydrocortisone during the immediate pre- and postoperative periods because of the possible presence of adrenal suppression. Reactive thrombocytosis usually occurs in the postoperative period, and generally disappears within a month. Antiplatelet therapy to prevent thrombosis is recommended for adults if the platelet count exceeds $1,000,000/mm^3$ (50). In children, however, reactive thrombocytosis is almost never associated with thrombotic complications and generally requires no treatment (52). Recurrent immune thrombocytopenia may occur if accessory splenic tissue is not removed along with the spleen (53).

Autoimmune Hemolytic Anemia

Splenectomy for autoimmune hemolytic anemia is associated with remission in less than 50% of cases in childhood (52). However, if corticosteroids, gammaglobulin, and immunosuppressive therapy fail to control the hemolysis, splenectomy should be tried.

HYPERSPLENISM

Hypersplenism due to an underlying non-hematologic disease should be treated with splenectomy if peripheral cytopenia is severe and the underlying disease cannot be treated. Hypersplenism can result from virtually any cause of splenic enlargement, including mechanical or vascular factors, infection, and infiltration by malignant, granulomatous or reticuloendothelial cells.

Congestive splenomegaly due to obstruction of venous drainage can be caused by thrombosis of the splenic veins, obstruction of portal or hepatic veins, or increased pressure in the inferior vena cava due to longstanding right heart failure. In such conditions splenomegaly is most often an incidental finding and requires no intervention. In some cases, however, cell counts may drop low enough to warrant splenectomy (28).

Splenic embolization using Gelfoam particles injected directly into the splenic artery offers an alternative to surgery for patients with hypersplenism (54,55). This technique has been used successfully in patients with biliary atresia, Gaucher's disease, and thalassemia. While embolization has the advantages of preserving splenic function and avoiding laparotomy, complications include recurrent hypersplenism, pleural effusion, pancreatitis, splenic rupture and splenic abscess. Splenic rupture and splenic abscess appear to be preventable if no more than 60 to 70% of the spleen is infarcted.

A massively enlarged spleen can be treated in stages, with 30 to 40% embolization at a time, repeated at two week intervals. Patients should receive antibiotics and effective analgesia during embolization to prevent splinting and consequent pulmonary problems. When performed correctly, splenic embolization offers the advantage of reducing the spleen size and correcting cytopenias, while preserving splenic function and avoiding a surgical procedure.

Partial splenectomy is another alternative for treatment of hypersplenism. This approach has been used in chronic Gaucher's disease in which there is a progressive splenic enlargement and pancytopenia (56). Since patients with Gaucher's disease are believed to have an especially high risk of infection because of reticuloendothelial cell infiltration of the spleen, avoidance of splenectomy is important. Moreover, total removal of reticuloendothelial storage sites of the spleen may result in accelerated accumulation of fat in the liver and bone marrow.

The problem with both partial splenectomy and splenic embolization is that over time residual splenic tissue will hypertrophy and hypersplenism may occur. When this happens, a repeat operation or repeat embolization may be technically difficult or dangerous because of adhesions and fibrosis from the first procedure. Follow-up studies on patients treated with splenic embolization or partial splenectomy will be important to determine how well immune function is preserved, and how soon hypersplenism recurs.

Other storage diseases in which splenectomy may be indicated for treatment of pancytopenia include Niemann-Pick disease, Hurler's disease, Wolman's disease, gangliosidosis, Tangier's disease, and primary amyloidosis (57).

MISCELLANEOUS CONDITIONS

Connective Tissue Disease

Connective tissue diseases may involve the spleen. Although more commonly seen in adults, the question of splenectomy sometimes arises in children with systemic lupus erythematosis (SLE) or polyarteritis nodosa. In SLE, splenectomy for treatment of the immune thrombocytopenia is much less effective than splenectomy in cases of idiopathic thrombocytopenic purpura. A series of patients with SLE and thrombocytopenia showed a remission rate of only 14% following splenectomy, as opposed to the remission rate of 80% reported in patients with ITP (58). Treatment with corticosteroids or alternative treatments should be tried before recommending splenectomy for SLE patients with thrombocytopenia.

Wiskott-Aldrich Syndrome

The use of splenectomy in Wiskott-Aldrich syndrome remains controversial. This X-linked immunodeficiency disorder is associated with a thrombocytopenia which often responds to splenectomy. Although splenectomy could cause an increase in the platelet count, the operation was previously felt to be contraindicated because of the co-existing immune deficiency. Many reported patients died of overwhelming infection within a few months following splenectomy (59). Splenectomies were performed only on selected patients whose dangerously low platelet counts made the risk of life-threatening hemorrhage more urgent than that of post-splenectomy sepsis.

A recent review of 16 patients with Wiskott-Aldrich syndrome who had splenectomy indicated that splenectomy should not be dismissed as a possible therapeutic alternative for these patients (60). Those maintained on prophylactic antibiotics showed a mean survival of 91.4 months. Two-thirds of these patients were alive 11 or more years after splenectomy. On the other hand, 5 out of 7 patients who did not take prophylactic antibiotics died within 33 months of surgery.

Perhaps high-dose gammaglobulin will prove to be useful in this group of patients, both in raising platelet counts and in increasing resistance to infection. At present, splenectomy in Wiskott-Aldrich syndrome should be tried if the degree of thrombocytopenia is felt to be life-threatening.

MALIGNANCY

Isolated splenic involvement can be seen in approximately 10% of patients with stage III Hodgkin's disease. Thus, splenectomy is recommended by the majority of cancer centers and oncology study groups in this country as part of the staging laparotomy for Hodgkin's disease. Debate continues as to whether total splenectomy is necessary in all cases. Review of histopathological material indicates that about 10% of involved spleens would not be detected if examinations of the spleen were limited to partial splenectomy (61). This would lead to a risk of understaging of about 2 to 3%. This number of cases with occult splenic involvement must be balanced against the risk of fatal sepsis in splenectomized Hodgkin's disease patients. In 1976, prior to the use of pneumococcal vaccine and prophylactic penicillin, the Children's Cancer Study Group (CCSG) reported a 10% incidence of fulminant septicemia in 200 children with Hodgkin's disease, half of whom died (62). In contrast, the Intergroup Hodgkin's Disease Childhood Study reported no cases of fatal sepsis in patients treated since February, 1978, when the use of pneumococcal vaccine and prophylactic penicillin became the recommended practice (63). The pneumococcal vaccine should be given as soon as possible after diagnosis and before institution of therapy, since antibody response is impaired in previously treated patients (64,65).

Only rarely is splenectomy indicated in other childhood malignancies. Although contraindicated in juvenile chronic myeloid leukemia (CML), splenectomy may be used in adult CML to eliminate discomfort of the patient due to massive splenic enlargement and to reduce transfusion requirements (66). Splenectomy does not delay blastic transformation, nor does it prolong survival time or improve response to chemotherapy as was previously suggested.

Primary tumors of the spleen are rare, but hemangioendothelioma, lymphosarcoma, and reticulum cell sarcoma may occur (67). Benign epidermoid cysts can enlarge to enormous size (68). These fluid-filled cysts are predisposed to traumatic rupture and infection if not removed. At surgery, viable splenic tissue should be preserved if possible. One case report describes removal of a football-sized cyst from a 9 year old boy's spleen. The bulk of uninvolved tissue was intact and functional on subsequent nuclear scan (69).

Benign hemangiomas, often presenting with thrombocytopenia due to consumptive coagulopathy, may be limited to the spleen or they may be associated with hemangiomatous lesions of the bone and skin (70). If hemangiomas are limited to the spleen, splenectomy will cure the coagulopathy.

INFECTION

Splenic abscess has always been associated with a high mortality rate, largely because of delayed or missed diagnosis. Prior to the use of the CT scan to aid early diagnosis, 37% of splenic abscesses were diagnosed post-mortem and the overall mortality was 40 to 47% (71). A much lower mortality rate of 17% was reported for splenic abscesses diagnosed earlier in the clinical course (72). Optimal treatment of splenic abscesses includes antibiotics, splenectomy, and irrigation and drainage of the left subdiaphragmatic space. However, with earlier diagnosis of splenic abscesses by CT scan, more cases are now being treated without splenectomy, using antibiotics and percutaneous drainage (74).

GENERAL CONSIDERATIONS

If splenectomy is advised for hemolytic disease, preoperative studies should include an ultrasound examination of the gallbladder. Cholecystectomy should be performed at the same operation if gallstones are present. Careful abdominal exploration at the time of surgery, or liver/spleen scan pre-operatively, should identify any accessory spleens so these can be removed. All splenectomized patients need preoperative counseling and regular post-operative follow-up (Table 2).

They should receive pneumococcal vaccine and *Hemophilus influenzae* vaccine if under 5 years of age. The vaccine should be administered before splenectomy, or before discharge after the operation so that the vaccination is not overlooked. Follow-up pneumococcal titers measured on vaccinated sickle cell patients indicated that a booster vaccination should be given 4 to 5 years following primary vaccination (75). The need for re-vaccination of other groups of splenectomized children is not yet established.

Prophylactic penicillin should be given at a dose of 250 mg twice daily for the rest of the patient's life. Probably most important, splenectomized patients must be educated about their increased risk for infection, and should be instructed to seek medical attention immediately in case of fever.

A large follow-up study of splenectomized patients given optimal preventative care will be necessary to determine accurate mortality rates for different conditions, and help guide decisions about splenectomy in the future. In all possible cases, the operation should be delayed until the child passes the age of 5 or 6 years. Traumatized spleens should be treated medically, or surgically repaired whenever possible.

Table 2 Measures to Reduce the Risk of Post-Splenectomy Sepsis

1. Administer Pneumococcal and *Hemophilus influenzae* B vaccine (prior to splenectomy if possible).
2. Prescribe prophylactic Penicillin (250 mg twice a day)
3. Educate patient/parents to seek prompt medical attention for fever
4. Schedule regular medical appointments to renew prophylactic antibiotics and reinforce precautions
5. Advise wearing a medi-alert emblem

Patients treated with new techniques such as splenic implantation, partial splenectomy or splenic embolization, should be followed over the long term to assess their immunologic competence and relapse rate. In all cases, the risks and benefits to each patient need to be weighed individually, and splenectomy recommended only after alternative therapies have failed.

REFERENCES

1. Puestow CB: *Surgery of the biliary tract, pancreas and spleen.* Chicago, Yearbook Medical Publishers, 1971:353-357.
2. Boles ET: The spleen. In: Welch KJ, Randolph JG, Ravitch MM eds: *Pediatric Surgery* ed 2; New York, Yearbook Medical Publishers, 1986;1107-1113.
3. King DR, Lobe TE, Haase GM, Boles ET: Selective management of the injured spleen. *Surgery* 1981;90:677-682.
4. Linne T, Eriksson M, Lannergren K, Tordai P, Czar-Weidhagen B, Swedberg K: Splenic function after nonsurgical management of splenic rupture. *J Pediatr* 1984;105(2):263-265.
5. Douglas GJ, Simpson JS: The conservative management of splenic trauma. *J Pediatr Surg* 1971;6:565-570.
6. Ein SH, Shandling B, Simpson JS, Stephens CA: Nonoperative management of traumatized spleen in children: How and why? *J Pediatr Surg* 1978;13:117-119.
7. Sherman R: Rationale for and methods of splenic preservation following trauma. *Surgical Clinics of North America* 1981;61:127-133.
8. Pearson HA, Johnston MT, Smith KA, Touloukian RJ: The born-again spleen: Return of splenic function after splenectomy for trauma. *N Engl J Med* 1978;298:1389-1392.
9. Singer DB. Postsplenectomy sepsis. In: *Perspectives in Pediatric Pathology* 1973;I:285-311.
10. Case records of the Massachusetts General Hospital (Case 36-1975). *N Engl J Med* 1975;293:547-553.
11. Pearson HA, Johnston D, Smith K, Touloukian RJ: Born-again spleens and resistance to infection. Letter. *N Engl J Med* 1978;299(15):832.
12. Velcek FT, Jongco GW, Shaftan GW, Klotz DH, Rao SP, Schiffman G, Kottmeier PK: Post-traumatic splenic replantation in children. *J Pediatr Surg* 1982;17(6):879-883.
13. Moore G, Stevens R, Moore E, Aragon G: Failure of splenic implants to protect against fatal postsplenectomy infection. *Am J Surg* 1983;146:413-414.
14. Livingston C, Levine B, Sirinek R: Preservation of splenic tissue prevents postsplenectomy pulmonary sepsis following bacterial challenge. *J Surg Res* 1982;33:356-361.
15. Roth H, Waldherr R: Problems in spleen autotransplantation: Comparative study of types of implantation in animal experiments. *Progress in Pediatric Surgery* 1985;18:182-189.

16. Chapman RG, McDonald LL: Red cell life-span after splenectomy in hereditary spherocytosis. *J Clin Invest* 1968;47:2263-2267.
17. Vaughn V, McKay R, Nelson W: *Textbook of Pediatrics* ed 10; Philadelphia, W. B. Saunders, 1975;1120.
18. Barker K, Martin FRR: Splenectomy in congenital microspherocytosis. *Br J Surg* 1969;56:561-564.
19. Bates GC, Brown CH: Incidence of gallbladder disease in chronic hemolytic anemia. *Gastroenterology* 1952;21:104-109.
20. Rutkow I: Twenty years of splenectomy for hereditary spherocytosis. *Arch Surg* 1981;116:306-308.
21. Wenckert A, Robertson B: The natural course of gallstone disease. *Gastroenterology* 1966;50:376.
22. Gracie WA, Ransohoff DF: The natural history of silent gallstones. *N Engl J Med* 1982;307:798-800.
23. McSherry CK, Glenn F: The incidence and causes of death following surgery for nonmalignant biliary trait disease. *Ann Surg* 1980;191:271.
24. Manno CS, Cohen AR: Splenectomy in spherocytosis: Is it worth the risk? Abstract. *Society for Pediatric Research* 1984;18(4):244A.
25. Kelleher J, Luban N, Mortimer P, Kamimura T: Human serum "parvovirus"; a specific cause of aplastic crisis in children with hereditary spherocytosis. *J Pediatr* 1982;102(5):720-722.
26. Croom RD, McMillan C, Orringer E, Sheldon GF. Hereditary spherocytosis: Recent experience and current concepts of pathophysiology. *Ann Surg* 1986;203(1):34-39.
27. MacKenzie FAF, Elliot DH, Eastcott HH, et al: Relapse in hereditary spherocytosis with proven splenunculus. *Lancet* 1962;i:1102-1104.
28. Mitchell A, Morris P: Surgery of the spleen. *Clin Haematol* 1983;121(2): 565-590.
29. Pearson H, McIntosh S, Ritchey A, et al: Developmental aspects of splenic function in sickle cell diseases. *Blood* 1979;53(3):358-365.
30. Pearson H, Ritchey A, Chilcote R, et al: The developmental pattern of splenic dysfunction in the sickle cell disorders. 1982; Cooperative Study of Sickle Cell Disease Publication. National Institutes of Health, Bethesda, Md.
31. Pearson H, Cornelius E, Schwartz A, et al: Transfusion-reversible functional asplenia in young children with sickle cell anemia. *N Engl J Med* 1970;283(7):334-337.
32. Rogers DW, Clarke J, Cupidore L, et al: Early deaths in Jamaican children with sickle cell disease. *Br Med J* 1978;i:1515-1516.
33. Topley J, Rogers D, Stevens M, Serjeant G: Acute splenic sequestration and hypersplenism in the first 5 years in homozygous sickle cell disease. *Arch Dis Child* 1981;56:765-769.
34. Charache S, Lubin B, Reid C, eds: Acute splenic sequestration and aplastic crisis. In: *Management and Therapy of Sickle Cell Disease*. NIH Publication No. 84-2117, September 1984, 22. Bethesda, Md.

35. Graziano JH, Piomelli S, Hilgartner M, et al: Chelation therapy in beta-thalassemia major. III. The role of splenectomy in achieving iron balance. *J Pediatr* 1981;99(5):695-699.
36. Cohen A, Markenson A, Schwartz E: Transfusion requirements and splenectomy in thalassemia major. *J Pediatr* 1980;97:100-102.
37. Piomelli S, Hart D, Graziano J, et al: Current strategies in the management of Cooley's anemia. Fifth Cooley's Anemia Symposium. Bank A, Anderson WF, Zaino EC (eds): *Annals of the New York Academy of Sciences* New York, 1985;445:256-257.
38. Modell B, Badoukas V: *The Clinical Approach to Thalassemia.* Grune & Stratton, New York, 1984; pp. 115-139.
39. Pootrakul P, Rugkiatsakul R, Wasi P: Increased transferrin iron saturation in splenectomized thalassemia patients. *Br J Haemat* 1980;46:143-145.
40. Van Wyck DB: Overwhelming postsplenectomy infection (OPSI): The clinical syndrome. *Lymphology* 1983;16:107-114.
41. Smith CH, Erlandson ME, Stern G: Postsplenectomy infection in Cooley's anemia. *Ann NY Acad Sci* 1964;119:748-757.
42. Pringle K, Spigos D, Tan W, et al: Partial splenic embolization in the management of thalassemia major. *J Pediatr Surg* 1982;17(6):884-891.
43. Ramos ME, Newman AJ, Gross S: Chronic thrombocytopenia in childhood. *J Pediatr* 1978;92:584.
44. Woerner SJ, Abildgaard CF, French BN: Intracranial hemorrhage in children with idiopathic thombocytopenic purpura. *Pediatrics* 1981;67:453.
45. Russell E, Maurer H: Alternatives to splenectomy in the management of chronic idiopathic thrombocytopenia in childhood. *Am J Pediatr Hemat/Oncol* 1984;6(2):175-178.
46. Bussell JB, Schulman I, Hilgartner MW, Barandum S: Intravenous use of gammaglobulin in the treatment of chronic immune thrombocytopenia as a means to defer splenectomy. *J Pediatr* 1983;103(4):651-655.
47. Fehr J, Hofmann V, Kappeler U: Transient reversal of thrombocytopenia in idiopathic thrombocytopenic purpura by high-dose intravenous gammaglobulin. *N Engl J Med* 1982;306(21):1254-1258.
48. Imback P, Barandum S, Hirt A, Wagner H: Intravenous immunoglobulin for ITP in childhood. *Am J Pediatr Hemat Oncol* 1984;6(2):171-174.
49. Simons SM, Main CA, Yaish HM, Rutzky J: Idiopathic thrombocytopenic purpura in children. *J Pediatr* 1975;87:16.
50. Schwartz S. Splenectomy for hematologic disease. *Surg Clin N Am* 1981; 61:117-125.
51. Miller D, Baehner R, McMillan C (eds): *Blood Diseases of Infancy and Childhood*; St. Louis, Mosby, 1984, pp. 242-243.
52. Aspnes GT, Pearson HA, Spencer RP: Recurrent idiopathic purpura with "accessory" splenic tissue. *Pediatrics* 1975;55:131-134.
53. Mozes M, Spigos DG, Pollak R. Partial splenic embolization, an alternative to splenectomy: Results of a prospective randomized study. *Surgery (St Louis)* 1984;96(4):694-701.

54. Stellin G, Kumpe DA, Lilly JR: Splenic embolization in a child with hypersplenism. *J Pediatr Surg* 1982;17(6):892-893.
55. Bar-Maor JA, Govrin-Yehudain J: Partial splenectomy in children with Gaucher's disease. *Pediatrics* 1985;76(3):398-401.
56. Bowdler A: Splenomegaly and hypersplenism. *Clin Hematol* 1983;12(2): 467-488.
57. Hall S, McCormick JL, Greipp PR: Splenectomy does not cure the thrombocytopenia of systemic lupus erythematosus. *Ann Intern Med* 1985;102: 325-328.
58. Weider PL, Blaese RM: Hereditary thrombocytopenia; relation to Wiskott-Aldrich syndrome with special reference to splenectomy: report of a family and review of the literature. *J Pediatr* 1972;80:226-234.
59. Lum LG, Tubergen DG, Corash L, Blaese RM: Splenectomy in the management of the thrombocytopenia of the Wiskott-Aldrich syndrome. *N Engl J Med* 1980;302(16):892-896.
60. Dearth JC, Gilchrist GS, Telander RL: Partial splenectomy for staging Hodgkin's disease; risk of false negative results. *N Engl J Med* 1979;299:345-346.
61. Chilcote RR, Baehner RE, Hammond GD, and the investigators and special studies committee of the Children's Cancer Study Group: Septicemia and meningitis in children splenectomized for Hodgkin's disease. *N Engl J Med* 1976;295:793-800.
62. Muraji T, Hays DM, Siegel S: Evaluation of the surgical aspects of staging laparotomy for Hodgkin's disease in children. *J Pediatr* 1982;17(6):843-847.
63. Levine AM, Overturf GP, Field RF: Use and efficacy of pneumococcal vaccine in patients with Hodgkin's disease. *Blood* 1979;54:1171-1175.
64. Addiego JE, Ammann AJ, Schiffman G: Response to pneumococcal polysaccharide vaccine in patients with untreated Hodgkin's disease. *Lancet* 1980;2:450.
65. Spiers ASD, Galton DAG, Catovsky D: Splenectomy for complications of chronic granulocytic leukemia. *Lancet* 1975;2:627-630.
66. Sutow WW, Fernback DJ, Vietti TJ: *Clinical Pediatric Oncology*. St. Louis, CV Mosby Co, 1984;801-802.
67. Blank E, Campbell JR: Epidermoid cysts of the spleen. *Pediatrics* 1973; 51(1):75-84.
68. Sink JD, Filston HD, Kirks DR: Removal of splenic cyst with salvage of functional splenic tissue. *J Pediatr* 1982;100(3):412-414.
69. Dadash-Zadeh M, Czapek EE, Schwartz AD: Skeletal and splenic hemangiomatosis with consumption coagulopathy: Response to splenectomy: Case Report. *Pediatrics* 1976;57(5):803-806.
70. Chun CS, Raff MJ, Contreras L: Splenic abscess. *Medicine (Baltimore)* 1980;59(1):50-65.
71. Linos DA, Nagorney DM, McIlrath DC: Splenic abscess: The importance of early diagnosis. *Mayo Clin Proc* 1983;58:261-264.

72. Gerzof S, Robbins A, Johnson W, Birkett D, Nabseth D: Percutaneous catheter drainage of abdominal abscesses. *N Engl J Med* 1981;305(12): 653-657.
73. Sones P: Percutaneous drainage of abdominal abscesses. *Am J Radiol* 1984; 142:35-39.
74. Weintraub PS, Schiffman G, Addiego JE: Long-term follow-up and booster immunization with polyvalent pneumococcal polysaccharide in patients with sickle cell anemia. *J Pediatr* 1984;105(2):261-263.

Part V

Perspectives

14

New Trends in Spleen Research

Reticuloendothelial Basis of the Clearance of Blood by the Spleen

LEON WEISS
School of Veterinary Medicine of the University of Pennsylvania, Philadelphia, Pennsylvania

The spleen provides alternative vascular pathways, it sorts and stores blood cells, and repairs and destroys impaired erythrocytes. It also supports phagocytosis, hematopoiesis and immunologic reactivity, contains microorganisms, and controls infectious diseases. These various activities depend upon the extraordinary capacity of the spleen to clear the blood; this ability of the spleen is dependent upon its reticuloendothelial nature and its unique vasculature.

In this chapter, I will discuss the circulation of the spleen and the reticuloendothelial character of the spleen. Then I will turn to the splenic clearance of blood and its derivative capacities. I will correlate structure and function of the spleen and will attempt to identify the fundamental cellular mechanisms upon which both normal and pathologic functions of the spleen depend.

THE INTERMEDIATE CIRCULATION OF THE SPLEEN

The spleen depends upon its unique intermediate circulation for its clearance capacity. The intermediate circulation consists of terminal arterial vessels, proximal venous and lymphatic vessels, and the specialized filtration beds interposed between the arterial and venous (and lymphatic) vessels (Figures 1-5) (2-5,13, 19,21,25,27,28,31-38). The intermediate circulation is anatomically open in that there is no endothelial continuity between terminal arterial vessels and proximal venous vessels. Instead, reticular meshworks, different in conformation

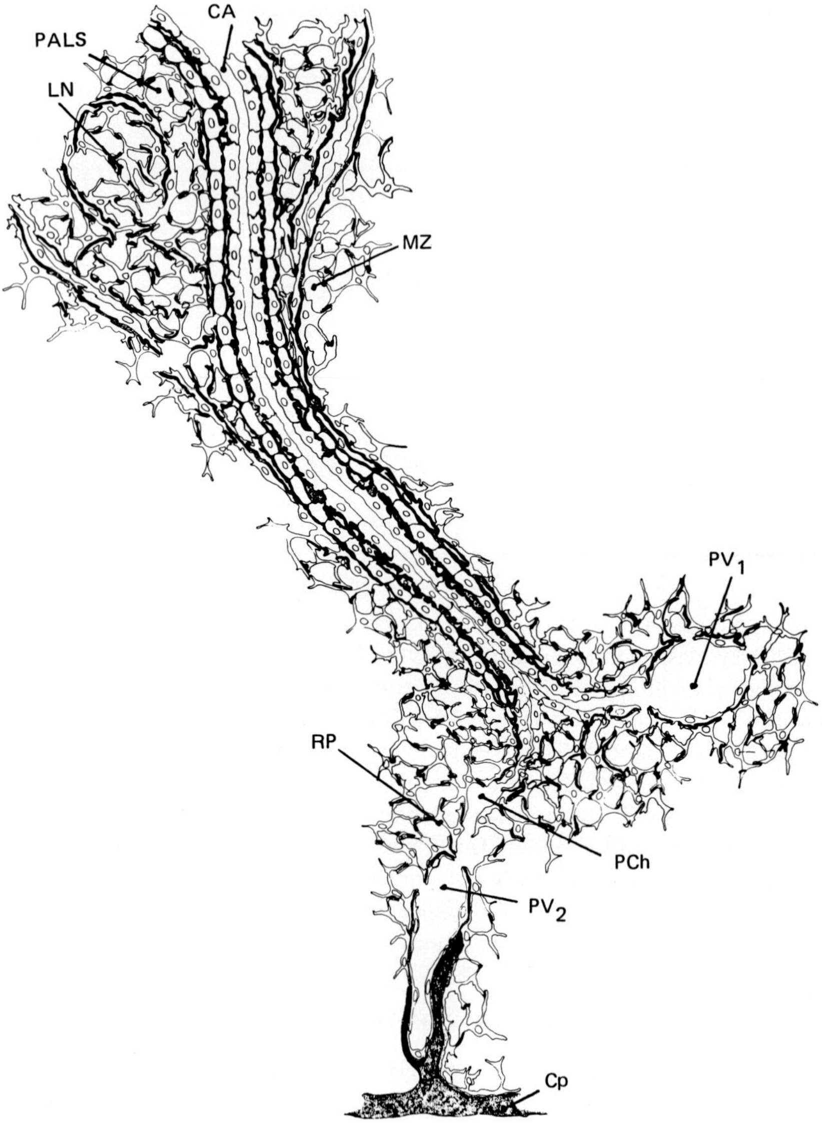
CA
PALS
LN
MZ
PV1
RP
PCh
PV2
Cp

in different parts of the spleen, are interposed between arterial and venous (and lymphatic) vessels (35-37).

These reticular meshworks are the means of splenic clearance. Accordingly, I have termed them filtration beds (37). These filtration beds are composed of an anatomically open circulation and the presence of an interposed filtration bed. In spite of this anatomic arrangement of open circulation more than 95% of the blood circulates as if the vasculature were anatomically closed, passing through the spleen in 30 seconds or less (17,27,28). This large component of the splenic circulation is, therefore, physiologically closed (35-37).

The existence of an anatomically open but physiologically closed circulation may be rationalized as follows: In some cases arterial terminals are quite close to the venous wall, even sharing a common basement membrane. Where the arterial ending is distant from the venous wall, the filtration bed may, nonetheless, convey blood efficiently from artery to vein by tubular structures fashioned from their sheet-like cytoplasmic processes. Furthermore, the filtration bed which intervenes between arterial and venous vessels may contract, pulling arterial endings against venous interendothelial slits. Indeed, filtration beds are able to contract not unlike blood vessels; their constituent reticular cells are rich in contractile filaments and are innervated by sympathetic nerves. In fact, as inferred by findings on scanning electron microscopic examination of plastic vascular casts, contracted spleens offer direct flow; on the other hand, relaxed spleens offer an open circulation (27,28,34).

Experiments were done in which blood was washed out of isolated spleen by vascular perfusates. These studies showed that the spleen does offer several types

---

Figure 1 Schematic drawing of a nonsinusal spleen. Only the vaculature and reticular cell stroma are shown; free cells, as lymphocytes, erythrocytes, etc., are left out. The reticular cell stroma of white pulp, marginal zone, and red pulp form meshworks of distinctive forms which constitute filtration beds.

The central artery (CA) emerges from the periarterial lymphatic sheaths (PALS), the T cell zones which, with lymphatic nodules (LN) comprise the white pulp (WP) of the spleen. Immediately surrounding the white pulp is the marginal zone (MZ). The white pulp is limited peripherally by reticular cells forming a circumferential reticulum (CR). The central artery continues into the red pulp (RP) and terminates in a bifurcation. One branch ends quite close to the wall of a pulp vein (PV_1), its termination placed in line with an aperture in the vein's wall. A second arterial branch terminates a greater distance from a venous wall, but a preferential channel (PCh) runs through the reticulum of red pulp (which constitutes the filtration bed) between the terminal arterial vessel and the pulp vein (PV_2). PV_2 continues into a trabecular vein. A section of capsule (Cp) is shown.

(a)

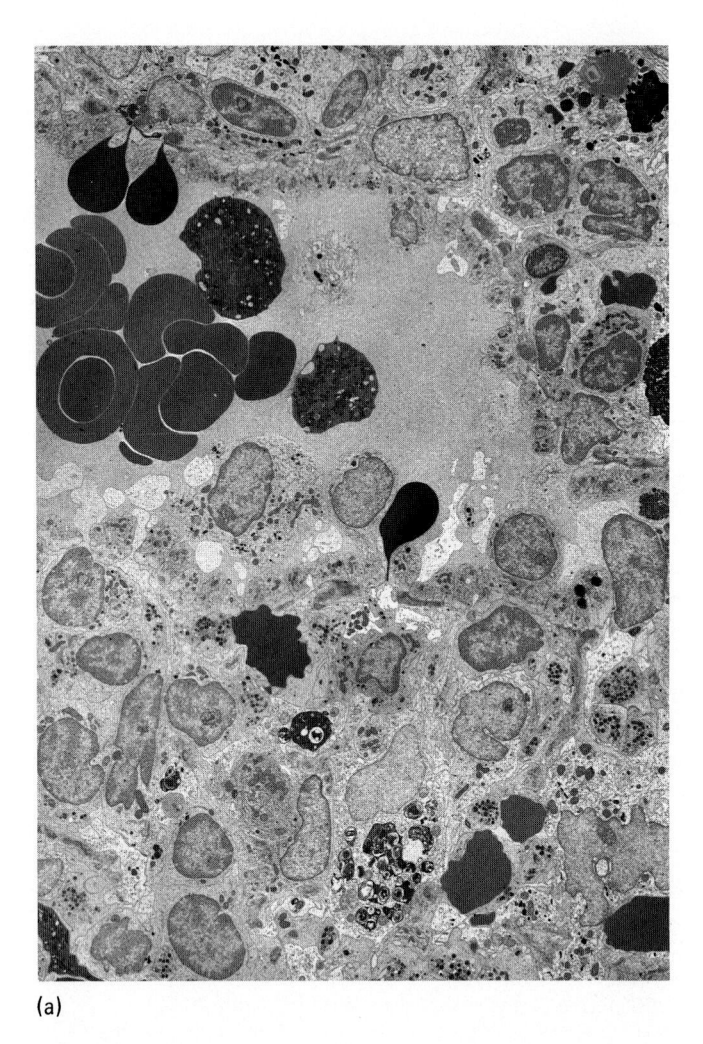

Figure 2 *Human Red Pulp.* (a) This field consists of a portion of a vascular sinus surrounded by a rather densely packed collection of cells. Please refer to the accompanying labelled tracing (b), which has been reduced. The persinusal tissue, often termed splenic cord, is the filtration bed of red pulp that receives terminating arterial vessels. Its stroma consists of adventitial reticular cells (ARC) lying on the outside surface of the sinus and extending outwards, merging into the reticular meshwork (or filtration bed) of the cord. This filtration bed is charged with a variety of free cells as is evident in this field. Many macrophages (Mo) are caught in this filtration bed, imparting a phagocytic function to it. These macrophages probably came into the splenic cords as monocytes and, held there, differentiated into macrophages. The venous sinus, its lumen labelled the most

(b)

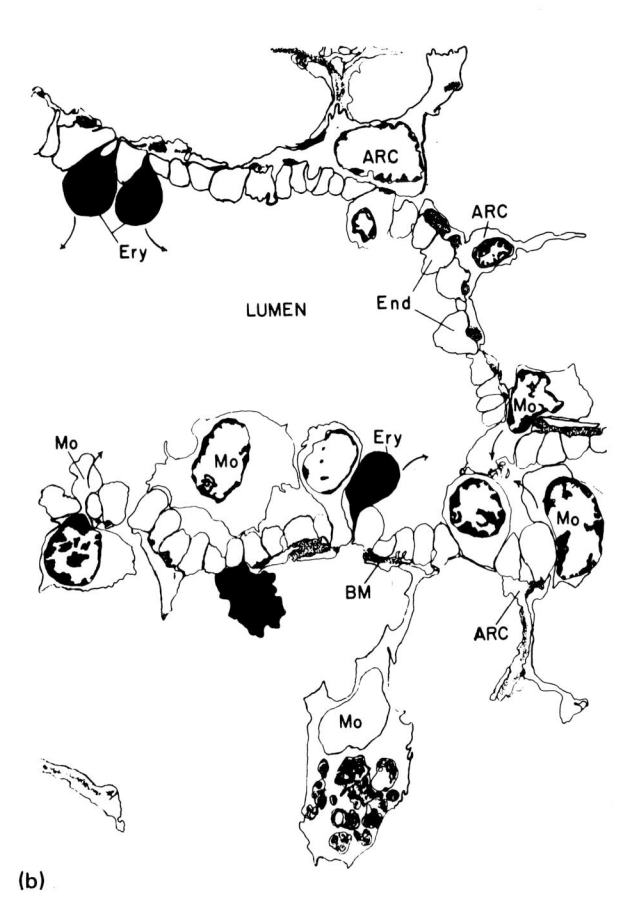

Figure 2 (continued) proximal to the venous vessels, is fully lined by a distinctive endothelium (End). Free circulating cells, as the labelled erythrocytes (Ery), must pass through the interendothelial slits of the endothelium. The erythrocytes in passage across the wall are drawn out into thin strands in the interendothelial slits. Only those erythrocytes plastic enough to thin down to this extent pass readily through the interendothelial slit. (X1450, H & E stain)

of delayed circulation where, presumably, blood is filtered by the filtration beds (17,27,28). Blood flow may be moderately delayed (for minutes), or may be considerably delayed (for up to an hour). Further studies, moreover, have shown a splenic circulation that was even more delayed (up to 12 hours) (1,23,24). This delay in circulation is comparable to that shown by Gowans and his colleagues (14,15) in lymph nodes, for circulation of lymphocytes of the recirculating lymphocyte pool (6,7,9,33). These several delayed circulations permit

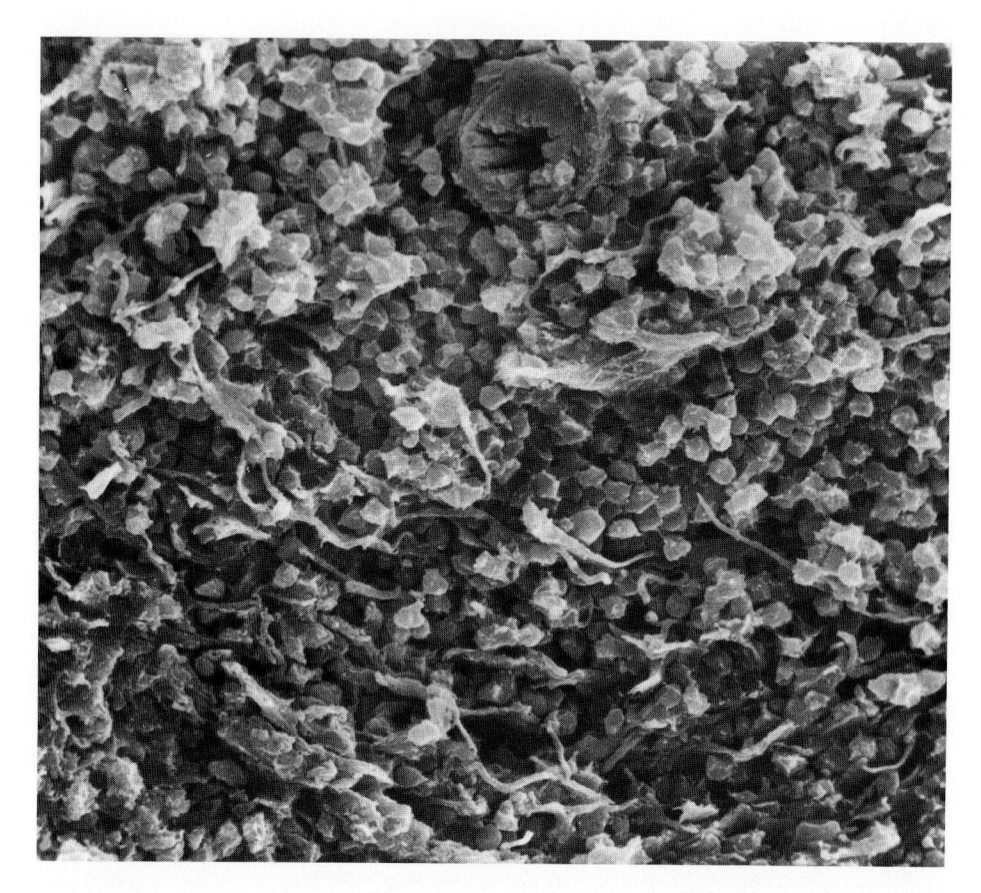

Figure 3 *Rat white pulp.* The organization of the white pulp, largely the periarterial lymphatic sheath, is displayed in this scanning electron micrograph. The central artery lies at the middle of the upper margin. The rest of the field is occupied by small, near-spherical lymphocytes (T cells) and reticular cells. The reticular cells are rather light, have extended processes which coalesce about threadlike reticular fibers. The reticular cell branches are arranged circumferentially about the central artery. (X2700) (From *Blood* 1974;43:605.)

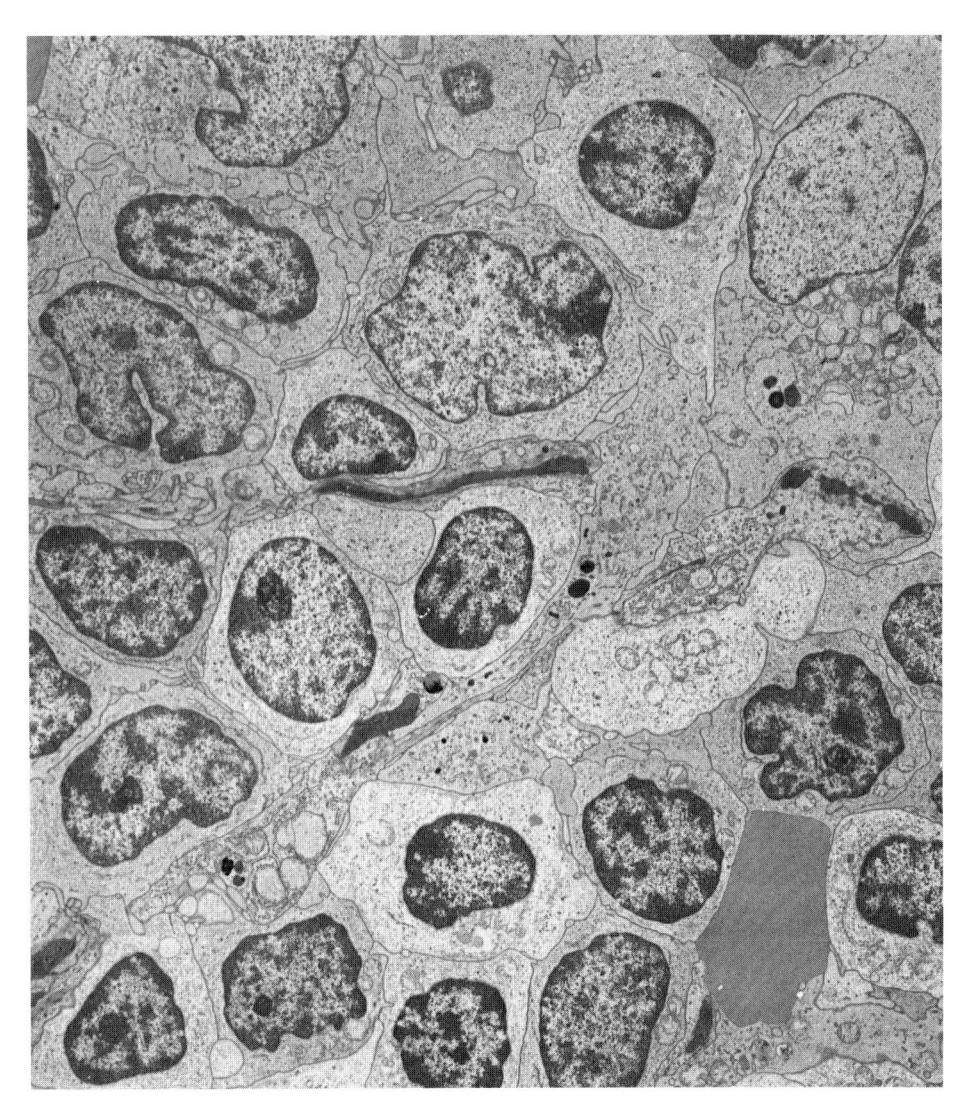

Figure 4 *Human white pulp.* In this transmission electron micrograph the top of the field is central and the bottom peripheral white pulp, verging into the marginal zone. The dense linear structures are reticular fibers of the circumferential reticulum. Each of the fibers is surrounded by the cytoplasm of reticular cells. Most of the field consists of lymphocytes and their associated cells. A few erythrocytes are present. (X3280)

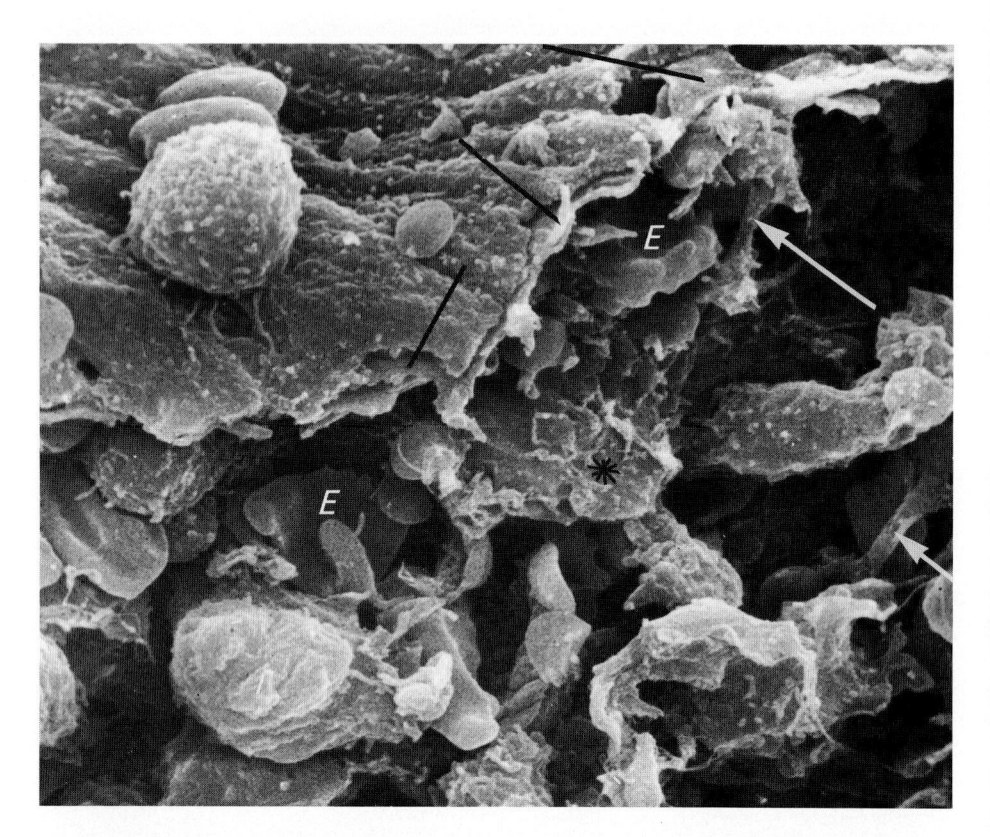

Figure 5 *Rat red pulp.* The luminal surface of a vascular sinus is shown in the left upper quadrant of this scanning electron micrograph. Note that the endothelial surface is formed by long endothelial cells lying side by side, the interendothelial slits marked by longitudinal grooves. Several blood cells lies upon the endothelium. The adventitial layer of reticular cells protrudes from the cut edge of the sinus and is marked by three black arrows. In the underlying cord the strandular process of two reticular cells are indicated by white arrows. Two crenulated erythrocytes (E) lie in the cord just under the shelter of the wall of the vascular sinus. (X2700) (From *Blood* 1975;43:665.)

blood cell storage, as well as time for erythrocyte conditioning, hematopoiesis, and immunological reactions to take place.

RETICULOENDOTHELIAL CHARACTER OF THE SPLEEN

The bold, useful, and imperfect concept of the reticuloendothelial system (RES) has engendered a unified and comprehensive view of several seemingly unrelated functions and disorders, including the control of infectious diseases, immunology, hematopoiesis, lipid metabolism and storage diseases, disorders of pigmentation, and tumorgenesis. This unified concept of the role of the RES in these various functions and disorders is obtained through understanding of cellular interactions, notably the interplay of macrophages, reticular cells, and endothelial cells of vascular sinuses. These various cells and their interactions are linked by their putative capacity for phagocytosis. In development of the RES, however, other cell types, such as mast cells and the cells of the Langerhans system of antigen-presenting cells, have been included. The reticuloendothelial system maintains macrophages, reticular cells, and vascular sinuses among its chief cellular and tissue components (12,18,29,34,41-43).

MACROPHAGES

Discoveries of macrophages, enriched by pathologic studies of the spleen and other hematopoietic tissues, stimulated formulation of the modern concept of the reticuloendothelial system (12,18,42,43). The macrophage dominated early conceptions of the RES and remains the salient cell. Indeed, most of the branched stromal cells of the hematopoietic tissues were initially thought to be macrophages; new cell types, such as interdigitating cells, were plucked out only as justifying criteria developed. In contrast, certain putative cell types initially differentiated from macrophages on the basis of one or another experimental system, are now recognized as likely macrophages. These cells appear to be variant only because of special methods or circumstances, as in the case of pyrrhol-blue cells, wandering cells, resting-wandering cells, clasmatocytes, rhagocrine cells, and polyblasts. These stromal cells which were free of phagosomes but deemed capable of phagocytosis, being a macrophage that "hasn't yet eaten," were classified as histiocytes. Monocytes were recognized as the bone marrow-produced precursors of macrophages. Likewise, epitheloid cells and multinucleate giant cells were considered as two cell forms into which macrophages readily differentiate.

While its prodigious phagocytic capacity has earned it the sobriquet "professional phagocyte," the macrophage is increasingly respected as possessing a wide repertoire of biological functions. This broad array of functions permits the macrophage to control inflammation, immunologic reactions, hematopoiesis,

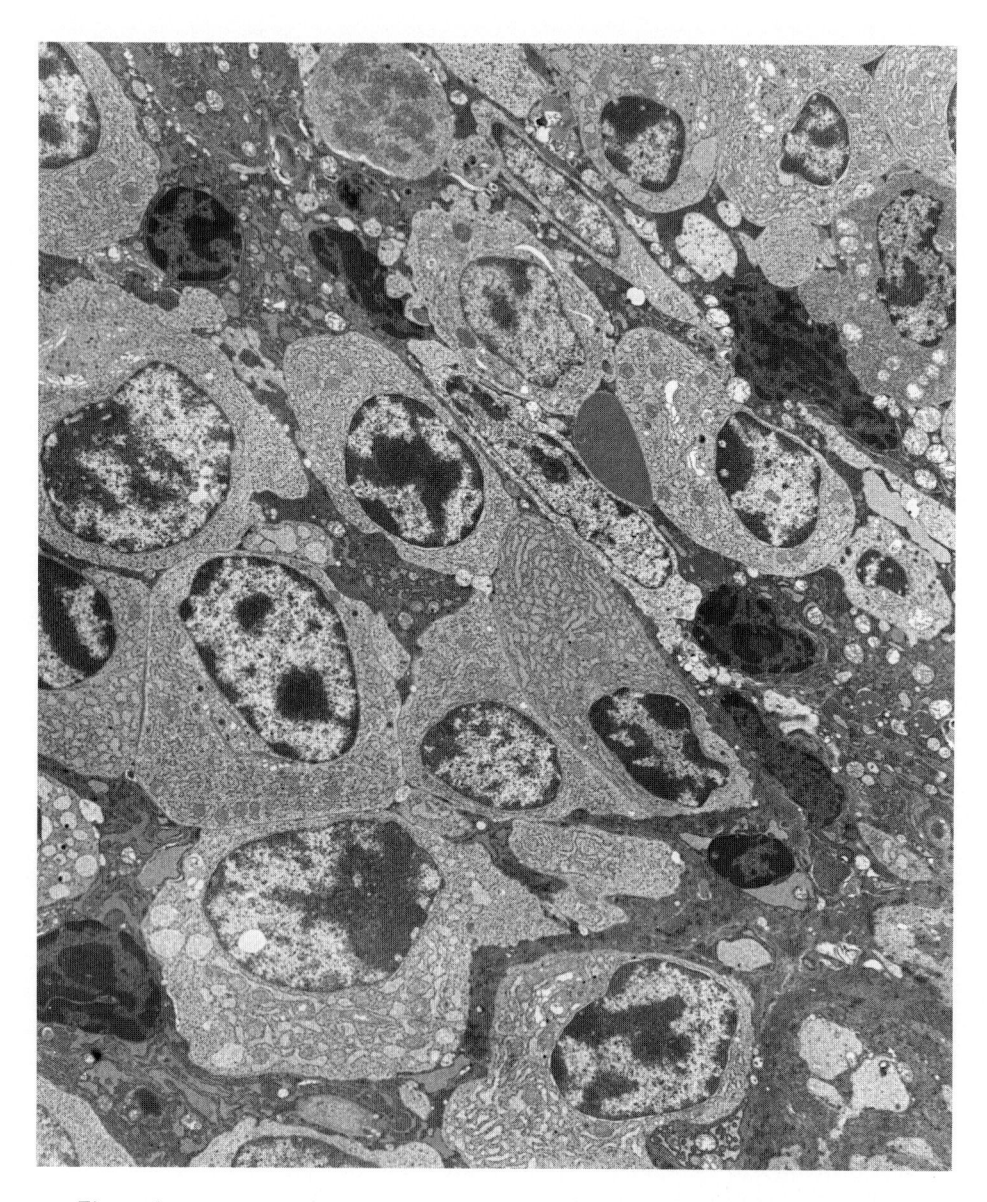

Figure 6 *Red pulp in murine malaria.* This field consists of free cells, most of which are plasma cells, and activated reticular cells. The latter, quite dense, are rich in endoplasmic reticulum and other organelles associated with high level protein synthesis and form a syncytial web pervading the red pulp, enclosing single free cells or clusters of them. (X5200) (See text and Weiss, Geduldig and Weidanz, *American Journal of Anatomy* 1986;176:257, for more information.)

and blood coagulation. It secretes hydrolytic enzymes, interferons, and hematopoietic colony stimulating factors, as well as components of complement, prostaglandins, and monokines. The macrophage controls the level of antigen, presents antigen, and appears to make antigen immunogenic. The macrophage is a major cell type recruited by lymphokines in cellular immunity, and it, in turn, through its secretions and interactions with other cell types, controls the expression of cellular immunity.

It is evident from examination of recent reviews on the reticuloendothelial system, that many functions of reticuloendothelial tissues, such as the clearance of the blood, continue to be attributed to macrophages. This is testimony to the great range of activity of these omnipresent cells. Attributing so many functions to the macrophage also may be due to the failure, even nowadays, to recognize the participation of other cell types which are difficult to demonstrate and hard to differentiate from macrophages.

THE ENDOTHELIUM OF VASCULAR SINUSES

The term vascular sinuses in this case refers to proximal venous vessels of hematopoietic tissues, of the liver and of many of the endocrine organs. These sinuses are wide-lumened, thin-walled vessels lined by an endothelium initially thought to be so unlike other endothelia that it was inappropriate to classify as "endothelium." The terms lining cells or littoral cells were advanced for these endothelial cells because they were considered both phagocytic and capable of differentiating into hematopoietic stem cells. The vascular sinuses of the liver are distinctive in containing a phagocytic cell type, the Kupffer cell, which originates in bone marrow, travels to hepatic venous sinuses, and insinuates itself into the endothelium.

Kupffer cells are as phagocytic as connective tissue macrophages. They may proliferate, thus maintaining their number without consistently depending upon immigrant precursors. They may leave the sinusal endothelium, especially when laden with phagosomes, and enter the circulation. In the circulation, they resume their migratory pattern, usually to be caught in the pulmonary circulation. But the endothelial cells of the hepatic venous sinuses of the spleen and bone marrow, are but reluctant phagocytes. These cells show slight to moderate phagocytosis only when presented long-term with large-scale phagocytic loads. Moreover, there is no modern evidence that sinusal endothelial cells are capable of differentiating into hematopoietic stem cells.

Sinusal endothelium surely is distinctive. In the venous sinuses of the spleen, for example, endothelial cells are rod-shaped, reinforced by basal bundles of intermediate and fine filaments. These endothelial cells are ensheathed by a basement membrane pierced by large, regular fenestrations that make the remaining substance of the basement membrane look like rectilinear fibers (2-5, 21,32,34,36). In the rabbit, this basement membrane may look like chicken wire; in humans, it may look like hardware cloth, with the annular component wide and the longitudinal component narrow. Moreover, sinusal endothelium has distinctive functions, which include the testing and pitting of erythrocytes. In fact, it is now evident that no endothelium is merely a mechanical lining. Every endothelium is distinctive and complex, possessing functions related to controlling the coaguability of blood, inflammation, selective passage of blood cells, etc. Since all endothelia are complex biological entities, it would appear unnecessary to apply other terms than "endothelium" to the lining of venous sinuses.

It is important to recognize, especially when one attempts to evaluate the intermediate circulation of the spleen, that while many spleens (including those of human beings, dogs, armadillos, and rabbits), contain venous sinuses and are therefore classified as sinusal (2-5,19,31,32). In nonsinusal spleens (i.e., cat, mouse, horse), the red pulp is made up of an extensive pulp space made up of reticular filtration beds. The veins do not honeycomb the pulp space, as do venous sinuses. Instead, pulp veins, the proximal veins, tend not to venture far into the pulp space but lie against trabeculae, draining into trabecular veins.

Physiologically closed circulations have been observed in cat spleen, which contains an anatomically open vasculature. This finding validates the conclusion that the intermediate circulation of the spleen is anatomically open and physiologically closed. Much work on the circulation of the spleen which showed a closed circulation, including Kniseley's pioneer work of the 1930s, was done on kittens and cats. Further support for the concept that the circulation of the spleen is anatomically open and physiologically closed comes from McCuskey's laboratory. In these studies, observations upon the living circulation of the spleen and fixed electron microscopic preparations of the same tissue were correlated (21).

RETICULAR CELLS

Reticular cells (RC) are classified as fibroblastic because they look like fibroblasts. These cells are closely associated with reticular fibers (now identified, in general, as consisting of collagen type III), and have, at most, only limited phagocytic functions (34,39). Reticular cells are therefore presumed to produce reticular fibers. For this purpose they joint company with connective tissue fibroblasts, osteoblasts, chondroblasts, odontoblasts, smooth muscle cells, adipocytes, and other cells that secrete extracellular matrix. Indeed, those reticular cells that provide the adventitial cover of vascular sinuses in bone marrow may accumulate lipid and become the adipocytes of marrow. This latter process is readily reversible by hematologic stress in axial bone marrow.

Reticular cells generally have received little attention in studies of the reticuloendothelial system. These cells are simply accorded their role in forming the stromal reticular meshwork that supports the free, migratory cells in its interstices. In most preparations, the associated reticular fibers can be sharply demonstrated with silver stains. In contrast, reticular cells simply do not stand out or possess, as do macrophages, a salient, vividly demonstrable function. But the "framers" of the reticulendothelial system (those who created our current concepts) did attribute important functions to reticular cells (18). Like the endothelial cells of the venous sinuses, reticular cells appear to be phagocytic. But, like the endothelium of the vascular sinuses, reticular cells appear phagocytic only when the phagocytic load is large and sustained.

Reticular cells were also considered as multipotent, needing only the stimulus of hematopoietic stress to round off the reticulum to become hemocytoblasts, or multipotent hematopoietic stem cells. This conclusion is not supported by modern work. The fatty modulation of reticular cells in bone marrow has been mentioned above (35). Reticular cells may become pigmented, becoming major bearers of malarial pigmentation. Furthermore, there are a few reports rather early in the studies of the reticuloendothelial system in which proliferation of the reticular cells, reticulosis, was recognized (18). In reticulosis, the reticular cells were characterized as large, dark, markedly vacuolated cells, associated with monocytoid cells. Such changes were interpreted as neoplastic, being a type of monocytic leukemia. More recent reports describe "dark" dendritic cells, closely associated with hematopoietic cells and of unclear identity and function. I will return to the matter of dark dendritic cells and reticulosis, and I will attempt to put these cells in a systemic, operative context.

INDUCTIVE CAPACITIES OF FIBROBLASTS

There is an important line of research, pertinent to hematopoiesis and splenic function, initiated by Grobstein in the 1940s. These studies established that fibroblastic cells induce the differentiation of other cells (8,11,16,26). Grobstein showed that the histiotypic formation of the murine salivary gland depends upon the inductive presence of surrounding mesenchyme. Without mesenchyme the epithelium grew only as indifferent sheets. Remote mesenchyme induced crude glandular formations. Similar results have been obtained with kidney, eye, skin, and many other tissues.

The influences of mesenchyme may not require cell-to-cell contact, often relying instead on extracellular factors passed by fine filters. Moreover, where hormones play a role in the induction, it appears, as in the development of seminal vesicles, that the hormones work through the intermediacy of fibroblasts. They do not act directly upon the differentiating epithelium. While many studies of the inductive capacities of mesenchyme are necessarily restricted to prenatal systems, there are important postnatal examples of the continuing influence of the connective tissues. The hematopoietic tissues retain many embryonal characteristics, there is turning over of cells and differentiating from stem cells throughout life. In studies using subrenal capsule implants in the guinea pig, the induction of hematopoietic tissues by fibroblasts, and the type of the hematopoiesis (lymphopoiesis vs. myelopoiesis), were all observed to be dependent upon the source of fibroblasts (11).

Fibroblasts in adult animals do show distinctive, although restricted, morphologic patterns and change. The ovarian theca undergoes cytomorphosis and steroid hormone production. Also, fibroblasts in the female reproductive system show decidual change in the progestational phase of the ovarian cycle, being quite marked during pregnancy. Kaye (22) showed that a particular race of fibroblasts immediately subtend the epithelium of the colon. These cells divided, migrated, and differentiated in parallel and in synchrony with the colonic epithelium. The fibroblastic adventitial reticular cells in the vascular sinuses of bone marrow are capable of undergoing transformation to adipocytes. By transforming, these cells thereby obtrude upon the hematopoietic compartment and reduce hematopoietic volume. But marrow adipocytes, in addition to such mechanical functions, aromatize testosterone to estrogen (affecting erythropoiesis and bone deposition) and induce granulocytopoiesis (35).

Fibroblasts of wound healing, unusually rich in contractile filaments are contractile. Splenic reticular cells in marginal and red pulp are the fibroblasts of wound healing. They contain contractile filaments and are innervated by sympathetic fibers. The meshworks that these dendritic cells form are thus set up not unlike vascular smooth muscle supplied by vasomotor nerves. The presence of these meshworks emphasizes the essential vascular character of the spleen.

HEGEMONIES OF THE RETICULOENDOTHELIAL SYSTEM: BARRIER-FORMING SYSTEMS OF ACTIVATED RETICULAR CELLS

The modern concept of the reticuloendothelial system originated when the monophyletic-vs.-polyphyletic controversy on blood cell origin gripped the field of experimental hematology. The major question was reduced to the potency of the lymphocyte. The monophyletists argued that the lymphocyte was the totipotent hematopoietic stem cell, equivalent to the hemocytoblast, and capable of differentiating into any of the blood cell types. The polyphyletists held that the lymphocyte was fully differentiated, thus incapable of differentiating into any of the other blood cell types. This controversy was an expression, in scientific terms, of a fundamental schism in human thinking, the "lumpers" vs. the "splitters." It was a controversy between those with one encompassing vision vs. those with a set of discrete, unrelated values. Isiah Berlin compared this situation to the dichtomy in the metaphor of the hedgehog and the fox, where the fox knows many things and the hedgehog knows one big thing. The controversy was posed before scientific methods were available to solve it. This controversy arose before stem cells could be labelled indubitably, innocuously, and indelibly, and followed in the course of their differentiation in the context of the body, and before there was any understanding of lymphocyte function.

The problem, of course, has now been solved. It turns out that there are several types of lymphocyte, not one type, as had been assumed by both the monophyletists and polyphyletists. T lymphocytes and B lymphocytes meet the polyphyletist standard of cells that are so fully differentiated that they are not capable of differentiating into other cell types. On the other hand, one of the null lymphocytes, the colony forming unit-spleen (CFU-S), does meet the monophyletic requirement, being a multipotent hematopoietic stem cell capable of differentiating into other blood cell types. While the conclusions of both monophyletist and polyphyletist have turned out to be both correct and incorrect, neither has been vindicated because neither's conclusions were reached by competent scientific means.

Without significant rigor, intuition and rhetoric ruled. To the damage of its scientific status, the reticuloendothelial system became the arena within which the dialectical problems of the monophyletic vs. polyphyletic schools of blood cell formation were played out. But so engaging was the issue of the origin of blood cells, and so little scientific discipline was brought to the discussion, that even on points of general agreement conclusions were often incorrect. For example, it was widely accepted that both sinusal endothelium and the reticular cell were hematopoietically multipotent. This point of view naively depended upon the notion that intermediate morphologic stages between putative stem cell and fully differentiated cell indicated a genuine developmental sequence. It is true that the differentiation of granulocytes from myeloblasts, and the development of erythrocytes from basophilic erythroblasts, was worked out this way. In the differentiation of erythroblasts and myeloblasts one deals with cells with such "natural" markers as hemoglobin or the presence of specific granules or nuclear polymorphism. In study of differentiation of other cells, experimental markers must be used, such as those employed to distinguish T cells from B cells.

The scientific status and value of the reticuloendothelial system was further diminished because its functions were interpreted and extrapolated too broadly. Many surmises of complex normal and pathological processes, such as lipid metabolism, storage disease, and pigment deposition, about which very little was known, were heaped upon it. Virtually all types of white blood cells and all the connective tissue cell types, including mast cells, have been included in the reticuloendothelial system. While this expansion in the classification has greatly increased the scope of the reticuloendothelial system, it has detracted from its neatness and coherence. The elegant correlation of structure and function of the early studies could not be sustained.

Attempts have been made to render the reticuloendothelial system manageable: hegemonies or dominant subsystems have been created from the overarching concept of the reticuloendothelial system. The mononuclear phagocytic system (MPS) (12) focuses on the macrophage and its attendant cells, and has engendered a flourishing literature. The lympho-reticular system, a pathological construct not as widely used as the MPS, puts attention on the lymphatic tissues and their stroma. Here, I advance the hegemony of barrier-forming systems (BFS) of activated reticular cells (ARC) as a useful concept to direct scientific studies onto an enormously versatile system of fibroblastic cells (whose name, reticular cell, inheres in the term reticuloendothelial system). These fibroblastic cells control a good deal of the activity of the reticuloendothelial system. I will make the case for this hegemony after discussion of the behavior of the spleen in the clearance of the blood.

CLEARANCE OF BLOOD BY THE SPLEEN

Nearly all of the functions of the spleen depend upon its extraordinary capacity to clear the blood (1,6,7,9,14,15,20,23,33,40). Clearance of the blood is the beginning of a complex sequence. The process includes sorting out cells and particles cleared from the blood, storing them, setting them up to interact with other cells, participating in hematopoietic differentiation and immunologic responses, destroying or containing pathogens, and controlling infectious diseases. The spleen also clears T and B lymphocytes, antigen, antigen-presenting cells and other accessory cells from the blood. The spleen sorts them out into T cell and B cell zones, and sets them up to engage in immune reactions. If the T and B lymphocytes fail to react immunologically, the cells are released, to recirculate to the spleen for another opportunity. The spleen clears microbes and other particles from the blood. It provides for the containment or destruction of microbes by phagocytosis, oxygen burst, immunological reactions, or other mechanisms.

The spleen receives reticulocytes and B cells from bone marrow and provides the final conditioning before they are released to the general circulation. Damaged erythrocytes are cleared from the blood by the spleen. They may be destroyed and re-utilized or pitted and sent back to the circulation as spherocytes. Platelets are stored in the spleen in large numbers in ready reserve. Monocytes are trapped from the blood and then differentiate into macrophages and, in certain circumstances, become epitheloid cells and multinucleate giant cells.

The spleen is especially effective in removing encapsulated bacteria from the blood and destroying them. After splenectomy, an individual is at risk from overwhelming infections with pneumococci, *Hemophilus influenzae*, or meningococci. The spleen plays a key role in the control of malaria (see below). The spleen, especially when it is enlarged, can effectively remove cells from the blood, removing such imperfect cells as phenylhydrazine-damaged erythrocytes. However, the process is not highly efficient, requiring many passes before the blood is cleared. Likewise, the spleen clears T cells and holds them in T cell zones, which are the periarterial lymphatic sheaths of white pulp. But most T cells entering the spleen are not cleared the first time through. The leave by way of veins, recirculating in the blood many times before they are cleared. Filtration capacity is functionally limited, even when it is greatly increased by anatomic enlargement of the spleen. But an enlarged spleen may become so aggressive a filter that it can reduce the levels of circulating blood cells to abnormally low levels. The consequent anemia, leukopenia and thrombocytopenia are the effects of this hypersplenism.

As one closely examines splenic clearance, it becomes evident, even in large spleens, that the filtration beds may be shut off. As a result, there is little or no clearance of the blood. Wyler and his colleagues (20,40) elegantly demonstrated this process in experimental *Plasmodium berghei* malaria. Early in the disease the filtration beds are open and the spleen clears the blood of parasitized erythrocytes (PE) quite effectively. The spleen becomes enlarged and the filtration capacity is above-normal. But then, remarkably, the filtration beds shut down, and the spleen fails to clear parasitized erythrocytes or other imperfect circulating cells, such as phenylhydrazine-damaged erythrocytes. As a result of the failure of splenic clearance, severe anemia develops and the parasitemia increases greatly. Then, at just short of 2 weeks of disease, a crisis occurs and the disease is resolved. The closed-down splenic filtration beds open and circulating parasitized erythrocytes are swept into them and destroyed.

In the pre-crisis spleen the filtration beds support massive erythropoiesis. With the opening of the filtration beds at the time of crisis, the reticulocytes produced within the closed-off beds are rapidly released to the circulation and ameliorate the anemia. In malaria the filtration beds are regulated: they may be opened to the circulation, or sealed off from it. When the beds are open in an enlarged spleen, as after a crisis, filtration is heightened (expressed as hypersplenism). But the precrisis spleen is asplenic, blood is shunted right through without clearance. In asplenia, blood-spleen barriers develop, sealing off filtration beds from the circulation (36,37).

The splenic responses in experimental malaria are not unique, instead they are expressive of general splenic capacities. The spleen's erratic clearance behavior causes the most troublesome problems in the management of sickle cell disease (30). Before the spleen is reduced to the fibrous nubbin of the adult with sickle cell disease, it is large. Such an enlarged spleen can swing from profound hypersplenism, trapping so many circulating erythrocytes so rapidly to produce life-threatening anemia: the acute sequestration syndrome. Or just as suddenly and just as unpredictably, the enlarged spleen may shut down its filtration beds, giving rise to functional asplenia. This failure to clear micro-organisms may result in severe infection.

Additional mechanisms controlling clearance are present. These control mechanisms normally exist to only a limited degree. But they are quite evident in the splenomegaly associated with damaged erythrocytes, presence of infections or metabolic diseases, in malaria (37), in sickle cell disease, in patients with spectrin-deficient erythrocytes, in patients receiving glucocorticoid therapy, and in Hodgkin's disease. These control mechanisms depend upon the activation of reticular cells (ARC). Activation of these cells, which is evident on electron microscopy, is associated with the appearance of high-level protein synthesis and secretion (Figure 6). These changes are similar to those induced in lymphocytes by antigen or mitogen.

Large nucleoli appear. Reticular cells turn over slowly; activated reticular cells, in contrast, divide actively. The hyaloplasm becomes dense and the perinuclear space is expanded. From the outer nuclear membrane, an extensive, branched, dilated system of endoplasmic reticulum (ER) extends deep into the cytoplasm, imparting a lacy character to the cell. In mice, reticular fibers disappear; in human beings they persist. (As activation subsides and the cells regain their unactivated appearance in the mouse, reticular fibers reappear.) In their fullest differentiations, activated reticular cells possess sheetlike cell processes which become more numerous and branched. These cell processes fuse with one another to form vast, broad, complex syncytial protoplasmic sheets.

In addition to activation of the reticular cells contributing to reticular meshworks, activated reticular cells originate from the surfaces of the trabeculae and the capsule, as well as from circulating reticular stem cells. The latter (reticular stem cells) may be observed within the lumen and in the wall of splenic blood vessels as dark round cells with prominent nucleoli, dilated endoplasmic reticulum and mitochondria, and dense hyaloplasm. Early in their extravascular differentiation, reticular stem cells form clusters of perivascular, small-branched cells, already engaged in syncytial fusing. These syncytia then move out into the pulp, their branches becoming more extended. They form extensive, irregular sheets which take on a variety of conformations, all of which appear to have barrier functions. I recognize these reticular cell-derived syncytial sheets as a reticuloendothelial system hegemony, a barrier forming system (BFS).

Barrier forming systems ensheathe blood vessels constituting the outermost layer of the adventitial tunic. They insinuate themselves into the circumferential reticulum which partially encloses the white pulp, making the enclosure more complete. In sinusal spleens the perivascular reticular meshworks, constituting the filtration beds, are well developed. By a combination of activation of reticular cells making up the filtration beds and the infiltration of blood-borne reticular stem cells, the filtration beds and the infiltration of blood-borne reticular stem cells, the filtration bed is augmented and comes to be made up of activated cells. Through branching and syncytial fusion, these activated cells form an extraordinarily fine-meshed extensive cytoplasmic meshwork. This meshwork constitutes a complex highly-branched syncytial cytoplasmic membrane, which tightly encloses single free cells and clusters of cells (Figure 6).

This system of cellular membranes appears to open and close locules of the filtration bed. In this way a dynamic blood-spleen barrier is formed which controls access to the filtration beds. In non-sinusal animals, in contrast to sinusal animals, the rather large pulp space contains few reticular cells, and the filtration beds tend to be rather poorly developed. In spleens of non-sinusal animals, barrier forming systems of activated reticular cells have a prominent role even under normal conditions.

The Mechanisms of Splenic Clearance of the Blood: A Synthesis

The spleen clears the blood using filtration beds fabricated of reticular cells. Reticular cells are the fibroblastic, contractile, innervated, dendritic cells of the reticuloendothelial system, which ensheathe argyrophilic reticular (collagen) fibers. The sheet-like processes of the reticular cells, reinforced by reticular fibers, form the locules of the filtration beds. Like the alveoli of the lung, these locules normally communicate with one another. Directly, or indirectly, arterial terminal vessels empty blood into the locules of these filtration beds and the filtered blood is drained by proximal venous vessels. Thus, the filtered blood is drained by sinuses in sinusal spleens, and it is drained by pulp veins in non-sinusal spleens.

The locules of the filtration bed are used to clear the blood, but these locules may be bypassed and blood may be shunted directly from artery to vein. In this case, blood circulates through the spleen as rapidly as through muscle and other tissues, possessing a physiologically closed circulation. This process probably occurs by contraction of the filtration bed, which brings the orifice of the terminal arterial vessel to proximity with an inter-endothelial slit or aperture in the wall of proximal venous vessels. But other mechanisms may well exist. While there is no endothelial continuity between the terminal arterial vessel and the proximal venous vessel, the arterial terminal may end quite close to the vein, even sharing a basement membrane for a short distance. Between arterial terminal and proximal vein, moreover, the sheet-like processes of the interposed reticular cells may form tubular structures which are capable of conveying blood as efficiently as bona fide blood vessels.

But in normal spleens to some extent, and in enlarged spleens to a great extent, barrier-forming systems made of activated reticular cells may both control clearance and contribute to activities consequent to clearance. Activated reticular cells are reticular cells activated to high level protein synthesis. Their salient morphological features are dense hyaloplasm, nucleoli, and extensive dilated endoplasmic reticulum which pervades the cytoplasm, imparting a lacy appearance to the cell. In the mouse, reticular cells forego the production of reticular fibers during their activation, but reassume it when activation wanes. Activated reticular cells originate not only from existing reticular cells but from circulating reticular stem cells which are cleared from the blood and accumulate initially in the perivascular filtration beds. Activated reticular cells fuse with one another, forming extensive, syncytial, complexly branched cellular membranes constituting barrier forming systems. The barriers may surround white pulp, insinuated into the activated circumferential reticulum. Barrier forming systems may ensheathe blood vessels, forming the outermost layer of the tunica adventitia. They may infiltrate the wall of locules of the filtration beds in position to seal off the locules, or allow them to remain open.

In the pulp spaces of nonsinusal spleens barrier forming systems may float in the circulating blood of the pulp, tethered to the outside surface of blood vessels or to trabeculae. They may enclose single blood cells or hematopoietic cells, or they may enclose multicellular hematopoietic colonies. These barrier forming systems thereby form a variety of blood-spleen barriers, having varied function. They may open or close the filtration beds, particularly in splenomegaly where normal mechanisms of contraction and tube formation may work only with difficulty. They may trap cells and infectious agents on their surface. By enclosing hematopoietic colonies, barrier forming systems concentrate colony regulating factors and protect the colonies against parasitization. They may close off the white pulp after the initiation of an immune response, protecting against epiphenomenal responses and the dissipation of the cellular immunologic resources.

SUMMARY

While the spleen provides rapid (as well as delayed) blood flow, its circulation is anatomically open, there being no endothelial continuity between distal arterial and proximal venous vessels. Filtration beds and the macrophages they hold are reticuloendothelial structures, interposed between terminal arterial and venous vessels. Because the character of the splenic circulations, the presence of blood-spleen barriers, the storage, sorting and modification of blood cells, the control of infectious disease, and the manifestations of disease are determined by the activity of the filtration beds, mechanisms controlling the filtration beds are becoming important foci of research. The management of sickle cell disease in infants and children, for example, is determined by the behavior of the splenic filtration beds. Thus, in the acute sequestration syndrome of sickle cell disease, a large spleen suddenly sequesters circulating blood cells, causing a lethal anemia, relieved by splenectomy. Just as unpredictably there occurs the paradox of a large spleen whose filtration beds are sealed off, functional asplenia, resulting, because it fails to clear the blood of microbes, in debilitating infection. Hypersplenism and asplenia occur in other hemolytic anemias and infections.

The macrophage and phagocytosis have dominated experimental studies of the reticuloendothelial system. In this chapter, I emphasize the fibroblastic reticular cell. Both macrophage and fibroblast have traditionally been viewed too narrowly: macrophages do much more than phagocytize, fibroblasts do much more than synthesize collagen. Reticular cells form the locules of the splenic filtration beds. To limited degree normally, and at high levels in the course of infectious disease, or in the course of clearing damaged blood cells, splenic reticular cells become intensely activated and augmented by proliferation and by immigration of circulating precursors. Activated reticular cells differentiate, branching extensively and fusing with one another to form extraordinarily extensive, complexly branched syncitial sheets. These sheets enwrap arteries and veins. They are intercalated into the reticulum, insinuated between established reticular cells and their reticular fibers, filling the large apertures in the circumferential reticulum bounding white pulp, sealing off or extending the filtration beds of red pulp and marginal zones.

The conception of the vasculature and filtration beds and their regulation by barrier systems of activated reticular cells, constitutes a most useful basis for understanding the physiology and pathology of the spleen and other reticuloendothelial tissues.

REFERENCES

1. Anderson ND, Weiss L: Lymphocyte traffic in the spleen. *Fed Proc* 1976; 35:608 (Abstract).
2. Blue J, Weiss L: Vascular pathways in nonsinusal red pulp; an electron microscope study. *Am J Anat* 1981;161:135.
3. Blue J, Weiss L: Periarterial macrophage sheaths (ellipsoids) in cat spleen; an electron microscope study. *Am J Anat* 1981;161:115.
4. Blue J, Weiss L: Species variation in the structure and function of the marginal zone; an electron microscope study of the cat spleen. *Am J Anat* 1981; 161:189.
5. Blue J, Weiss L: Electron microscopy of the red pulp of the dog spleen including vascular arrangements, periarterial sheaths (ellipsoids), and the contractile, innervated meshwork. *Am J Anat* 1981;161:189.
6. Butcher EC, Weissman IL: Lymphoid tissues and organs. In, Paul W, (Ed): *Fundamental Immunology*. Raven Press, New York, p. 109.

7. Chin JW, Pearson JD, Hay JB: Cells in sheep lymph and their migratory characteristics. In, Johnston MG, (ed): *Experimental Biology of the Lymphatic Circulation*. Research Monographs in Cell and Tissue Physiology. Elsevier Science Publishing, Amsterdam, 1985.
8. Croissant R, Gunther H, Slavkin HC: How are embryonic preameoloblasts instructed by odontoblasts to synthesize enamel? In, Slavkin HC, Greulich RC, (eds); *Extracellular Matrix Influences on Gene Expression*. Academic Press, New York, 1975, pp. 515-522.
9. DeSousa MAB: *Lymphocyte Circulation. Experimental and Clinical Aspects*. John Wiley, New York, 1981.
10. Ford WL: The kinetics of lymphocyte recirculation within the rat spleen. *Tissue Kinet* 1969;2:171.
11. Friedenstein AJ, Chailakhan RK, Latsinik NV, et al: Stromal cells responsible for transferring the microenvironment of hematopoietic tissue. *Transplantation* 1974;17:331-340.
12. Friedman H, Escobar MR, Reichard SM: In 10 volumes 1979-1988 (continuous) *The Reticuloendothelial System: A Comprehensive Treatise*. Plenum Press, New York.
13. Fujita T, Kashimura M, Adachi K: Scanning electron microscopy and terminal circulation. *Experientia* 1985;40:167-168.
14. Gowans JL: The recirculation of lymphocyte from blood to lymph in the lymph in the rat. *J Physiol* 1959;146:54.
15. Gowans JL, Knight EJ: The route of recirculation of lymphocytes in the rat. *Proc R Soc London (Biol)* 1964;159:257.
16. Grobstein C: Developmental role of the intercellular matrix; retrospection and prospection. In, Slavkin HC, Greulich RC (eds); *Extracellular Matrix Influences on Gene Expression*. Academic Press, New York, 1975;pp. 9-16.
17. Groom AC, Song SH: Effects of norepinephrine on washout of red cells from the spleen. *Am J Physiol* 1971;22:255-258.
18. Jaffe RH: The reticulo-endothelial system. In, Downey H, (ed): *The Handbook of Hematology*. Hoeber, New York, 1988, pp. 973-1272.
19. Knisely MH: Spleen studies. I. Microscopic observations of the circulatory system of living unstimulated mammalian spleen. *Anat Rec* 1936;65:23.
20. Looareesuwan S, Ho M, Wattanagoon Y, et al: Dynamic alteration in splenic function during acute Falciparum malaria. *N Engl J Med* 1987;317(11):675.
21. McCuskey Rs, McCuskey RP: In vivo and electron microscopic studies of the splenic microvasculature in mice. *Experientia* 1985;40:179.
22. Parker FG, Barnes EN, Kaye GI: The pericryptal fibroblast sheath. *Gastroenterology* 1974;67:607.
23. Pellas TC, Weiss L: Deep splenic lymphatic vessels in the mouse; a route of lymphocyte recirculation. *Anat Rec*. In press, 1988.
24. Pellas TC, Weiss L: Lymphocyte migration and recirculation in the mouse; migratory pathways of thoracic duct-derived B cells, L3T4+ and Lyt 2+ T cell subsets in lymphatic and nonlymphatic tissues. *Cell Tiss Res*. In press, 1988.

25. Reilly FD: Innervation and vascular pharmacodynamics of the mammalian spleen. *Experientia* 1985;40:187.
26. Saxen L: Transmission and spread of kidney induction. In, Slavkin HC, Greulich RC, (eds); *Extracellular Matrix Influences on Gene Expression.* Academic Press, New York, 1975, pp. 523-529.
27. Schmidt EE, MacDonald LC, Groom AC: Circulatory pathways in the sinusal spleen of the dog, studied by scanning electron microscopy of microcorrosion casts. *J Morphol* 1983;178:111-123.
28. Schmidt EE, MacDonald IC, Groom AC: The intermediate circulation in the nonsinusal spleen of the cat; studied by scanning electron microscopy of microcorrosion casts. *J Morphol* 1983;178:125.
29. Seifert MF, Marks SC: The regulation of hemopoiesis in the spleen. *Experientia* 1985;41:192.
30. Serjeant GR: *Sickle Cell Disease.* Oxford, London, 1986.
31. Tablin F, Weiss L: Equine spleen; an electron microscopic analysis. *Am J Anat* 1983;166:393.
32. Tischendorf F: On the evolution of the spleen. *Experientia* 1985;41:199.
33. van Ewijk W, Nieuwenhius P: Compartments, domains and migration pathways of lymphoid cells in the splenic pulp. *Experientia* 1985;41:199.
34. Weiss L: New trends in spleen research; conclusion. *Experientia* 1985;41:243.
35. Weiss L: The spleen. In, *Histology* 6th Ed. Urban and Schwarzenburg, Munich. In press, 1988.
36. Weiss L: The anatomy of the spleen. In, Bowdler AJ, (ed): *The Spleen: Structure, Functions, and Clinical Significance.* Oxford, London. In press, 1988.
37. Weiss L, Geduldig U, Weidanz WP: Mechanisms of splenic control of malaria; reticular cell activation and the development of a blood-spleen barrier. *Am J Anat* 1986;176:251.
38. Weiss L, Powell R, Schiffman FJ: Terminating arterial vessels in red pulp of the spleen. *Experientia* 1985;41:233.
39. Weiss L, Sakai H: The hematopoietic stroma. *Am J Anat* 1984;170:447.
40. Wyler DJ: The spleen in malaria. In, Evered D, Whelan J, (eds): *Malaria and the Red Cell.* Ciba Foundation Symposium, London. Pitman Books Ltd. London, 1983.
41. Male D, Champion B, Cooke A, (eds): *Advanced Immunology* J. B. Lippincott Company, Philadelphia, 1987.
42. Halpern PN, Benecerraf B, Delafresnaye JF, (eds): *Physiology of the Reticuloendothelial System.* A Symposium. The Council for International Organizations of Medical Sciences. UNESCO and W.H.O., Paris, France, Blackwell, Oxford, 1957.
43. Heller JH (ed); *Reticuloendothelial Structure and Function.* Third International Symposium. The International Society for Research of the Reticuloendothelial System. Rapallo, Italy, Ronald Press, New York, 1958.

Index

Abnormalities of the spleen, imaging in the diagnosis of, 371-399
  asplenia and polysplenia syndromes, 376-378
  benign and malignant tumors, 397-399
  functional asplenia, 378-379
  herniation of the spleen through the diaphragm, 371
  hypersplenism and accessory spleens, 371-372
  postsplenectomy sepsis, 386-388
  splenic cysts and abscesses, 388-396
  splenic-gonadal fusion, 372-376
  trauma, 379-386
  wandering spleen, 378
Abscesses, 253-256
  imaging in the diagnosis of, 388-396
Accessory spleens, 42-43
  imaging in the diagnosis of, 371-372

Acquired immunodeficiency syndrome (AIDS), 246
Acute infections, splenomegaly and, 173
Acute lymphoblastic leukemia, 80-81, 127
Acute lymphocytic leukemia (ALL), 274
Acute pulmonary histoplasmosis, 247
Acute splenic sequestration, 175-177
Acute viral hepatitis, 246
Adult spleen, relationships and appearance of, 4-7
Agnogenic myeloid metaplasia, 177
Amyloidosis, 64-65, 175, 345-346
  systemic, 128
Analphalipoproteinemia (Tangier disease), 175, 325-326
Anatomic hyposplenism, 110-113
Anatomic localization of splenic diseases, 38

Anatomy of the spleen, 1-19, 239-240
  the adult spleen, relationships and appearance, 4-7
  development, 1-4
  microscopic organization, 7-17
    capsule and trabeculae, 7
    open versus closed circulation, 17
    splenic pulp, 7-15
    splenic vasculature, 14, 16-17
Angiosarcoma as cause of splenomegaly, 300-302
Anisosplenia, 42
Antibody-mediated cell clearance, 187-192
  role of IgG in, 188-192
Antibody production, 218-219
  hyposplenism and, 151-152
Anti-tumor immunity, 266-268
Aplastic anemia, 178-179
Asplenia, functional, 378-379
Asplenia syndrome, 113-114
  imaging in the diagnosis of, 376-378
  management of, 154-157
Autoimmune disorders, 62-71, 187-213
  associated with hyposplenism, 119-123
  autoimmune hemolytic anemia, 198-201
  autoimmune neutropenia, 201-202
  immune thrombocytopenic purpura, 49, 57, 62-64, 194-198
  spleen as immune clearance organ, 192-194
Autoimmune hemolytic anemia (AIHA), 198-201
  autoantibody in, 199-201
  splenectomy for, 201, 418
  splenic destruction of red blood cells and, 201
Autoimmune neutropenia, 201-202

Benign tumors, 38, 72-73
  causing splenomegaly, 266
  imaging in the diagnosis of, 397-399
Biologic substances removed by the spleen, 222
Blood clearance by the spleen, 446-450
Bone marrow transplantation (BMT), 279-280
"Born-again spleen" syndrome, 130
Brucellosis, 172, 256-257

Carbohydrate metabolism disorders, 321-323
  diabetes mellitus, 323
  glycogen storage disorders, 175, 321, 322
Cat-scratch disease, 257
Chemotherapy, 276-278
Childhood splenectomy, 407-427
  conditions associated with, 408
  connective tissue diseases and, 420
  general considerations for, 422-423
  hematologic indications (red cell disorders) for, 410-418
    autoimmune hemolytic anemia, 418
    enzyme deficiencies, 413
    hemoglobinopathies, 413-417
    hereditary spherocytosis, 410-413
    idiopathic thrombocytopenic purpura, 417-418
    other membrane disorders, 413
  hypersplenism and, 418-419
  infection and, 421-422
  malignancy and, 420-421
  measures to reduce risk of postsplenectomy sepsis, 422
  for traumatic rupture, 407-410

INDEX 457

[Childhood splenectomy]
  Wiskott-Aldrich syndrome and, 420
Cholesteryl ester storage disease (CESD), 344-345
Chronic lymphocytic leukemia (CLL), 26, 81, 273
Chronic myelogenous leukemia (CML), 26, 49
Chronic myeloid leukemia (CML), 86-89, 274-275
Circulatory disturbances, 42-46
Collagen-vascular disorders, 173-174
Computer-assisted tomography (CAT) scanning, 224, 226, 271, 370-371, 407
Congenital heart disease, splenic syndromes occurring with, 42
Congenital hyposplenism, 113-132
  associated with gastrointestinal disorders, 123-127
  associated with old age, 115
  due to impaired vascular supply to the spleen, 119
  due to in situ splenic congestion, 115-119
  immunologic or autoimmune disorders associated with, 119-123
  malignancies and, 127-128
  miscellaneous conditions associated with, 128-132
Congenital (TORCH) infections, 240-245
Congestive splenomegaly, 228
  hypersplenism and, 174-175
Connective tissue diseases, splenectomy for, 420
Corticosteroids, 130
Cystinosis, 346
Cysts, imaging in the diagnosis of, 388-396
Cytomegalovirus (DMV), 240-245

Diabetes mellitus, 323

Ectopic spleen, 3, 4
Endemic malaria, 258
Endothelium of vascular sinuses, 441-442
Enzyme deficiencies, splenectomy for, 413
Epinephrine stimulation test for hypersplenism, 169
Epstein-Barr virus (EBV), 245

Familial erythrophagocytic lymphohistiocytosis (FEL), 202
Fanconi's anemia, 114
Felty's syndrome, 173
Fibroblasts, inductive capacities of, 443-444
Fibronectin, 131
Filtration function of the spleen, 219-220
Fucosidosis, 342-343
Functional asplenia, 378-379
Functional hyposplenism, 110-113
Functions of the spleen, 218-222, 355, 356
  antibody formation, 218-219
  filtration, 219-220
  hematopoiesis, 220-222
  hyposplenism and, 145-166
    blood function, 147
    destruction of blood, 147-148
    infection, 149-154
    management of the asplenic state, 154-157
    pitting function, 148-149
    reservoir function, 146
  measurement of, 222
  phagocytosis, 220, 356

Gamma globulin, 129, 407
Gangliosides, 338-339

Gastrointestinal disorders, hyposplenism in association with, 123–127
Gaucher's disease, 56–59, 175, 326–329
Giant splenomegaly, 230
Glycogen storage diseases, 175, 321, 322
Glycoprotein degradation disorders, 342–343
  fucosidosis, 342–343
  mannosidosis, 342
  sialidosis, 343
Gold thiomolate (sodium aurothiomolate), 129

Hairy cell leukemia (HCL), 81–83, 273–274
Hematologic changes, detection of hyposplenism by, 105–110
Hematologic disorders:
  as cause of hypersplenism, 175–179
  differential features of splenic abnormalities found in, 88
Hematopoiesis, 21–24, 220–222, 356
  in disease, 25–27
  hyposplenism and, 147
  in man, 24–25
  phylogenesis and ontogenesis, 21–23
  regulation of, 27–29
Hemochromatosis, 346–347
Hemodialysis, hypersplenism and, 179–180
Hemoglobinopathies, splenectomy for, 413–417
Hereditary elliptocytosis, 413
Hereditary spherocytosis (HS), 46, 47
  splenectomy for, 410–413
Hereditary stomatocytosis, 413
Herniation of the spleen through the diaphragm, 371

Herpes simplex, 240–245
High-dose gamma globulin, 407
Histiocytic disorders causing splenomegaly, see Splenomegaly, neoplastic and histiocytic disorders causing
Histiocytosis-X (HX), 66–67, 178, 294–300
  organ involvement in, 295
Hodgkin's disease, 77–81
  imaging in the diagnosis of, 397–399
  splenectomy for, 420–421
  splenomegaly in, 281–284
Human fetal spleen, hematopoiesis in, 24–25
Human immunodeficiency virus (HIV) infection, 246–247
Hunter syndrome, 335–336
Hurler's syndrome, 333–335
Hyperchylomicronemia (type I hyperlipoproteinemia), 323–325
Hypersplenism, 167–186
  in association with splenomegaly, 231–234
  congestive splenomegaly and, 174–175
  disorders associated with, 231
    hematologic diseases, 175–179
    inflammatory and collagen-vascular disorders, 173–174
    storage diseases, 175
  etiologies of, 170–173
  imaging in the diagnosis of, 371–372
  laboratory evaluation of, 169–170
  miscellaneous conditions associated with, 179–180
  neoplastic conditions associated with, 179
  pathophysiology of, 168–169
  splenectomy for, 418–419
  treatment of, 180
Hyposplenism, 99–144

INDEX 459

[Hyposplenism]
  causes of functional and anatomic hyposplenism, 110-113
  congenital hyposplenism, 113-132
  diseases associated with, 220
  laboratory techniques for evaluation of, 110
  methods to evaluate adequacy of splenic function, 99-110
    hematologic changes, 105-110
    radiologic studies, 100-105
  spleen function and, 145-166
    blood function, 147
    destruction of blood, 147-148
    infection, 149-154
    management of the asplenic state, 154-157
    pitting function, 148-149
    reservoir function, 146

I-cell disease (mucolipidosis II), 339
Idiopathic thrombocythemia (IT), 26
Idiopathic thrombocytopenic purpura (ITP), splenectomy for, 417-418
IgG (immunoglobulin G), 188-192
  use in ITP of, 198
IgM, 190-192
Imaging the spleen, 355-405
  anatomy and embryology, 360
  clinical applications in diagnosing abnormalities, 371-399
    asplenia and polysplenia syndromes, 376-378
    benign and malignant tumors, 397-399
    functional asplenia, 378-379
    herniation of the spleen through the abdomen, 371
    hypersplenism and accessory spleens, 371-372
    postsplenectomy sepsis, 386-388
    splenic cysts and abscesses, 388-396

[Imaging the spleen]
    splenic-gonadal fusion, 372-376
    trauma, 377-386
    wandering spleen, 378
  in detecting splenomegaly, 223-227
  techniques, 361-371
    computed tomography, 370-371
    radionuclide scans, 364-370
    sonography, 361-363
    variations in size, 360-361
Immune clearance organ, role of the spleen as, 192-194
Immune disorders, 62-71
  associated with hyposplenism, 119-123
Immune thrombocytopenic purpura (ITP), 49, 57, 62-64, 194-198
  morphological considerations, 194-195
  platelet kinetics in, 195-196
  splenectomy in, 197-198
  splenetic production of antiplatelet antibody in, 196-197
  use of intravenous immunoglobulin in, 198
Impaired vascular supply to the spleen, hyposplenism due to, 119
Increased splenic uptake, 365
Inductive capacities of fibroblasts, 443-444
Infection-associated hemophagocytic syndrome (IAHS), 53, 55
Infectious diseases, 38, 50-56, 364
  causing hyposplenism, 149-154
  causing splenomegaly, 173, 239-264
    acute viral hepatitis, 246
    cat-scratch disease, 257
    congenital (TORCH) infections, 240-245
    human immunodeficiency virus (HIV) infection, 246-247

[Infectious diseases]
    infections in travelers and immigrants, 258-259
    infectious mononucleosis syndromes, 245-246
    infective endocarditis, 253
    ornithosis, 252
    rickettsial infections, 251-252
    spirochettsial infections, 250-251
    splenic abscesses, 253-256
    systemic mycoses, 247-250
    tapeworm infestations, 257-258
    tuberculosis, 252-253
    zoonoses, 256-257
  splenectomy and, 421-422
Infectious etiologies of hypersplenism, 170-173
Infectious mononucleosis syndromes, 53, 54, 245-246
Infective endocarditis, 253
Inflammatory disorders, hypersplenism and, 173-174
In situ splenic congestion, hyposplenism due to, 115-119
Interferon, 278-279
Intermediate circulation of the spleen, 431-439
Intravenous gamma globulin, 129
Isolated congenital asplenia, 113

Leismaniasis (kala-azar), 170-172
Leukemias as causes of splenomegaly, 272-282
  treatment of, 276-280
Lipoprotein metabolism disorders, 323-326
  analphalipoproteinemia (Tangier disease), 175, 325-326
  type I hyperlipoproteinemia, 323-325
Lymphomas:
  as causes of splenomegaly, 281-284

[Lymphomas]
  differential featuers of splenic abnormalities found in, 88
  malignant, 38, 73-89
Lymphomatous disorders, 177
Lymphoproliferative disorders, 177

Macrophages, 439-441
Magnetic resonance imaging, (*see* Nuclear magnetic resonance imaging)
Malaria, 170, 258
Malignancies, 364
  hyposplenism in association with, 127-128
  splenectomy and, 420-421
Malignant fibrous histiocytoma (MFH), 300
Malignant histiocytosis, 288-294
  organ involvement in, 295
Malignant lymphoma, 73-89
Malignant tumors:
  causing splenomegaly, 266
  imaging in the diagnosis of, 397-399
Mannosidosis, 342
Maroteaux-Lamy disease, 336
Methyldopa, 129
Microscopic organization of the spleen, 7-17
  capsule and trabeculae, 7
  open versus closed circulation, 17
  splenic pulp, 7-15
  splenic vasculature, 14, 16-17
Mucolipidosis II (I-cell disease), 339
Mucopolysaccharidoses, 333-337
  Hunter syndrome, 335-336
  Hurler syndrome, 333-335
  Maroteaux-Lamy disease, 336
  Sanfilippo disease, 336
  Sly syndrome, 337
Multiple sulfatase deficiency sulfatidosis, 337-338

INDEX

Myelofibrosis:
  as cause of splenomegaly, 284–287
  with myeloid metaplasia (MMM), 26, 86–89
Myeloproliferative disorders, 38, 73–89, 177

Neonates, hyposplenism in, 110–113
Neoplastic conditions:
  associated with hypersplenism, 179
  associated with splenomegaly, 265–318
Neutral lipid storage diseases, 343–345
Neutrophils, destruction in autoimmune neutropenia of, 202
Niemann-Pick disease, 59–62, 175, 330–333
Non-Hodgkin's lymphoma (NHL):
  imaging in the diagnosis of, 397, 399
  splenomegaly in, 281–284
Nuclear magnetic resonance imaging (MRI), 224, 226, 271

Old age, hyposplenism and, 115
Ontogenesis of splenic hematopoiesis, 21–23
Ornithosis, 252
Overwhelming infection (OPSI) syndrome, 149–150

Pathology of the spleen, 37–95
  benign tumors, 38, 72–73
  examination, 37–41
  immune and autoimmune disorders, 62–71, 187–213
  infectious diseases, 38, 50–54, 364
  malignancy and myeloproliferative disorders, 38, 73–89, 177
  red blood cell abnormalities, 46–49
  storage diseases, 56–62, 364

[Pathology of the spleen]
  structural abnormalities and circulating disturbances, 42–46
Peliosis of the spleen, 43–44
Penicillin, prophylactic, 422
Phagocytosis, 220, 356
  hyposplenism and, 152–153
Phylogenesis of splenic hematopoiesis, 21–23
Physiology of the spleen, 239–240
"Pitting" of red blood cells, 356
  hyposplenism and, 148–149
Platelet destruction, 356
Polycythemia vera (PV), 26, 177
Polysplenia syndrome, 42, 114
  imaging in the diagnosis of, 376–378
Postsplenectomy sepsis, 131
  imaging in the diagnosis of, 386–388
  splenectomy to reduce risk of, 422
Primary hypersplenism, 231
Prophylactic penicillin, 422

Radio-isotope scans, 407
Radiologic studies to evaluate splenic function, 100–105
Radionuclide scanning, 169–170, 224, 364–370
Red blood cell disorders, 46–49
  splenectomy for, 410–418
    autoimmune hemolytic anemia, 418
    enzyme deficiencies, 413
    hemoglobinopathies, 413–417
    hereditary spherocytosis, 410–413
    idiopathic thrombocytopenic purpura, 417–418
    other membrane disorders, 413
  splenic destruction of cells, 201

Replantation of the spleen, 156-157
Research trends, 431-453
  clearance of blood by the spleen, 446-450
  endothelium of vascular sinuses, 441-442
  hegemonies of the reticuloendothelial system, 444-446
  inductive capacities of fibroblasts, 443-444
  intermediate circulation of the spleen, 431-439
  macrophages, 439-441
  reticular cells, 442-443
  reticuloendothelial character of the spleen, 439
Reticular cells (RC), 442-443
Reticuloendothelial system (RES), 439
  hegemonies of, 444-446
Rickettsial infections, 251-252
Roentgenographic examination, 224
Rubella, 240-245

Sanfilippo disease, 336
Sarcoidosis, 173-174
Schistosomiasis, 259
Sea-blue histiocytosis, 175, 333
Secondary hypersplenism, disorders associated with, 231
Septicemia, 114
Sialidosis, 343
Sickle cell disease, 43, 44, 48-49, 175-177
  hyposplenism and, 116-118
  splenectomy for, 413-415
Single-photon-emission computed tomography (SPECT), 224-225
Sly syndrome, 337
Sodium aurothiomolate (gold thiomolate), 129
Sonography, 361-363
Sphingolipid metabolism disorders, 326-333

[Sphingolipid metabolism disorders]
  Gaucher's disease, 56-59, 175, 326-329
  Niemann-Pick disease, 59-62, 175, 330-333
  sea-blue histiocyte disease, 175, 333
Spirochettsial infections, 250-251
Splenectomy:
  in AIHA, 201, 418
  hyposplenism and, 154-157
  indications for, 39, 40
  in ITP, 197-198
  (see also Childhood splenectomy)
Splenic embolization, 407, 423
Splenic-gonadal fusion, 43
  imaging in the diagnosis of, 372-376
Splenic hamartoma, 70, 72
Splenic implantation, 407, 423
Splenic infarcts, 45-46
Splenic pulp, 7-15
Splenic vasculature, 5, 6, 14, 16-17
Splenomegaly, 167, 217-238, 364
  acute infection and, 173
  congestive, as cause of hypersplenism, 174-175
  definition of, 222-227
    diagnostic imaging, 223-227
    physical examination, 222-223
  diagnostic overview, 227-236
    approach to, 234-236, 259-261
    background, 227-230
    disorders accompanied by splenomegaly, 229-230
    giant splenomegaly, 230
    hypersplenism, 231-234
  infections causing, 173, 239-264
    acute viral hepatitis, 246
    cat-scratch disease, 257
    congenital (TORCH) infections, 240-245
    human immunodeficiency virus (HIV) infection, 246-247

INDEX 463

[Splenomegaly]
  infections in travelers and immigrants, 258-259
  infectious mononucleosis syndromes, 245-246
  infective endocarditis, 253
  ornithosis, 252
  rickettsial infections, 251-252
  spirochettsial infections, 250-251
  splenic abscesses, 253-256
  systemic mycoses, 247-250
  tapeworm infestations, 257-258
  tuberculosis, 170, 252-253
  zoonoses, 256-257
 neoplastic and histiocytic disorders causing, 265-318
  angiosarcoma, 300-302
  clinical presentation, 268-269
  diagnosis, 270-272
  Hodgkin's disease, 281-284
  leukemia, 272-280
  lymphomas, 281-284
  miscellaneous, 302-304
  myelofibrosis, 284-287
  non-Hodgkin's lymphoma, 281-284
 pathophysiology of, 240
 storage disorders causing, 319-352
  amyloidosis, 64-65, 175, 345-346
  carbohydrate metabolism, 321-323
  cystinosis, 346
  glycoprotein metabolism, 342-343
  hemochromatosis, 346-347
  lipoprotein metabolism, 323-326
  mucolipidosis, 339
  mucopolysaccharidoses, 333-337
  neutral lipid storage diseases, 343-345
  sphingolipid metabolism, 326-333

[Splenomegaly]
  sulfatide lipidosis, 337-339
  tropical, 179
Splenosis, 43, 130
Storage disorders, 50-56, 364
  causing hypersplenism, 175
  causing splenomegaly, 319-352
  amyloidosis, 345-346
  carbohydrate metabolism, 321-323
  cystinosis, 346
  glycoprotein metabolism, 342-343
  hemochromatosis, 346-347
  lipoprotein metabolism, 323-326
  mucolipidosis, 339
  mucopolysaccharidoses, 333-337
  neutral lipid storage diseases, 343-345
  sphingolipid metabolism, 326-333
  sulfatide lipidosis, 337-339
Structural abnormalities, 42-46
Sulfatide lipidosis, 337-339
Syphilis, 240-245, 250-251
Systemic amyloidosis, 128
Systemic candidiasis, 50, 51, 52, 247
Systemic lupus erythematosis, 174
Systemic mycoses, 247-250

Tangier disease, 175, 325-326
Tapeworm infestations, 257-258
Technetium-99m sulfur-colloid scanning, 104-105
Thalassemia, splenectomy for, 413, 415-417
Toxoplasmosis, 240-245
Trauma of the spleen:
  imaging in the diagnosis of, 379-386
  splenectomy for traumatic rupture, 407-410

Tropical splenomegaly, 179
Tuberculosis, 170, 252–253
Tularemia, 256
Tumors:
  role of the spleen in anti-tumor immunity, 266-268
  (*see also* Benign tumors; Malignant tumors)
Type I glycogenosis, 321
Type I hyperlipoproteinemia, 323–325
Type III glycogenosis, 321
Type IV glycogenosis, 321, 322
Typhoid fever, 258

Ultrasound imaging, 225

Vascular sinuses, endothelium of, 441–442
Vascular system, impaired, hyposplenism due to, 119

Wandering spleen, 378
Wilms' tumor, 127
Wiskott-Aldrich syndrome, 420
Wolman's disease, 343–344

X-rays, 224

Zoonoses, 256–257